QUICK
Access

QUICK Access

Patient Information on Conditions, Herbs & Supplements

INTEGRATIVMEDICINE

Integrative Medicine Communications
www.onemedicine.com

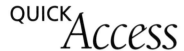

QUICK Access

Patient Information on Conditions, Herbs & Supplements

First edition 2000
Printed in the United States of America
ISBN 0-9670772-8-1
Library of Congress Catalog Card Number 99-096341

Integrative Medicine Communications
1029 Chestnut St., Newton, MA 02464
Phone: 617-641-2300
Fax: 617-641-2301
www.onemedicine.com

Disclaimer

No responsibility is assumed by the publisher for any injury and/or damage to any person or property as a matter of product liability, negligence, or otherwise, or from any use or operation of any methods, products, instructions, or ideas contained in any material herein. This publication contains information relating to general principles of medical care that should not in any event be construed as specific instructions for individual patients. The reader is advised to check product information (including package inserts) for changes and new information regarding dosage, precautions, and contraindications before administering any drug. No claim or endorsements are made for any drug or compound currently in investigative use.

ADVISORY BOARD

WELCOME TO QUICK ACCESS!

Let us tell you something about us and this important product.

OUR COMPANY: *Quick Access* has been developed by Integrative Medicine Communications (IMC), a company founded by people with a wealth of experience in professional and consumer publishing and information management, serving the continuing needs of modern health care providers. IMC strives to be the recognized source of high quality and scientifically sound information integrating conventional medicine with safe and efficacious complementary and alternative therapies.

OUR PRODUCT: In developing *Quick Access*, we first built an information base for health professionals providing them access to a complete armamentarium of approaches used to maintain health, treat disease, or manage conditions. We then adapted the professional content for the patient, adjusting for scope, language, and reading level—the monographs found in this book. Building *Quick Access* required a respect for the evidence to support the use of "conventional" and "non-conventional" therapeutic modalities, and the ability to utilize the talents of advisors, researchers, writers, fact checkers, proofreaders, and project managers in synthesizing the information into a tightly formatted and well-balanced final work.

OUR FOCUS: Our intention was to develop essential, accurate, practical, referenced, and formatted information. Whether it be with conditions, herbs, or dietary supplements, health care providers and patients can be assured that each monograph reflects a consistent organization and scope.

HOW TO USE *QUICK ACCESS*: The work contains monographs that allow quick answers to a wide range of questions—you may photocopy these monographs for distribution to patients, clients, or customers. This monograph system is comprised of the following three broad categories.

1) Condition Monographs—provide the patient with information on standard medical care with additional information on nutritional support and the use of alternative and complementary modalities. We include what the best evidence allows as safe and productive adjuncts to conventional medical care. As a result, herbs and dietary supplements receive a relatively larger share of coverage.

2) Herb Monographs—provide important information on the use of herbs in maintaining health or in treating conditions. The user may be searching for a particular herb, and use this section first, or may be looking here for more substance, having seen reference to the herb's use in a condition monograph.

3) Supplement Monographs—provide substantive information on the use of dietary supplements in maintaining health or in support of condition management. Vitamins, minerals, trace elements, micro-nutrients, and food supplements are included.

A comprehensive Quick Reference Guide allows for a quick search of category lists drawn from the *Quick Access* monographs. At a glance, you can review the herbs or supplements used in treating a particular condition, the contraindications of using a particular herb or supplement, and much more. Once you have found what you are looking for in the Quick Reference Guide, refer to the appropriate monograph for detail. There are 13 separate lists that can be searched in this Quick Reference Guide, allowing easy and targeted access to the information you are looking for:

- Conditions: By Medical Category
- Conditions: By Signs and Symptoms
- Conditions: By Herb or Supplement Treatment Options
- Herbs: By Uses/Indications
- Herbs: By Warnings, Precautions, Contraindications
- Herbs: By Side Effects
- Herbs: By Interactions With Other Drugs, Herbs, Supplements
- Herbs: By Taxonomic Cross Reference
- Supplements: By Uses/Indications
- Supplements: By Warnings, Precautions, Contraindications
- Supplements: By Side Effects

- **Supplements: By Interactions With Other Drugs, Herbs, Supplements**
- **Combined Herb/Supplement Treatments By Condition**

PRODUCT INTEGRITY: All of the information in *Quick Access* is well-researched, succinctly presented, and consistently formatted. References in *Quick Access* are original to the professional monographs and are current and clinically significant. A panel of health professionals representing the intended audience of pharmacists, physicians, nurses and nurse practitioners, nutritionists, dietitians, chiropractors, herbalists, naturopathic physicians, and other health practitioners have helped us shape the product and reviewed the information for appropriateness.

We have built this product for you and your patient, and pledge to be responsive to your existing and future information needs. We welcome your feedback.

CONDITIONS

CONDITIONS (continued)

HERBS

HERBS (continued)

SUPPLEMENTS

SUPPLEMENTS (continued)

QUICK Access

MEDICAL CONDITIONS

Allergic Rhinitis
Alopecia
Amenorrhea
Anemia
Angina
Anorexia Nervosa
Anxiety
Asthma
Atherosclerosis
Attention Deficit
Hyperactivity Disorder
Benign Prostatic Hyperplasia
Bronchitis
Burns
Bursitis
Candidiasis
Chronic Fatigue Syndrome
Chronic Obstructive Pulmonary
Disease
Cirrhosis Of The Liver
Common Cold
Congestive Heart Failure
Conjunctivitis
Constipation
Cough
Cutaneous Drug Reactions
Dementia
Depression
Dermatitis
Diabetes Mellitus
Diarrhea
Dysmenorrhea
Dysphagia
Eczema

Edema
Endocarditis
Endometriosis
Fever Of Unkown Orgin
Fibromyalgia
Food Allergy
Gallbladder Disease
Gastritis
Gastroesophageal Reflux Disease
Gout
Headache, Migraine
Headache, Sinus
Headache, Tension
Hemorrhoids
Hepatitis, Viral
Herpes Simplex Virus
Herpes Zoster (Varicella-Zoster) Virus
HIV and AIDS
Hypercholesterolemia
Hyperkalemia
Hypertension
Hyperthyroidism
Hypoglycemia
Hypothyroidism
Infantile Colic
Influenza
Insect Bites and Stings
Insomnia
Intestinal Parasites
Irritable Bowel Syndrome
Laryngitis
Low Back Pain
Menopause
Motion Sickness

Myocardial Infarction
Obesity
Osteoarthritis
Osteomyelitis
Osteoporosis
Otitis Media
Parkinson's Disease
Peptic Ulcer Disease
Peridcarditis
Pertussis
Pharyngitis
Preeclampsia
Primary Pulmonary Hypertension
Prostatitis
Psoriasis
Pulmonary Edema
Raynaud's Phenomenon
Reiter's Syndrome
Rheumatoid Arthritis
Roseola
Seizure Disorders
Sexual Dysfunction
Sinusitis
Sleep Apnea
Sprains and Strains
Tendinitis
Thyroiditis
Ulcerative Colitis
Urethritis
Urinary Incontinence
Urinary Tract Infections In Women
Urolithiasis
Vaginitis
Warts

■ ALLERGIC RHINITIS

Allergic rhinitis (also called hay fever) is the most common form of allergy. Symptoms often vary with the seasons.

■ SIGNS AND SYMPTOMS
- Stuffy, runny nose
- Sneezing
- Itchy nose, eyes, and throat
- "Sinus" symptoms—headache, feeling of pressure behind the eye, pain above the cheekbones and on the lower forehead, aching teeth
- Skin rashes or hives
- Diarrhea or frequent urination

■ WHAT CAUSES IT?
Your body's immune system is overreacting to irritants in the environment, such as the following.
- Pollens, grasses, or ragweed (in certain seasons and areas)
- Dust and household mites
- Changes in temperature or humidity
- Spicy foods
- Smoking or prolonged exposure to second-hand smoke

■ WHAT TO EXPECT AT YOUR PROVIDER'S OFFICE
Your health care provider will examine your nose and nasal secretions. You may be instructed to use a nasal spray, a decongestant, or an antihistamine. You may also be referred to an allergist, a physician who can pinpoint what you are allergic to by performing skin or blood tests.

■ TREATMENT OPTIONS
- Corticosteroid nasal sprays may take one to two weeks to work.
- Over-the-counter antihistamines can be taken every day. However, they may cause drowsiness.
- Oral decongestants (such as Sudafed) relieve the stuffiness but can have side effects.

Complementary and Alternative Therapies
Allergic rhinitis may be successfully treated with alternative therapies, beginning with dietary changes. Use the tincture and homeopathic remedies for acute allergic reactions.

NUTRITION
- Do not eat foods that trigger your allergies.
- Eat fewer foods and additives that are likely to cause inflammation and allergic reactions, such as saturated fats (meats and dairy products), refined foods, eggs, citrus, bananas, chocolate, peanuts, shellfish, food coloring, preservatives, caffeine, alcohol, tobacco, and sugar.
- Eat fresh fruits and vegetables, whole grains, nuts, and seeds.
- Drink plenty of water and fresh juices.

The following nutritional supplements can help your symptoms.
- Vitamin A (10,000 to 15,000 IU per day)
- Zinc (20 to 30 mg per day)
- Vitamins B_6 (50 to 100 mg per day) and B_5 (50 to 75mg/day)
- Vitamin C (1,000 mg three to four times per day)
- Vitamin E (400 IU per day)
- N-acetylcysteine (200 mg three times per day)

HERBS
Herbs may be used as dried extracts (capsules, powders, teas), glycerites (glycerine extracts), or tinctures (alcohol extracts). Unless otherwise indicated, teas should be made with 1 tsp. herb per cup of hot water. Steep covered 5 to 10 minutes for leaf or flowers, and 10 to 20 minutes for roots. Drink 2 to 4 cups per day.

Plants high in bioflavonoids (quercetin, *curcuma,* rose hips, bilberry) are especially useful because they reduce your body's production of histamines (substances that cause allergy symptoms) and strengthen connective tissue. Rose hips *(Rosa canina)* can be used as an infusion or solid extract. Nettles *(Urtica urens)* are traditionally used for hay fever and may be drunk as an infusion, 2 cups a day.

A tincture of equal parts of coneflower *(Echinacea),* goldenseal *(Hydrastis canadensis),* cleavers *(Gallium asparine),* eyebright *(Euphrasia officinalis),* ginger root *(Zingiber officinalis),* and elderberry *(Sambucus nigra)* will strengthen your immune system, increase circulation, and help your respiratory system work better. Take 30 drops two or three times per day.

HOMEOPATHY
Some of the most common remedies used for allergic rhinitis are listed below. Usually, the dose is 12X to 30C every one to four hours until your symptoms get better.
- *Allium cepa* for a lot of irritating nasal discharge and tearing eyes
- *Euphrasia* for bland nasal discharge, with stinging, irritating tears
- *Sabadilla* for sneezing with watery discharge from nose and eyes
- *Wyethia* for an itchy nose, throat, and soft palate

PHYSICAL MEDICINE
Use a nasal rinse made with water and salt to taste like tears. Rinse each nostril and, with your head over a sink, hold your head sideways and let the water run from your upper nostril to your lower nostril. Keep your nostrils lower than your throat to prevent the salt water from draining into the back of your throat. This rinse shrinks your sinus membranes and increases drainage.

ACUPUNCTURE
Treatment with acupuncture can help promote both immune system function and drainage of lymphatic fluid.

MASSAGE
Therapeutic massage can assist drainage of lymphatic fluid.

■ FOLLOWING UP
Take steps at home to eliminate allergens (such as covering your pillows and mattress with plastic covers and using an air purifier).

■ SPECIAL CONSIDERATIONS
Extended use of antihistamines or nasal sprays can make your allergic rhinitis worse. If you are pregnant, do not take high doses of vitamins A and C.

■ ALOPECIA

Alopecia is the absence or slowing of hair growth in an area of the body where hair formerly grew. It may be caused by physical damage to the hair itself or to the hair follicles, but it is most often the result of changes in the natural growth cycle of hair. In some types of alopecia, the growth cycle is disrupted by some temporary situation such as a chemical imbalance or stress. However, the vast majority (95 percent) of cases of hair loss in both men (male pattern baldness) and women (female diffuse baldness) are genetic in origin. This is called androgenetic alopecia.

■ SIGNS AND SYMPTOMS

- Male pattern baldness. Thinning or absence of hair at the hairline and top of the head.
- Female diffuse baldness. A gradual thinning of hair, especially on the top of the head. Hairline generally remains intact.
- Broken hairs, or hairs easily removed
- One or more round or oval bald patches

■ WHAT CAUSES IT?

Androgenetic alopecia is caused by a genetic tendency for certain hair follicles to produce a substance that reacts with male hormones. As you get older, this reaction eventually causes the follicle to shut down. Female diffuse baldness progresses more slowly than male pattern baldness because of the small amount of male hormones in a woman's body. A hormone imbalance may make the problem worse.

Temporary hair loss may result from any shock to the body's systems, including starvation, systemic infection, childbirth, thyroid or immunologic disorders, drugs (especially chemotherapy for cancer), or stress. Hair follicles can be destroyed permanently by scarring from burns, severe scalp infections, X-ray therapy, or skin disorders. Damage may also result from tight hairstyles over a long period of time, chemical treatments such as hair coloring or permanents, or the habitual pulling out of the hair. A fungal condition called tinea capitis ("ringworm of the scalp") also results in hair loss. The causes of alopecia areata, or patchy hair loss, are not well understood. It tends to happen in times of stress.

■ WHAT TO EXPECT AT YOUR PROVIDER'S OFFICE

If the cause of your hair loss is uncertain, your provider may suggest thyroid function tests or a blood test to rule out immune system problems. A biopsy, in which a small sample of scalp tissue is taken to be examined microscopically, is occasionally recommended.

■ TREATMENT OPTIONS

Minoxidil lotion (Rogaine) is usually the first treatment to try. It is sold over the counter. Men also have the option of taking the prescription drug finasteride (Propecia). Either medication must be used indefinitely to maintain regrown hair. If you use these medications, your health care provider should monitor you for side effects.

The most effective treatments for alopecia areata involve steroid drugs such as cortisone. Tinea capitis is treated with antifungal medications taken by mouth, in combination with antifungal shampoo used two to three times per week. Surgical options include hair transplants, scalp reduction, and strip or flap grafts.

Complementary and Alternative Therapies

These therapies have limited success in treating male pattern baldness.

NUTRITION

- Reduce your intake of pro-inflammatory foods (saturated fats, dairy products, and other animal products) and eat more fresh vegetables, whole grains, essential fatty acids, and, in particular, protein (non-animal sources of protein include nuts, legumes, and soy).
- Biotin (300 mcg per day) and trace minerals, such as those found in blue-green algae (2 to 6 tablets per day), help hair growth.
- Androgenetic alopecia: vitamin B_6 (50 to 100 mg per day), zinc (30 mg per day), and gamma linolenic acid (1,000 mg twice a day) helps to inhibit 5-alpha reductase.
- Hormone imbalance: essential fatty acids (1,000 mg twice a day), B_6 (50 to 100 mg per day), vitamin E (400 IU per day), and magnesium (200 mg twice a day) enhance hormone production.

HERBS

Herbs may be used as dried extracts (capsules, powders, teas), glycerites (glycerine extracts), or tinctures (alcohol extracts). Teas should be made with 1 tsp. herb per cup of hot water. Steep covered 5 to 10 minutes for leaf or flowers, and 10 to 20 minutes for roots.

- Combine the following in equal parts and use as tea (2 to 3 cups per day) or tincture (20 to 30 drops two to three times per day): ginkgo (*Ginkgo biloba*), rosemary (*Rosemarinus officinalis*), prickly ash bark (*Xanthoxylum clava-herculis*), black cohosh (*Cimicifuga racemosa*), yarrow (*Achillia millefolium*), and horsetail (*Equisetum arvense*)
- Androgenetic alopecia: Green tea (*Camelia sinensis*), 2 cups per day, and saw palmetto (*Serenoa repens*), 100 mg twice a day
- Hormone imbalance: Chaste tree (*Vitex agnus-cactus*), 200 to 300 mg per day, has a normalizing effect on the pituitary.
- Viral origin or immune system cause: Herbs that support immune function can help treat the underlying cause of this type of alopecia. Echinacea (*Echinacea angustifolia*), astragalus (*Astragalus membranaceus*), and Siberian ginseng (*Eluthroccus senticosus*)

PHYSICAL MEDICINE

Stress reduction techniques can increase blood flow to the scalp.

MASSAGE

Therapeutic massage increases circulation and reduces stress. Scalp massage using essential oils of rosemary, lavender, sage, thyme, and cedarwood may be helpful in increasing circulation. Add 3 to 6 drops of essential oil to 1 tbsp. of jojoba or grapeseed oil. Massage into scalp daily.

■ SPECIAL CONSIDERATIONS

A small percentage of men using finasteride may experience a decreased sex drive or difficulty in achieving an erection.

If you are pregnant, postpone treatment until after your baby is born.

■ AMENORRHEA

Amenorrhea is the absence of menstruation. When a girl reaches age 16 and has not begun menstruating, she may have primary amenorrhea. When a woman who has had menstrual cycles misses three periods in a row, she is considered to have secondary amenorrhea. A hormone balance can cause hypoestrogenemic amenorrhea.

■ SIGNS AND SYMPTOMS

Symptoms sometimes related to primary amenorrhea include headaches; abnormal blood pressure; vision problems; acne; excessive hair growth, and perhaps either a short, stubby physique or extremely tall stature.

Symptoms sometimes related to secondary amenorrhea include nausea, swollen breasts, headaches, vision problems, unusual thirst, goiter (an enlarged thyroid gland), skin darkening, extreme weight loss, alcoholism, liver disease, and kidney failure. Hot flushes, mood changes, depression, and vaginal dryness are common with estrogen deficiency.

■ WHAT CAUSES IT?

Generally, the causes of amenorrhea include certain genetic defects, body structure abnormalities, or endocrine disorders. Specific causes include the following.

- Developmental problems, such as the absence of the uterus or vagina
- Hormone imbalance produced by the endocrine system
- Excessive amounts of the male hormone testosterone
- Improper functioning of the ovaries
- Intrauterine infection or endometritis
- Menopause, usually between the ages of 40 and 55
- Pregnancy or breast feeding
- Discontinuation of oral contraceptives
- Disease (such as diabetes mellitus or tuberculosis)
- Stress or psychological disorders
- Malnutrition, extreme weight loss, anorexia nervosa
- Extreme obesity (overweight)
- Extreme exercise (such as long-distance running)
- Drug abuse

■ WHAT TO EXPECT AT YOUR PROVIDER'S OFFICE

Your provider will conduct a physical examination, which will include an internal pelvic examination. Laboratory tests may include analysis of mucus from the cervix and uterus, blood tests, and computer assisted tomography (CAT) scan, magnetic resonance imaging (MRI), or ultrasound.

■ TREATMENT OPTIONS

Your provider may suggest the following drugs.
- Oral contraceptives or hormones to cause menstruation to start
- Estrogen replacement for low levels of estrogen caused by ovarian disorders, hysterectomy, or menopause.
- Progesterone to treat ovarian cysts and some intrauterine disorders

Complementary and Alternative Therapies

Alternative therapies may help the body metabolize hormones while ensuring that the nutritional requirements for hormone production are met.

NUTRITION

Eat fewer refined foods and limit animal products. Limit the cruciferous family of vegetables (cabbage, broccoli, brussel sprouts, cauliflower, kale).

Eliminate methylxanthines (coffee, chocolate). Eat more whole grains, organic vegetables, and omega-3 fats (cold-water fish, nuts, and seeds). In addition, you may take the following supplements.
- Calcium (1,000 mg per day), magnesium (600 mg per day), vitamin D (200 to 400 IU/day), vitamin K (1 mg per day), and boron (1 to 3 mg per day).
- Iodine (up to 600 mcg per day), tyrosine (200 mg one to two times per day), zinc (30 mg per day), vitamin E (800 IU per day), vitamin A (10,000 to 15,000 IU per day), vitamin C (1,000 mg three times per day), and selenium (200 mcg per day).
- B$_6$ (200 mg per day) may reduce high prolactin levels.
- Essential fatty acids: Flax seed, evening primrose, or borage oil (1,000 to 1,500 mg one to two times per day).

HERBS

Herbs may be used as dried extracts (capsules, powders, teas), glycerites (glycerine extracts), or tinctures (alcohol extracts). Unless otherwise indicated, teas should be made with 1 tsp. herb per cup of hot water. Steep covered 5 to 10 minutes for leaf or flowers, and 10 to 20 minutes for roots. Drink 2 to 4 cups per day. .
- Chaste tree (*Vitex agnus-cactus*) helps normalize pituitary function but must be taken for 12 to 18 months. Use under the supervision of your provider if you take hormone therapy.
- Black cohosh (*Cimicifuga racemosa*), licorice (*Glycyrrhiza glabra*), and squaw vine (*Mitchella repens*) help to balance estrogen levels. Do not take licorice if you have high blood pressure.
- Chaste tree, wild yam (*Dioscorea villosa*), and lady's mantle (*Alchemilla vulgaris*) help balance progesterone levels.
- Kelp (*Nereocystis luetkeana*), bladderwrack (*Fucus vesiculosis*), oatstraw (*Avena sativa*), and horsetail (*Equisetum arvense*) are rich in minerals that support the thyroid.
- Milk thistle (*Silybum marianum*), dandelion root (*Taraxecum officinalis*), and vervain (*Verbena hastata*) support the liver.

HOMEOPATHY

Homeopathy may be useful as a supportive therapy.

PHYSICAL MEDICINE

The following help increase circulation and relieve pelvic congestion.
- Castor oil pack. Apply oil to skin of abdomen, cover with a clean soft cloth and plastic wrap. Place a hot water bottle or heating pad over the pack and let sit for 30 to 60 minutes. Use for three days.
- Contrast sitz baths. Use two basins that you can comfortably sit in. Sit in hot water for three minutes, then in cold water for one minute. Repeat this three times to complete one "set." Do one to two sets per day, three to four days per week.

ACUPUNCTURE

May help normalize hormone production and endocrine function.

MASSAGE

Therapeutic massage may improve endocrine function by relieving stress.

■ SPECIAL CONSIDERATIONS

Becoming pregnant may be difficult or impossible. Amenorrhea also may cause pregnancy complications.

■ ANEMIA

Anemia is characterized by a deficiency in red blood cells or in the concentration of hemoglobin (iron-containing portions of red blood cells). These deficiencies are caused by either decreased production or increased destruction of red blood cells. Anemia is most common among women in their reproductive years (5.8 percent), infants (5.7 percent), and the elderly (12 percent). Because one of the major functions of red blood cells is to transport oxygen, a decrease in red blood cells decreases the amount of oxygen delivered to the body's tissues, which results in the symptoms of anemia.

■ SIGNS AND SYMPTOMS

There is tremendous variability among individuals as to when the following symptoms of anemia develop.

- Tiredness
- Shortness of breath
- Paleness
- Lightheadedness
- Headache
- Heart palpitations and chest pain

■ WHAT CAUSES IT?

Anemia may have the following causes.

- Pregnancy and breast-feeding
- Iron, folic acid, vitamin B_{12}, or other vitamin deficiencies
- Certain chronic conditions
- Gastrointestinal blood loss (caused by ulcers, cancer, parasites)
- Genitourinary blood loss (such as from heavy menstruation)
- Excessive blood loss (after surgery or regular blood donations)
- Excessive alcohol or drug use
- Malabsorption syndromes (for example, celiac disease)
- Congenital diseases (for example, sickle cell anemia)
- Malnutrition

■ WHAT TO EXPECT AT YOUR PROVIDER'S OFFICE

Anemia is often the result of an underlying disease. Laboratory tests to examine your blood will be ordered. If you are anemic, your health care provider will determine why in order to begin treatment.

■ TREATMENT OPTIONS

Treatment depends on the cause and severity of the anemia. Because anemia is often the result of nutritional deficiencies, your health care provider can help you outline a diet that contains all of the nutrients you need for healthy blood formation such as vitamin B_{12}, iron, and folic acid. If your anemia is the result of an underlying disease, that disease must first be successfully treated.

Complementary and Alternative Therapies

Most cases of anemia will respond well to nutritional therapy. Note that excess iron is toxic and you should not take supplements unless lab tests indicate iron deficiency and your health care provider recommends them. Herbal and nutritional treatments may be helpful when used along with medical treatment.

NUTRITION

- Ferrous fumerate, glycerate, or glycinate (100 mg per day for three to six months) are the most absorbable forms of iron. Ferrous sulfate (325 mg per day) is poorly absorbed and more frequently causes problems with GI upset and constipation. Dietary sources of iron include meat, beans, green leafy vegetables, beet greens, blackstrap molasses, almonds, and brewer's yeast.
- Vitamin C—up to 1,000 mg three times per day to aid in absorption of iron.
- Vitamin B_{12}—cyanocobalamine, 1,000 IU via injection twice a day for one week, then weekly for a month, then every two to three months. Dietary sources include organ meats, meats, eggs, fish, and cheese.
- Folic acid (1 to 2 mg per day)—for folic acid deficiency. Good food sources include green leafy vegetables and grains.
- Omega-3 and omega-6 essential fatty acids (1,000 to 1,500 IU) have been shown to decrease the frequency of sickle-cell crisis. EFAs can increase clotting times, so if you are taking anticoagulants, your health care provider will need to check these times.

HERBS

Herbs are generally a safe way to strengthen and tone the body's systems. As with any therapy, it is important to work with your provider on getting your problem diagnosed before you start any treatment. Herbs may be used as dried extracts (capsules, powders, teas), glycerites (glycerine extracts), or tinctures (alcohol extracts). Unless otherwise indicated, teas should be made with 1 tsp. herb per cup of hot water. Steep covered 5 to 10 minutes for leaf or flowers, and 10 to 20 minutes for roots. Drink 2 to 4 cups per day. Tinctures may be used singly or in combination as noted.

You may be treated with the following herbal therapies for one to three months and then reassessed.

- Blackstrap molasses, also known as pregnancy tea (1 tbsp. per day in a cup of hot water), is a good source of iron, B vitamins, minerals, and is also a very gentle laxative.
- Spirulina, or blue-green algae, has been used successfully to treat both microcytic and macrocytic anemias. Dose is 1 heaping tsp. per day.
- Alfalfa *(Medicago sativa)*, dandelion *(Taraxacum officinale)* root or leaf, burdock *(Arctium lappa)*, and yellow dock *(Rumex crispus)* have long been used to fortify and cleanse the blood. For mild cases of anemia, they may help bring levels of hemoglobin into normal range. Dosage is 1 tbsp. per cup of water. Simmer roots for 20 minutes and leaves for 5 minutes. A single herb, or a combination of these four herbs, may be used.

HOMEOPATHY

A common remedy used for this condition is listed below. Usually, the dose is 12X to 30C every one to four hours.

- *Ferrum phosphoricum* 12C once a day for iron-deficiency anemia

■ FOLLOWING UP

Maintaining a normal balanced diet is very important if the cause of your anemia is nutritional. Also, avoid drugs that can have adverse effects on your gastrointestinal system and avoid excessive alcohol intake if one or both of these are the cause of your anemia.

■ SPECIAL CONSIDERATIONS

Complications from anemia can range from loss of productivity due to weakness and fatigue to coma and death. Some neurologic changes caused by anemia are irreversible. Pregnant women need three or four times as much iron as normal. A folic acid deficiency during pregnancy can result in infants being born with neural-tube defects, such as spina bifida.

■ ANGINA

Angina is chest pain caused by coronary heart disease, a partial block-age of the coronary arteries. If you have angina, your heart may not get enough blood, especially when you exercise or are under stress. If you have chest pain when you are resting, or the pain doesn't go away after a few minutes, call 911 or your local emergency number. You may be having a heart attack.

■ SIGNS AND SYMPTOMS
- Pressing or squeezing pain in the chest
- Pain lessens in a few minutes when you rest or take medication prescribed by your health care provider

■ WHAT CAUSES IT?
Coronary heart disease is the root cause of angina. Some risk factors for developing angina are older age, male sex, menopause, family history of angina, diabetes, smoking, high cholesterol, high blood pressure, obesity, sedentary lifestyle, and stress.

■ WHAT TO EXPECT AT YOUR PROVIDER'S OFFICE
You will have an electrocardiogram (EKG), during which electrodes will be fastened to your chest with a sticky gel. Your health care provider may also suggest a stress test, in which the EKG is taken while you walk on a tread-mill or use a stationary bicycle. Your health care provider may recommend coronary arteriography, where a catheter is inserted through a small incision to inject a dye that makes your blood flow visible on an x-ray image. Any blockages in and around your heart will appear.

■ TREATMENT OPTIONS
There are two main goals in treating angina. The first is to allow you to perform moderate exercise without pain. The second is to treat the underlying heart disease and prevent it from getting worse.

Drug Therapies
Your health care provider may prescribe medications such as nitroglycerin or aspirin to make blood flow more easily. Beta-blockers and calcium-channel blockers reduce the amount of blood the heart needs by lowering the blood pressure, the heart rate, or the heart's pumping force.

Surgical Procedures
If drugs are ineffective, you may need surgery. There are many different types of surgery to remove blockages from blood vessels or widen blood vessels so blood flows more easily.

Complementary and Alternative Therapies
Specific herbs and nutrients can help treat angina.

NUTRITION
Avoid saturated fats (meat and full-fat dairy products), refined foods, caffeine, and alcohol. Eat more fresh vegetables, whole grains, and essen-tial fatty acids (cold-water fish, nuts, and seeds).

The following supplements may help reduce symptoms of angina by strengthening heart muscle, lowering cholesterol, supporting connective tissue, and helping blood cells function normally.
- Coenzyme Q10 (50 to 100 mg one to two times per day)
- L-carnitine (330 mg two to three times per day)
- Vitamin E (400 to 800 IU per day)
- Essential fatty acids (1,000 to 1,500 mg one to two times a day)
- L-taurine (100 mg twice a day) and magnesium (200 mg two to three times per day)
- Vitamin C (1,000 mg two to three times per day)
- Bromelain (400 to 1,000 mg per day)

HERBS
Herbs may be used as dried extracts (capsules, powders, teas), glycerites (glycerine extracts), or tinctures (alcohol extracts). Unless otherwise indi-cated, teas should be made with 1 tsp. of herb per cup of hot water. Steep, covered, 5 to 10 minutes for leaf or flowers, and 10 to 20 minutes for roots. Drink 2 to 4 cups per day.

Hawthorn *(Crataegus oxyacantha)*, linden flowers *(Tilia cordata)*, and motherwort *(Leonorus cardiaca)* may be used long-term as teas with a high degree of safety.

A cardiac tonic that contains herbs to stimulate circulation and strengthen the cardiovascular system includes hawthorn *(Crataegus oxyacantha)*, ginkgo *(Ginkgo biloba)*, linden flowers *(Tilia cordata)*, mistletoe *(Viscum album)*, Indian tobacco *(Lobelia inflata)*, and motherwort *(Leonorus cardiaca)*. A tincture made from equal parts of these herbs should be taken in 20 drops three times a day.

For acute relief of symptoms use a tincture made from equal parts of the following herbs: yellow jasmine *(Gelsemium sempervirens)*, Indian tobacco *(Lobelia inflata)*, monkshood *(Aconite napellus)*, night-blooming cereus *(Cactus grandiflorus)*, and ginger *(Zingiber offici-nalis)*. Take 10 to 20 drops every 15 minutes when necessary, up to eight consecutive doses.

HOMEOPATHY
Some of the most common remedies used for angina are listed below. Usually, the dose is 12X to 30C every one to four hours until your symptoms get better.
- *Aconite* for panic and fear of death with tachycardia.
- *Cactus* for constriction in chest, pains down the left arm.
- *Glonoine* for rapid pulse, violent palpitations, cardiac pains that radiate to arms, and waves of pounding headache.

ACUPUNCTURE
Acupuncture can relieve symptoms and help treat underlying causes.

MASSAGE
Massage can improve circulation to peripheral tissues.

■ FOLLOWING UP
Keep track of what causes your angina pain, what it feels like, how often you get it, and how long it lasts. If there's a change in your pattern, let your health care provider know right away.

■ SPECIAL CONSIDERATIONS
Hawthorn, linden, and motherwort are safe during pregnancy. Stronger herbs should not be used without provider supervision.

■ ANOREXIA NERVOSA

Anorexia is a serious eating disorder in which people deliberately starve themselves to lose weight. No matter how thin they become, they still believe they are overweight. Without proper treatment, the disorder can be fatal. More than 90 percent of people with anorexia are females, though a growing number of males now have the disorder. It usually begins between the ages of 13 and 18 and is often triggered by a severe emotional shock.

■ SIGNS AND SYMPTOMS

- Extreme weight loss due to self-imposed starvation
- Compulsive exercising
- A number of symptoms associated with starvation including anemia, brittle hair and nails, dry skin, hypothermia, constipation, and the appearance of soft, downy hair on the torso
- Depression, withdrawal, irritability, sleeplessness, low sex desire
- Obsession with food, such as collecting recipes; hoarding food
- Unwillingness to eat in public
- Inflexible thinking; strictly controlled emotional responses
- The loss of menstrual periods for three months or more
- An irrational fear of gaining weight

■ WHAT CAUSES IT?

- An overwhelming sense of being out of control, and attempting to take control of one's life by regulating food intake
- Unrealistic fear of developing an adult body
- Severe trauma or emotional shock during puberty or pre-puberty
- Anorexia is known to run in families.
- Abnormal levels of certain chemicals in the brain may exist.
- Frequent dieters stand an 8-times greater chance of anorexia.
- Society's unrealistic emphasis on thinness places certain individuals such as cheerleaders, dancers, runners, models, jockeys, wrestlers, and actresses and actors at higher risk for anorexia.

■ WHAT TO EXPECT AT YOUR PROVIDER'S OFFICE

Your health care provider will ask you questions about your eating habits—how much and what you eat—and your exercise routine. He or she will do blood and other diagnostic tests to eliminate the possibility that your weight loss is caused by medical problems. You will most likely be referred to a therapist or psychiatrist who understands eating disorders.

■ TREATMENT OPTIONS

It is best to get treatment as soon as symptoms appear. There are several forms of treatment for anorexia, including therapy with a psychiatrist specially trained in both treating the disorder and in nutritional counseling. Your health care provider will help you "relearn" how to eat correctly. He or she may also recommend protein supplements, relaxation techniques, and antidepressant drugs. In severe cases, hospitalization may be needed.

Complementary and Alternative Therapies

Alternative therapies may be especially helpful in people who have fixated on avoiding anything "artificial."

NUTRITION

- Zinc (15 mg per day increased to 50 mg twice a day)—may improve mood and appetite.

- Protein supplements (1 to 3 servings a day)—will help ensure sufficient amino acids and help prevent wasting.
- A multivitamin will help compensate for dietary deficiencies.

HERBS

Herbs may be used as dried extracts (capsules, powders, teas), glycerites (glycerine extracts), or tinctures (alcohol extracts). Unless otherwise indicated, teas should be made with 1 tsp. herb per cup of hot water. Steep covered 5 to 10 minutes for leaf or flowers, and 10 to 20 minutes for roots. Drink 2 to 4 cups per day. Tinctures may be used singly or in combination as noted.

- Goldenseal *(Hydrastis canadensis)*—a strong digestive stimulant, and tonic to the digestive tract; is a specific to anorexia nervosa
- Condurango *(Marsdenia condurango)*—digestive stimulant for diminished appetite or dietary abuse; is a specific to anorexia nervosa
- Licorice *(Glycyrrhiza glabra)*—antidepressant effects, heals mucous membranes of the digestive tract. Do not take if you have high blood pressure. May cause peripheral edema (fluid retention), which goes away when licorice is stopped.
- Wild yam *(Dioscorea villosa)*—hormone balancing, antidepressant.
- Valerian *(Valeriana officinalis)*—sedative, digestive bitter, and appetite stimulant
- Lemon balm *(Melissa officinalis)*—mild sedative, spasmolytic, may gently help regulate thyroid-stimulating hormone and thyroid function
- Oatstraw *(Avena sativa)*—nerve tonic, antidepressant, relieves irritation of mucous membranes. This herb is slow to start acting but is long-lasting.
- St. John's wort *(Hypericum perforatum)*—for depression or anxiety leading to fatigue and adrenal gland exhaustion
- Fenugreek *(Trigonella foenum-graecum)*—nutritive and digestive tonic used where there is digestive debility and poor nutrition.
- Saw Palmetto *(Serenoa repens, S. serrulatta, S. serrullatum)*—digestive tonic and connective-tissue rebuilder.
- Siberian ginseng *(Eleuthrocuccus senticosus)*—a supportive adaptogen used to improve vitality and stamina.

HOMEOPATHY

Homeopathy may be useful as a supportive therapy.

ACUPUNCTURE

May be helpful in restoring energy and reducing stress.

MASSAGE

May be helpful if the patient is willing to be touched. Essential oils (lavender, rosemary, verbena) can be added to increase the relaxing effect.

■ FOLLOWING UP

Long-term monitoring and support is necessary.

■ SPECIAL CONSIDERATIONS

- Seek care from professionals specializing in eating disorders.
- Because the disorder is primarily psychological and not simply due to appetite loss, psychotherapy is usually necessary.
- Anorexia causes difficulties in conceiving and carrying a baby to term.
- The common medical complications of anorexia include osteoporosis, kidney damage, and heart failure.

■ ANXIETY

Anxiety is a general feeling of being worried. Everyone experiences anxiety from time to time as a result of life experiences, but those with generalized anxiety disorder feel anxious frequently or excessively, not necessarily as a result of a particular situation.

■ SIGNS AND SYMPTOMS

- Muscle tension, trembling
- Fast heart beat (tachycardia)
- Fast or troubled breathing (dyspnea)
- Dizziness or impaired concentration
- Palpitations
- Sweating
- Fatigue
- Irritability
- Sleep disturbances

■ WHAT CAUSES IT?

Anxiety can result from many specific causes, such as an underlying medical condition or drugs you are taking. However, there may be no specific cause. Factors such as genetics and early life experiences may play a role.

■ WHAT TO EXPECT AT YOUR PROVIDER'S OFFICE

Your health care provider will talk to you about when you feel anxious, what it feels like, and your medical history. He or she will give you a physical examination and may take blood or urine samples for laboratory tests. In some cases, you will have an electrocardiogram (EKG) to rule out heart problems.

■ TREATMENT OPTIONS

If your health care provider finds a specific physiological cause for your anxiety, he or she will treat that condition. For anxiety without a physical cause, your health care provider will work with you to find other ways to treat your anxiety. Usually, this means first trying a method of relaxation, and if this does not work, prescribing medication. Treatment may also include short-term counseling to help you feel better about your life and cope with stress better.

Complementary and Alternative Therapies

Mind-body techniques, nutrition, and herbs may be an effective way to treat anxiety. Progressive muscle relaxation, diaphragmatic breathing, biofeedback, meditation, and self-hypnosis can help you relax and reduce your anxiety. Talk with your health care provider about these techniques.

NUTRITION

- Avoid caffeine, alcohol, sugar, refined foods, and cut down on foods that are known to cause allergies (common food allergens are dairy, soy, citrus, peanuts, tree nuts, wheat, fish, wheat, fish, eggs, corn, food colorings, and additives). Fresh vegetables, whole grains, and protein nourish the nervous system, so eat more of these.
- Calcium (1,000 mg per day), magnesium (400 to 600 mg per day), and B complex (50 to 100 mg per day) help support the nervous system and minimize the effects of stress.

HERBS

Herbs are generally a safe way to strengthen and tone the body's systems. As with any therapy, it is important to work with your provider on getting your problem diagnosed before you start any treatment. Herbs may be used as dried extracts (capsules, powders, teas), glycerites (glycerine extracts), or tinctures (alcohol extracts). Unless otherwise indicated, teas should be made with 1 tsp. herb per cup of hot water. Steep covered 5 to 10 minutes for leaf or flowers, and 10 to 20 minutes for roots. Drink 2 to 4 cups per day. Tinctures may be used singly or in combination as noted.

A tea (3 to 4 cups per day) or tincture (10 to 20 drops four to six times per day) from the following herbs will help to reduce anxiety and strengthen the nervous system.

- Kava kava *(Piper methysticum)* for mild to moderate anxiety.
- St. John's wort *(Hypericum perforatum)* for anxiety associated with depression.
- Passionflower *(Passiflora incarnata)* for anxiety with insomnia.
- Oatstraw *(Avena sativa)* nourishes the nervous system.
- Lemon Balm *(Melissa officinalis)* for anxiety with depression and heart palpitations.
- Lavender *(Lavendula officinalis)* for nervous exhaustion and restoring the nervous system.
- Skullcap *(Scutellaria laterifolia)* relaxes and revitalizes the nervous system.

Kava kava (100 to 200 mg two to four times a day) and St. John's wort (300 mg two to three times per day) may be taken as dried extracts to maximize effectiveness in moderate anxiety.

Essential oils of lemon balm, bergamot, and jasmine are calming and may be used as aromatherapy. Place several drops in a warm bath or atomizer, or on a cotton ball.

HOMEOPATHY

Some of the most common remedies used for anxiety are listed below. Usually, the dose is 12X to 30C every one to four hours until your symptoms get better.

- *Aconite* for anxiety with palpitations, shortness of breath, and fear of death
- *Arsenicum* for anxiety with restlessness, especially after midnight
- *Phosphorus* for anxiety when alone and fearing that something bad will happen

MASSAGE

Therapeutic massage can be helpful in reducing anxiety and alleviating stress.

■ FOLLOWING UP

Follow your health care provider's instructions, and practice relaxation techniques as needed.

■ SPECIAL CONSIDERATIONS

Be sure to tell your health care provider if you are pregnant. Call your provider if you experience any significant side effects from prescribed medications.

While the herbal tea suggested above is safe during pregnancy, you avoid the dried extracts of kava kava and St. John's wort if you are pregnant.

■ ASTHMA

Asthma is chronic inflammation of the airways resulting from swelling and excessive mucus. The airways may be further blocked when an irritant, or trigger, causes spasms of the bronchial passage. This can cause coughing, wheezing, and difficulty breathing.

■ SIGNS AND SYMPTOMS

- Shortness of breath, difficulty breathing, or wheezing
- Chest tightness or constriction
- Cough (can be the only symptom)
- Skin turning blue (cyanosis)

■ WHAT CAUSES IT?

- Sensitivity to allergens in the air, such as dust, cockroach waste, animal dander, mold, pollens
- Food allergies
- Respiratory infections
- Air pollutants, such as tobacco, aerosols, perfumes, fresh newsprint, diesel particles, sulfur dioxide, elevated ozone levels, and fumes from paint, cleaning products, and gas stoves
- Changes in the weather, especially in temperature and humidity
- Behaviors that affect breathing (exercising, laughing, crying)

■ WHAT TO EXPECT AT YOUR PROVIDER'S OFFICE

Your health care provider will probably check your blood pressure, listen to your chest and back with a stethoscope, and take blood samples. He or she may also order an electrocardiogram (EKG) or chest or sinus X-rays to make sure your asthma is not a symptom of a more serious condition.

■ TREATMENT OPTIONS

You can help control your asthma in the following ways.
- Avoid your "triggers."
- Take anti-inflammatory drugs or antibiotics prescribed by your provider. These can help you breathe more easily.
- Use the inhaler prescribed by your provider if you have an asthma attack. An asthma attack is a serious situation. It can result in critical health problems, even death. If your inhaler does not stop the attack, call your provider or go to the nearest health care facility.
- Your provider may also prescribe oxygen for severe asthma attacks.

Complementary and Alternative Therapies

Asthma may relate to stress and anxiety. Mind-body techniques such as deep breathing, meditation, tai chi, yoga, and stress management can help.

NUTRITION

Note: Lower doses are for children.
- Eliminate all food allergens from your diet. Common food allergens are dairy, soy, citrus, peanuts, tree nuts, wheat, fish, shellfish, eggs, corn, food colorings, and additives. An elimination trial may help determine food sensitivities. Remove suspected allergens from your diet for two weeks. Re-introduce one food every three days. Watch for reactions such as gastrointestinal upset, mood changes, headaches, and worsening of asthma. Check with your health care provider before doing this test.
- Reduce pro-inflammatory foods in your diet, including saturated fats (meats, especially poultry, and dairy), refined foods, and sugar.
- Increase intake of vegetables, grains, legumes, onions, and garlic.

- Vitamin C (250 to 1,000 mg two to four times per day) taken one hour before exposure to an allergen may reduce allergic reactions. Rose hips or palmitate do not cause allergic reactions.
- B_6 (50 to 200 mg per day) may improve symptoms. Pyridoxal-5-phosphate (P5P), a form of B_6, may be more readily used by your body.
- Magnesium (200 mg two to three times per day) relaxes bronchioles.
- Consider hydrochloric acid supplementation to decrease the number and severity of food sensitivities and aid absorption of some nutrients.
- B_{12} deficiency may increase reactivity to sulfites.
- N-acetyl cysteine (50 to 200 mg three times per day) and selenium (50 to 200 mcg per day) protect lung tissue from damage.

HERBS

Herbs may be used as dried extracts (capsules, powders, teas), glycerites (glycerine extracts), or tinctures (alcohol extracts). Teas should be made with 1 tsp. herb per cup of hot water. Steep covered 5 to 10 minutes for leaf or flowers; 10 to 20 minutes for roots. Drink 2 to 4 cups per day.
- Green tea *(Camellia sinensis)* is a powerful antioxidant.
- For long-term lung support, combine equal parts of the following herbs in a tea. Licorice root *(Glycyrrhiza glabra)*, coltsfoot *(Tussilago farfara)*, wild cherry bark *(Prunus serotina)*, elecampane *(Inula helenium)*, plantain *(Plantago major)*, and skullcap *(Scutellaria laterifolia)*. Do not take licorice if you have high blood pressure. Prolonged use of coltsfoot can damage the liver; look for a "pyrrolizidine alkaloid-free" label.
- Essential oils that may help are elecampane, frankincense, lavender, mint, and sage. Add 4 to 6 drops in a bath, atomizer, or humidifier.

HOMEOPATHY

Some of the most common remedies used for asthma are listed below. Usually, the dose is 12X to 30C every one to four hours until your symptoms get better.
- *Arsenicum album* for asthma with restlessness and anxiety
- *Ipecac* for constant constriction in the chest with a bad cough
- *Pulsatilla* for asthma with pressure in chest and air hunger
- *Sambucus* for asthma that wakes you with a sensation of suffocation

PHYSICAL MEDICINE

Cold compresses to the chest during acute attacks may lessen severity.

Contrast hydrotherapy may decrease inflammation, relieve pain, and aid healing. Alternate three minutes hot application to the chest with one minute cold. Repeat three times for one set; do two to three sets per day.

Castor oil pack. Apply oil directly to chest, cover with a clean soft cloth and plastic wrap. Apply a heat source on top; let sit 30 to 60 minutes.

ACUPUNCTURE

Acupuncture may reduce frequency and intensity of asthma attacks.

MASSAGE

Massage may reduce stress, easing reactions to allergens.

■ FOLLOWING UP

Your provider may give you a peak-flow meter to use at home to closely monitor your condition.

■ ATHEROSCLEROSIS

Atherosclerosis, or hardening of the arteries, occurs when the inside walls of an artery become thicker and less elastic. The thickening reduces the area available for blood flow. Although atherosclerosis reveals few symptoms at first, the damaged artery eventually cannot carry enough blood to supply the necessary amount of oxygen. The result is often a stroke or heart attack. About 1 million people die as a result of atherosclerosis each year in the United States.

■ SIGNS AND SYMPTOMS

- Pain and cramps at the site of the narrowed artery (chest, leg, etc.)
- Gradual or sudden increase in the severity of symptoms
- Hardened feel of arteries in forearms or carotid arteries in neck
- Lowered or absent pulses
- In more severe cases, muscle wasting, ulcer, or gangrene

■ WHAT CAUSES IT?

Cholesterol and similar substances called lipoproteins attach themselves to the inside linings of the arteries. There, they gradually thicken into a substance called plaque. Plaque causes the artery to become tougher and less flexible. As plaque grows, it narrows the artery more and more, in some cases blocking it entirely. A sudden obstruction, as when a blood clot gets wedged in the blocked artery, can lead to immediate problems, such as stroke and heart attack.

■ WHAT TO EXPECT AT YOUR PROVIDER'S OFFICE

Your health care provider will examine your neck, abdomen, and groin area for "bruits"—blowing sounds that indicate turbulence in blood flow. The provider will also take further blood samples. He or she may recommend X-rays, ultrasound or computed tomography (CAT scans). You may have a stress test, in which you run or jog for several minutes while providers monitor your blood pressure. For arteriography, you are X-rayed after a dye is injected into your bloodstream.

■ TREATMENT OPTIONS

Some risks for atherosclerosis, such as being male or a postmenopausal woman, are beyond your control. But you can control other risks. Eat a healthy diet low in fat and sugar, learn to manage stress, exercise regularly, quit smoking, control diabetes and high blood pressure, and maintain a healthy weight.

Cholestyramine and colestipol, nicotinic acid, gemfibrozil, probucol, and a class of medications called statins, can reduce the amount of cholesterol and other fats in your blood. Your health care provider may recommend endarterectomy, in which a surgeon scrapes plaque from the inside of the carotid artery in your neck. This surgery has a high rate of success, although it has some risks.

Complementary and Alternative Therapies

Nutritional supplements can be very effective. Hawthorn has an important role in both treating and preventing atherosclerosis. Yoga, meditation, relaxation, and biofeedback show promise.

NUTRITION

- Vegetarian diet can help stop or possibly reverse the hardening process.
- Antioxidants: vitamin C (1,000 mg three times a day), vitamin E (400 IU a day), coenzyme Q10 (30 to 50 mg three times a day), selenium (200 mcg a day), lipoic acid (50 mg twice a day)
- Essential fatty acids (1,500 mg twice a day): While there has been much emphasis on low-fat diets, it may be more important to alter the types of fat in the diet, decreasing saturated fats and trans fatty acids, and replacing them with poly- and mono-unsaturated fats.
- Diet: garlic, ginger and onions all have a beneficial effect on platelet aggregation. Increase fiber (especially water-soluble), fruits, vegetables, and vegetarian sources of protein.
- Homocystiene metabolism: folic acid (800 mcg a day), B$_6$ (50 mg a day), B$_{12}$ (400 mcg a day), betaine (200 to 1,000 mg a day)
- Chromium (200 mcg a day): may result in plaque reduction
- Magnesium (500 mg): decreases arrhythmias, angina, and death rates following heart attack, especially when given with potassium
- Bromelian (150 to 250 mg four times a day away from meals): stops platelets from sticking together and breaks down plaque
- Carnitine (750 to 1,500 mg twice a day): important in fatty acid metabolism, depleted in cardiac muscle during acute heart attacks

HERBS

Herbs may be used as dried extracts (capsules, powders, teas), glycerites (glycerine extracts), or tinctures (alcohol extracts). Unless otherwise indicated, teas should be made with 1 tsp. herb per cup of hot water. Steep covered 5 to 10 minutes for leaf or flowers, and 10 to 20 minutes for roots. Drink 2 to 4 cups per day.

- Hawthorn *(Crataegus oxycantha)*: prevents cholesterol deposits and improves blood flow. Take 3 to 5 g as either dried herb, solid extract, or liquid extract.
- Ginkgo *(Ginkgo biloba)*: helps keeps arteries clear and keeps platelets from sticking together (250 mg three times a day)
- Mistletoe *(Viscum album)*: keeps arteries flexible and reduces high blood pressure (can be toxic; use under a practitioner's care)
- Linden *(Tilia cordata)*: atherosclerosis, historically used to lower blood pressure, especially with digestive problems and nervousness
- Rosemary *(Rosemariana officinalis)*: increases coronary artery blood flow (used to stimulate digestion and relieve tension)
- Gentian *(Gentiana lutea)*: bitter, digestive tonic, historically used for smoking cessation, avoid with ulcers

Hawthorn or ginkgo are recommended for treating atherosclerosis. Concentrated extracts may be required to achieve the recommended doses. In addition, a tincture (30 to 60 drops three times a day) or tea (1 cup three times a day) of one to four of the above herbs, taken before meals, may be helpful.

HOMEOPATHY

Homeopathy may be useful as a supportive therapy.

ACUPUNCTURE

May be helpful in decreasing tension, stimulating proper digestion and elimination, and increasing a sense of well-being.

MASSAGE

May be helpful at relieving tension.

■ FOLLOWING UP

Take measures to prevent the conditions that lead to this disease. Have your blood pressure and cholesterol levels measured regularly.

■ ATTENTION-DEFICIT/HYPERACTIVITY DISORDER (ADHD)

Attention-deficit/hyperactivity disorder (ADHD) is a complicated behavioral disorder that affects 3 to 5 percent of school-age children—90 percent of whom are boys. ADHD is a biological disorder caused by irregularities in brain chemistry, and it usually continues throughout life. Diagnosis is difficult, particularly in adults, because symptoms are similar to those seen in other illnesses. In order to be classified as ADHD, symptoms must have appeared before the age of 7 years, and must be causing significant disruption across several settings such as at home, school, or socially for at least six months.

■ SIGNS AND SYMPTOMS

The following are indications of a person with ADHD.
- Fails to give close attention to details or makes careless mistakes
- Easily distracted when playing or doing tasks
- Does not seem to listen when spoken to
- Does not follow through on instructions and fails to finish work
- Difficulty organizing tasks and activities
- Avoids or dislikes tasks that require a lot of concentration
- Loses things; forgetful
- Fidgets with hands or feet or squirms in seat; leaves seat
- Runs or climbs excessively in inappropriate situations, restless
- Difficulty playing quietly
- Acts as if "driven by a motor;" acts without thinking first
- Talks excessively
- Blurts out answers before questions are completed
- Has a hard time waiting for a turn; interrupts others

■ WHAT CAUSES IT?

ADHD is not caused by poor parenting, poor teachers, too much television, or excess sugar. The following are some likely causes.
- Biological factors having to do with brain activity
- Environmental factors including low birth weight, lack of oxygen (hypoxia) at birth, and fetal exposure to toxins such as lead or mercury, alcohol, cocaine, and nicotine.
- Children of fathers with ADHD are more likely to have ADHD.
- Nutritional factors; many specialists believe allergies to food, food colorings or additives, or sugar, as well as low levels of certain vitamins and other nutrients, can cause or aggravate symptoms.

■ WHAT TO EXPECT AT YOUR PROVIDER'S OFFICE

Your child's provider will ask for a detailed history from you and others who spend time with the child, and will review your child's report cards for comments on behavior. He or she may also spend time observing your child in a comfortable setting, such as a playroom.

■ TREATMENT OPTIONS

Treatment is most effective with a combination of medicine and behavioral therapies. Behavioral modification techniques include the following.
- Rewarding good behavior instead of punishing bad
- Specific and positive incentives or rewards
- Exercises and activities to improve learning deficits
- Designing an individual educational program
- Activities such as sports, music, games, or other special interests

Drug Therapies

Medications used to treat ADHD include Dexedrine, Cylert, and Ritalin. Antidepressants may be prescribed in some cases.

Complementary and Alternative Therapies

Many parents seek alternative treatment for ADHD, because of concerns with the effects of chronic drug therapy in young children. Some, but not all, children respond dramatically to dietary changes. The doses listed are for children. For adults, increase the dose by $1^1/_2$ to 2 times.

NUTRITION
- Essential fatty acids help regulate inflammation and nervous irritability. Reduce animal fats and increase fish and vegetable oil intake, especially olive and grapeseed oils. A mix of omega-6 (evening primrose) and omega-3 (flaxseed) may be best (2 tbsp. oil per day or 1,000 to 1,500 mg twice per day). For children under 10, cod liver oil may be the most effective (1 tsp. per day).
- Foods containing salicylates (almonds, apples, berries, tomatoes, oranges) may be another dietary factor affecting ADHD. A possible mechanism is related to prostaglandin metabolism. Common food sensitivities are dairy, corn, wheat, soy, and eggs.
- Vitamins: C (1,000 mg twice per day), E (400 IU per day), B-complex (50 to 100 mg per day)
- Minerals: Calcium/magnesium (250 to 500 mg per day), especially before bed

HERBS

Herbs may be used as dried extracts (capsules, powders, teas), glycerites (glycerine extracts), or tinctures (alcohol extracts). Unless otherwise indicated, teas should be made with 1 tsp. herb per cup of hot water. Steep covered 5 to 10 minutes for leaf or flowers, and 10 to 20 minutes for roots. Drink 2 to 4 cups per day.
- Lemon balm (*Melissa officinalis*): mild sedative, relieves spasms
- Lavender (*Lavendula angustifolia*): mild sedative and blood purifier
- Chamomile (*Matricaria recutita*): reduces swelling and spasms
- Passionflower (*Passiflora incarnata*): relieves nervous gastrointestinal complaints
- Linden (*Tilia cordata*): mild sedative, antispasmodic
- Catnip (*Nepeta cataria*): helps you relax and relieves spasms
- Kava kava (*Piper methysticum*): anti-anxiety

A combination of four to six of the above herbs (1 cup tea two to three times per day, or 30 to 60 drops tincture) can be helpful.

HOMEOPATHY

Some of the more common remedies for ADHD are listed below.
- *Chamomilla* for a person who is irritable and easily distracted
- *Arsenicum album* for anxiety, especially with stomach pains and insomnia or restless sleep
- *Argentum nitricum* for anxious children that may be very cheerful

ACUPUNCTURE

Adults, and some children, respond well to acupuncture to treat ADHD.

MASSAGE

Parents can be taught massage techniques to use on their children.

■ SPECIAL CONSIDERATIONS

ADHD can affect people throughout their lives. A team approach to care and emotional support is necessary to help you cope with its impact.

■ BENIGN PROSTATIC HYPERPLASIA

Benign prostatic hyperplasia (BPH), a noncancerous growth of the prostate gland, makes urination difficult and uncomfortable. The expanding prostate squeezes the urethra, the channel that carries urine from the bladder. BPH affects only men. Symptoms usually develop around age 50. At age 60, you'll most likely have BPH. At age 80, you'll have an 80 percent chance of experiencing urination problems caused by BPH.

■ SIGNS AND SYMPTOMS
- The need to urinate frequently
- Inability to sleep through the night without getting up to urinate
- Difficulty starting urine stream or complete inability to urinate
- Decreased strength and force of the urine stream
- Dribbling after urination ends
- Blood in the urine (BPH can cause small blood vessels to burst)

■ WHAT CAUSES IT?
Nobody knows the basic cause of BPH. Research shows that testosterone, the male hormone, or dihydrotestosterone, a chemical produced when testosterone breaks down in a man's body, may cause the prostate to keep growing. Since it surrounds the urethra, the prostate gland squeezes the urethra as it expands. Some over-the-counter medications for colds or allergies can drastically worsen BPH.

■ WHAT TO EXPECT AT YOUR PROVIDER'S OFFICE
Your health care provider will feel your prostate gland directly by putting a gloved finger in your rectum. He or she will also order blood tests and possibly a urine sample. Your health care provider may also ask you to urinate into a device that measures the flow of urine. In intravenous pyelogram, your health care provider injects a dye into a vein to make the flow of urine visible on an X ray. In cystoscopy, your provider uses a small probe, passed through your urethra, to directly view the inside of your urethra and bladder. Your penis will be numbed before this procedure.

■ TREATMENT OPTIONS
One-third of mild BPH cases clear up by themselves.

Drug Therapies
Alpha-blockers can relieve urination problems by relaxing the muscles at the outlet from the bladder. Another drug, finasteride, can shrink the prostate, but it can take up to three months to work.

Surgical Procedures
Balloon urethroplasty uses a balloon to widen the urethra and improve the flow of urine. Prostatic stents do the same thing with a spring-like device. Transurethral microwave therapy and transurethral hyperthermia are new treatments that use microwaves or heat to destroy prostate tissue.

Transurethral resection of the prostate, used on 90 percent of patients undergoing BPH surgery, removes pieces of the enlarged prostate through the urethra. A less invasive method, transurethral incision of the prostate, makes small cuts in the prostate and the neck of the bladder. Laser surgery vaporizes excess tissue in the prostate.

Complementary and Alternative Therapies
Your health care provider may want to keep a close eye on your condition as part of the management of BPH.

NUTRITION
- Zinc (60 mg per day)—to reduce the size of the prostate.
- Selenium (200 mcg per day)—anti-oxidant in the prostate
- Essential fatty acids (1,000 to 1,500 IU one to two times per day)—anti-inflammatory, for optimum prostaglandin concentrations
- B_6 (100 to 250 mg per day)—reduces the elevated levels of prolactin found in people who have BPH
- Amino acids glycine, glutamic acid, and alanine (200 mg per day of each)—provide relief from symptoms
- Avoid alcohol, especially beer, and saturated fats.
- Pumpkin seeds can help maintain a healthy prostate.

HERBS
Herbs may be used as dried extracts (capsules, powders, teas), glycerites (glycerine extracts), or tinctures (alcohol extracts). Unless otherwise indicated, teas should be made with one teaspoon herb per cup of hot water. Steep covered 5 to 10 minutes for leaf or flowers, and 10 to 20 minutes for roots. Drink 2 to 4 cups per day.
- Saw palmetto *(Serenoa ripens)*—160 mg twice a day is difficult to achieve in tea or tincture; extract standardized for 85 percent to 95 percent of fatty acids and sterols is recommended. Saw palmetto is widely used in Europe.
- Stinging nettle root *(Urticae radix)*—Increases urinary flow and volume. Daily dose of 4 to 6 g of drug or equivalent preparation.

HOMEOPATHY
Some of the most common remedies used for this condition are listed below. Usually, the dose is 12X to 30C every one to four hours until your symptoms get better.
- *Chimaphila umbellata* is specific for retention of urine with an enlarged prostate
- *Conium* for BPH with a feeling of heaviness in the pelvic area, especially with premature ejaculation
- *Pareira* for urinary retention with BPH, especially with painful urging or pain in the bladder
- *Selenium* for BPH with dribbling, impotence, and constipation
- *Thuja occidentalis*, specifically if there is a forked stream of urine

PHYSICAL MEDICINE
- Kegel exercises (contracting and releasing the pelvic muscles)
- Contrast sitz baths. You will need two basins that can be comfortably sat in. Sit in hot water for three minutes, then in cold water for one minute. Repeat this three times to complete one set. Do one to two sets per day, three to four days per week.

■ FOLLOWING UP
Whatever your treatment, have regular checkups. After prostate surgery, drink plenty of water, eat a balanced diet, avoid heavy lifting and operating machinery, and don't strain when you move your bowels.

■ BRONCHITIS

Bronchitis is a respiratory tract infection (viral or bacterial) that causes inflammation of the mucous lining of the bronchial tubes. Acute bronchitis generally is reversible. Chronic bronchitis, often referred to as smoker's cough, is not usually reversible.

■ SIGNS AND SYMPTOMS

Acute bronchitis:
- Cough that produces mucus or pus
- Burning sensation in the chest
- Sore throat and fever (with some types)
- Fatigue
- Blue-tinted lips
- Wheezing
- Weight gain

Chronic bronchitis:
- Chronic cough that produces excessive amounts of mucus or pus
- Wheezing, shortness of breath
- Present for three consecutive months, two years in a row

■ WHAT CAUSES IT?

Acute bronchitis is usually caused by a virus, but can also be caused by bacteria. Generally, acute bronchitis is passed from person to person. The main causes of chronic bronchitis are cigarette smoking and prolonged exposure to air pollution or other irritants such as dust and grain.

■ RISK FACTORS

- Cigarette smoking
- Severe pneumonia early in life
- Being a man over age 50

■ WHAT TO EXPECT AT YOUR PROVIDER'S OFFICE

Your provider will listen to your chest and back, look at your throat, and may draw blood and take a culture of the secretions from your lungs.

■ TREATMENT OPTIONS

Your health care provider may prescribe antibiotics to help treat your bronchitis if it is caused by bacteria. He or she may also suggest using a humidifier, taking a cough medicine that contains an expectorant (something that helps you "bring up" secretions), and drinking plenty of fluids.

Complementary and Alternative Therapies

Alternative therapies can be useful in treating chronic bronchitis.

NUTRITION

- Eliminate known allergenic foods (for example, eggs, milk, nuts, peanuts, soy), food coloring, preservatives, and additives. Reduce intake of mucus-producing foods such as dairy, citrus, wheat, and bananas. Onions and garlic help to thin mucus.
- Vitamin C (1,000 mg three to four times per day), zinc (30 mg per day), and beta-carotene (50,000 to 100,000 IU per day) support the immune system. Some studies suggest that smokers do not use beta-carotene. N-acetyl cysteine (200 mg twice a day between meals) protects lung tissue from damage and helps break up mucus.

HERBS

Herbs may be used as dried extracts (capsules, powders, teas), glycerites (glycerine extracts), or tinctures (alcohol extracts). Herbs can be used in combination. Tincture combinations should be taken at 30 drops three to four times per day. Make infusions with 1 heaping tsp. of herbal combination, steep covered for 10 minutes, and drink 3 to 4 cups per day. Substitute grindelia *(Grindelia robusta)* for licorice root if you have high blood pressure.

- Acute bronchitis: Thyme leaf *(Thymus vulgaris)*, licorice root *(Glycyrrhiza glabra)*, coneflower *(Echinacea purpura)*, ginger *(Zingiber officinalis)*, and linden flowers *(Tilia cordata)*. Smokers should substitute Indian tobacco *(Lobelia inflata)* for the linden flowers. White horehound *(Marrabium vulgare)* is a gentle stimulating expectorant (helps you cough up mucus) that relaxes spasms of the bronchi airway (passages in the lungs). Sundew *(Drosera rotundifolia)* helps you cough up mucus and relaxes spasms.
- Chronic bronchitis: Pleurisy root *(Asclepias tuberosa)*, Indian tobacco *(Lobelia inflata)*, elecampane *(Inula helenium)*, licorice root, lungwort *(Sticta pulmonaria)*, and lomatium *(Lomatium dissectum)*. Boneset *(Eupatorium perfoliatum)*, is an herb that helps to sweat out impurities and relax spasms. Pill bearing spurge *(Euphorbia hirta)*, is an herb that breaks up mucus and relaxes spasms.
- Garlic *(Allium sativum)* and ginger tea can be used long-term (2 cloves of garlic and 2 to 3 slices of ginger root). Simmer in 1 cup of water for 15 minutes. Drink 3 to 4 cups per day. Add honey or lemon to flavor.

HOMEOPATHY

Some of the most common remedies used for bronchitis are listed below. Usually, the dose is 12X to 30C every one to four hours until your symptoms get better.
- *Antimonium* tart for rattling cough with dizziness
- *Hepar sulphuricum* for later stages of bronchitis with wheezing, small amounts of phlegm, and coughing when you get cold
- *Ipecacuanha* for first stages of bronchitis with deep, wet cough
- *Phosphorus* for painful cough, and if you are thirsty and chilly

PHYSICAL MEDICINE

- Castor oil pack. Apply oil directly to skin, cover with a clean soft cloth and plastic wrap. Place a heat source (hot water bottle or heating pad) over the pack and let sit for 30 to 60 minutes.
- Chest rubs with 3 to 6 drops of essential oil in 1 tbsp. of food-grade oil. Thyme, eucalyptus, and pine oils can ease bronchial spasm and thin mucus.
- Running a humidifier with essential oils such as eucalyptus, tea tree, or marjoram at night may help thin mucus and ease cough.
- Postural drainage can be of great help in relieving congestion.

ACUPUNCTURE

Acupuncture can bring relief to bronchial spasm and enhance immune function. Smoking cessation through acupuncture can be very successful.

MASSAGE

Therapeutic massage can increase circulation and loosen mucus.

■ FOLLOWING UP

It can take from one to eight weeks to recover completely. To help prevent getting bronchitis again, do not smoke and try to avoid pollutants in the air. Getting an annual flu shot can also help.

■ BURNS

Eighty percent of burns occur in the home, and about 5 percent require hospitalization. Most burns can be managed at home or with a trip to your health care provider's office. Sunburn, scalding, electrical burns, and chemical burns are cared for in similar ways.

■ SIGNS AND SYMPTOMS

You can assess burns by their appearance and cause.

- The skin is red and painful, but there are no blisters or oozing. You can generally handle this type of burn at home.
- Besides the redness and pain, there are also blisters and oozing. You may want a health care provider's help.
- The skin looks charred, white or brownish yellow, and leathery, but without blisters and often without pain. You need immediate care.
- The burned area is more than superficial and involves the face, neck, shoulders, elbows, hands, genital area, ankles, or feet, where the skin is thin. You need immediate care.
- The burn was caused by a chemical. See a health care provider right away, especially if your eyes were affected.
- The burn was caused by electricity. You need immediate care.

■ WHAT CAUSES IT?

The causes of burns are listed below.

- Fires
- Hot water or steam
- The sun
- Electricity
- Chemicals

■ WHAT TO EXPECT AT YOUR PROVIDER'S OFFICE

Before you reach your health care provider's office, cool the burned area with cold water or ice, and cover the area loosely with dry gauze. Don't pop any blisters or apply butter or other greasy substance.

Your health care provider will estimate how serious the burn is. He or she may cleanse the area, open blisters, and remove dead skin. Next he or she will apply antibiotic cream and a soft covering. Your health care provider may tell you to do the following.

- Keep the burned area elevated above your heart whenever possible.
- For moderate swelling and redness, use warm moist bandages. If you develop a fever or swelling, call your provider.
- For itching, use a moisturizing cream.

■ TREATMENT OPTIONS

Antibiotic creams for burns are available over the counter. Reapply the cream and change the bandage twice a day until the burn is healed.

Complementary and Alternative Therapies

Herbs can help speed wound healing, reduce the risk of infection, and may help prevent scarring. Homeopathic remedies can provide excellent pain relief.

NUTRITION

- Hydration is important in managing moderate to severe burns. Drink plenty of juices, water, and electrolyte replacement drinks.
- Vitamin C (1,000 to 1,500 mg three times per day), zinc (30 to 50 mg per day), and beta-carotene (100,000 IU per day) to support immune function and enhance skin healing.
- Vitamin E (1,200 IU d-alpha tocopherols three times a day) is a strong antioxidant and reduces scarring.

- Bromelain (250 to 500 mg four times a day between meals) can help decrease inflammation. Use with turmeric (*Curcuma longa*, 500 mg four times a day) to heighten effects.
- L-glutamine (3 to 10 grams three times a day) provides amino acids that may be necessary to prevent damage caused by severe burns.

HERBS

Herbs may be used as dried extracts (capsules, powders, teas), glycerites (glycerine extracts), or tinctures (alcohol extracts).

- To stimulate the immune system and reduce risk of infection during the period right after the injury, combine equal parts of tinctures of coneflower (*Echinacea purpura*) and goldenseal (*Hydrastis canadensis*). Take 30 to 60 drops every three to four hours.
- Daily application of gotu kola (*Centella asiatica*) to the burn site prevents or limits the shrinking and swelling of the skin, inhibits scar formation, and increases healing.
- Some herbs enhance circulation to the skin. Combine equal parts of the following in a tea (1 cup four to six times a day) or tincture (30 to 60 drops three to four times a day): yarrow (*Achillea millefolium*), cleavers (*Gallium aparine*), prickly ash bark (*Xanthoxyllum clava-herculis*), marigold (*Calendula officinalis*), plantain (*Plantago major*), and ginger root (*Zingiber officinalis*).
- For relief of severe pain combine equal parts of tincture of Jamaican dogwood (*Piscidia erythrina*), valerian (*Valeriana officinalis*), St. John's wort (*Hypericum perforatum*), and California poppy (*Escholzia californica*) with one-half part of gelsemium (*Gelsemium sempiverens*). Take 10 to 15 drops every 15 minutes for up to eight doses, when you are in pain.
- Aloe vera: Cut a fresh leaf and apply the gel to burn, or peel leaf, blend pulp, then apply to burn.
- Comfrey leaf (*Symphytum officinalis*): Make a strong tea with 1 heaping tsp. herb per cup. Use as a wash for the burned area.
- Combine powders of slippery elm (*Ulmus rubra*), marshmallow root (*Althea officinalis*), goldenseal, and comfrey root. Apply to burns to speed healing and reduce risk for infection.

HOMEOPATHY

Common remedies for burns are listed below. Usually, the dose is 12X to 30C every one to four hours.

- *Cantharis* for burns and scalds with cutting, burning, or smarting pains that are relieved with cold applications.
- *Carbolic acid* for fainting following a burn, with coldness of the skin and rapid progression to shock and collapse.
- *Carbo vegetabilis* for burns with severe lightheadedness and sluggishness of circulation.

Topical homeopathic preparations for burns may provide relief of acute pain. Do not apply over broken skin.

■ FOLLOWING UP

Your health care provider may want to check you periodically. Most burns heal in three to five weeks. If the burn is large, he or she may refer you for physical therapy or reconstructive surgery.

■ SPECIAL CONSIDERATIONS

Electrical burns often affect the nervous system and muscles, so emergency cardiopulmonary resuscitation (CPR) and life support may be needed.

■ BURSITIS

Bursitis is an inflammation of a bursa, a small structure inside every joint that helps to lubricate and cushion it. Usually bursitis occurs in the larger joints, such as the shoulder, hip, knee, or elbow. It can happen once or can recur over time. Without seeing your health care provider, you usually can't easily tell the difference between bursitis and pain caused by a strain or arthritis.

■ SIGNS AND SYMPTOMS
- Pain in the joint that gets worse when you move the joint (the pain may come all at once or develop gradually over time)
- Swelling
- Redness
- Fever and warm joint area (if an infection is present)

■ WHAT CAUSES IT?
Typically the bursa becomes irritated or injured when the area is overused with repetitive motion or strenuous activity. It may also be caused by a bacterial infection. Certain other medical conditions, such as gout or rheumatoid arthritis, can also cause bursitis.

■ WHAT TO EXPECT AT YOUR PROVIDER'S OFFICE
Your health care provider will ask you to identify exactly where the joint hurts and feel the joint for swelling or particular areas of tenderness. Your health care provider may remove some fluid from the bursa with a small needle to check for signs of infection. You may also be given a blood test to check for other medical conditions.

■ TREATMENT OPTIONS
In some cases the only treatment needed is to rest the joint to let the area heal. A splint, sling, or other device can support the joint and keep it from moving. Applications of heat or cold may help relieve pain and swelling.

Drug Therapies
You may be instructed to take aspirin, acetaminophen, or ibuprofen for a few days to ease the pain. In more severe or long-lasting cases, your provider may give you an injection of a corticosteroid directly into the joint. This will help reduce the inflammation. The injection may also include a local anesthetic to ease the pain. If tests show that the bursa was infected, your health care provider will also prescribe an antibiotic.

Complementary and Alternative Therapies
Alternative therapies may be useful in reducing the pain and inflammation of bursitis while supporting healthy connective tissue.

NUTRITION
Include in your diet anti-inflammatory oils such as those found in cold-water fish, nuts, and seeds. The following supplements may help.
- Glucosamine sulfate (500 mg two or three times a day), for connective tissue support
- Omega-3 oils (1,000 mg two or three times a day), such as flaxseed oil, as an anti-inflammatory agent
- Vitamin C with bioflavonoids (1,000 mg three times a day), for connective tissue repair
- Proteolytic enzymes such as bromelain (250 mg twice a day), to reduce inflammation
- Bioflavonoids and oral digestive enzymes for inflammation

HERBS
Herbs are generally a safe way to strengthen and tone the body's systems. As with any therapy, it is important to work with your provider on getting your problem diagnosed before you start any treatment. Herbs may be used as dried extracts (capsules, powders, teas), glycerites (glycerine extracts), or tinctures (alcohol extracts). Unless otherwise indicated, teas should be made with 1 tsp. herb per cup of hot water. Steep covered 5 to 10 minutes for leaf or flowers, and 10 to 20 minutes for roots. Drink 2 to 4 cups per day. Tinctures may be used alone or in combination as noted.
- Herbs that reduce swelling include meadowsweet *(Filipendula ulmaria)*, white willow *(Salix alba)*, Jamaican dogwood *(Piscidia erythrina)*, and turmeric *(Curcuma longa)*. A tincture of one, or a combination of these, may be taken at 15 drops every 15 minutes up to four doses for acute pain relief, or 30 drops four times per day for general pain relief. Turmeric increases the effects of bromelain.
- For bursitis with muscle spasm, add valerian *(Valeriana officinalis)*.
- For chronic bursitis, add hawthorn *(Crataegus oxyanthoides)*.

HOMEOPATHY
Some of the most common remedies are listed below. Usually, the dose is 12X to 30C every one to four hours.
- *Arnica* gel applied topically (to the skin) as directed gives excellent short-term pain relief.
- *Arnica* for bursitis occuring after an injury to the joint
- *Ruta graveolons* for rheumatic pains in the joint
- *Bellis perennis* for injury with a great deal of bruising
- *Rhus-toxicodendron* for pain that gets better with movement
- "Traumeel" injections as an alternative to corticosteroids

ACUPUNCTURE
Acupuncture can be helpful in reducing swelling and inflammation, and especially in relieving pain.

MASSAGE
You should not use massage if your bursitis is caused by an infection. Otherwise, massage (especially myofascial release therapy) can be used for general relaxation and to reduce discomfort from inflammation and from compensating for a sore joint.

■ FOLLOWING UP
Tell your health care provider if your symptoms are not relieved by your treatment. Be sure to follow your provider's instructions for resting the joint to allow the swelling to subside before returning to your usual routines. You can help prevent bursitis from recurring by avoiding repetitive motions, resting between periods of intense activity, and doing stretching exercises before starting an activity.

■ SPECIAL CONSIDERATIONS
Do not take aspirin, acetaminophen, or ibuprofen for more than a few days unless so directed by your provider. Be sure to tell your health care provider if you are pregnant.

■ CANDIDIASIS

Candidiasis is an infection caused by a yeastlike fungus called candida. It can infect the mouth, vagina, skin, stomach, and urinary tract. Approximately 75 percent of women will get candidiasis of the vagina during their lifetime, and 90 percent of all people with HIV/AIDS develop candida infections.

■ SIGNS AND SYMPTOMS
- Creamy white patches in the mouth or on the throat
- Painful cracks at the corners of the mouth
- Skin rashes, patches, and blisters found most commonly in the groin, between fingers and toes, and under the breasts
- Vaginal itching and irritation with a curdlike discharge

■ WHAT CAUSES IT?
Normal amounts of candida existing in the mouth, stomach, and vagina do not cause infections. Candidiasis occurs when there is a buildup of candida. This may be caused by taking certain drugs (especially antibiotics), pregnancy, being overweight, bacterial infection, or by several health conditions (for example, immune disorders, diabetes, and psoriasis).

■ WHAT TO EXPECT AT YOUR PROVIDER'S OFFICE
Your health care provider may take samples for testing (for example, a vaginal wet smear) and do extensive tests (such as a CT scan or test of your stool) if it appears that the infection has spread. Your provider will probably prescribe an antifungal medication. He or she may also recommend changes in your diet. These treatments usually cure candidiasis. If you have recurrent bouts of candidiasis, your provider will explore the possibility of an immune deficiency or some other disease.

■ TREATMENT OPTIONS
Drug Therapies
A number of antifungal medications are available to treat the many forms of candidiasis. These include oral rinses, oral tablets, vaginal tablets and suppositories, and creams. Most treatments last from two or three days to two weeks. Follow your provider's orders as prescribed. If you do not complete the treatment regimen, infection could return or you may be reinfected by a different strain of candida.

Complementary and Alternative Therapies
The "candida diet" allows no alcohol, no simple sugars, and very limited amounts of refined foods. Alternative therapies aim to "starve" the yeast and use natural antifungals.
- Vitamin C (500 to 1,000 mg per day), vitamin E (200 to 400 IU per day), and selenium (200 mcg per day) are anti-inflammatory.
- Essential fatty acids: anti-inflammatory, a mix of omega-6 (evening primrose) and omega-3 (flaxseed) may be best (2 tbsp. oil per day or 1,000 to 1,500 mg twice a day). Reduce animal fats in your diet and increase fish and nuts.
- Biotin (300 mcg) inhibits a form of candida that is the most irritating to membranes
- B-complex: B_1 (50 to 100 mg), B_2 (50 mg), B_3 (25 mg); B_5 (100 mg); B_6 (50 to 100 mg), B_{12} (100 to 1,000 mcg), folate (400 mcg per day)
- Calcium (1,000 to 1,500 mg per day) to correct deficiency often found in people with yeast infections, and magnesium (750 to 1,000 mg per day) to balance calcium intake

- Lactobacillus acidophilus (2 to 5 million organisms three times per day) to help restore normal balance of bowel and mucous membranes.
- Caprylic acid (1 gram with meals) is an antifungal fatty acid
- Avoid simple carbohydrates including fruit juice, yeast, and fermented foods; limit fruit to one serving per day, increase garlic (fungicidal), nuts (essential fatty acids), whole grains (B vitamins), oregano, cinnamon, sage, and cloves (antifungal spices)

HERBS
Herbs may be used as dried extracts (capsules, powders, teas), glycerites (glycerine extracts), or tinctures (alcohol extracts). Teas should be made with 1 tsp. herb per cup of hot water. Steep covered 5 to 10 minutes for leaf or flowers; 10 to 20 minutes for roots. Drink 2 to 4 cups per day.
- Pau d'arco bark (lapacho or taheebo): antifungal, best used as a tea (2 tbsp. boiled in 1 quart of water; 3 to 6 cups per day), or use the cooled tea as a vaginal douche
- Goldenseal *(Hydrastis canadensis),* Oregon grape root *(Mahonia nervosa),* and barberry *(Berberis vulgaris)* are digestive and immune stimulants. Chamomile *(Matricaria recicuta)* and licorice *(Glycyrrhiza glabra)* are anti-inflammatory. Use a tea or tincture of the four herbs listed above (1 cup tea three times per day or 30 to 60 drops tincture three times per day) for six weeks. Do not take licorice if you have high blood pressure.
- Topical treatments include tea tree oil *(Melaleuca alternifolia)* or lavender essential oil *(Lavendula species)* two to three times a day; apply full strength to skin infections (discontinue if skin irritation develops); marigold *(Calendula officinalis)* apply three to five times per day in a salve for rashes.
- Fireweek *(Epilobium parviflorum):* take as a tea for oral, vaginal, and intestinal candidias

HOMEOPATHY
Some of the most common remedies used for candidiasis are listed below. Usually, the dose is 12X to 30C every one to four hours until your symptoms get better.
- *Borax* for bleeding oral mucosa, especially with diarrhea
- *Belladonna* for bright red, inflamed skin that is not raw or oozing, but is painful, especially with irritability
- *Chamomilla* for "diaper" rash, especially with irritability
- *Arsenicum album* for burning, itching rashes, especially with anxiety
- *Graphites* for thick, cracked skin (corners of mouth or heels)
- *Kreosotum* for leukorrhea that causes itching and swelling

ACUPUNCTURE
May be helpful to stimulate immune system, digestion, and relieve stress.

■ FOLLOWING UP
You can prevent another yeast infection by taking lactobacillus acidophilus when you take antibiotics, avoiding antibiotics that act against a wide variety of bacteria when possible, wearing cotton or silk underwear, maintaining good hygiene, and staying at the proper weight. Women should avoid douches (except when medically necessary), vaginal deodorants, and bubble baths.

■ SPECIAL CONSIDERATIONS
Tell your health care provider if you are pregnant.

■ CHRONIC FATIGUE SYNDROME

With chronic fatigue syndrome (CFS), you feel so worn out that you are unable to do even half of your normal daily activities—and the feeling doesn't go away. This syndrome affects twice as many women as men. It may last a month, a couple of years, or many years.

■ SIGNS AND SYMPTOMS
- Severe fatigue that comes on suddenly, especially after you've had the flu
- Low-grade fever (100.4° Fahrenheit) and chills
- Sore throat and swollen glands
- Muscle and joint aches
- Headaches
- Feeling of being in a fog and unable to concentrate or remember

■ WHAT CAUSES IT?
No one knows what causes CFS, but a virus may be responsible. Risk factors include extreme stress or anxiety, flu-like illness that doesn't completely go away, and poor eating habits.

■ WHAT TO EXPECT AT YOUR PROVIDER'S OFFICE
Your health care provider will go over your symptoms, check your medical history, and do a physical examination. He or she may use laboratory tests, such as a blood or urine test, to rule out other problems. If you have CFS, your health care provider will prescribe drugs to treat your symptoms, or will suggest herbs, vitamins, or dietary changes to help you. Usually these treatments and time will be enough to cure the problem.

If the usual treatments do not work, your doctor may check for other conditions, such as a psychiatric illness, muscle disease, or exposure to a toxic agent, that can cause symptoms similar to those of CFS.

■ TREATMENT OPTIONS
Drug Therapies
Many drugs can improve your symptoms, including antidepressants and drugs to boost your immune system. Pain relievers and anti-inflammatories can help relieve muscle and joint aches.

Complementary and Alternative Therapies
Following nutritional guidelines and using herbs and homeopathic remedies as recommended, may alleviate the debilitating symptoms of CFS and improve overall vitality. Counseling, support groups, meditation, yoga, and progressive muscle relaxation are stress-management techniques that may help as well.

NUTRITION
Avoid refined foods, sugar, caffeine, alcohol, saturated fats, dairy products, and gluten-containing grains. Eat more fresh vegetables, legumes, whole grains (non-gluten), protein, and essential fatty acids (found in nuts, seeds, and cold-water fish).

The following supplements may help reduce symptoms of CFS.
- Beta carotene (50,000 IU per day) to strengthen immune function.
- Vitamin C (1,000 mg three to six times per day) to increase endurance.
- B complex (50 to 100 mg per day or 2 ml by injection one to two times per week) with additional B_6 (100mg per day) and B_5 (100 to 250 mg per day) to reduce the effects of stress.
- Pantothenic acid (4 to 7 mg per day).
- Magnesium aspartate (400 to 1,000 mg per day) to support energy production.
- L-carnitine (330 mg one to three times per day) to support energy production in the cells.

HERBS
Herbs are generally a safe way to strengthen and tone the body's symptoms. As with any therapy, it is important to work with your provider on getting your problem diagnosed before you start any treatment. Herbs may be used as dried extracts (capsules, powders, teas), glycerites (glycerine extracts), or tinctures (alcohol extracts). Unless otherwise indicated, teas should be made with 1 tsp. herb per cup of hot water. Steep covered 5 to 10 minutes for leaf or flowers, and 10 to 20 minutes for roots. Drink 2 to 4 cups per day. Tinctures may be used singly or in combination as noted.

A tincture of Siberian ginseng *(Eleuthrococcus senticosus)*, schizandra berry *(Schizandra chinensis)*, ashwaganda root *(Withania somnifera)*, gotu kola *(Centella asiatica)*, and astragalus root *(Astragalus membranaceus)*. Take 20 to 30 drops two to three times per day. These are safe to take long-term and may need to be taken for four to six months for maximum benefit.

Herbs that support overall vitality and relieve exhaustion include licorice root *(Glycyrrhiza glabra)*, lomatium root *(Lomatium dissectum)*, skullcap *(Scutellaria laterifolia)*, passionflower *(Passiflora incarnata)*, lavender *(Lavendula officinalis)*, and rosemary leaf *(Rosemarinus officinalis)*. Take 20 to 30 drops two to three times per day. Do not take licorice if you have high blood pressure.

Essential oils of jasmine, peppermint, and rosemary are calming and restorative and may be used in aromatherapy. Place several drops in a warm bath or atomizer, or on a cotton ball.

HOMEOPATHY
Homeopathy may be useful as a supportive therapy.

ACUPUNCTURE
Chronic fatigue syndrome is related to deficiencies in multiple organ systems that can be addressed with acupuncture treatment.

MASSAGE
Therapeutic massage can reduce stress-related symptoms, improve circulation, and increase your overall sense of well-being.

■ FOLLOWING UP
Your health care provider will do routine checkups while you are taking the drugs or treatments he or she has prescribed. Contact him or her if new symptoms develop.

■ SPECIAL CONSIDERATIONS
The effects of herbs in pregnancy have not been fully investigated and they should be used only under the careful supervision of your health care provider. Avoid high doses of vitamin C if you are pregnant.

■ CHRONIC OBSTRUCTIVE PULMONARY DISEASE

Chronic obstructive pulmonary disease (COPD) causes severe shortness of breath, which can result from chronic bronchitis, emphysema, or both. Chronic bronchitis is defined as a constant cough and excessive mucus production that lasts for at least three months for more than two consecutive years. Emphysema is characterized by damage to the lungs, which causes them to lose their elasticity. COPD is the fifth leading cause of death in the United States.

■ SIGNS AND SYMPTOMS

- Cough (often with phlegm that is hard to "bring up")
- Shortness of breath during exertion (and eventually, at rest)
- Excessive mucus production and impaired mucus elimination
- Wheezing
- Recurrent respiratory infections

■ WHAT CAUSES IT?

Smoking is the number one cause of COPD. It can also be caused be exposure to pollutants. One rare form is inherited.

■ WHAT TO EXPECT AT YOUR PROVIDER'S OFFICE

Your health care provider will listen to your chest for wheezes, crackles, and decreased breath sounds. If your symptoms are severe, your provider will order a chest X-ray and lung-function tests. He or she will measure levels of blood gases in your arteries to determine if your condition might be hereditary. He or she will urge you to quit smoking immediately.

■ TREATMENT OPTIONS

Quitting smoking is the key to both preventing COPD and keeping it from getting worse. Your health care provider may also recommend antibiotics, supplemental oxygen, bronchodilators and corticosteroids (inhalers), and other prescription drugs to help relieve your symptoms.

Your provider will probably talk with you about lifestyle changes you can make to help relieve the symptoms of COPD. These include exercising, and eating a healthy diet. He or she may also suggest support groups and therapy to help make living with the condition easier.

Complementary and Alternative Therapies

Complementary and alternative therapies can help decrease your symptoms and prevent infections. Some also can help you quit smoking.

NUTRITION

- Dairy products and bananas increase mucus buildup and should be avoided. Garlic, onions, and horseradish may actually decrease mucus production.
- Some essential fatty acids: as an anti-inflammatory, dose is 1,000 to 2,000 IU, mixed omega-3 and omega-6 oils (flaxseed, fish, borage, and evening primrose oil; avoid vegetable oils and saturated fats)
- Coenzyme Q10 , makes it easier for you to exercise without getting short of breath. Dose is 10 to 50 mg three times a day.
- Other important antioxidants: selenium (200 mcg per day), vitamin E (400 IU per day), vitamin C (1,000 mg three times per day), L-carnitine (750 mg twice a day). Note that beta-carotene may increase the risk of lung cancer in smokers.
- Bromelain helps reduce mucus production (250 to 500 mg three times per day, on an empty stomach). You may be sensitive to this if you are allergic to pineapple. Bromelain may also aggravate gastritis.
- N-acetyl cysteine reduces mucus (400 mg three times a day).
- Magnesium promotes muscle relaxation in your lungs and blood vessels (100 to 500 mg twice a day). Magnesium may cause diarrhea if you are sensitive to it. An intravenous infusion of magnesium can also be very helpful, but must be done by a health care provider).

HERBS

Herbs may be used as dried extracts (capsules, powders, teas), glycerites (glycerine extracts), or tinctures (alcohol extracts). Unless otherwise indicated, teas should be made with 1 tsp. herb per cup of hot water. Steep covered 5 to 10 minutes for leaf or flowers, and 10 to 20 minutes for roots. Drink 2 to 4 cups per day.

- Mullein (*Verbascum thaspis*): brings up phlegm, soothes irritation
- Ginger (*Zingiber officinalis*): dissolves secretions, relieves bronchial spasms
- Fennel (*Foeniculum fructus*): dissolves secretions, mild anti-spasmodic, calming digestive stimulant
- Coltsfoot (*Tussilago farfara*): soothes and reduces inflammation. Prolonged use may cause liver damage due to pyrrolizidine alkaloids.
- Licorice (*Glycyrrhiza glabra*): antiviral, antidepressant, soothing, reduces swelling. Do not take if you have high blood pressure.
- Hawthorne (*Cretaegus oxycanthus*): protects blood vessels.

Mix equal parts of herb, or tincture of four to six of the above herbs. Dose is 1 cup tea three times per day, or 30 to 60 drops tincture three times per day.

- Essential oils: eucalyptus, thyme, rosemary, and lavender: place 3 to 5 drops in 2 cups of water in a humidifier to prevent infection.

HOMEOPATHY

Homeopathy may be useful as a supportive therapy.

PHYSICAL MEDICINE

- Castor oil pack. Used externally, castor oil is a powerful anti-inflammatory. Apply oil directly to skin, cover with a clean soft cloth and plastic wrap. Place a heat source (hot water bottle or heating pad) over the pack and let sit for 30 to 60 minutes. For best results use for three consecutive days in one week. When placed over the lungs, castor oil packs decrease inflammation and stimulate drainage.
- Postural drainage, yogic breathing, and pulmonary rehabilitation programs may all be helpful.

ACUPUNCTURE

Has been shown to have great benefit in smoking cessation.

■ FOLLOWING UP

Your health care provider will want you to come back once or twice a year to monitor your lung function; however, if your symptoms become more severe, you should see your provider immediately so that life-threatening respiratory failure does not occur.

■ SPECIAL CONSIDERATIONS

If you have COPD, you are prone to respiratory infections. Your health care provider will most likely tell you to get a flu shot every year.

■ CIRRHOSIS OF THE LIVER

Cirrhosis is irreversible chronic injury of the liver. It often has no symptoms. Your health care provider will diagnose cirrhosis based on your medical history, a physical examination, and laboratory tests.

■ SIGNS AND SYMPTOMS

The signs and symptoms of cirrhosis can range from an absence of symptoms (in 10 to 20 percent of patients) to liver failure. Cirrhosis can also have symptoms such as jaundice (yellowing of the skin), weight loss, abdominal pain, testicular atrophy (in men), menstrual irregularity (in women), swelling and fluid in the abdomen, and enlarged veins.

■ WHAT CAUSES IT?

The most common cause of cirrhosis is alcoholism. Consuming a lot of alcohol daily (32 to 48 oz. of beer, 4 to 8 oz. of liquor, 16 to 32 oz. of wine) for 10 years or more increases your chances of developing cirrhosis. How much alcohol you drink and for how long are more important than the type of alcohol ingested. Between 5 and 10 percent of people in the United States are alcoholics. Of these, 10 to 15 percent will develop liver disease. Cirrhosis can also be caused by the ingestion of drugs and toxins, infections, inherited medical conditions, and cardiovascular diseases. About 10 percent of cases have no known cause.

■ WHAT TO EXPECT AT YOUR PROVIDER'S OFFICE

Your health care provider will take a detailed history in order to differentiate your liver disease from other conditions (obesity, hepatitis, diabetes mellitus, biliary obstruction, drug toxicities, infections, and other types of cirrhosis). Your provider will order a complete blood count and liver function tests; in addition he or she may order a liver biopsy. And finally, if your cirrhosis is caused by alcoholism, your provider will strongly urge you to stop drinking and will counsel you as to the risks you are taking by continuing to drink. He or she may suggest Alcoholics Anonymous as a good place to start your rehabilitation.

■ TREATMENT OPTIONS

Your health care provider will treat you to try to slow the progression of the cirrhosis and also to treat any complications it causes.

Drug Therapies

Your health care provider may prescribe drugs to slow the progression of the disease, such as Colchicine, diuretics, Neomycin, and Lactulose.

Complementary and Alternative Therapies

Have much to offer in the treatment of liver disease.

NUTRITION

- B-complex: B_1 (50 to 100 mg), B_2 (50 mg), B_3 (25 mg); B_5 (100 mg); B_6 (50 to 100 mg), B_{12} (100 to 1,000 mcg), folate (400 mcg per day) to reduce deficiencies common in liver disease
- Antioxidants: Vitamin C (1,000 to 3,000 mg per day), vitamin E (400 to 800 IU per day), and selenium (200 mcg per day) reduce toxic effects of alcohol and drugs and prevent tissue damage.
- Essential fatty acids are anti-inflammatory; dietary manipulation includes reducing animal fats and increasing fish and nuts. A mix of omega-6 (evening primrose) and omega-3 (flaxseed) may be best (1 tbsp. oil per day or 1,000 to 1,500 mg per day).
- Choline, lecithin, methionine (1 g each per day) for fat absorption

- Carnitine (300 mg per day) prevents fatty liver.
- Glutathione (500 mg twice a day) helps remove ammonia from the brain, a complication of cirrhosis.
- Vitamin K is necessary for blood clotting; often depleted in cirrhosis
- Desiccated liver (500 mg three times per day) helps provide nutrition to promote liver repair.
- Restrict intake of protein to 45 g per day as long as a minimum of 400 g of carbohydrates is ingested daily.
- A change from animal to vegetable protein may be helpful.

HERBS

As with any therapy, it is important to work with your health care provider on getting your problem diagnosed before you start any treatment. Herbs may be used as dried extracts (capsules, powders, teas), glycerites (glycerine extracts), or tinctures (alcohol extracts). Unless otherwise indicated, teas should be made with 1 tsp. herb per cup of hot water. Steep covered 5 to 10 minutes for leaf or flowers, and 10 to 20 minutes for roots. Drink 2 to 4 cups per day.

Due to the high doses required and the need to avoid alcohol, the preferred form of these herbs is powdered.

- Milk thistle *(Silybum marianum)*: 100 mg three times per day prevents free radical damage in the liver.
- Barberry *(Berberis vulgaris)*: 250 to 500 mg per day corrects metabolic abnormalities in liver cirrhosis.
- Catechin *(Uncaria gambir)*: 400 mg three times per day, is antioxidant, antiviral, and helps regenerate liver tissue.

HOMEOPATHY

Homeopathy may be useful as a supportive therapy.

PHYSICAL MEDICINE

Castor oil pack. Used externally, castor oil is a powerful anti-inflammatory. Apply oil directly to skin, cover with a clean soft cloth (for example, flannel) and plastic wrap. Place a heat source (hot water bottle or heating pad) over the pack and let sit for 30 to 60 minutes. For best results, use for three consecutive days. Apply pack over liver. Preliminary study shows immune enhancement in healthy patients; was historically used to stimulate liver function.

ACUPUNCTURE

May be helpful to alleviate symptoms and increase physiological functioning.

MASSAGE

May help alleviate stress and lymph congestion.

■ FOLLOWING UP

Your health care provider will supervise and manage your condition over the long term because cirrhosis can have serious and life-threatening complications, particularly if you continue to drink.

■ SPECIAL CONSIDERATIONS

Survival and management of cirrhosis is possible, especially with proper treatment. Your health care provider will use caution when prescribing medications if you have cirrhosis because many medications cause complications in someone with a weakened liver.

■ COMMON COLD

The common cold is an upper respiratory infection caused by a virus. In the United States, adults have between 3 and 5.6 colds a year, and children have as many as 8.3.

■ SIGNS AND SYMPTOMS

- Sneezing and nasal congestion
- Sore throat, cough, or hoarseness
- Fever
- In children, sudden onset of fever (lasting two to three days), irritability, restlessness, and sneezing
- Headache

■ WHAT CAUSES IT?

More than 200 different types of viruses cause colds. You can get a cold by touching a person with a cold or by shaking hands with a person with a cold and then touching your nose or eyes. Colds are also transmitted through the air. Exposure to cold outdoor air and fatigue do not make you more likely to get a cold, although psychological stress may. People in large families are more likely to catch colds, as are children at day care centers and workers in office buildings.

■ WHAT TO EXPECT AT YOUR PROVIDER'S OFFICE

Most people diagnose and treat their own colds and do not see a doctor. Antibiotics and antihistamines cannot help cure your cold. Colds go away on their own after about 5 to 7 days for adults and 10 to 14 days for children.

■ TREATMENT OPTIONS

Drug Therapies

- Nasal decongestants: may help prevent sinus and ear infections. Do not take if you have a heart condition or high blood pressure.
- Nasal sprays: Use only for the recommended amount of time (usually three to five days). You can become reliant on them, and they can make your symptoms worse if used for too long.
- Aspirin and other pain relievers: can be used for fever or aches. They may cause the immune system to respond more slowly or increase nasal symptoms (runny and stuffy nose). Take only if necessary. Do not give aspirin to children under 18 because of the risk of Reye's syndrome.

Complementary and Alternative Therapies

Alternative therapies offer effective symptom relief. Also be sure to rest and drink plenty of fluids.

NUTRITION

- Vitamin C (1,000 mg three to six times per day) enhances immune function
- Zinc (23 mg lozenges taken every two hours) may shorten the duration of a cold, and may also protect against the development of usual symptoms. This high dose is for short-term use only.

- Vitamin A (25,000 IU per day) maintains integrity of mucous membranes and stimulates antibody response. This high dose is for short-term use only.
- Beta-carotene (200,000 IU per day) stimulates the immune system and is an antioxidant; safe for women of childbearing age
- Avoid dairy and bananas. They increase mucus production.
- Garlic and onions have antiviral properties.

HERBS

Herbs are generally a safe way to strengthen and tone the body's systems. As with any therapy, it is important to work with your provider on getting your problem diagnosed before you start any treatment. Herbs may be used as dried extracts (capsules, powders, teas), glycerites (glycerine extracts), or tinctures (alcohol extracts). Unless otherwise indicated, teas should be made with 1 tsp. herb per cup of hot water. Steep covered 5 to 10 minutes for leaf or flowers, and 10 to 20 minutes for roots. Drink 2 to 4 cups per day. Tinctures (solutions made from herb and alcohol, or herb, alcohol, and water) may be used singly or in combination as noted.

- Coneflower (*Echinacea angustifolia*): helps your immune system function properly; controversy exists about whether to use it for longer than two to six weeks at a time and whether to use in people with autoimmune disorders or AIDS.
- Goldenseal (*Hydrastis canadensis*): antiviral, antibacterial
- Astragulus (*Astragulus membraneceus*): shortens duration of colds
- Licorice (*Glycyrrhiza glabra*): antiviral, soothing to mucous membranes
- Elderberry (*Sambuccus canadensis*): antiviral, increases bronchial secretions

A mix of the above every two to four hours (1 cup tea or 30 to 60 drops tincture)

HOMEOPATHY

Some of the most common remedies used for this condition are listed below. Usually, the dose is 12X to 30C every one to four hours until your symptoms get better.

- *Allium cepa* for colds with a lot of watery nasal discharge that burns and irritates the nostrils
- *Euphrasia* for colds with a lot of watery nasal watery discharge that is irritating to the eyes
- *Aconite* for colds that come on suddenly, with fever and anxiety
- *Mercurius* for a lot of irritating nasal discharge and general weakness

■ FOLLOWING UP

Be sure to see your health care provider if you are not feeling better after 7 to 10 days or have developed new symptoms.

■ SPECIAL CONSIDERATIONS

Tell your health care provider if you are pregnant or think you are pregnant. Some decongestants can be harmful to your baby.

■ CONGESTIVE HEART FAILURE

Congestive heart failure (CHF) occurs when the heart cannot pump out enough blood to meet the needs of the body. Any form of heart disease may lead to CHF, which results in a reduced ability to exercise and in severe cases can impair daily function. CHF is the most common cause of death for people over age 65.

■ SIGNS AND SYMPTOMS

- Shortness of breath
- Fatigue, exercise intolerance
- Rust-colored sputum
- Distended neck veins
- Cough—especially when waking
- Excessive nighttime urination
- Excessive protein in the urine
- Insomnia
- Nausea, vomiting
- Anorexia
- Anxiety
- Swelling in the extremities

■ WHAT CAUSES IT?

CHF can be the result of any type of heart disease or condition. The following factors make it more likely that you will get CHF.

- Smoking
- High-fat diet, excess body weight
- Alcohol abuse
- High sodium intake
- Influenza, pneumonia
- Noncompliance with prescribed medications or recommended diet

■ WHAT TO EXPECT AT YOUR PROVIDER'S OFFICE

Your health care provider will focus on identifying the cause and precipitating factors for CHF. Procedures include blood tests and electrocardiograms (ECG). Surgery may be needed if you have severe CHF.

■ TREATMENT OPTIONS

Drug Therapies

- Vasodilators—reduce narrowing of vessels; cornerstone of treatment; for example, angiotensin-converting enzyme (ACE) inhibitors; side effects include kidney failure, cough, low blood pressure
- Diuretics—main types of diuretics include thiazide, loop diuretics, and potassium-sparing diuretics
- Digitalis glycosides—increase the ability of the heart muscle to properly contract properly; prevent heart rhythm disturbances

Complementary and Alternative Therapies

Nutrition and herbal medicine can play an important role in increasing the strength of the heart without also increasing its workload.

NUTRITION

- Antioxidants: vitamin C (1,000 mg three times a day), vitamin E (400 IU per day), selenium (200 mcg per day)
- Coenzyme Q10 (30 to 50 mg twice a day): antioxidant, increases oxygenation of tissue, including heart muscle
- Essential fatty acids (1,500 mg twice a day): anti-inflammatory
- Diet: garlic, ginger and onions all have a beneficial effect on circulation. Increase fiber (especially water-soluble), fruits, vegetables, and vegetarian sources of protein. Increase potassium and decrease sodium in the diet.
- Homocysteine metabolism: Folic acid (800 mcg per day), B_6 (50 mg per day), B_{12} (400 mg per day), betaine (200 to 1,000 mg per day)
- Magnesium (500 mg): mild vasodilation (dilates blood vessels)
- Taurine (500 mg twice a day): helps your heart work more efficiently

- Carnitine (750 to 1,500 mg twice a day): important in fatty acid metabolism, increases efficiency of cardiac function

HERBS

Herbs may be used as dried extracts (capsules, powders, teas), glycerites (glycerine extracts), or tinctures (alcohol extracts). Unless otherwise indicated, teas should be made with 1 tsp. of herb per cup of hot water. Steep covered 5 to 10 minutes for leaf or flowers, and 10 to 20 minutes for roots. Drink 2 to 4 cups per day.

- Hawthorn (*Crataegus oxyacantha*): increases blood vessel integrity; dose is 3 to 5 g. This dose is difficult to achieve in tea or tincture. Supplements or solid extract are used.
- Mistletoe (*Viscum album*): protects against high blood pressure and hardening of the arteries, historically for exhaustion and nervousness
- Linden (Tilia cordata): historically used to lower blood pressure
- Rosemary (*Rosemariana officinalis*): increases coronary artery blood flow, used to stimulate digestion and relieve nervous tension
- Mother wort (*Leonorus cardiaca*): regulates heart rhythm
- Dandelion (*Taraxacum officinalis*): potassium-sparing diuretic
- Indian tobacco (*Lobelia inflata*): helps reduce spasm, stimulates respiratory function, used in smoking cessation. May be toxic if used above recommended doses.
- Lily of the valley (*Convallaria majalis*): specific for cardiac insufficiency; exceeding recommended doses may lead to nausea, vomiting, headache, stupor. Use no more than 30 drops per day.
- Horsetail herb (*Equisetum arvense*): diuretic

Hawthorn should be included in any treatment. In addition, use a combination of four to six of the above herbs at 1 cup tea three times per day or 30 to 60 drops tincture three times per day.

HOMEOPATHY

Homeopathy may be useful as a supportive therapy.

PHYSICAL MEDICINE

Castor oil pack. Apply oil directly to chest, cover with a clean soft cloth and plastic wrap. Place a heat source over the pack and let sit for 30 to 60 minutes. For best results use three consecutive days.

Contrast hydrotherapy. Alternate hot and cold applications to the chest. Alternate three minutes hot with one minute cold and repeat three times. This is one set. Do two to three sets per day. For very sick patients, use cool and warm applications to decrease the contrast.

ACUPUNCTURE

May be helpful for increasing circulation and cardiac strength.

MASSAGE

May help increase lymphatic drainage and reduce swelling.

■ FOLLOWING UP

It is very important to prevent the heart disease from getting worse by getting plenty of exercise, eating a proper diet, and avoiding health risks.

■ SPECIAL CONSIDERATIONS

CHF is dangerous during pregnancy. The first two weeks after giving birth is particularly dangerous for women with CHF.

■ CONJUNCTIVITIS

Conjunctivitis is an inflammation of the membrane covering the inside of your eyelids and the outer part of your eyeball. Commonly called "pink eye," conjunctivitis is generally not serious but can be highly contagious.

■ SIGNS AND SYMPTOMS

Conjunctivitis causes the following symptoms in one or both eyes.

- Redness
- Itching
- Tearing
- Discharge (watery or thick)
- Crust that forms overnight
- Sensitivity to light
- Gritty feeling

■ WHAT CAUSES IT?

Conjunctivitis is most often the result of viruses, like those that cause the common cold. Conjunctivitis can also be caused by bacterial infections, allergies, chemicals, irritation from contact lenses, or eye injury. Viral and bacterial conjunctivitis are very contagious.

■ WHAT TO EXPECT AT YOUR PROVIDER'S OFFICE

If both eyes are affected, with itching and a clear discharge, it's likely that allergies are the cause. Swollen glands usually indicate a virus, and a thick, crusty discharge is a sign of a bacterial infection.

Your provider may use a lamp for closer examination, or gently swab a stain across the surface of your eye. He or she may test your vision or measure the pressure in your eye, to rule out glaucoma.

■ TREATMENT OPTIONS

Conjunctivitis is generally not a serious problem and often will go away by itself. But it is still important to consult your health care provider. Chronic conjunctivitis, left untreated, can cause permanent eye damage.

Bacterial conjunctivitis is generally treated with antibiotics such as Polytrim drops or Polysporin ointment. Forms of conjunctivitis caused by viruses do not respond to antibiotics, but antihistamines and anti-inflammatory medications may help relieve your symptoms.

Complementary and Alternative Therapies

Alternative therapies can help relieve your symptoms. If you have a mild case of conjunctivitis, begin with compresses. For a moderate infection, use an eyewash as well.

NUTRITION

Doses listed are for adults. Decrease by one-half to two-thirds for children, at the recommendation of a health care provider. Vitamin A (10,000 IU/day), vitamin C (1,000 mg three to four times per day), and zinc (30 to 50 mg/day) strengthen your immune system and help you heal faster.

HERBS

Herbs may be used as dried extracts (capsules, powders, teas), glycerites (glycerine extracts), or tinctures (alcohol extracts).

Compresses and eye washes are external treatments. A compress is made with a clean cloth, gauze pads, or cotton balls soaked in a solution and then applied over the eyes. Eye washes may be administered with an eye cup or a sterile dropper.

Compress: Use five drops of tincture in $1/4$ cup water or steep 1 tsp. herb in 1 cup hot water for 5 to 10 minutes and strain. Soak cloth or gauze in solution and apply to the eyes for 10 minutes, three to four times a day.

- Eyebright *(Euphrasia officinalis):* helps fight infection and dry up excess fluid, specific for eyes
- Chamomile *(Matricaria recutita):* helps fight infection
- Fennel seed *(Foeniculum vulgare):* helps fight infection
- Marigold *(Calendula officinalis):* soothes irritation
- Plantain *(Plantago lanceolata, P. Major):* astringent and soothing. The fresh leaves are the most effective plant part.
- Flax *(Linum usitatissimum):* as a soothing poultice made with 1 oz. of bruised flax seed steeped for 15 minutes in 4 oz. of water, wrapped in cheesecloth then applied directly to the affected eye.
- Grated fresh potato has astringent (drying and disinfecting) properties. Wrap in cheesecloth and apply.

Use above herbs singly or in combination: Mix equal parts together then steep 1 tsp. herb in 1 cup of hot water to make a tea. Cool before administering to the eye.

Eyewash: goldenseal *(Hydrastis canadensis)* and boric acid: 10 drops of goldenseal tincture with 1 tsp. of boric acid in 1 cup of water.

HOMEOPATHY

Some of the most common remedies used for conjunctivitis are listed below. Usually, the dose is 12X to 30C every one to four hours until your symptoms get better.

- *Aconite* for after exposure to wind or cold; for thin discharge
- *Apis mellifica* for red, burning and swollen eyelids
- Combination remedies containing *Apis, Euphrasia,* and *Sabadilla* may be effective for allergic conjunctivitis
- *Allium cepa* for red, burning, tearing eyes that are sensitive to light

ACUPUNCTURE

Treatment may be administered for pain relief and relieving congestion.

■ FOLLOWING UP

Viral and bacterial conjunctivitis are both very contagious. Family members should use separate towels. Wash your hands often. Children should generally be kept home from school and day care.

Be sure to follow your health care provider's advice about using any medications, particularly if you have been given antibiotics or corticosteroids. If you wear contact lenses, keep them clean to avoid further irritation and future infections. Do not wear them until your eyes have healed.

People with allergy-related conjunctivitis sometimes develop a severe form with a stringy discharge, swollen eyelids, scaly skin, and significant discomfort. This needs aggressive treatment to prevent scarring of the cornea.

■ SPECIAL CONSIDERATIONS

In most U.S. hospitals, medication such as silver nitrate is routinely administered to the eyes of newborns to prevent conjunctivitis from developing from bacteria in the birth canal.

■ CONSTIPATION

Constipation is a condition that causes you to have difficulty passing stools. Normally, people have anywhere from two or three bowel movements a week to two or three a day. Constipation can occur at any age, but it is more frequent in infancy and old age.

■ SIGNS AND SYMPTOMS

- Infrequent, difficult passage of stools (fewer than three bowel movements a week)
- Sudden decrease in frequency of bowel movements
- Stools harder than normal
- Bowel still feels full after bowel movement
- Bloated sensation

■ WHAT CAUSES IT?

Most cases of constipation are caused by changes in diet or physical activity, including not drinking enough fluids. Psychological factors, particularly depression, may cause constipation. Chronic abuse of laxatives can also lead to chronic constipation. Certain drugs can cause it, as can physical abnormalities in the bowel or intestinal tract.

■ WHAT TO EXPECT AT YOUR PROVIDER'S OFFICE

Your health care provider will perform a physical exam and may feel your abdomen or give you a rectal examination. You may have tests on your blood and stool, or a barium enema.

■ TREATMENT OPTIONS

Chronic constipation can usually be prevented with a combination of dietary changes, extra fluid intake, exercise, and, when necessary, short-term use of a laxative. Your health care provider may talk with you about proper bowel habits (consistent, unhurried elimination practices). He or she may have you use a laxative or stool softener over the short term or suggest a bulk-forming agent, such as psyllium, bran, or methylcellulose. You can purchase these bulk-forming agents over the counter.

Complementary and Alternative Therapies

Lifestyle and dietary changes along with nutritional support can contribute to the long-term resolution of constipation. You can use herbs to help tone and strengthen bowel function. Use laxative herbs with caution because they may become less effective with habitual use.

NUTRITION

- Take time to eat, breathe slowly and chew food thoroughly.
- Eat smaller, more frequent meals and avoid overeating at one sitting.
- Eliminate refined foods, sugars, caffeine, alcohol, and dairy products from your diet.
- Decrease intake of saturated fats (animal products) and increase essential fatty acids (cold-water fish, nuts, and seeds).
- Eat more fresh vegetables and whole grains.
- Drink more water.
- Stewed or soaked prunes, 1 to 3 a day, have a slightly laxative effect.
- Flax meal, 1 heaping tsp. in 8 oz. of apple juice, provides fiber and soothes the digestive tract. Follow with an additional 8 oz. of water.
- Warm lemon water taken before meals stimulates digestion.
- Consider digestive enzymes for chronic constipation.
- Vitamin C, 1,000 mg, two to three times per day
- Magnesium, 250 mg, two to three times per day

HERBS

Herbs may be used as dried extracts (capsules, powders, teas), glycerites (glycerine extracts), or tinctures (alcohol extracts). Unless otherwise indicated, teas should be made with 1 tsp. herb per cup of hot water. Steep covered 5 to 10 minutes for leaf or flowers, and 10 to 20 minutes for roots. Drink 2 to 4 cups a day. Tinctures may be used singly or in combination as noted.

A combination of herbs to tone digestion and relieve constipation includes the following in equal parts as a tea or tincture: licorice root *(Glycyrrhiza glabra)*, cascara sagrada *(Rhamnus purshiana)*, dandelion root *(Taraxacum officinalis)*, yellow dock *(Rumex crispus)*, fennel seed *(Foeniculum vulgare)*, and ginger *(Zingiber officinalis)*. Steep tea for 20 minutes. Drink 1 cup, three times a day, before meals. You may take 15 to 20 drops of a tincture, three times a day, before meals. For long-term use (more than two weeks), eliminate cascara and substitute burdock *(Arctium lappa)*. Do not take licorice if you have high blood pressure.

HOMEOPATHY

Some of the most common remedies used for constipation are listed below. Usually, the dose is 12X to 30C every one to four hours until your symptoms get better.

- *Calcarea carbonica* for constipation without urge to pass stool
- *Nux vomica* for constipation with constant, yet ineffectual, urge to pass stool
- *Silica* for constipation with the sensation that stool remains in the rectum after bowel movements

PHYSICAL MEDICINE

Castor oil packs to the abdomen may be useful in resolving constipation. Apply oil directly to skin, cover with a clean, soft cloth (for example, flannel) and plastic wrap. Place a heat source (hot water bottle or heating pad) over the pack and let sit for 30 to 60 minutes. For best results, use for three consecutive days in one week.

Contrast hydrotherapy may help to tone and strengthen bowel function. Apply hot and cold towels to the abdomen. Alternate three minutes hot with one minute cold and repeat three times. This is one set. Do two to three sets a day.

ACUPUNCTURE

Acupuncture can stimulate and tone digestive function.

MASSAGE

Therapeutic massage can help reduce stress and relieve constipation due to spasm and nervous tension.

■ FOLLOWING UP

If you have chronic constipation, you may need to work regularly with your provider. Left untreated, it can cause serious health problems.

■ SPECIAL CONSIDERATIONS

Constipation is common in pregnancy and is usually relieved by changing your diet and drinking more water. If you are pregnant, do not take herbs that are stimulating to the digestive tract since they can induce contractions. Do not use laxative herbs in pregnancy without a provider's supervision.

◼ COUGH

Cough is one of the most common reasons for visits to health care providers. Normal coughing is important to keep your throat and airways clear. However, excessive coughing may mean you have an underlying disease or disorder. Coughs generally fall into one of the two following categories.

Acute coughs (typically lasting no longer than three weeks) usually begin suddenly because of a cold, flu, or sinus infection.

Chronic coughs (lasting longer than three weeks) are most commonly caused by cigarette smoke, airborne pollutants, postnasal drip, asthma, and bronchitis.

◼ SIGNS AND SYMPTOMS

Depending on the condition causing it, a cough may be accompanied by the following.

- Upper respiratory tract infection (URI)
- Postnasal drip
- Wheezing (possible asthma)
- Heartburn
- Vomiting
- Fever, chills, night sweats
- Edema, or fluid retention

◼ WHAT CAUSES IT?

- Upper respiratory tract infection
- Irritants inhaled into the airway passages
- Postnasal drip
- Certain heart disease or blood pressure medications
- Aspiration (foreign matter drawn into the lungs)
- Congestive heart failure

◼ WHAT TO EXPECT AT YOUR PROVIDER'S OFFICE

Your health care provider will conduct a physical examination, including a careful, detailed history of your symptoms. He or she will examine your nasal passages, throat, and lungs.

◼ TREATMENT OPTIONS

Your health care provider may suggest the following.

- Stay away from cigarette smoke and airborne irritants that may be present in your home or workplace.
- Stop taking medications that trigger the cough reflex.
- Take a trial period of medication to treat suspected illnesses.

Your provider may prescribe medications such as cough suppressants, inhalers, antibiotics, anithistamines, or expectorants, depending on the type of cough you have and its cause. The goal of treatment is not only to soothe your cough, but to treat its underlying cause.

Complementary and Alternative Therapies

While coughs due to severe underlying causes require medical treatment, alternative therapies can be useful in treating coughs secondary to viral URI, allergens, irritants, and asthma. In addition, alternative therapies can be used at the same time as conventional medications to optimize your recovery.

NUTRITION

- Avoid foods that you are allergic to. Food allergy testing can help determine your food allergies.
- Eat less mucus-producing foods such as dairy, citrus, wheat, and bananas. Eat more fresh vegetables, fruits, and whole grains.
- Take Vitamin C (1,000 mg three or four times a day), zinc (30 mg per day), and beta-carotene (100,000 IU per day) to support your immune system.

HERBS

Herbs are generally a safe way to strengthen and tone the body's systems. As with any therapy, it is important to work with your provider on getting your problem diagnosed before you start any treatment. Herbs may be used as dried extracts (capsules, powders, teas), glycerites (glycerine extracts), or tinctures (alcohol extracts). Unless otherwise indicated, teas should be made with 1 tsp. herb per cup of hot water. Steep covered 5 to 10 minutes for leaf or flowers, and 10 to 20 minutes for roots. Drink 2 to 4 cups per day. Tinctures may be used singly or in combination as noted.

- Strong expectorants: horehound (*Marrubium vulgare*), thyme (*Thymus vulgaris*), and mullein (*Verbascum densiflorum*)
- Gentle expectorants: fennel (*Foeniculum vulgare*), sweet violet (*Viola odorata*), ginger (*Zingiber officinalis*), and balm of Gilead (*Populus candicans*)
- Cough suppressants: wild cherry bark (*Prunus serotina*), coltsfoot (*Tussilago farfara*), and linden flowers (*Tilea europea*)
- Immune support: purple coneflower (*Echinacea purpura*), licorice root (*Glycyrrhiza glabra*), garlic (*Allium sativum*), and onion (*Allium cepa*). Avoid licorice root (*Glycyrrhiza glabra*) if you have high blood pressure.
- Toning: Indian tobacco (*Lobelia inflata*)--especially useful for smokers, elderberry (*Sambucus nigra*), elecampane (*Inula helenium*), plantain (*Plantago lancelota*), and gumweed (*Grindelia camporum*)

Thyme (*Thymus vulgaris*), eucalyptus, and pine oils can be applied to the skin to help with a cough. Make a chest rub with 2 to 4 drops of essential oil in 1 tbsp. of food-grade oil (olive, flax, sesame, almond, and the like). Or, make a castor oil pack with 4 to 6 drops of essential oil. Note that exposure to essential oils may keep homeopathic remedies from working.

HOMEOPATHY

Some of the most common remedies used for cough are listed below. Usually, the dose is 12X to 30C every one to four hours until your symptoms get better.

- *Aconite* for sudden onset of cough or croup (difficult, noisy breathing with a hoarse cough)
- *Spongia toasta* for harsh, barking cough
- *Drosera* for dry, spasmodic cough
- *Rumex crispus* for dry, shallow, tickling cough
- *Ipecac* for deep, wet cough with gagging from the cough
- *Phosphorous* for tight chest with cough
- *Causticum* for cough with raw painful feeling in chest
- *Antimonium tart* for rattling cough with dizziness

◼ FOLLOWING UP

Use the remedies that work best for you and follow the instructions of your health care provider. Be sure to get rest and drink plenty of water.

◼ SPECIAL CONSIDERATIONS

Severe coughing can cause rib fractures, in which case your provider will investigate the possibility of bone disorders, such as osteoporosis.

■ CUTANEOUS DRUG REACTIONS

Cutaneous drug reactions are adverse responses to drugs that appear on the skin. A red, itchy rash and hives are the most common reactions, however there are many different types, and some are life-threatening. Drugs that most frequently cause problems include sulfa drugs, antibiotics such as penicillins and tetracyclines, and phenytoin (a drug that prevents convulsions).

■ SIGNS AND SYMPTOMS

- Red, itchy rash or blotches
- Hives
- Acne-like eruptions
- Pigmentation changes (may appear as brown or grey blotches)
- Dry, cracked skin, as in eczema
- Peeling skin
- Tissue death (necrosis)

■ WHAT CAUSES IT?

Some drugs that might cause cutaneous reactions include the following.

- Allopurinol (gout medication)
- Antibiotics (penicillins, tetracyclines)
- Aspirin
- Barbiturates
- Chemotherapeutic agents (cancer treatments)
- Cortisones and other steroids
- Diuretics (water pills)
- Heavy metals (gold, copper)
- Nonsteroidal anti-inflammatory drugs (NSAIDs)
- Phenothiazines (antihistamines and sedatives)

■ WHAT TO EXPECT AT YOUR PROVIDER'S OFFICE

Your health care provider will examine your skin, mouth, and throat. He or she will ask you to list the drugs (prescription, nonprescription, and illegal) and herbal and vitamin supplements you've taken over the last four weeks. Your provider may have you stop taking the suspected drug and prescribe something else.

■ TREATMENT OPTIONS

Symptoms will often disappear once you stop taking the suspected drug, however, you may need treatment to recover. Your health care provider may prescribe drugs to help stop the reaction, such as epinephrines, corticosteroids, antihistamines, or topical ointments.

Complementary and Alternative Therapies

Mild to moderate reactions may be safely and effectively treated with alternative therapies.

NUTRITION

- Vitamin C (1,000 mg three to four times per day) stabilizes certain types of skin cells and stops reactions.
- B complex with extra B$_{12}$ (1,000 mcg per day) aids in skin health.
- Vitamin E (400 to 800 IU per day) improves circulation to your skin.
- Zinc (30 to 50 mg per day) supports the immune system.
- Bromelain (125 to 250 mg two to three times per day) reduces inflammation.
- Magnesium (400 to 800 mg per day) may help prevent spasms in the bronchial passages.

HERBS

Herbs may be used as dried extracts (capsules, powders, teas), glycerites (glycerine extracts), or tinctures (alcohol extracts). Unless otherwise indicated, teas should be made with 1 tsp. herb per cup of hot water. Steep covered 5 to 10 minutes for leaf or flowers, and 10 to 20 minutes for roots. Drink 2 to 4 cups per day. Tinctures may be used singly or in combination as noted.

- Turmeric (*Curcuma longa,* 100 mg two to three times per day)
- Quercetin (up to 1,000 mg three times per day)
- Hesperidin (200 mg three to four times per day)

An infusion of equal parts of coneflower (*Echinacea augustifolia*), yarrow (*Achillea millefolium*), chamomile (*Matricaria recutita*), peppermint (*Mentha piperita*), and red clover (*Trifolium pratense*) will strengthen your immune system, reduce swelling, and help with lymph drainage (fluid that is part of immune system).

To relieve itching, use one or more of the following herbs brewed as a tea, 1 tsp. of herb per cup of water: peppermint (*Mentha piperata*), chickweed (*Stellaria media*), or chamomile (*Matricaria recutita*). Be sure the tea is cool, and apply to the affected area as needed. To help your skin heal, add one or more of the following: marigold (*Calendula officinalis*), comfrey (*Symphytum officinale*), or coneflower (*Echinacea angustifolia*).

For open sores use powdered slippery elm (*Ulmus fulva*), goldenseal (*Hydrastis canadensis*), and marshmallow root (*Althea officinale*). Add enough skin wash to make a paste. Apply to affected area as needed.

Aloe vera gel applied to your skin can soothe burning and reduce swelling. For further skin relief, add powdered oatmeal (or 1 cup of oatmeal in a sock) to a lukewarm bath. Or, make a skin balm from flaxseed oil (2 tbsp.) plain or with 5 drops of oil of chamomile (*Matricaria recutita*) or marigold (*Calendula officinalis*).

HOMEOPATHY

Some of the most common remedies used for cutaneous drug reactions are listed below. Usually, the dose is 12X to 30C every one to four hours until your symptoms get better.

- *Apis* for acute swelling with burning pains that are relieved by cold applications
- *Graphites* for eczema or urticaria (hives) with tremendous itching
- *Ledum* for cellulitis or eczema with severe inflammation
- *Rhus tox* for burning and itching that are relieved by hot applications
- *Urtica urens* for burning and itching

■ FOLLOWING UP

It is important to stay in touch with your health care provider until the reaction is completely cleared up. If you have severe reactions, wear medical-alert jewelry stating what drugs you are allergic to.

■ SPECIAL CONSIDERATIONS

If you have any questions about any drug—whether it is prescribed by your health care provider or purchased over the counter—ask your pharmacist or health care provider.

■ DEMENTIA

Dementia is a mental disorder that includes memory impairment and at least one of the following: difficulty speaking, impaired movement, and inability to plan and initiate appropriate behaviors socially or at work. Dementia usually occurs in elderly people. It is rare in children. Approximately 2 to 4 percent of the population over age 65 has dementia caused by Alzheimer's disease.

■ SIGNS AND SYMPTOMS
- Memory impairment
- Language problems
- Motor skills impairment (such as balance and walking)
- Impaired ability to recognize objects
- Inability to think abstractly
- Spatial disorientation (e.g., judging distances)
- Depression and suicidal behavior
- Uninhibited behavior
- Anxiety, mood, and sleep problems
- Hallucinations

■ WHAT CAUSES IT?
Alzheimer's disease accounts for half to two thirds of all dementia cases. Other causes of dementia are listed below.
- Vascular disease
- General medical conditions, like traumatic brain injury
- Parkinson's, Huntington's, Creutzfeldt-Jakob, and other diseases
- Brain tumor
- Vitamin B deficiencies
- Drug or alcohol abuse, medications, or exposure to toxic substances

■ WHAT TO EXPECT AT YOUR PROVIDER'S OFFICE
Your health care provider will go over your symptoms and will do a physical examination. However, since there is no definitive test for dementia, your provider will rely greatly on interviews with you and your family, especially to discover noticeable declines in mental and physical abilities.

■ TREATMENT OPTIONS
Treatments are aimed at reversing or lessening the symptoms. A combination of drug and psychiatric or behavioral therapies will be used. Your health care provider may also closely evaluate current medications if you are elderly and have dementia, since older people are extremely sensitive to drugs. Exercise, both physical and mental, can slow the progress of dementia.

Complementary and Alternative Therapies
Alternative therapies may offer great promise in treating dementia without the side effects of pharmaceuticals. Treatment with nutrition can provide rapid results in some people with nutritional deficiencies. Herbal treatment is widely used in Europe with promising results.

NUTRITION
- Antioxidants are key—vitamin E (400 to 800 IU per day), vitamin C (1,000 mg three times per day), and coenzyme Q10 (10 to 50 mg three times per day)
- Vitamins: biotin (300 mcg); B_1 (50 to 100 mg), B_2 (50 mg), B_6 (50 to 100 mg), B_{12} (100 to 1,000 mcg). B_{12} may need to be administered through injection for best results.

- Minerals: calcium and magnesium (1,000 and 500 mg per day, respectively), zinc (30 to 50 mg per day); excess of manganese and copper can increase the risk for dementia
- Intravenous chelating agents such as ethylenediaminetetraacetic acid (EDTA) may help restore normal circulation in the brain.
- Essential fatty acids regulate certain types of blood cells, stabilize arterial walls and have anti-inflammatory properties. Dietary changes include reducing intake of animal fats and increasing that of fish.

HERBS
Herbs may be used as dried extracts (capsules, powders, teas), glycerites (glycerine extracts), or tinctures (alcohol extracts). Unless otherwise indicated, teas should be made with 1 tsp. herb per cup of hot water. Steep covered 5 to 10 minutes for leaf or flowers, and 10 to 20 minutes for roots. Drink 2 to 4 cups per day.

Choose four to six herbs from the most appropriate category and use one cup or 30 to 60 drops three times per day.
- Ginkgo *(Ginkgo biloba)* is specific for preventing and treating Alzheimer's and senile dementia. May be taken in a standardized extract of 40 to 50 mg three times per day. If you are taking an anticoagulant drug, use ginkgo only under the supervision of your provider.
- Hawthorn *(Crataegus oxyacantha)* is a circulatory stimulant .
- Rosemary *(Rosemarinus officinalis)* stimulates circulation, improves digestion, relieves depression.
- Siberian ginseng *(Eleuthrococcus senticosus)* increases endurance and increases cerebral circulation. Use this herb with caution if you have high blood pressure.
- Lemon balm *(Melissa officinalis)* reduces spasms and anxiety .
- Ginger *(Zingiber officinale)* helps with general weakness.
- St. John's wort *(Hypericum perforatum)* helps relieve depression and anxiety.

HOMEOPATHY
Some of the most common remedies used for dementia are listed below. Usually, the dose is 12X to 30C every one to four hours until your symptoms get better.
- *Alumina* for dullness of mind, vagueness, slow answers to questions
- *Argentum nitricum* for dementia with irritability, especially with lack of control over impulses
- *Cicuta* for dementia after head injuries, especially with convulsions
- *Helleborus* for stupefaction, when a person answers questions slowly and stares vacantly
- *Silica* for mental deterioration with anxiety over small details

■ FOLLOWING UP
Someone with dementia probably will require continuous care and monitoring by both your health care provider and family members.

■ SPECIAL CONSIDERATIONS
Caregiver and patient education focusing on knowledge of the disease, health, and the patient's well-being results in better patient care. Caregivers must also closely monitor patients to make sure they are taking medications appropriately.

■ DEPRESSION

Depression, also called unipolar mood disorder, is characterized by depression symptoms that last at least two weeks. It affects emotions, thinking, behavior, and physical well-being. It occurs most often in people between the ages of 25 and 44. Depression is rated in terms of severity (mild, moderate, severe) and is classified by how frequently it occurs.

■ SIGNS AND SYMPTOMS

Significantly depressed mood, lowered interest or pleasure in activities (including sex), and at least four of the following are signs of depression.

- feelings of worthlessness
- self-criticism
- inappropriate guilt
- significant weight loss or weight gain
- lack of sleep or excessive amounts of sleep
- hyperactivity or inactivity
- fatigue or loss of energy
- poor concentration
- frequent thoughts of death or suicide

■ WHAT CAUSES IT?

Stressful life events and genetic predisposition are causes of depression. Here are some other factors that can put you at risk.

- family history of depression
- prior suicide attempt
- being female
- age (usually occurs under the age of 44)
- having just had a baby
- stressful life events (especially loss of a loved one) or lack of a social support system
- current or past alcohol or drug abuse

■ WHAT TO EXPECT AT YOUR PROVIDER'S OFFICE

Your health care provider will perform a physical examination. You may be asked questions to find out what symptoms of depression you are experiencing. Your provider may also give you blood tests or psychological tests.

■ TREATMENT OPTIONS

Depending on the type of depression you have and how severe it is, your health care provider may recommend drugs or psychotherapy. If your case is severe, hospitalization might also be recommended. If your depression is seasonal, your provider may recommend light therapy. Yoga, exercise, and tai chi may also be helpful.

Drug Therapies

You may be prescribed an antidepressant, such as one of the following. These medications vary in terms of dosage and side effects. Be sure to follow your health care provider's instructions for taking them.

- selective serotonin reuptake inhibitors (SSRIs), such as fluoxetine (Prozac) or sertraline (Zoloft)
- monoamine oxidase inhibitors (MAOIs), such as phenelzine (Nardil)
- tricyclic antidepressants, such as amitriptyline (Elavil)

Complementary and Alternative Therapies

Usually a combination of nutrition and herbs will provide relief.

NUTRITION

- B_{12} and folate. Particularly the elderly are at risk for this deficiency. Dose is 800 mcg per day for folate and 100 to 500 mcg per day for B_{12}.
- Other vitamins shown to be low in people with depression are vitamin C (1,000 mg three times a day), biotin (300 mcg per day), B_1 (50 to 100 mg per day), B_2 (50 mg), B_6 (50 to 100 mg per day). Minerals shown to be deficient in people with depression are calcium (800 to 1,200 mg per day), iron (15 to 30 mg per day), and magnesium (400 to 800 mg per day). A good multivitamin can efficiently address these deficiencies. In addition, chromium (200 to 500 mcg per day) helps stabilize mood changes associated with hypoglycemia.
- Essential fatty acids: depleted in depression (1,000 to 1,500 IU per day)

HERBS

Herbs may be used as dried extracts (capsules, powders, teas), glycerites (glycerine extracts), or tinctures (alcohol extracts). Unless otherwise indicated, teas should be made with 1 tsp. herb per cup of hot water. Steep covered 5 to 10 minutes for leaf or flowers, and 10 to 20 minutes for roots. Drink 2 to 4 cups per day. Tinctures may be used singly or in combination as noted.

- St. John's wort (*Hypericum perforatum*): Numerous studies support its use in mild to moderate depression; side effects may include sensitivity to sunlight, stomach upset, headaches and rash. Dose is 1 to 4 ml tincture per day, or 250 mg three times per day when it is the only herb you are taking. It may take four to six weeks to become effective. If you are taking an antidepressant medication, do not take St. John's wort except under the close supervision of your health care provider.
- Valerian (*Valeriana officinalis*): sedative, with digestive problems
- Black cohosh (*Cimicifuga racemosa*): chronic depression, especially when caused by hormonal problems
- Ginkgo (*Ginkgo biloba*): circulatory stimulant, especially with decreased circulation or memory loss
- Oat straw (*Avena sativa*): nerve tonic, gentle, slow acting
- Siberian ginseng (*Eleuthrococcus senticosus*): improves ability to withstand stress
- Licorice (*Glycyrrhiza glabra*): antidepressant, especially for long-term stress with a digestive or hormonal component. Do not take licorice if you have high blood pressure.
- Passionflower (*Passiflora incarnata*): especially for emotional upheaval with nervousness and insomnia
- Lemon balm (*Melissa officinalis*): mild sedative and spasmolytic

A combination of equal parts of four to six herbs (1 cup tea three times a day, or 30 to 60 drops tincture) listed above can be very helpful.

HOMEOPATHY

Homeopathy may be useful as a supportive therapy.

ACUPUNCTURE

Recent studies show that acupuncture can be effective at relieving symptoms, at times statistically comparable to antidepressants or psychotherapy.

MASSAGE

Therapeutic massage has been shown to be effective in increasing circulation and promoting general well-being.

■ FOLLOWING UP

Your health care provider will probably schedule a follow-up appointment with you to check on how your treatment is going. If your depression gets worse, and especially if you are having thoughts of suicide, call your provider right away.

■ DERMATITIS

Dermatitis (also called eczema) is an itchy inflammation of the skin. There are many types of dermatitis.

■ SIGNS AND SYMPTOMS
- Itching, pain, stinging, or burning
- Blisters, thick or scaly skin, red skin, sores from scratching

■ WHAT CAUSES IT?
- Allergic reactions (for example, to poison oak or ivy)
- Low humidity or soaps and detergents
- Chemicals, such as nickel and cobalt
- Working with chemicals or wetting hands often
- Genetic make up

■ WHAT TO EXPECT AT YOUR PROVIDER'S OFFICE
Your health care provider will try to determine the cause of your dermatitis and make sure you have dermatitis and not a similar disease, such as psoriasis, skin cancer, or some psychological conditions.

■ TREATMENT OPTIONS
- Some corticosteroids, such as prednisone, are taken internally to reduce swelling. Others, such as hydrocortisone, are applied directly to the skin to relieve discomfort.
- Antihistamines relieve itching; some may also help you sleep.
- Antibiotics, either topical (to put on your skin) or in pill form, are prescribed if there is an infection.

Complementary and Alternative Therapies
Following nutritional guidelines and using herbal support may help reduce inflammation and hypersensitivity. Hypersensitivity associated with stress and anxiety may be helped by mind-body techniques such as meditation, tai chi, yoga, and stress management.

NUTRITION
Note: Lower doses are for children.
- Eliminate or reduce exposure to environmental or food allergens. Common allergenic foods are dairy, soy, citrus, peanuts, wheat (sometimes all gluten-containing grains), fish, eggs, corn, and tomatoes.
- Reduce pro-inflammatory foods in the diet including saturated fats (meats, especially poultry, and dairy), refined foods, and sugar.
- Increase intake of fresh vegetables, whole grains, and essential fatty acids (cold-water fish, nuts, and seeds).
- Flaxseed, borage, or evening primrose oil (1,000 to 1,500 mg one to two times per day) are anti-inflammatory. Children should be given cod liver oil (1 tsp. per day) or omega-3 oils (fish oils).
- Beta-carotene (25,000 to 100,000 IU per day), zinc (10 to 30 mg per day), and vitamin E (200 to 800 IU per day) support immune function and skin healing.
- Vitamin C (1,000 mg two to four times per day) inhibits histamine release. Rose hips or palmitate are citrus-free and hypoallergenic.
- Selenium (100 to 200 mcg per day) helps regulate fatty acid metabolism and is a co-factor in liver detoxification.
- Bromelain (100 to 250 mg two to four times per day) helps reduce inflammation.

HERBS
Herbs may be used as dried extracts (capsules, powders, teas), glycerites (glycerine extracts), or tinctures (alcohol extracts). Unless otherwise indi-

cated, teas should be made with 1 tsp. herb per cup of hot water. Steep covered 5 to 10 minutes for leaf or flowers; 10 to 20 minutes for roots.

Flavonoids, a substance found in dark berries and some plants, have anti-inflammatory properties, strengthen connective tissue, and reduce hypersensitivity. The following bioflavonoids may be taken in dried extract form.
- Catechin (25 to 150 mg two to three times per day), quercetin (50 to 250 mg two to three times per day), hesperidin (50 to 250 mg two to three times per day), and rutin (50 to 250 mg two to three times per day).
- Rose hips *(Rosa canina)* are also high in bioflavonoids and may be used as a tea. Drink 3 to 4 cups per day.

The following herbs support skin healing and lymphatic drainage; use in combination as a tincture (15 to 30 drops three times per day) or tea (2 to 4 cups per day). Peppermint *(Mentha piperita)*, red clover *(Trifolium pratense)*, cleavers *(Gallium aparine)*, yarrow *(Achillea millefolium)*, and prickly ash bark *(Xanthoxylum clava-herculis)*.

Sarsaparilla *(Smilax species)* helps heal hot, red, inflamed skin, and gotu kola *(Centella asiatica)* is good for dry, scaly, crusty skin. Use 3 ml sarsaparilla and 2 ml gotu kola tincture daily, or 3 cups tea per day.

Oregon grape *(Mahonia aquafolium)* or red alder bark *(Alnus rubra)* taken as tincture (20 to 30 drops three times a day) helps the liver process waste.

Creams and salves containing one or more of the following herbs may help relieve itching and burning, and promote healing. Chickweed *(Stellaria media)*, marigold *(Calendula officinalis)*, comfrey *(Symphytum officianale)*, and chamomile *(Matricaria recutita)*.

Peppermint leaf tea *(Mentha piperita)* may be cooled and applied to relieve itching and burning. An external menthol ointment can also help.

HOMEOPATHY
Some of the most common remedies used for dermatitis are listed below. Usually, the dose is 12X to 30C every one to four hours until your symptoms get better.
- *Apis mellifica* for hot, swollen vesicles
- *Rhus toxicodendron* for intense itching and burning
- *Urtica urens* for burning, stinging pains

ACUPUNCTURE
Acupuncture may help restore normal immune function and reduce the hypersensitivity response.

MASSAGE
Massage may help reduce stress, which makes dermatitis worse.

■ FOLLOWING UP
Carefully avoid whatever gives you dermatitis and prevent infection and scarring by not scratching.

■ SPECIAL CONSIDERATIONS
Check with your provider before using any medication if you are pregnant.

■ DIABETES MELLITUS

Diabetes mellitus results when your body doesn't adequately regulate the sugar levels in your blood. More than a half million new cases are diagnosed in the U.S. each year. Up to 50 percent of the people who have diabetes do not know it. It affects people of all ages, races, and income levels. There are two major forms.

Type 1 (insulin-dependent diabetes mellitus [IDDM]) usually occurs before age 30. Only about 10 percent of diabetes cases are type 1.

Type 2 (non-insulin-dependent diabetes mellitus [NIDDM]) usually occurs over age 40 and accounts for about 90 percent of cases.

■ SIGNS AND SYMPTOMS

- Frequent urination, thirst that does not go away, frequent eating, rapid weight loss, and high blood sugar levels occurring together
- Increased susceptibility to infection
- Fatigue or weakness
- Blurred vision
- Itching, numbness, and tingling in the hands and feet
- Leg cramps

■ WHAT CAUSES IT?

You are more likely to have type 1 diabetes if you have a family history of diabetes, thyroid disease, other endocrine diseases, or an autoimmune disease. Drinking cow's milk in infancy has been linked to juvenile diabetes.

The following factors put you more at risk for type 2 diabetes.

- Being overweight
- Leading a sedentary lifestyle
- Eating a diet high in fat and calories
- Being over age 40
- Having a family history of diabetes or endocrine diseases

■ WHAT TO EXPECT AT YOUR PROVIDER'S OFFICE

Your health care provider will take a blood test to measure your blood sugar level. He or she may talk to you about starting an exercise program and changing your diet.

■ TREATMENT OPTIONS

Your health care provider will create a treatment program that might include modified diet, exercise, blood sugar (glucose) self-monitoring, and oral hypoglycemic medication, or regular injections of insulin (a substance produced by the body that helps regulate blood sugar), as well as alternative therapies.

Complementary and Alternative Therapies

Alternative therapies can play an important role in preventing some of the serious complications that may be caused by diabetes. A combination of herbs and nutrition can be quite helpful. Regular exercise is very important.

NUTRITION

- The classic diet to control diabetes is high in complex carbohydrates and fiber. Some people, however, achieve better glucose control with a high-protein diet with very few carbohydrates.
- Essential fatty-acids can help your body use insulin better and can help prevent cardiovascular and neurological complications of diabetes.

Evening primrose oil (2,000 mg twice a day) or fish oil (1,200 mg bid) is the best way to get these fatty acids.

- OPCs (oligomeric procyanidins) such as pycnogenol or grape seed extracts help support vascular health.
- B-complex vitamins—biotin (300 mcg), B_1 (50 to 100 mg), B_2 (50 mg), B_3 (100 mg), B_6 (50 to 100 mg), B_{12} (100 to 1,000 mcg), and folate (400 mcg per day)—help control blood sugar levels.
- Vitamin C (2 to 3 g per day) may prevent certain complications.
- Vitamin E (400 IU per day) may reduce insulin requirements. Start at 100 IU and gradually increase the dose.
- Brewer's yeast contains chromium, which may improve glucose tolerance, and glutathione, an antioxidant (9 g or 3 tbsp. brewer's yeast per day and/or 200 mcg chromium).
- Magnesium (400 mg per day) may help the arteries.
- Manganese (500 to 1,000 mcg) may help stabilize blood sugar levels.
- Zinc (30 mg per day) may decrease glucose levels.
- Coenzyme Q10 (50 to 100 mg twice a day) is depleted in people with diabetes. It also helps your body use fatty acids better.
- Vanadium (5 to 10 mg per day) can normalize cholesterol.
- Chromium picolinate (200 mcg) may normalize sugar metabolism.

HERBS

Herbs may be used as dried extracts (capsules, powders, teas), glycerites (glycerine extracts), or tinctures (alcohol extracts). Unless otherwise indicated, teas should be made with 1 tsp. herb per cup of hot water. Steep covered 5 to 10 minutes for leaf or flowers, and 10 to 20 minutes for roots. Drink 2 to 4 cups per day. Tinctures may be used alone or in combination as noted. Herbs for diabetes include the following.

- Garlic *(Allium sativum)*
- Onion *(Allium cepa)*
- Bilberry *(Vaccinium myrtillus)*
- Fenugreek *(Trigonella foenum-graecum)*

Bilberry and fenugreek, equal parts, can be used as 1 cup tea three times per day, or 30 to 60 drops tincture three times per day.

Cayenne *(Capsicum annum):* 0.075 percent capsaicin cream on the skin can decrease pain from nerve damage in two to four weeks.

HOMEOPATHY

Homeopathy may be useful as a supportive therapy.

ACUPUNCTURE

Acupuncture can relieve your symptoms and increase your vitality.

MASSAGE

Massage may be helpful in relieving stress, which can stabilize your blood sugar level, and maintain healthy circulation.

■ FOLLOWING UP

Successful treatment of diabetes requires working with your provider.

■ SPECIAL CONSIDERATIONS

Glucose control is important before becoming pregnant. Do not take oral hypoglycemic medicines during pregnancy. In addition, gestational diabetes can occur during pregnancy and cause complications if left untreated. Gestational diabetes usually goes away after the baby is born.

For additional information supporting this handout, please refer to our website: www.onemedicine.com/public/products/access

29

DIARRHEA

Diarrhea is an increase in the wateriness, volume, or frequency of bowel movements. Although uncomfortable, most diarrhea is not serious and will go away in a few days without treatment. See a health care provider, however, if the feces contains blood, if the diarrhea is particularly severe, or if the diarrhea lasts more than a few days.

SIGNS AND SYMPTOMS

Diarrhea is a symptom of another ailment. Symptoms you might experience with diarrhea include the following.

- Frequent need to defecate
- Abdominal pain, cramping
- Fever, chills, general sick feeling
- Weight loss

WHAT CAUSES IT?

Most diarrhea is caused by an infection (viral, bacterial, or parasitic) or intestinal disorders such as inflammatory bowel disease. Other common causes include viruses and food poisoning. Eating local food and drinking local water during foreign travel can result in "traveler's diarrhea." Exposure to people who have diarrhea can also result in diarrhea.

WHAT TO EXPECT AT YOUR PROVIDER'S OFFICE

Your health care provider will question you about your symptoms. Your provider will also check if you are dehydrated and may feel your abdomen to see if it is tender, listen to your abdomen with a stethoscope, and give you a rectal exam.

TREATMENT OPTIONS
Drug Therapies

Your health care provider may suggest drugs for your diarrhea, including the following.

- Opioid derivatives: Lomotil and Imodium
- Adsorbents: Pepto-Bismol (for traveler's diarrhea) and Kaopectate
- Bulk-forming medications: Metamucil, Knosyl

Complementary and Alternative Therapies

Work with your provider to find remedies that are right for you.

NUTRITION

- Avoid coffee, chocolate, dairy products, strong spices, and solid foods. Introduce clear soup, crackers, white bread, rice, potatoes, applesauce, and bananas as diarrhea gets better.
- Rice or barley water, fresh vegetable juices (especially carrot and celery), miso broth, or other clear broths help restore proper fluid and electrolyte balance. Make rice and barley water using 1 cup of raw grain to 1 quart of boiling water. Let steep for 20 minutes. Strain and drink throughout the day.
- Lactobacillus taken as powder or in capsules helps normalize bowel flora and may help cure your diarrhea. Take as directed.
- Vitamin C (1,000 mg three to four times per day) and vitamin A (10,000 to 20,000 IU per day) help your immune system function well. However, high doses of vitamin C may cause diarrhea. High doses of vitamin A should not be taken for a long time without health care provider supervision.
- Glutamine (3,000 mg three times per day) is helpful in treating diarrhea that is caused by irritation of the intestinal lining rather than infection.

HERBS

Do not use herbs to treat diarrhea without talking to your health care provider first. If your diarrhea is caused by certain types of infections, herbal treatments could make it worse. The most common herbal remedies for diarrhea are described below. They are best used as teas unless otherwise noted. Teas should be made with 1 tsp. herb per cup of hot water. Steep covered 5 to 10 minutes for leaf or flowers, and 10 to 20 minutes for roots. Drink 2 to 4 cups per day.

Swelling reducers:
- Quercetin (250 to 500 mg two to four times per day)
- Chamomile *(Matricaria recutita)*
- Marshmallow root *(Althea officinalis)* as cold-water tea. Soak 2 tbsp. root in 1 quart of water overnight. Strain; drink throughout the day.

Infection fighters:
- Barberry *(Berberis vulgaris)* 250 to 500 mg three times per day
- Goldenseal *(Hydrastis canadensis)* 250 to 500 mg three times per day
- Licorice root *(Glycyrrhiza glabra).* Do not take if you have high blood pressure.

Antidiarrheal herbs:
- Blackberry leaf *(Rubus fruticosus)* or raspberry leaf *(Rubus idaeus)* 1 heaping tsp. per cup. Drink $1/2$ cup per hour.
- Carob powder; use 4 tsp. per 4 oz. of water or mix in applesauce. Take $1/2$ to 1 tsp. every 30 to 60 minutes.
- Slippery elm powder *(Ulmus rubra)* or marshmallow root powder *(Althea officinalis);* use 1 oz. powder to 1 quart of water. Make a paste with the powder and a small amount of water. Gradually add in the rest of the water and then simmer down to 1 pint. Take 1 tsp. every 30 to 60 minutes.

HOMEOPATHY

Some of the most common remedies used for diarrhea are listed below. Usually, the dose is 12X to 30C every one to four hours.
- *Arsenicum album:* weak, chilly, anxious, and restless with diarrhea.
- *Podophyllum:* yellow, explosive, painless diarrhea
- *Chamomilla:* greenish, frothy stool with severe colicky pains
- *Mercurius vivus:* strong urging with offensive, bloody diarrhea.
- *Aloe:* colicky, cramping pains before and during stool
- *Veratrum album:* diarrhea and vomiting; collapsed states

FOLLOWING UP

If your diarrhea does not stop in three to five days, contact your health care provider.

SPECIAL CONSIDERATIONS

If you are pregnant, tell your doctor. Dehydration can cause you to go into labor early. Also, the spasms that diarrhea causes may cause you to have contractions. Do not take goldenseal *(Hydrastic canadensis),* barberry *(Berberis vulgaris),* or high doses of vitamin A if you are pregnant.

Diarrhea can be serious, even fatal, for infants and elderly people because of dehydration and the loss of electrolytes.

DYSMENORRHEA

Dysmenorrhea is pain associated with menstruation. Primary dysmenorrhea affects young women in their teens and early twenties. Pain usually begins a day or two before menstrual flow, and may continue through the first two days of menstruation. Discomfort tends to decrease over time and after pregnancy. Secondary dysmenorrhea is caused by underlying physical problems.

SIGNS AND SYMPTOMS

Symptoms and degree of pain vary, but may include the following.

- Abdominal cramping or dull ache that moves to lower back and legs
- Heavy menstrual flow
- Headache
- Nausea
- Constipation or diarrhea
- Frequent urination
- Vomiting (not common)

WHAT CAUSES IT?

Primary dysmenorrhea is caused by the following.

- Strong uterine contractions stimulated by increased production of the hormone prostaglandin by the lining of the uterus (endometrium)
- Anxiety and stress
- Blood and tissue being discharged through a narrow cervix
- Displaced uterus
- Lack of exercise

Secondary dysmennorhea can be caused by the following.

- Endometriosis (inflammation of the lining of the uterus)
- Blood and tissue being discharged through a narrow cervix
- Uterine fibroid or ovarian cyst
- Infections of the uterus
- Pelvic inflammatory disease (PID)
- Intrauterine device (IUD)

WHAT TO EXPECT AT YOUR PROVIDER'S OFFICE

A pelvic examination may include an internal examination, laparoscopy, and ultrasound. You may need a Pap test or D&C to analyze tissue. Blood and urine samples may be required.

TREATMENT OPTIONS

Drug Therapies

Your provider may suggest the following drugs.

- Anti-inflammatory agents such as ibuprofen (800 mg to start; 400 to 600 mg every six hours).
- Gonadotropin-releasing hormone (GnRH) or oral contraceptives
- Antibiotics will cure PID
- Estrogen or oral progestins (for example, norethindrone for 12 months brings relief in 80 percent of patients, however, there may be side effects).

Complementary and Alternative Therapies

Dysmenorrhea may be effectively treated with nutritional support and mind-body techniques such as meditation, yoga, tai chi, and exercise.

NUTRITION

- Increase intake of essential fatty acids, which are found in cold-water fish, nuts, and seeds. Reduce intake of saturated fats (meat and dairy products). Eliminate refined foods, sugar, dairy products, and methylxanthines (coffee and chocolate). Increase intake of fresh fruits and vegetables, proteins, and whole grains.
- Magnesium (400 mg per day) with B_6 (100 mg per day) throughout cycle to promote hormone production and induce relaxation. Can be used at higher doses during your period (magnesium up to 600 mg per day, and B_6 up to 300 mg per day) for pain relief.
- Vitamin E (400 to 800 IU per day) to improve blood supply to muscles
- B-complex (50 to 100 mg per day) to reduce the effects of stress
- Omega-3 oils such as flax seed, evening primrose, or borage oil (1,000 to 1,500 mg one to two times per day), to reduce inflammation and support hormone production
- Niacinamide (50 mg twice a day) to reduce pain. Begin seven days before your period until the end of flow. Add rutin (60 mg per day) and vitamin C (300 mg per day) to increase effects.

HERBS

Herbs may be used as dried extracts (capsules, powders, teas), glycerites (glycerine extracts), or tinctures (alcohol extracts). Teas should be made with 1 tsp. herb per cup of hot water. Steep covered 5 to 10 minutes for leaf or flowers; 10 to 20 minutes for roots. Drink 2 to 4 cups per day.

- Chaste tree *(Vitex agnus-cactus)* and black cohosh *(Cimicifuga racemosa),* 30 drops each, twice a day, to reduce dysmenorrhea.
- Red raspberry *(Rubus idaeus)* tea strengthens uterine tissue.
- Tea of chamomile *(Matricaria recutita)* and ginger root *(Zingiber officinalis)* can help reduce ovarian cyst pain.
- Tinctures of cramp bark *(Viburnum opulus),* black cohosh, Jamaican dogwood *(Piscidia erythrina),* and wild yam *(Dioscorea villosa)* can be used together in equal parts to relieve pain and cramping. Use 20 drops every half hour for four doses, then as needed up to eight doses per day for seven days.

HOMEOPATHY

Homeopathy may be useful as a supportive therapy.

PHYSICAL MEDICINE

The following methods can relieve pelvic pain.

- Castor oil pack. Apply oil directly to skin, cover with a clean soft cloth (for example, flannel) and plastic wrap. Place a heat source (hot water bottle or heating pad) over the pack and let sit for 30 to 60 minutes. For best results use three consecutive days in one week.
- Contrast sitz baths. Use two basins that you can comfortably sit in. Sit in hot water for three minutes, then in cold water for one minute. Repeat this three times to complete one set. Do one to two sets per day three to four days per week.

ACUPUNCTURE

Dysmenorrhea may respond to acupuncture, particularly for pain relief.

MASSAGE

Therapeutic massage is helpful in reducing the effects of stress.

FOLLOWING UP

If your symptoms change, or treatment does not help, tell your provider.

SPECIAL CONSIDERATIONS

Avoid caffeine, alcohol, and sugar prior to onset of your period.

■ DYSPHAGIA

Dysphagia is the medical term for difficulty swallowing, or the feeling that food is "sticking" in your throat or chest. The feeling is actually in your esophagus, the tube that carries food from your mouth to your stomach. You may experience dysphagia when swallowing solid foods, liquids, or both. Oropharyngeal dysphagia involves difficulty moving food from your mouth into your upper esophagus. Esophageal dysphagia involves difficulty moving food through your esophagus to your stomach. Dysphagia can affect you at any age, although the likelihood increases as you grow older.

■ SIGNS AND SYMPTOMS

The following are symptoms of oropharyngeal dysphagia.
- Difficulty trying to swallow
- Choking or breathing saliva into your lungs while swallowing
- Coughing while swallowing
- Regurgitating liquid through your nose
- Breathing in food while swallowing
- Weak voice
- Weight loss

The following are symptoms of esophageal dysphagia.
- Pressure sensation in your mid-chest area
- Sensation of food stuck in your throat
- Weight loss
- Chest pain
- Pain with swallowing
- Belching
- Chronic cough
- Sore throat
- Bad breath

■ WHAT CAUSES IT?

Dysphagia in children is often due to malformations, conditions such as cerebral palsy or muscular dystrophy, or gastroesophageal reflux disease (GERD). Dysphagia in adults is often due to tumors (benign or cancerous), conditions that cause the esophagus to narrow, neuromuscular conditions, or GERD. Other causes include smoking, excessive alcohol use, certain medications, and teeth or dentures in poor condition.

■ WHAT TO EXPECT AT YOUR PROVIDER'S OFFICE

Your health care provider may ask about your symptoms and eating habits. For infants and children, the health care provider may want to observe them eating. Your provider may also listen to your heart, take your pulse, and will want to know your medical history.

A variety of tests can be used for dysphagia.
- In endoscopy or esophagoscopy, a tube is inserted into your esophagus to help your provider evaluate the condition of your esophagus, and to try to open any parts that might be closed off.
- In esophageal manometry, a tube is inserted into your stomach to measure pressure differences in various regions.
- In endoscopic ultrasonography, ultrasound is used to evaluate the condition of your esophagus.
- X rays of your neck, chest, or abdomen may be taken.
- In a barium swallow, moving picture or video X rays are taken of your esophagus as you swallow barium, which is visible on an X ray.

■ TREATMENT OPTIONS

Dysphagia generally is treated with drugs, procedures that open up the esophagus, or surgery. Your treatment will depend the cause, the seriousness, and any complications you may be experiencing. In most cases, you can be treated without hospitalization as long as you are able to eat enough and have a low risk of complications. If your esophagus is severely obstructed, however, you may be hospitalized. Infants and children with dysphagia often are hospitalized.

Complementary and Alternative Therapies

Herbs can be effective at decreasing spasms and healing an inflamed esophagus. Homeopathic remedies may be used at the same time.

HERBS

Herbs may be used as dried extracts (capsules, powders, teas), glycerites (glycerine extracts), or tinctures (alcohol extracts).
- Licorice *(Glycyrrhiza glabra):* reduces spasms and swelling and is a pain reliever specifically for the gastrointestinal tract. Do not take licorice for a long period of time or if you have high blood pressure. The dose is 380 to 1,140 mg per day. Chewable lozenges may be the best form of licorice for treating GERD.
- Slippery elm *(Ulmus fulva):* demulcent (protects irritated tissues and promotes their healing); dose is 60 to 320 mg per day. One tsp. powder may be mixed with water and drunk three to four times a day.

In addition, a combination of four of the following herbs may be used as either a tea or tincture. Use equal parts of the herbs, either 1 tsp. of each per cup of water and steep 10 minutes three times a day, or equal parts of tincture 30 to 60 drops three times a day.
- Valerian *(Valeriana officinalis):* improves digestion and helps you relax, especially if you feel anxious or depressed
- Wild yam *(Dioscorea villosa):* reduces spasms and swelling, especially where there is fatigue
- St. John's wort *(Hypericum perforatum):* relieves pain, depression
- Skullcap *(Scutellaria lateriflora):* antispasmodic, sedative, relaxant
- Linden flowers *(Tilia cordata):* antispasmodic, mild diuretic

HOMEOPATHY

Some of the most common remedies used for dysphagia are listed below. Usually, the dose is 12X to 30C every one to four hours until your symptoms get better.
- *Baptesia* if you can swallow only liquids; especially with a red inflamed throat that is relatively pain-free
- *Baryta carbonica* if you have huge tonsils
- *Carbo vegatabilis* for bloating and indigestion that is worse when lying down; especially with flatulence and fatigue
- *Ignatia imara* for "lump in the throat," back spasms, cough; especially when symptoms appear after you have experienced grief
- *Lachesis* if you cannot stand to be touched around the throat (including by clothing that is tight at the neck)

■ FOLLOWING UP

Dysphagia should not limit your activities, but your health care provider may restrict your diet.

■ ECZEMA

Eczema, also called dermatitis, is a patch of itchy skin where blisters form, then dry and become crusty. There is no cure, but treatments can make you comfortable and help prevent outbreaks.

■ SIGNS AND SYMPTOMS
- Itching
- Red bumps
- Blisters
- Crusts
- Swelling
- Oozing
- Scaliness

■ WHAT CAUSES IT?
- Allergies to plants, chemicals, foods
- Certain drugs
- Vitamin or mineral deficiencies
- Certain physical or psychological disorders

■ WHAT TO EXPECT AT YOUR PROVIDER'S OFFICE
Your health care provider will look at your skin rash. He or she may ask about stress in your life, your diet, drugs you are taking, and chemicals or materials you may be exposed to at work, to find the cause of your rash.

■ TREATMENT OPTIONS
Your health care provider may prescribe a skin cream to relieve itching and dryness. He or she may also suggest that you do the following.
- Stay away from things that irritate your skin
- Avoid alcohol and tobacco
- Don't spend too much time in the sun

Complementary and Alternative Therapies
Discovering which foods you are allergic to and avoiding them is important. Following nutritional guidelines and using herbs as needed may help reduce swelling and allergic reactions. Eczema may be associated with stress and anxiety, so mind-body techniques such as meditation, tai chi, yoga, and stress management may help prevent it. Starch, oatmeal, and other baths may temporarily relieve the symptoms.

NUTRITION
Note: Lower doses are for children.
- Avoid foods you are allergic to. Common allergenic foods are dairy products, soy, citrus, peanuts, wheat, fish, eggs, corn, and tomatoes.
- A rotation diet, in which the same food is not eaten more than once every four days, may be helpful in treating chronic eczema.
- Eat fewer foods that cause inflammation, such as saturated fats (meats, especially poultry, and dairy), refined foods, and sugar.
- Increase intake of fresh vegetables, whole grains, and essential fatty acids (cold-water fish, nuts, and seeds).
- Flaxseed (3,000 mg twice a day), borage (1,500 mg twice a day), or evening primrose oil (1,500 mg twice a day) to reduce swelling. Children can be supplemented with cod liver oil ($1/2$ to 1 tsp. per day), or any of the above oils, 500 mg, twice a day.
- Beta carotene (25,000 to 100,000 IU/day), zinc (10 to 30 mg per day), and vitamin E (100 to 400 IU per day) to strengthen your immune system and help your skin heal.
- Zinc spray can heal the affected tissue in some patients.
- Vitamin C (250 to 1,000 mg two to four times per day) reduces your body's reponse to substances that cause allergies. Vitamin C from rose hips or palmitate is citrus-free and hypoallergenic.
- Selenium (50 to 200 mcg per day) helps regulate fatty acid metabolism and keeps your liver healthy.
- Bromelain (250 mg two to four times per day, taken between meals) reduces swelling.

Bioflavonoids, found in dark berries and some plants, help reduce swelling, strengthen connective tissue, and help reduce allergic reactions. The following are bioflavonoids that may be taken in dried extract form.
- Catechin (25 to 150 mg two to three times per day), quercetin (100 to 250 mg two to three times per day), hesperidin (100 to 250 mg two to three times per day), and rutin (100 to 250 mg two to three times per day).
- Rose hips (*Rosa canina*) are also high in bioflavonoids and may be used as a tea. Drink 3 to 4 cups per day.

HERBS
Herbs may be used as dried extracts (capsules, powders, teas), glycerites (glycerine extracts), or tinctures (alcohol extracts).
- Herbs that help your skin heal and increase lymphatic drainage are useful for relieving eczema. Use the following herbs in combination as a tincture (15 to 30 drops three times per day) or tea (2 to 4 cups per day): burdock root (*Arctium lappa*), yellow dock (*Rumex crispus*), red clover (Trifolium pratense), cleavers (*Gallium aparine*), yarrow (*Achillea millefolium*), peppermint (*Mentha piperita*), and nettles (*Urtica dioica*). To prepare a tea, steep the root elements for 10 minutes, then add the rest of the herbs and steep an additional 5 to 10 minutes.
- Skin creams and salves containing one or more of the following herbs may help relieve itching and burning, and promote healing: chickweed (*Stellaria media*), marigold (*Calendula officinalis*), comfrey (*Symphytum officinalis*), and chamomile (*Matricaria recutita*).
- Marshmallow root tea (*Althea officinalis*) may soothe and promote healing of gastrointestinal inflammation that is often found with eczema. Soak 1 heaping tbsp. of marshmallow root in 1 quart of cold water overnight. Strain and drink throughout the day.

HOMEOPATHY
The use of homeopathic remedies may make eczema worse.

ACUPUNCTURE
Acupuncture may help your immune system function better and reduce the allergic reactions that cause your eczema.

■ FOLLOWING UP
Eczema is usually just an annoyance, but it does recur and can become severe. Call your provider if it comes back frequently or grows worse.

■ SPECIAL CONSIDERATIONS
Starting an infant on solid foods conservatively and gradually may help prevent the food sensitivities that can cause eczema.

■ EDEMA

Edema (also known as dropsy or fluid retention) is swelling caused by the accumulation of abnormally large amounts of fluid in the spaces between the body's cells. It is a symptom rather than a disease or disorder. Widespread, long-term edema can indicate a serious underlying disorder.

■ SIGNS AND SYMPTOMS

These will vary and may include the following.
- Swollen limbs (possibly accompanied by pain, redness, heat)
- Facial puffiness; abdominal bloating
- Shortness of breath, extreme difficulty breathing, coughing up blood
- Sudden change in mental state or coma
- Muscle aches and pains

■ WHAT CAUSES IT?

Imbalance in the body's fluid transfer can be caused by the following.
- Sitting or standing for long periods
- Certain medications
- Hormonal changes during menstruation and pregnancy
- Infection or injury to a blood vessel; blood clots; varicose veins
- Allergies to food or insect bites
- Kidney, heart, liver, or thyroid disease
- High or low blood pressure; high salt intake
- Brain tumor or head injury
- Exposure to high altitudes or heat, especially when combined with heavy physical exertion

■ WHAT TO EXPECT AT YOUR PROVIDER'S OFFICE

Your health care provider will look for varicose veins, blood clots, wounds, or infections. An X ray, computed tomography scan, magnetic resonance imaging, urine test, or blood test may be necessary. Edema caused by organ failure or high altitude sickness may require hospitalization.

■ TREATMENT OPTIONS

Complete decongestive therapy (CDT) involves compression bandages and pressure "sleeves" tightened over swollen limbs to help force fluid through other channels for reabsorption by the body. Other options include a salt-reduction diet, daily exercise, resting with legs elevated above heart level, wearing support hose, and massage.

Drug Therapies

Drugs for edema include diuretics to reduce fluid levels, morphine, and medications to treating the underlying disorder.

Surgical Procedures

Surgery may be required to remove fat and fluid deposits associated with a certain type of edema called lipedema, or to repair damaged veins or lymphatic glands to reestablish lymph and blood flow.

Complementary and Alternative Therapies

The following nutritional and herbal support guidelines may help relieve edema, but the underlying cause must be addressed.

NUTRITION
- Eliminating food allergens from your diet decreases inflammation.
- A low-salt, high-protein diet may help edema. (However, you should not eat a high-protein diet if you have kidney disease.) You should also reduce your intake of sugar and refined carbohydrates.
- If you use diuretics, add more potassium to your diet.
- Natural diuretics: asparagus, parsley, beets, grapes, green beans, leafy greens, pineapple, pumpkin, onion, leeks, and garlic.
- Vitamin B_6 (50 to 100 mg per day) is a diuretic. The B vitamin thiamine may be supplemented (200 mg per day).
- Vitamins C (1,000 to 1,500 mg 3 times per day), E (400 to 800 IU per day), and Coenzyme Q10 (50 to 100 mg 2 times per day)
- Potassium aspartate (20 mg per day) if you are using diuretics
- Magnesium (200 mg two to three times per day) and calcium (1,000 mg per day) help maintain fluid exchange in the body.

HERBS
Herbs may be used as dried extracts (capsules, powders, teas), glycerites (glycerine extracts), or tinctures (alcohol extracts). Teas should be made with 1 tsp. herb per cup of hot water. Steep covered 5 to 10 minutes for leaf or flowers, and 10 to 20 minutes for roots.

A herbal diuretic is are best taken as a cooled tea (4 to 6 cups per day), although a tincture may also be used (30 to 60 drops four times a day). Combine three of these herbs with equal parts of two to three additional herbs from the following categories, as indicated: cleavers *(Gallium aparine)*, yarrow *(Achillea millefolium)*, oatstraw *(Avena sativa)*, elder *(Sambucus canadensis)*, red clover *(Trifolium pratense)*, and red root *(Ceonothus americanus)*

For cyclic edema, such as swelling from menstruation:
- Ginkgo *(Ginkgo biloba)* strengthens the integrity of blood vessels.
- Bilberry *(Vaccinium myrtillus)* is a gentle diuretic.
- Topical applications of creams containing one or more of the following may help strengthen your blood vessels: horse chestnut *(Aesculus hippocastanum)*, butcher's broom *(Ruscus asuleatus)*, sweet clover *(Melilotus officinalis)*, and rue *(Ruta graveolens)*.

HOMEOPATHY
Homeopathy may be useful as a supportive therapy.

PHYSICAL MEDICINE
- Dry skin brushing. Before bathing, briskly brush the entire skin surface with a rough washcloth, loofa, or soft brush. Begin at your feet and work up. Always stroke in the direction of your heart.
- Cold compresses made with yarrow tea.
- Contrast hydrotherapy involves alternating hot and cold applications. Alternate three minutes hot with one minute cold and repeat three times. This is one set. Do two to three sets per day.

ACUPUNCTURE
Acupuncture may improve fluid balance.

MASSAGE
Therapeutic massage can assist with lymph drainage.

■ SPECIAL CONSIDERATIONS

Excessive fluid retention during pregnancy (toxemia) is potentially dangerous to both you and your baby.

◾ ENDOCARDITIS

Endocarditis is an inflammation of the endocardium, a membrane that covers connective tissue in heart valves and lines heart chambers. Most cases are caused by a bacterial infection. Endocarditis is a serious ailment that can lead to severe medical complications, and can even be fatal if not treated.

◾ SIGNS AND SYMPTOMS

The most common symptom of endocarditis is fever. The fever may be high or low, and it may seem to come and go. Other common symptoms include the following.

- Skin sores
- Night sweats
- Chills
- Discomfort or uneasiness
- Muscle, joint, back pain
- Muscle weakness
- Stiff neck
- Headache
- Seizures
- Stroke
- Heart attack
- Difficulty speaking
- Paralysis
- Numbness
- Cold, painful hands and feet
- Small purplish spots on skin
- Bloody urine
- Bloody phlegm
- Painful tips of fingers or toes
- Shortness of breath
- Cough
- Unnatural pallor

◾ WHAT CAUSES IT?

Most of the causes of endocarditis are related to a bacterial infection. Heart conditions that increase your risk include having mechanical heart valves, a previous case of endocarditis, heart defects and dysfunctions, and degenerative heart disease. Dental and surgical procedures that increase your risk of infective endocarditis include dental procedures that irritate the gums, tonsillectomy, adenoidectomy, intestinal and respiratory surgery, gallbladder surgery, cystoscopy, bronchoscopy, and vaginal delivery with an infection present.

◾ WHAT TO EXPECT AT YOUR PROVIDER'S OFFICE

Your health care provider will listen to your heart and lungs, take your pulse, and check your eyes and skin. Your provider likely will order a number of tests, which could include blood tests, urine analysis, an echocardiogram, a computed tomography scan, and a cinefluoroscopy (a motion-picture type heart scan). In most cases, your provider will admit you to the hospital, possibly in intensive care, until your condition is better understood and your symptoms are under control.

◾ TREATMENT OPTIONS

Endocarditis is treated with antibiotics, almost always intravenously. In some cases, surgery is also required.

Drug Therapies

Infective endocarditis is usually treated with a combination of two or even three antibiotics, such as penicillin, gentamicin, vancomycin, cefazolin, ceftriaxone, nafcillin, oxacillin, rifampin, and ampicillin. Treatment generally takes two to six weeks.

Complementary and Alternative Therapies

Endocarditis has serious ramifications and requires aggressive medical treatment. Alternative therapies may be used concurrently to help reduce severity, duration, and progression of disease.

NUTRITION

- To support immune function, include vitamins C (1,000 mg up to three times a day), E (400 to 800 IU a day), A (10,000 IU/day) or beta carotene (100,000 IU a day), selenium (200 mcg a day), and zinc (30 mg a day).
- Coenzyme Q10 (100 mg twice a day) protects the heart.
- Magnesium (200 to 500 mg two to three times a day) for normal cardiac function. Do not take if you have kidney damage.
- Bromelain (250 to 500 mg three times a day between meals) is a proteolytic enzyme that may increase the effectiveness of antibiotic therapy.

HERBS

Herbs may be used as dried extracts (capsules, powders, teas), glycerites (glycerine extracts), or tinctures (alcohol extracts). Teas should be made with 1 tsp. herb per cup of hot water. Steep covered 5 to 10 minutes for leaf or flowers; 10 to 20 minutes for roots. Drink 2 to 4 cups per day.

- For long-term cardiac support combine the following herbs in a tea (3 cups per day) or tincture (30 to 60 drops three times a day): 2 parts hawthorn (*Crataegus oxyacantha*) with 1 part each motherwort (*Leonorus cardiaca*) and linden flowers (*Tilia cordata*). Use additional herbs from the following categories as needed.
- Cardiac arrhythmias: Add 1 part each lily of the valley (*Convalleria majus*) and night-blooming cereus (*Cactus grandiflorus*) to the cardiac formula above. These herbs must be used with caution and under a health care provider's supervision.
- Hawthorne berry can be helpful in decreasing arrhythmias. Use $^1/_2$ tsp. of the solid extract, or 1,000 mg three times per day.
- Infection: Combine equal parts of four to six of the following herbs: coneflower (*Echinacea purpura*), goldenseal root (*Hydrastis canadensis*), wild indigo (*Baptisia tinctoria*), myrrh (*Commiphora molmol*), garlic (*Allium sativum*), rosemary (*Rosemariana officinalis*). For acute infection take 60 drops of tincture every two hours. For chronic infections or for prophylaxis, take 30 to 60 drops three times per day.
- Renal involvement: Combine equal parts of bearberry (*Arctostaphylos uva ursi*), cleavers (*Galium aparine*), dandelion leaf (*Taraxecum officinalis*), black cohosh (*Cimicifuga racemosa*), yarrow (*Achillea millefolium*), and corn silk (*Zea mays*). Drink 3 cups per day.

HOMEOPATHY

Some of the most common remedies for this condition are listed below.

- *Aconite* if you fear death, have rapid heartbeat (tachycardia) with full, hard bounding pulse of sudden onset
- *Cactus grandiflorus* for endocarditis with mitral insufficiency. You may have a feeble, irregular pulse and feel a chest constriction.
- *Digitalis* if you have an irregular pulse with a sensation as if your heart would stop if you moved
- *Spongia* if you have a sensation of the heart swelling

ACUPUNCTURE

Acupuncture may help improve immunity and strengthen cardiac function.

◾ FOLLOWING UP

In addition to monitoring your condition while you are in the hospital, your health care provider will order follow-up procedures, such as blood tests, to determine how well the prescribed treatment is working.

■ ENDOMETRIOSIS

Endometriosis occurs when endometrial cells—the cells that make up the lining of your uterus—travel outside the uterus to other parts of your body. These misplaced cells are stimulated by hormones, just like the cells within your uterus, and bleed during your period (menstruation). Blood from these cells must be absorbed by your body. With each period, deposits build up and form scar tissue, which can be painful. Endometriosis affects 10 to 20 percent of American women of childbearing age. It is found in 30 percent of infertile women.

■ SIGNS AND SYMPTOMS

One third of women with endometriosis have no symptoms. The most common symptoms include the following.

- Pelvic pain, especially when you have your period
- Heavy or irregular menstruation
- Pain during sexual intercourse
- Infertility or miscarriage
- Pain with bladder or bowel function, or intestinal pain

■ WHAT CAUSES IT?

The cause is unknown, but there are three theories.

- Abnormal functioning of your immune system
- Retrograde (or reflux) menstruation, in which some menstrual blood flows backward through your fallopian tubes
- Genetic or heredity factors

■ WHAT TO EXPECT AT YOUR PROVIDER'S OFFICE

A physical examination may include gentle pushing on your abdomen and an internal examination. Definitive diagnosis is made with laparoscopy.

■ TREATMENT OPTIONS

Because there is no cure, treatment is to relieve symptoms.

Drug Therapies

The following drugs can relieve the symptoms of endometriosis.

- Nonsteroidal anti-inflammatory drugs (such as ibuprofen)
- Oral contraceptives
- Hormone-suppressing drugs (which stop menstruation)

Surgical Procedures

Laparoscopic laser techniques help shrink lesions. Total hysterectomy (removal of your uterus and ovaries) is recommended only when necessary but does not guarantee an end to your symptoms.

Complementary and Alternative Therapies

Providing liver support is the backbone of alternative treatment.

NUTRITION

- Eliminate all known food allergens.
- Eliminate alcohol, caffeine, chocolate, refined foods, food additives, sugar, and saturated fats (meats and dairy products).
- Eat only organic poultry and produce.
- Increase intake of whole grains, fresh vegetables, essential fatty acids, and vegetable proteins. Include liver-supporting foods such as beets, carrots, onions, garlic, leafy greens, artichokes, apples, and lemons.
- Vitamin C (1,000 mg three times per day) decreases inflammation.
- Zinc (30 to 50 mg per day) and beta-carotene (50,000 to 100,000 IU per day) support immune function and enhance healing.

- Vitamin E (400 IU per day) is necessary for hormone production.
- Selenium (200 mcg per day) is needed for fatty acid metabolism.
- Iron supplementation may be necessary if bleeding is severe.
- Calcium (1,000 to 1,500 mg per day) and magnesium (200 mg two to three times per day) are needed for hormone metabolism.
- Essential fatty acids (1,000 to 1,500 mg twice a day).

HERBS

Herbs may be used as dried extracts (capsules, powders, teas), glycerites (glycerine extracts), or tinctures (alcohol extracts).

Chaste tree (*Vitex agnus-cactus*) taken long-term (12 to 18 months) for maximum effectiveness. Combine 2 parts of chaste tree with 1 part of two herbs from each category. Drink 3 cups of tea per day or take 30 to 60 drops of tincture per day.

For liver support (include milk thistle and one other herb): Milk thistle (*Silybum marianum*), dandelion root (*Taraxacum officinalis*), vervain (*Verbena hastata*), or blue flag (*Iris versicolor*).

For reducing pelvic congestion: Squaw vine (*Mitchella repens*), motherwort (*Leonorus cardiaca*), red root (*Ceonothus americanus*), red raspberry (*Rubus idaeus*).

For management of severe pain and extensive endometriosis, Turska's formula is the preferred combination and should be used only under a health care provider's supervision.

HOMEOPATHY

Some of the most common remedies are listed below. Usually, the dose is 12X to 30C every one to four hours.

- *Belladonna* for menstruation with sensation of heaviness and heat
- *Calcarea phosphoricum* for excessive periods with backache
- *Chamomilla* for heavy menses with dark clotted blood and pains
- *Cimicifuga racemosa* for unbearable pain radiating from hip to hip

PHYSICAL MEDICINE

- Contrast sitz baths. You will need two basins that you can comfortably sit in. Sit in hot water for three minutes, then in cold water for one minute. Repeat this three times to complete one set. Do one to two sets per day, three to four days per week. (Do not perform this during menstrual flow.)
- Castor oil pack. Apply oil directly to abdomen, cover with a clean soft cloth and plastic wrap. Place a heat source over the pack and let sit for 30 to 60 minutes. Use for three consecutive days.
- Kegel exercises (contracting and releasing the pelvic muscles).

ACUPUNCTURE

Acupuncture may be helpful for endometriosis.

MASSAGE

Therapeutic massage may help resolve pelvic congestion.

■ SPECIAL CONSIDERATIONS

Endometriosis often resolves during pregnancy.

■ FEVER OF UNKNOWN ORIGIN

When health care providers cannot diagnose the cause of a patient's temperature that reaches 101 degrees Fahrenheit on and off for at least three weeks, they call it a fever of unknown origin (FUO). If the fever persists, your health care provider will continue to carry out tests to narrow down the causes. But in 5 to 15 percent of cases, they fail to find the reason for the fever.

Your health care provider may prefer not to give you medication for your fever while it remains undiagnosed. Research suggests that fever helps fight off infections, so treating the fever without knowing the cause might reduce the body's ability to deal with the possible infection. However, providers will prescribe drugs to reduce fever in children who suffer seizures induced by fever. Because a higher temperature increases a person's need for oxygen, your provider may prescribe fever-reducing drugs if you have heart or lung problems.

■ SIGNS AND SYMPTOMS
- Fever of more than 101°F (38.3°C), either continuous or intermittent, for at least two weeks
- Fever above 101°F whose cause remains unknown even after extensive diagnostic testing

■ WHAT CAUSES IT?
By carrying out a series of tests, health care providers try to narrow down the list of possible reasons for a high temperature.

■ WHAT TO EXPECT AT YOUR PROVIDER'S OFFICE
A provider trying to diagnose the cause of a fever of unknown origin must seek out every possible clue. He or she may ask you questions such as:
- Your work, because some workplaces contain organisms that can cause fever
- Places you have visited recently. Locations overseas, and even areas in the United States, can harbor diseases that can cause fever.

Your health care provider will also examine you closely, paying particular attention to your skin, eyes, nails, lymph nodes, heart, and abdomen. He or she will also take blood and urine samples. You may have an ultrasound examination, as well as computed tomography (CT scan) and magnetic resonance imaging (MRI). If the cause of the fever still can't be found, your provider may want to inject you with "labeled white blood cells." These are white blood cells that contain a harmless radioactive compound. Once injected, the white blood cells travel to infected parts of your body. The radioactivity allows your provider to see on an X-ray just where they have moved and thus locate the infection responsible for your fever. If that fails, your provider may want to perform minor surgery to take biopsy samples of, for example, your liver or bone marrow.

■ TREATMENT OPTIONS
Your health care provider will advise you to rest and drink plenty of fluids, and may even take you off medications for other ailments, because those

medications may be causing your fever. If you have a heart or lung condition, or if your child has seizures as a result of the fever, your provider will probably prescribe over-the-counter remedies to bring down the temperature. The most popular are acetaminophen (Tylenol) and aspirin.

Complementary and Alternative Therapies
General immune support with nutrition and herbs may alleviate fevers.

NUTRITION
- Eliminate alcohol, caffeine, refined foods, and sugar.
- Drink water or electrolyte replacement (sports) drinks.
- Vitamin C (250 to 1,000 mg two to three times per day), beta-carotene (15,000 to 50,000 IU per day), and zinc (10 to 30 mg per day) help your immune system work better and reduce inflammation.

HERBS
Herbs may be used as dried extracts (capsules, powders, teas), glycerites (glycerine extracts), or tinctures (alcohol extracts). Unless otherwise indicated, teas should be made with 1 tsp. herb per cup of hot water. Steep covered 5 to 10 minutes for leaf or flowers, and 10 to 20 minutes for roots. Drink 2 to 4 cups per day.

The following herbs may be helpful in reducing fever and improving immune response: coneflower *(Echinacea purpura)*, yarrow *(Achillea millefolium)*, white willow bark *(Salix alba)*, lemon balm *(Melissa officinalis)*, spearmint *(Mentha spicata)*, catnip *(Nepeta cateria)*, and elder *(Sambucus canadensis)*. Combine 1 part coneflower and 1 part white willow bark with equal parts of two or more herbs. Drink 3 to 4 cups per day, 2 to 4 oz. three to four times per day for children.

HOMEOPATHY
Some of the most common remedies used for fever of unknown origin are listed below. Usually, the dose is 12X to 30C every one to four hours until your symptoms get better.
- *Aconite* when fever comes on suddenly and alternates with chills, heat, and flushing of the face. Use if you feel anxious and thirsty for cold drinks.
- *Apis mellifica* for fever with alternating sweats and dry heat.
- *Belladonna* for sudden onset of high fever with hot, red face, glassy eyes, thirstlessness, and hot body with cold hands.
- *Bryonia* for fever with marked aggravation from the slightest movement.

ACUPUNCTURE
Acupuncture may be helpful in supporting immune function.

■ SPECIAL CONSIDERATIONS
Fever can be dangerous if you are pregnant. Nutritional, herbal, and homeopathic treatments for fevers are generally safe in pregnancy, yet use with caution.

■ FIBROMYALGIA SYNDROME

Fibromyalgia syndrome (FMS) is characterized by pain in the muscles and bones, trouble sleeping (or waking up feeling tired), and multiple tender points on the body. FMS, while different for everyone who has it, tends to come and go throughout life. It is not deforming, degenerative, life-threatening, or imaginary.

■ SIGNS AND SYMPTOMS

- Fatigue
- Morning stiffness
- Paresthesia (tingling)
- Raynaud's phenomenon
- Skin sensitivity
- Headaches
- Psychological disturbances
- Pain after exertion
- Memory lapses
- Sleep disorders
- Restless leg syndrome
- Dizziness
- Irritable bowel syndrome
- Joint pain and swelling

■ WHAT CAUSES IT?

The tendency to get FMS may be inherited. Illness or physical trauma such as an accident often precedes FMS symptoms. Many patients report a history of psychological problems, such as depression or anxiety.

■ WHAT TO EXPECT AT YOUR PROVIDER'S OFFICE

Although FMS does not show up in laboratory and imaging tests, your provider must perform them to rule out other causes of your symptoms. Your provider will also perform a physical examination of your joints. Be sure to tell your provider about all of your symptoms.

■ TREATMENT OPTIONS

The goal is to help you function as well as possible on a day-to-day basis; it is not possible to get rid of all pain and other symptoms.

Drug Therapies

The following drugs may be prescribed.

- Sleep disturbances are often treated successfully with low doses of tricyclic antidepressants. Benzodiazapines may also be used.
- Psychological disturbances can be treated with tricyclic antidepressants and sedative-hypnotics.
- Pain in the bones and muscles can be treated with lidocaine or procaine (injected into trigger points) or with capsaicin (used topically).

Complementary and Alternative Therapies

Nutritional support, herbs, and mind-body techniques may help reduce symptoms.

NUTRITION

- Eliminate all food allergens from the diet. Common allergenic foods are dairy, soy, citrus, peanuts, wheat, fish, eggs, corn, and tomatoes. Try an elimination trial: Remove suspected allergens from the diet for two weeks. Reintroduce one food every three days. Watch for reactions such as gastrointestinal upset, mood changes, flushing, fatigue, and worsening of symptoms. A rotation diet, in which the same food is not eaten more than once every four days, may reduce sensitivities.
- Decrease carbohydrate intake; increase protein; fats in moderation.
- Eliminate inflammatory foods such as refined foods, sugar, saturated fats (meat and dairy products), alcohol, and caffeine.
- Eat whole foods such as vegetables, whole grains, fruits, protein, and essential fatty acids (cold-water fish, nuts, and seeds).
- Vitamin C (1,000 mg three to four times per day) reduces swelling and helps your immune system function better.

- Coenzyme Q10 (50 to 100 mg one to two times per day) improves oxygen delivery to tissues and has antioxidant activity.
- Chromium picolinate (200 mcg with meals) may reduce reactive hypoglycemia which may make your symptoms worse.
- Magnesium (200 mg two to three times per day) with malic acid (1,200 mg one to two times per day) relieves pain and fatigue.
- 5-Hydroxytryptophan (100 mg three times per day) may help with depression and insomnia.
- B vitamins help reduce the effects of stress: B-complex (50 to 100 mg per day), niacinamide (100 mg per day), and B_6 (100 mg per day).
- Melatonin (0.5 to 3 mg one time before bed) may help sleep.
- Zinc (30 mg per day) is essential for proper immune function.
- Phosphatidyl choline and phosphatidyl serine (300 mg per day) may help depression and improve memory.

HERBS

Herbs may be used as dried extracts (capsules, powders, teas), glycerites (glycerine extracts), or tinctures (alcohol extracts). Teas should be made with 1 tsp. herb per cup of hot water. Steep covered 5 to 10 minutes for leaf or flowers; 10 to 20 minutes for roots. Drink 2 to 4 cups per day.

The following herbs may help increase resistance to stress and strengthen the immune system. Siberian ginseng (*Eleutherococcus senticosus*), schizandra berry (*Schizandra chinensis*), ashwaganda root (*Withania somnifera*), gotu kola (*Centella asiatica*), and astragalus root (*Astragalus membranaceus*). Use ginseng alone or with equal parts of two to three herbs. Take 20 to 30 drops two to three times per day. These may need to be taken for four to six months for maximum benefit.

Herbs that alleviate pain and nervous tension include the following: black cohosh (*Cimicifuga racemosa*), kava kava (*Piper methysticum*), skullcap (*Scutellaria laterifolia*), passionflower (*Passiflora incarnata*), lavender (*Lavendula officinalis*), and valerian (*Valeriana officinalis*). Combine equal parts and take as a tincture 20 to 30 drops two to three times per day.

Essential oils of jasmine, lemon balm, rosemary, and clary sage relieve nervous exhaustion and may be used in aromatherapy. Place several drops in a warm bath or atomizer, or on a cotton ball, and inhale.

HOMEOPATHY

Homeopathy may be useful as a supportive therapy.

PHYSICAL MEDICINE

Two to four cups of Epsom salts in a warm bath can soothe aching muscles.

ACUPUNCTURE

Acupuncture treatment may be helpful in stimulating circulation and promoting a sense of well-being.

MASSAGE

Massage may reduce stress and improving circulation.

■ FOLLOWING UP

Education and support groups may help you manage your condition.

■ FOOD ALLERGY

As many as two out of five Americans believe that they have allergies to certain foods. In fact, fewer than 2 percent have true food allergies. A food allergy occurs when the body's immune system reacts to otherwise harmless proteins in certain foods. While most food allergies are mild, in some cases they can cause anaphylactic shock, a serious, sometimes life-threatening, reaction. Food allergies affect mostly young children. With the exception of peanut allergy, the majority of children outgrow their allergic sensitivities.

■ SIGNS AND SYMPTOMS

- Swelling or itching lips, tongue, and mouth
- Dermatitis or hives
- Runny and itchy nose
- Headache
- Stomach pain or upset

The following symptoms should be treated as a medical emergency.

- Immediate and extreme facial swelling and itching
- Breathing difficulties
- Rapid increase in heart rate
- Rapid drop in blood pressure
- Itching or tightening of the throat
- Sudden hoarseness

■ WHAT CAUSES IT?

The foods that most commonly cause allergic reactions are peanuts, tree nuts (walnuts, pecans, almonds), milk, eggs, soy, fish, shellfish, and wheat. In most cases, allergies occur when an individual who has a genetic sensitivity to certain allergens is exposed to the substance.

■ WHAT TO EXPECT AT YOUR PROVIDER'S OFFICE

Your health care provider may use one or more of the following tests.

- Blood tests
- Skin tests—small punctures made with needles containing tiny amounts of allergens
- Challenge or provocative testing—your provider may place food extracts under your tongue or inject them.

■ TREATMENT OPTIONS

Antihistamines available either by prescription or over the counter are usually recommended to relieve mild itching, swelling, rash, runny nose, or headache. The most serious allergic reaction, anaphylactic shock, can come on suddenly and accelerate quickly. In some instances, survival may depend on an injection of epinephrine. If you have history of anaphylactic shock, you should keep a preloaded syringe of epinephrine with you.

Complementary and Alternative Therapies

Alternative therapies reduce inflammation, minimize hypersensitivity reactions, and heal the digestive tract.

NUTRITION

Note: Lower doses are for children.

- An elimination/challenge trial may help uncover sensitivities. Remove suspected foods from the diet for two weeks. Reintroduce one at a time and watch for reactions. Do not perform a challenge with peanuts if there is history of anaphylactic shock.
- A rotation diet, in which the same food is not eaten more than once every four days, may be helpful in minimizing allergic reactions.

- Reduce pro-inflammatory foods in the diet including saturated fats (meats, especially poultry, and dairy), refined foods, and sugar. If you are sensitive to antibiotics, eat only organic meats.
- Increase intake of vegetables, whole grains, and essential fatty acids [cold-water fish, nuts (unless allergic to them), and seeds].
- Flax seed, borage, or evening primrose oil (1,000 to 1,500 mg one to two times per day) are anti-inflammatory. Children should be supplemented with cod liver oil ($^1/_2$ to 1 tsp. per day).
- Zinc (10 to 30 mg per day) and beta-carotene (25,000 to 50,000 IU per day) support immune function.
- Vitamin C (250 to 1,000 mg two to four times per day) inhibits histamine release. Vitamin C from rose hips or palmitate is citrus-free and does not cause allergic reactions.
- B-complex vitamins (25 to 100 mg per day) help immune function.
- Selenium (50 to 200 mcg per day) helps metabolism.
- Bromelain (100 to 250 mg between meals) decreases inflammation.
- Pancreatin (8X USP) one to two tablets with meals for digestion.
- Pro-flora supplements (one to three capsules per day) can help normalize bowel flora.

HERBS

Herbs may be used as dried extracts (capsules, powders, teas), glycerites (glycerine extracts), or tinctures (alcohol extracts). Unless otherwise indicated, teas should be made with 1 tsp. herb per cup of hot water. Steep covered 5 to 10 minutes for leaf or flowers, and 10 to 20 minutes for roots. Drink 2 to 4 cups per day.

- Quercetin (100 to 250 mg three times per day before meals) minimizes reactions to food.
- Rose hips *(Rosa canina)* tea is anti-inflammatory, high in hypoallergenic vitamin C, and healing to the digestive tract. Drink 3 to 4 cups per day, 4 oz. three to four times per day for children.
- Marshmallow root tea *(Althea officinalis)* may soothe and promote healing of gastrointestinal inflammation. Soak 1 heaping tbsp. of marshmallow root in 1 qt. of cold water overnight. Strain and drink throughout the day.
- Dandelion *(Taraxacum officinale),* milk thistle *(Silybum marianum),* celandine *(Chelidonium majus),* and chicory *(Cichorium intybus)* stimulate liver function.
- To enhance digestion and reduce spasm, choose three or more of the following to make a tea to sip before meals. Chamomile *(Matricaria recutita),* peppermint *(Mentha piperita),* passionflower *(Passiflora incarnata),* meadowsweet *(Filependula ulmaria),* fennel *(Foeniculum vulgare),* and catnip *(Nepeta cataria).*

HOMEOPATHY

Homeopathy may be useful as a supportive therapy.

ACUPUNCTURE

Acupuncture may help restore normal immune function.

MASSAGE

Therapeutic massage may help reduce the effects of stress.

■ SPECIAL CONSIDERATIONS

If you have allergies, there is a greater likelihood that your baby will develop food allergies. Studies show that breastfeeding can delay development of food allergies.

■ GALLBLADDER DISEASE

Gallbladder disease is swelling of the gallbladder, a pear-shaped organ under the liver that secretes bile, a fluid that helps with digestion. Gallbladder disease often occurs with gallstones. You can have gallstones and never have any symptoms, although if the stones are large, they can be painful and require treatment.

■ SIGNS AND SYMPTOMS
- Pain, mostly on the upper right side of the abdomen
- Pain following meals, intolerance of fatty foods
- Nausea, vomiting
- Loss of appetite

■ WHAT CAUSES IT?
A gallbladder attack is caused by inflammation of the gallbladder. This usually happens because a stone is blocking a passageway in the gallbladder. Gallstones develop in the gallbladder when substances in bile form hard particles. They can be as small as a grain of sand or as large as a golf ball.

■ WHAT TO EXPECT AT YOUR PROVIDER'S OFFICE
If you are having a gallbladder attack, you will feel tenderness when the upper right side of your abdomen is touched. Jaundice (yellowing of the skin) occurs when the bile duct (a tube between the liver and gallbladder) is also blocked. If your health care provider thinks you have a gallstone, you will probably have an ultrasound. During an ultrasound, sound waves take pictures of your gallbladder. This test is painless and can be performed quickly, which is important if you are in a lot of pain.

■ TREATMENT OPTIONS
Gallbladders that cause pain are usually removed. Most gallbladder surgery today is performed with a laparoscope, an instrument that shows the surgeon pictures of your gallbladder as it is being removed and allows for a smaller incision and a shorter hospital stay than traditional surgery.

Some drugs can dissolve stones, avoiding the need for surgery. It can take two years for a stone to dissolve.
- Oral bile acids can dissolve cholesterol stones that are quite small (less than 15mm in diameter). It works for 40 percent of people within two years. There are two types of oral bile acids: chenodeoxycholic acid and ursodeoxycholic acid. Chenodeoxycholic acid has more side effects.
- Methyl tert-butyl ether—a strong solvent; 95 percent of the stone's mass dissolves in 12.5 hours

Complementary and Alternative Therapies
It is important to see your provider for tests before you start any alternative treatment, so that you will use the remedies that are right for the size of your stone and your condition.

NUTRITION
- Decrease total fat intake, especially saturated fats (meat and dairy products).
- Eliminate food allergens. Eggs, in particular, may irritate the gallbladder.
- Eat more fiber. Consider fiber supplements such as flax meal (1 tsp. one to three times per day). Combine 1 heaping tsp. of flax meal in 8 oz. of apple juice for a drink high in fiber and pectin.
- Lecithin (1,000 to 5,000 mg per day) for cholesterol excretion
- Choline (1,000 mg per day) and lipase (10,000 NF units with meals) stimulate gallbladder function.
- Vitamin E (400 to 800 IU/day) and vitamin C (1,000 mg two to three times per day) promote bile production.

HERBS
Herbs are generally a safe way to strengthen and tone the body's systems. As with any therapy, it is important to work with your provider on getting your problem diagnosed before you start any treatment. Herbs may be used as dried extracts (capsules, powders, teas), glycerites (glycerine extracts), or tinctures (alcohol extracts). Unless otherwise indicated, teas should be made with 1 tsp. herb per cup of hot water. Steep covered 5 to 10 minutes for leaf or flowers, and 10 to 20 minutes for roots. Drink 2 to 4 cups per day. Tinctures may be used singly or in combination as noted.
- Choleretic herbs stimulate bile production and increase bile solubility. Especially useful are milk thistle (*Silybum marianum*), dandelion root (*Taraxecum officinalis*), greater celandine (*Chelidonium majus*), globe artichoke (*Cynara scolymus*), and turmeric. (*Curcuma longa*). Use these herbs singly or in combination as a tea or tincture (15 to 20 drops), two to three times per day before meals.
- Enteric-coated peppermint oil may help dissolve stones (0.2 to 0.4 ml three times a day between meals).

HOMEOPATHY
Some of the most common remedies are listed below. Usually, the dose is 12X to 30C every one to four hours until your symptoms get better.
- *Colocynthis* for colicky abdominal pains that are lessened by pressure or bending double
- *Chelidonium* for abdominal pain that moves to right shoulder area
- *Lycopodium* for abdominal pain that is worse with deep breaths

PHYSICAL MEDICINE
Castor oil pack. Apply oil directly to skin, cover with a clean soft cloth (such as flannel) and plastic wrap. Place a heat source (hot water bottle or heating pad) over the pack and let sit for 30 to 60 minutes. For best results, use for three consecutive days. Apply to abdomen, especially the gallbladder area, to help reduce swelling.

ACUPUNCTURE
Acupuncture may prove especially helpful in pain relief, reducing spasm, and easing bile flow and proper liver and gallbladder function.

■ FOLLOWING UP
Early surgery usually ends symptoms and recurrence; stones may recur in the bile duct, however.

■ SPECIAL CONSIDERATIONS
If you have diabetes or are pregnant, there is a higher chance of complications from gallbladder attacks. If you are pregnant, use choleretic herbs with caution. Milk thistle and dandelion root are safe in pregnancy. Talk with your health care provider before you take any medication or supplement.

■ GASTRITIS

Gastritis is an inflammation of the lining of your stomach. It is not a single disease but rather a group of disorders. Gastritis can "eat away" the stomach lining and cause bleeding. In some cases, gastritis does not damage the stomach lining and does not have a specific cause.

■ SIGNS AND SYMPTOMS

The following are symptoms of gastritis.

- Indigestion and heartburn
- Nausea
- Loss of appetite
- Abdominal pain that is often worse after eating
- Gastrointestinal bleeding (signs of this are vomiting material that looks like coffee-grounds, or having very dark stools)

■ WHAT CAUSES IT?

The causes of gastritis include the following.

- Aspirin use
- Alcohol and tobacco use
- Serious illness
- Reflux injury (such as bile backing up into the stomach and esophagus)
- Trauma (for example, surgery, radiation, chemotherapy, severe vomiting, having swallowed a foreign object)
- Bacterial, viral, fungal, and parasitic infections
- Pernicious anemia
- Systemic disease (for example, Crohn's disease)

■ WHAT TO EXPECT AT YOUR PROVIDER'S OFFICE

Your health care provider will take your medical history and conduct a physical examination. Your provider will refer you to a gastroenterologist if you need further examination, such as an endoscopy or a gastroscopy. A biopsy may be taken of the tissues of your esophagus or stomach to determine the cause of your discomfort.

■ TREATMENT OPTIONS

Gastritis treatment depends on the cause of the problem.

- *Helicobactor pylori* infestation, a common bacterial cause of gastritis and ulcers, is treated with a three-drug combination for two weeks: Pepto-Bismol, metronidazole, and tetracycline (or amoxicillin if you cannot take tetracycline).
- For some types of gastritis, you must stop ingesting all irritating substances, including alcohol, tobacco, aspirin, and spicy foods.

Complementary and Alternative Therapies

Nutritional and herbal support help to heal the stomach lining, fight infection, and reduce recurrence.

NUTRITION

- Avoid dairy products, caffeine, alcohol, and sugar. Coffee, even decaffeinated, should be eliminated because it contains potentially irritating oils.
- Eliminate any known food allergens from your diet.
- Include sulfur-containing foods such as garlic, onions, broccoli, cabbage, Brussels sprouts, and cauliflower in the diet. Sulfur is the basis for forming glutathione, which provides antioxidant protection to the stomach lining. N-acetyl cysteine (200 mg twice a day between meals) is also the basis for forming glutathione.
- Vitamin C (1,000 mg three times per day) decreases nitrosamines, substances that have been linked to stomach cancer.
- Zinc (30 to 50 mg per day) helps you heal.

HERBS

Herbs are generally a safe way to strengthen and tone the body's systems. As with any therapy, it is important to work with your provider on getting your problem diagnosed before you start any treatment. Herbs may be used as dried extracts (capsules, powders, teas), glycerites (glycerine extracts), or tinctures (alcohol extracts). Unless otherwise indicated, teas should be made with 1 tsp. herb per cup of hot water. Steep covered 5 to 10 minutes for leaf or flowers, and 10 to 20 minutes for roots. Drink 2 to 4 cups per day.

- DGL (deglycyrrhizinated licorice), 250 mg four times per day 15 to 20 minutes before meals and one to two hours after the last meal of the day, increases circulation and healing to stomach lining. This preparation is safe for people with high blood pressure or to take long-term. If you have high blood pressure, talk with your health care provider before taking any medications.
- Powders of slippery elm (*Ulmus fulva*) and marshmallow root (*Althea officinalis*) may be taken singly or together, 1 tsp. two to three times per day, to decrease inflammation and encourage healing.
- Ginger root tea (*Zingiber officinalis*) increases circulation and enhances digestion. Drink 2 to 3 cups per day with meals.
- For *H. pylori*, bismuth subcitrate (120 mg four times per day for eight weeks) may be helpful in eliminating the bacteria and reducing recurrence of gastritis. Do not use this long-term. Be sure to take it under the supervision of your health care provider, since you may still need antibiotics if the *H. pylori* is not gone after eight weeks.

HOMEOPATHY

Homeopathy may be useful as a supporting therapy. There are three remedies to consider: *nux vomica, aresenicum album,* and *lycopodium.*

ACUPUNCTURE

Acupuncture may be helpful in reducing stress and improving overall digestive function.

MASSAGE

Therapeutic massage can reduce stress and increase your sense of well-being.

■ FOLLOWING UP

Return to your health care provider if your symptoms do not get better or if they get worse.

■ SPECIAL CONSIDERATIONS

Do not ignore potentially life-threatening symptoms such as vomiting blood or blood in your stool. Be sure to see your health care provider regularly, and call him or her if there is any change in your symptoms. If you are pregnant, nutritional guidelines and herbal support are safe, but talk with your health care provider before taking any medicine or supplements. Do not take bismuth subcitrate if you are pregnant.

■ GASTROESOPHAGEAL REFLUX DISEASE (GERD)

Gastroesophageal reflux disease (GERD) occurs when material from your stomach or small intestine repeatedly enters your esophagus. Some individuals have GERD for many years. Complications, such as serious damage to the esophagus, respiratory diseases, and ear, nose, and throat conditions can occur, but are more likely with older people.

■ SIGNS AND SYMPTOMS

Heartburn—a burning sensation in the chest, throat, neck, or back—is the primary symptom of GERD. Other symptoms include:

- Regurgitation
- Difficulty or pain with swallowing
- A full sensation in the neck
- Belching
- Chest pain (similar to angina)
- Laryngitis
- Chronic cough
- Wheezing
- Hoarseness
- Sore throat
- Bad breath

■ WHAT CAUSES IT?

GERD has many possible causes.

- Spicy foods, tomato-based foods, citrus fruits, fatty foods, chocolate, coffee, alcohol, and certain medications
- Overeating, burping intentionally, wearing tight-fitting clothes, bending over frequently, lying down soon after eating, and smoking
- Physical condition (particularly being overweight)
- The effectiveness of the valve at the bottom of your esophagus in preventing material from your stomach from entering the esophagus
- Medical conditions

■ WHAT TO EXPECT AT YOUR PROVIDER'S OFFICE

Your health care provider can generally diagnose GERD by discussing your symptoms, what you eat and drink, medications you are taking, and your lifestyle. Your provider also may order diagnostic tests.

■ TREATMENT OPTIONS

Treatment options include the following.

- Avoiding food, drinks, and medications that can cause GERD
- Modifying your lifestyle as needed
- Raising the head of your bed about six inches
- Taking antacids and other medication to relieve symptoms as needed

In rare instances, your health care provider may recommend surgery, but usually only if drug therapy is unsuccessful.

Drug Therapies

For mild cases of GERD, your provider will likely recommend drugs you can take when you need to relieve symptoms. For moderate and severe cases of GERD, your provider may prescribe drugs that you must take two to four times a day. Your provider may also recommend that you take a "maintenance" drug dose to prevent GERD from recurring.

Complementary and Alternative Therapies

Changes in your diet can help decrease the irritation of GERD. Herbs may be very effective at healing esophagitis (inflammation of the esophagus).

NUTRITION
- Digestive enzymes may help if you have heartburn.
- Avoid sweets, oils, fats, and caffeine.

HERBS
Herbs may be used as dried extracts (capsules, powders, teas), glycerites (glycerine extracts), or tinctures (alcohol extracts). Unless otherwise indicated, teas should be made with 1 tsp. herb per cup of hot water. Steep covered 5 to 10 minutes for leaf or flowers, and 10 to 20 minutes for roots. Drink 2 to 4 cups per day.

Some herbs typically used to help digestive problems actually make GERD worse. The following herbs can be used to treat GERD.
- Licorice (*Glycyrrhiza glabra*) is an anti-inflammatory and antispasmodic, and relieves pain in the gastrointestinal tract. Chewable lozenges may be the best form for treating GERD. Take 380 to 1,140 mg a day. Do not take licorice if you have high blood pressure or use it for a prolonged period of time.
- Slippery elm (*Ulmus fulva*) protects irritated tissues and promotes their healing. Take 60 to 320 mg a day. You may mix 1 tsp. powder with water three to four times a day.

In addition, a combination of four of the following herbs may be used as either a tea (1 cup three times a day) or tincture (30 to 60 drops three times a day).
- Valerian (*Valeriana officinalis*)—bitter, sedative, especially for anxiety or depression or poor digestion
- Wild yam (*Dioscorea villosa*)—antispasmodic, anti-inflammatory, especially for fatigue from long-term stress and poor digestion
- St. John's wort (*Hypericum perforatum*)—pain reliever, antidepressant
- Skullcap (*Scutellaria laterifolia*)—antispasmodic, sedative, calming, especially for disturbed sleep
- Linden flowers (*Tilia cordata*)—antispasmodic, mild diuretic, gentle bitter, especially for dyspepsia (gas)

HOMEOPATHY
Some of the most common remedies used for GERD are listed below. Usually, the dose is 12X to 30C every one to four hours until your symptoms get better.
- *Arsenicum album* for burning pain that feels better with warmth
- *Carbo vegatabilis* for bloating and indigestion that is worse when lying down, especially with flatulence and fatigue
- *Lycopodium* for heartburn that feels worse with eating
- *Nux vomica* for heartburn with cramping and constipation

ACUPUNCTURE
May be helpful to normalize digestion and relieve stress

■ FOLLOWING UP

Contact your health care provider if the medication does not help or if you experience side effects, such as cramping or diarrhea.

■ SPECIAL CONSIDERATIONS

GERD is quite common during pregnancy, particularly in the third trimester. Chewable papaya tablets may provide relief and are safe to use.

■ GOUT

Gout usually affects men over age 30 with a family history of gout, but it can occur at any time and also affects women, especially after menopause. Recent food and alcohol excess, surgery, infection, physical or emotional stress, or the use of certain drugs can lead to the development of gout symptoms.

■ SIGNS AND SYMPTOMS

- Extreme pain in a single joint, usually the base of the big toe, but other joints can also be affected (such as the feet, fingers, wrists, elbows, knees, or ankles)
- Joint is shiny red-purple, swollen, hot, and stiff
- Fever as high as 39°C (102.2° F) with or without chills
- Attack develops over a matter of hours and may get better over a few days or weeks
- In later attacks, you may see lumps (called tophi) just under the skin in the outer ear, hands, feet, elbow, or knee

■ WHAT CAUSES IT?

The body either produces too much uric acid, doesn't excrete enough uric acid, or both, so that the acid accumulates in tissues in the form of needle-like crystals that cause pain. Gout generally occurs because of a predisposition to the condition, but it can result from blood disorders or cancers, such as leukemia, or the use of certain drugs.

■ WHAT TO EXPECT AT YOUR PROVIDER'S OFFICE

Your health care provider will examine the affected joint, evaluate how painful it is, and may ask if there is any history of gout in your family. Your provider may take a sample of fluid from the affected joint, draw blood for a blood test, or take X-rays to rule out other possibilities.

■ TREATMENT OPTIONS

Your health care provider may give you ibuprofen or another nonsteroidal anti-inflammatory drug (NSAID) to help with the pain and swelling. You must avoid drinking alcoholic beverages and avoid the foods that trigger your attacks. Besides NSAIDs, you may be given other drugs.

Complementary and Alternative Therapies

A combination of therapies can be very effective at decreasing both the length and frequency of attacks.

NUTRITION

- Maintain a healthy weight. However, it is important to avoid crash dieting and rapid weight loss.
- Drink plenty of water because dehydration may make gout worse.
- Restrict purines in your diet. Purines increase lactate production, which competes with uric acid for excretion. Foods with a high purine content include beef, goose, organ meats, sweetbreads, mussels, anchovies, herring, mackerel, and yeast. Foods with a moderate amount of purines include meats, poultry, fish and shellfish not listed above. Spinach, asparagus, beans, lentils, mushrooms, and dried peas also contain moderate amounts of purines.
- Do not drink alcohol, especially beer.
- Cherries—One half pound of cherries per day (fresh or frozen) for two weeks lowers uric acid and prevents attacks. Cherries and other dark red berries (hawthorn berries and blueberries) contain anthocyanadins that increase collagen integrity and decrease inflammation. Cherry juice (8 to 16 ounces of per day) is also helpful.

- Vitamin C—8 grams per day can lead to decreased blood uric acid levels. Note that there is a small subset of people with gout who will actually get worse with this level of vitamin C.
- Folic acid—10 to 75 mg per day inhibits xanthine oxidase, which is required for uric acid production.
- EPA (eicosapentaenoic acid) inhibits pro-inflammatory leukotrienes. Dose is 1,500 mg per day.
- Niacin—Avoid niacin in doses greater than 50 mg per day. Nicotinic acid may bring on an attack of gout.
- Vitamin A—There is some concern that elevated retinol levels may play a role in some attacks of gouty arthritis.

HERBS

Herbs may be used as dried extracts (capsules, powders, teas), glycerites (glycerine extracts), or tinctures (alcohol extracts). Unless otherwise indicated, teas should be made with one teaspoon herb per cup of hot water. Steep covered 5 to 10 minutes for leaf or flowers, and 10 to 20 minutes for roots. Drink two to four cups per day.

- Devil's claw *(Harpagophytum procumbens)* reduces pain and inflammation. Dose is one to two grams three times per day of dried powdered root, four to five ml three times per day of tincture, or 400 mg three times per day of dry solid extract during attacks.
- Bromelain *(Ananas comosus)*—proteolytic enzyme (anti-inflammatory) when taken on an empty stomach. Dose is 125 to 250 mg three times per day during attacks.

HOMEOPATHY

Some of the most common remedies used for gout are listed below. Usually, the dose is 12X to 30C every one to four hours until your symptoms get better.

- *Aconite* for sudden onset of burning pain, anxiety, restlessness, and attacks that come after a shock or injury
- *Belladonna* for intense pain that may be throbbing; pain is made worse by any motion and better by pressure; joint is very hot
- *Bryonia* for pain made much worse by any kind of motion; pain is better with pressure and with heat
- *Colchicum* for pains made worse by motion and changes of weather, especially if there is any nausea associated with the attacks
- *Ledum* when joints become mottled, purple and swollen; pain is much better with cold applications and is worse when overheated

PHYSICAL MEDICINE

- Hot and cold compresses—three minutes hot alternated with 30 seconds cold provide pain relief and increase circulation.
- Bed rest for 24 hours after acute attack. However, prolonged bed rest may make the condition worse.

■ FOLLOWING UP

If you have had several attacks and the joint has suffered damage, your provider may refer you to an orthopedist.

■ SPECIAL CONSIDERATIONS

People who have had gout have an increased risk of developing kidney stones, high blood pressure, kidney disease, diabetes mellitus, high levels of triglycerides, and atherosclerosis.

■ HEADACHE, MIGRAINE

Migraines are pounding or throbbing headaches that start suddenly, last for hours and usually occur with other symptoms such as nausea. The headaches usually occur between ages 10 and 30, often vanishing after age 50 or, in women, after menopause. More women than men have migraines.

■ SIGNS AND SYMPTOMS

- Throbbing or pounding pain on one side of your head (or both)
- Nausea and vomiting
- Disturbances in your hearing or vision (such as flashes of light) that often start 10 to 30 minutes before the headache
- Parts of your body may feel numb, weak, or tingly
- Light, noise, and movement—especially bending over—make your head hurt worse; you want to lie down in a dark, quiet room
- Your feet and hands feel cold and may look bluish

■ WHAT CAUSES IT?

No one knows for certain what causes migraine. They can run in families. Researchers do know that something triggers blood vessels in the head to tighten and then expand, a process that irritates the nerves surrounding those blood vessels. Things that can trigger migraine include the following.

- Abnormal blood levels of the neurotransmitter serotonin
- Medicines for high blood pressure, angina, and arthritis
- Certain foods and alcohol; missing meals; too much sun; sleeping too little or too much
- Hormones and menstruation
- Certain odors, such as perfume or cigarette smoke
- Stress

■ WHAT TO EXPECT AT YOUR PROVIDER'S OFFICE

Your health care provider will ask questions to help identify the cause of your headaches. He or she will teach you how to use painkillers so the medicine doesn't cause a "rebound headache."

■ TREATMENT OPTIONS

- Avoid known migraine triggers if possible.
- Try aspirin, ibuprofen, and naproxen for mild migraine, or prescription medicines for moderate to severe migraine.
- Put an ice pack on your forehead when headache strikes.
- Ask your provider about lidocaine nasal spray for quick relief.
- Blood pressure medicines known as beta-blockers or calcium-channel blockers work by controlling blood vessel expansion and contraction. They can prevent migraine in some people.
- Regular aerobic exercise can reduce the frequency and intensity of migraine episodes.

Complementary and Alternative Therapies

A combination of drugs for pain relief and complementary therapies to reduce recurrence can offer effective management of migraines. Biofeedback to control vascular contraction and improve stress management may influence the frequency and intensity of attacks.

NUTRITION

- Avoid food allergens. Some common allergens are alcohol (especially red wine), cheese, chocolate, citrus, cow's milk, wheat, eggs, coffee, tea, beef, pork, corn, tomato, rye, yeast, shellfish, food additives (preservatives and coloring), and nitrates.
- Avoid caffeine because it is a vasodilator.
- Essential fatty acids (1,500 to 3,000 mg per day) may be helpful. Supplementing with fish oil or flax seed oil (1 to 3 mg twice a day) may also be helpful.
- Magnesium (500 mg per day) increases muscle relaxation.
- Injection of one gram of magnesium by a physician can terminate an acute migraine headache within minutes.
- Injection of folic acid (15 mg) in one study achieved total relief of acute headache within one hour in 60 percent of patients.
- Omega-3 oils (EPA and DHA, average dose 14 grams daily) greatly reduce intensity and frequency of migraines.
- Vitamin B_2 (riboflavin) (400 mg/day for three months) has been shown to reduce migraine frequency by two-thirds.
- Vitamin C (2,000 mg per day), vitamin E (400 to 600 IU per day), vitamin B_6 (100 mg per day), choline (100 to 300 mg per day) and mixed bioflavonoids (1,000 mg per day).
- 5-hydroxytryptophan (300 mg twice a day) for migraine prevention, enhanced by taking with 25 mg of vitamin B_6.

HERBS

Herbs may be used as dried extracts (capsules, powders, teas), glycerites (glycerine extracts), or tinctures (alcohol extracts). Feverfew *(Tanacetum)* can help with both frequency and intensity of migraines. Take two fresh leaves daily, 250 to 300 mg dried herb (capsules) twice a day, or 30 drops of tincture three times per day. Use feverfew by itself.

Use the following herbs in combination. Put 1 tsp. of each herb in one cup of water; steep for 10 minutes, and take two to four times a day. For tinctures, use 60 drops of each herb, two to four times a day. Jamaican dogwood *(Piscidia piscipula)*; skullcap *(Scutellaria lateriflora)*; gingko *(Gingko biloba)*; ginger *(Zingiber officinalis)*; meadowsweet *(Filipendula ulmaria)*.

HOMEOPATHY

Some of the most common remedies used for migraines are listed below. Usually, the dose is 12X to 30C every one to four hours until your symptoms get better.

- *Iris versicolor:* for periodic migraines that begin with blurred vision
- *Lac defloratum:* for a migraine in the front of your head that starts with an aura of dim vision, nausea, vomiting, and chills
- *Natrum muriaticum:* for migraines that feel like "hammers beating the head," that are better when you lie down alone in the dark
- *Sanguinaria:* for right-sided migraines that begin in your neck and move up, and migraines that make you vomit

ACUPUNCTURE

May be helpful, especially if migraines are hormonally influenced.

MASSAGE

Massage may help release chronic neck and shoulder tension and maintain an even blood flow to the head.

PHYSICAL MEDICINE

Chiropractic adjustments or craniosacral therapy may be helpful.

■ SPECIAL CONSIDERATIONS

Call your provider if you suddenly develop new symptoms.

■ HEADACHE, SINUS

Sinus headaches cause a dull, deep, or severe pain in the front of your head and in your face. They are caused by an infection in the passages behind the cheeks, nose, and eyes. Bending down or leaning over makes the pain worse, as does cold and damp weather. Sinus headaches are often worse in the morning, and better by afternoon.

■ SIGNS AND SYMPTOMS

Sinus headaches produce the following symptoms.
- Dull or severe pain in one area at the front of your head
- Yellow or green discharge from your nose
- Red and swollen nasal passages
- Mild to moderate fever
- General sense of not feeling well

■ WHAT CAUSES IT?

Colds or respiratory viruses leave sinuses vulnerable to bacterial infection. Microorganisms can get into your sinuses and cause your mucous membranes to swell. This blocks normal drainage, and the increase in pressure results in a headache.

■ WHAT TO EXPECT AT YOUR PROVIDER'S OFFICE

Your health care provider may look in your nose and press spots on your face to check for soreness. Your provider may want you to have a computed tomography (CT) scan of your sinuses.

■ TREATMENT OPTIONS

The goal of the treatments listed below is to stop your headaches by clearing up your sinus infection.
- Use a vaporizer or inhale steam to help shrink swollen passages and promote drainage.
- Use a nasal spray to breathe easier, but do not take more doses or use longer than prescribed.
- If your health care provider prescribes antibiotics, follow the instructions carefully. It is very important to take all of your medicine.

Complementary and Alternative Therapies

These can be very helpful at minimizing the discomfort, treating the infection, stimulating the immune system, clearing the congestion, and decreasing the frequency of sinus headaches and infections.

NUTRITION

Use the same general nutrition for fighting infections—vitamin C (1,000 mg three times a day), zinc (30 to 60 mg a day), beta-carotene (15,000 IU a day).

HERBS

Herbs are generally a safe way to strengthen and tone the body's systems. As with any therapy, it is important to work with your provider on getting your problem diagnosed before you start any treatment. Herbs may be used as dried extracts (capsules, powders, teas), glycerites (glycerine extracts), or tinctures (alcohol extracts). Unless otherwise indicated, teas should be made with 1 tsp. herb per cup of hot water. Steep covered 5 to 10 minutes for leaf or flowers, and 10 to 20 minutes for roots. Drink 2 to 4 cups per day.

Use a combination of the herbs listed below, in equal parts. Use 1 tbsp. of dried herb per 1 cup water. Drink 4 to 6 cups per day. Or, use equal parts of tincture and take 60 drops every two to four hours. These herbs promote sinus drainage, relieve pain, and strengthen your immune system.
- Wild indigo *(Baptisia tinctoria)*
- Eyebright *(Euphrasia officinalis)*
- Licorice *(Glycyrrhiza glabra)*
- Coneflower *(Echinacea)*
- Goldenseal *(Hydrastis canadensis)*
- Jamaican dogwood *(Piscidea piscipula)* or St. John's wort *(Hypericum perforatum)*, in equal parts, may be added for pain relief
- Garlic *(Allium sativum)* and ginger *(Zingiber officinalis)*, as a tea—use 2 to 3 cloves of garlic and 2 to 3 slices of fresh ginger, steep 5 to 15 minutes and drink, breathing in the steam.

HOMEOPATHY

Some of the most common remedies used for sinus headache are listed below. Usually the dose is 12X to 30C every one to four hours until symptoms improve.
- *Arsenicum album* for sinusitis with thin, watery, irritating discharge, especially when sneezing does not relieve nasal stuffiness
- *Kali bichromium* for sinusitis with post-nasal drip, especially with ulcerations of the septum and weakness
- *Mercurius* for raw, ulcerated nostrils with swelling, may have bloody discharge and exhaustion
- *Pulsatilla* for sinusitis with thick, bland discharges, especially with weepiness, a lack of thirst, and wanting to be constantly comforted

PHYSICAL MEDICINE

You can also try other techniques to relieve pain from sinus headaches.
- Alternate hot and cold compresses. Place a hot compress across your sinuses for three minutes, and then a cold compress for 30 seconds. Repeat this procedure three times for a single treatment, two to six times a day.
- Try eucalyptus, lavender, rosemary, or thyme essential oils in steam or in a hot bath. To inhale steam, place 2 to 5 drops in a pot, simmer, and hold your head over the pot. For a bath, close windows and doors, and add 5 to 10 drops of oil to a full tub of hot water.
- Use a nasal rinse made with water and salt to taste like tears. Rinse each nostril and, with your head over a sink, hold your head sideways and let the water run from your upper nostril to your lower nostril. Keep your nostrils lower than your throat to prevent the salt water from draining into the back of your throat. This rinse shrinks your sinus membranes and increases drainage.

ACUPUNCTURE

May be useful to stimulate immune system and increase drainage.

■ FOLLOWING UP

If you're taking medicines, be sure you follow instructions.

■ SPECIAL CONSIDERATIONS

Do not use over-the-counter nasal sprays that contain phenylephrine for more than three days, and do not use prescription nasal sprays for more than seven days. They can be addictive.

■ HEADACHE, TENSION

Tension headaches usually start at the back of your head and move forward, covering your whole head with a steady, dull pain.

■ SIGNS AND SYMPTOMS

- The headache starts at the back of your head and spreads.
- Dull pressure or a squeezing pain lasts from half an hour to several hours or days.
- Muscles in your neck, shoulders, and jaw are tight and sore.
- Aching usually continues through the day.
- Your headache does not feel worse if you move about.

■ WHAT CAUSES IT?

When you feel tense, the muscles in your shoulders, neck, and jaw tighten up and press on blood vessels surrounded by nerves, making those nerves send pain messages to your brain. Causes include the following.

- Sitting too long or in an uncomfortable position
- Premenstrual syndrome (PMS)
- Low blood sugar
- Food allergy
- Not enough sleep; not enough fluids
- Clenching your jaw or grinding your teeth
- Pain that originates from other areas, such as your sinuses
- Stress
- Depression or anxiety

■ WHAT TO EXPECT AT YOUR PROVIDER'S OFFICE

Your health care provider will ask questions about your headaches, such as when they occur and how long they last. Your provider may run tests to rule out medical problems that could be causing your headaches.

■ TREATMENT OPTIONS

Over-the-counter pain relievers work for most people. Your provider may prescribe painkillers if you need them.

Complementary and Alternative Therapies

Main emphasis of therapies is muscle relaxation and stress management.

NUTRITION

- Replacing micronutrients depleted in times of stress is essential; the most critical are the vitamins C, E, beta-carotene, B-complex, and the minerals magnesium, potassium, calcium, zinc, manganese, and selenium. Magnesium (aspartate or glycinate, up to 750 mg per day) is especially critical because of its antispasmodic action.
- Avoid caffeine.
- Essential fatty acids can improve blood flow. Reduce animal fats and increase fish. A mix of omega-6 (evening primrose) and omega-3 (flax seed) may be best (2 tbsp. oil per day or 1,000 to 1,500 IU twice a day).
- Vitamin E: 400 to 800 IU/day may decrease muscle cramping.
- Elimination diet: Some tension headaches respond dramatically to this approach. The most common allergic foods are wheat, dairy products, corn, soy, and chocolate. Eliminate these foods completely for 2 weeks, then reintroduce the foods one at a time, every 3 days, and note reactions. Citrus, alcohol, red meat, flour products, spices, and carbonated drinks may also aggravate headaches.

- Calcium/magnesium: 1,000/500 mg per day may help regulate muscle contraction and relaxation.

HERBS

Herbs may be used as dried extracts (capsules, powders, teas), glycerites (glycerine extracts), or tinctures (alcohol extracts). Unless otherwise indicated, teas should be made with 1 tsp. herb per cup of hot water. Steep covered 5 to 10 minutes for leaf or flowers, and 10 to 20 minutes for roots. Drink 2 to 4 cups per day.

- Peppermint *(Mentha piperata)* oil is effective against tension. Add two drops of peppermint essential oil to 1 cup of water. Soak a cloth in the solution and apply as a compress.
- White willow bark *(Salix alba)* contains salicin, the pain reliever in aspirin. Do not use if you cannot take aspirin.
- Meadowsweet *(Filipendula ulmaria)* relieves pain, reduces nausea and heartburn, and helps relieve tension and digestive discomfort.
- Valerian *(Valeriana officinalis)* helps you relax and reduces spasms, and helps relieve tension with anxiety or digestive discomfort.
- Jamaican dogwood *(Piscidia piscipula)* helps you relax and relieves pain and spasms.
- Ginkgo *(Gingko biloba)* increases blood circulation to your brain, and can help relieve tension.
- Combine white willow *(Salix alba)*, meadowsweet *(Fillipendula ulmaria)* and two of the above herbs. Herbs—1 tbsp. in 1 cup water three times a day. Tincture—60 drops three times a day.
- Kava kava *(Piper methysticum)*—45 to 60 mg of kavalactone content three times a day, has a calming effect if anxiety is prominent.

HOMEOPATHY

Some of the most common remedies used for tension headache are listed below. Usually, the dose is 12X to 30C every one to four hours until your symptoms get better.

- *Aconite* is for tension headaches that appear suddenly, with anxiety, following shock, or with fever.
- *Bryonia* is recommended for congestive headaches that feel worse when you move and better with pressure or with your eyes closed.
- *Gelsemium* is recommended for heavy-feeling headaches.
- *Belladonna* is recommended for throbbing headaches.

PHYSICAL MEDICINE

You can do other things to avoid tension headaches or relieve pain.

- Biofeedback to control muscle tension.
- Acupuncture can help relieve pain.
- Using small circular motions, press acupressure points at the web between your thumb and index finger.
- Practice gentle neck stretches to ease tightness.
- Put an ice pack on your forehead. To increase the pain-relieving effect, soak your feet in hot water at the same time.
- Breathe deeply or try other relaxation exercises, such as yoga.
- Get regular exercise, especially for your back and abdomen.

■ FOLLOWING UP

Tension headaches may keep occurring if you do not treat the underlying causes. Exercise and stress reduction techniques will help.

■ HEMORRHOIDS

Hemorrhoids are a condition in which veins in the rectal or anal area become swollen and painful and may bleed. Hemorrhoids may occur inside the entrance to the anus (interior hemorrhoids) or outside the entrance to the anus (exterior hemorrhoids). A blot clot (thrombosis) may form in the vein, making the hemorrhoid more painful and sometimes requiring treatment.

■ SIGNS AND SYMPTOMS
- Constipation
- Straining while defecating
- Discomfort, itching, pain
- Tender swollen lumps in rectum
- Bleeding
- Sensation of fullness
- Mucus in stool

■ WHAT CAUSES IT?
Hemorrhoids are a type of varicose veins that simply occur with age. Being constipated or passing large, hard stools may contribute to the formation of hemorrhoids. In most cases, however, there is no obvious cause. In addition to age and constipation, other contributing factors include the following.
- Family history of hemorrhoids
- Certain medical conditions
- Pregnancy
- Sitting for prolonged periods of time
- Diet low in fiber or fluids

■ WHAT TO EXPECT AT YOUR PROVIDER'S OFFICE
Your provider will do an examination. If you have had significant bleeding or other symptoms, your provider may perform a procedure called sigmoidoscopy, or colonoscopy. In this procedure a small instrument is inserted into the rectum for inspection of tissues to check for other diseases.

■ TREATMENT OPTIONS
Medications can ease the pain and discomfort during the time it takes for the hemorrhoids to heal. In addition to medications, you can help prevent or heal hemorrhoids by doing the following.
- Prevent pressure on the area (for example, sit on an inflatable ring)
- Avoid straining during bowel movements
- Limit the amount of time sitting on the toilet
- Sit in warm baths with soapy water or Epsom salts 2 to 3 times daily for 15 to 20 minutes

Drug Therapies
- Stool softeners help reduce straining and prevent hard stools.
- Bulk laxatives help prevent hard stools and constipation.
- Rectal preparations relieve itching and discomfort.
- Topical anesthetics and systemic analgesics relieve pain.

Complementary and Alternative Therapies
NUTRITION
- Eat in a relaxed atmosphere, breathing and chewing food thoroughly.
- Eat smaller, more frequent meals and avoid overeating at one sitting.
- Eliminate refined foods, sugars, caffeine, alcohol, and dairy products.
- Decrease saturated fats (animal products) and increase polyunsaturated fats (cold-water fish, nuts, and seeds).
- Increase fresh vegetables and whole grains, as well as water intake.
- Stewed or soaked prunes, one to three/day have a slightly laxative effect and may help soften stools.
- Flax meal, one heaping teaspoon in eight ounces of apple juice, provides fiber and essential fatty acids to help relieve constipation. Follow with an additional eight ounces of water.
- Vitamin C (1,000 mg two to three times per day) supports the integrity of connective tissue.
- Vitamin E (400 to 800 IU per day) promotes healing.

HERBS
Bioflavanoids, a constituent found in dark berries and some plants, help restore the integrity of the vasculature. The following are bioflavanoids that may be taken in dried extract form as noted.
- Catechin (150 mg two to three times per day), quercetin (250 mg three to four times per day), hesperidin (250 mg three to four times per day), and rutin (250 mg three to four times per day).
- Rose hips *(Rosa canina)* and green tea *(Camelia sinensis)* are also high in bioflavanoids and either one may be used as a tea. Drink three to four cups/day.
- Stone root *(Collinsonia canadensis)* and horse chestnut *(Aesculus hippocastanum)* can be used to strengthen blood vessel walls (60 drops tincture twice a day).

Topical applications may relieve itching and burning, as well as promote healing. Apply one of the following two to four times a day.
- Witch hazel *(Hamamelis virginiana)* is an astringent that may reduce swelling (commercially available as Tuck's pads).
- A salve containing comfrey *(Symphytum officinalis)* and/or marigold *(Calendula officinalis)* soothes and promotes healing.
- A poultice made from grated potato is astringent and soothing.

HOMEOPATHY
Some of the most common remedies used for hemorrhoids are listed below. Usually, the dose is 12X to 30C every one to four hours.
- *Aesculus* for burning hemorrhoids with a sensation of a lump in anus that feels worse when walking
- *Aloe* for a sensation of pulsation in the rectum with large, external hemorrhoids
- *Collinsonia* for chronic, itchy hemorrhoids with constipation
- *Hamamelis* for large bleeding hemorrhoids with a raw feeling

PHYSICAL MEDICINE
Fill one basin with hot water, one with cold water. Sit in hot water for three minutes, then in cold water for one minute. Repeat this three times to complete one set. Do one to two sets per day three to four days per week.

ACUPUNCTURE
Acupuncture may be effective in resolving stagnant, congestive conditions.

■ FOLLOWING UP
Talk with your provider if the hemorrhoids are still a problem after one to two weeks. If you frequently have hemorrhoids, talk with your provider about diet and lifestyle changes to help prevent them in the future.

■ HEPATITIS, VIRAL

Hepatitis is a serious inflammation of the liver. Viral hepatitis, the most common form, usually appears as type A, B, or C. Type A (HAV), the most common, often affects schoolchildren. Type B (HBV) and Type C (HCV) affect people of all ages.

■ SIGNS AND SYMPTOMS

- Jaundice (yellow discoloration of skin and whites of eyes)
- Abdominal discomfort or uneasiness
- Fatigue, loss of weight
- Nausea, vomiting
- Dark urine, colorless stool
- Aversion to cigarettes

■ WHAT CAUSES IT?

- HAV: usually transmitted from feces on unwashed hands (putting dirty hands into the mouth) and by ingesting contaminated food and water.
- HBV: usually transmitted by injection of contaminated blood, through intravenous (IV) drug use, and through sexual activity.
- HCV: usually transmitted in a blood transfusion, through IV drug use, and possibly during sexual activity.

■ WHAT TO EXPECT AT YOUR PROVIDER'S OFFICE

Your health care provider will feel and tap your chest and back to determine if your liver or spleen is enlarged or tender. Your provider will request a blood test, possibly a urine test, and, in a few cases, a liver biopsy. Tell your provider if any of the following apply to you.

- Work in health care, such as in a medical laboratory or in dialysis
- Have a parent, sibling, or child infected with hepatitis
- Engage in unprotected sex
- Inject drugs
- Live in or are exposed to unsanitary conditions
- Consume possibly contaminated food or water
- Eat or handle raw shellfish

■ TREATMENT OPTIONS

Your provider will tell you to rest, drink a lot of fluids, and eat a well-rounded diet. Benadryl, compazine, metoclopramide, or hydroxyzine can help nausea. Acetaminophen (Tylenol) can help abdominal discomfort. If you have chronic viral hepatitis, your provider will treat you with corticosteroids or immunomodulators.

Complementary and Alternative Therapies

Alternative therapies can help support and protect the liver.

NUTRITION

- Reduce or eliminate alcohol, caffeine, refined foods, sugar, food additives, and saturated fats (meat and dairy products).
- Small, frequent meals are suggested to optimize digestion.
- Increase intake of grains, vegetables, fruits, vegetable proteins (legumes such as soy), and essential fatty acids (cold-water fish, nuts, and seeds). Foods that support the liver are beets, artichokes, yams, onions, garlic, green leafy vegetables, apples, and lemons.
- Green tea can decrease inflammation. 2 to 3 cups per day.
- Acidophilus supplements (one capsule with meals) helps keep healthy levels of the "good" bacteria in your body. Low vitamin K levels may be supplemented with 100 to 500 mg per day.
- Vitamin C (1,000 to 1,500 mg per day), beta-carotene (100,000 IU per day), vitamin E (400 to 800 IU per day), and zinc (30 to 50 mg

per day) strengthen your immune system. B-complex (50 to 100 mg per day), especially folic acid (800 to 1,000 mcg per day) and B_{12} (1,000 mcg per day) are needed for good liver function.
- Selenium (200 mcg per day) is needed to keep your liver healthy.
- Desiccated liver and thymus extracts can improve liver regeneration.
- Glutathione (500 mg twice a day) or N-acetyl cysteine (200 mg two to three times per day) provide liver cleansing and antioxidant support.

HERBS

Unless otherwise indicated, teas should be made with one teaspoon herb per cup of hot water. Steep covered 5 to 10 minutes for leaf or flowers, and 10 to 20 minutes for roots. Three to four liver-supportive herbs should be combined with two to three antiviral and immune-stimulating herbs. The high doses of single herbs suggested may be best taken as dried extracts (in capsules), although tinctures (60 drops four times per day) and teas (4 to 6 cups per day) may also be used.

Herbs for liver support include the following.

- Milk thistle (*Silybum marianum*, 200 to 250 mg three times per day) protects the liver. It may also be used as phosphatidylcholine-bound silymarin (100 to 150 mg three times per day).
- Chinese thoroughwax (*Bupleurum falcatum*) contains steroid-like substances that reduce inflammation.
- Globe artichoke (*Cynara scolymus*) promotes liver regeneration.
- Schizandra berry (*Schizandra chinensis*) protects liver health.
- *Eclipta alba*, usually used with phyllanthus.
- *Phyllanthus amarus* (200 mg three times per day).
- Turmeric (*Curcuma longa*, 250 to 500 mg three times per day). Combine with bromelain (250 to 500 mg three times per day between meals) to enhance its effects.

Immune support and antivirals include the following.

- Licorice root (*Glycyrrhiza glabra*, 250 to 500 mg three times per day). Do not take licorice if you have high blood pressure.
- Astragalus root (*Astragalus membrinaceus*)
- Coneflower (*Echinacea purpurea*)
- Goldenseal (*Hydrastis canadensis*)

HOMEOPATHY

Homeopathy may be useful as a supportive therapy.

PHYSICAL MEDICINE

Castor oil pack. Apply the oil directly to your right upper abdomen, cover with a cloth, plastic wrap, and a heat source; let sit for 30 to 60 minutes.

ACUPUNCTURE

Acupuncture may help support your liver function.

MASSAGE

Therapeutic massage may be helpful to your immune system.

■ FOLLOWING UP

If you have jaundice, it should disappear in two to eight weeks.

■ SPECIAL CONSIDERATIONS

HBV and HCV can be transmitted during pregnancy or childbirth.

■ HERPES SIMPLEX VIRUS

Herpes simplex virus (HSV) infections are very common worldwide. HSV-1 (oral-facial herpes) is transmitted through kissing or sharing drinking utensils, and HSV-2 (genital herpes) through sexual contact. Both HSV-1 and HSV-2 can cause infections around the face, mouth, and genitals. The infection may not show symptoms for a long time, and then become activated by ultraviolet light, fever, menstruation, emotional stress, a weakened immune system, and trauma to the skin or nerves. Herpes infections in infants and in people who have weak immune systems or herpes infections that affect the eyes are serious and potentially life-threatening.

■ SIGNS AND SYMPTOMS

You may experience swelling and redness in your face and mouth areas, including your gums and throat. You may feel tired, have a fever, and feel pain in your face and muscles. Blisters may appear on your lips, face, gums, tongue, inside your mouth, and on your genitals. You may also have vaginal (in women) or urethral (in men) discharge.

■ WHAT CAUSES IT?

You can get herpes simplex if you come in close contact with an individual infected with HSV-1 or HSV-2, such as a family member or sexual partner. Herpes simplex can also be transmitted through certain occupations (such as dentistry) or sports (such as wrestling). You can get herpes simplex from an infected person even if he or she does not have active symptoms. A mother can also pass the infection to her baby during vaginal birth.

■ WHAT TO EXPECT AT YOUR PROVIDER'S OFFICE

Your provider will explain that there is no cure for herpes simplex but that you can treat the symptoms.

■ TREATMENT OPTIONS

Antiviral medicines treat initial herpes infections and recurrences.
- Intravenous acyclovir—for herpes in newborns and for HSV encephalitis
- Oral acyclovir—for oral-facial herpes
- Oral acyclovir, oral valacyclovir, and oral famciclovir—for genital lesions
- Oral famciclovir and acyclovir—to reduce frequency and severity
- Idoxuridine, trifluridine, topical vidarabine, acyclovir, and interferon—for herpetic keratitis
- Intravenous foscarnet—for acyclovir-resistant HSV

Complementary and Alternative Therapies

Nutritional and herbal support can help you fight the herpes infection and strengthen your immune system.

NUTRITION
- Avoid alcohol, caffeine, refined foods, sugars, saturated fats, and arginine-containing foods (seeds, grains, nuts, nut butters, chocolate).
- Increase intake of high lysine-containing foods (fish, chicken, eggs, potatoes, and dairy products) during active herpes infection.
- Vitamin C (1,000 mg three times per day) and acidophilus (one capsule with meals) may reduce the length of outbreaks.
- Beta-carotene (50,000 to 100,000 IU per day) slows viral activity.
- Zinc (30 mg per day) slows viral reproduction.
- L-lysine (500 to 1,000 mg per day for prevention, 2,000 mg two to four times per day during an outbreak)

- Thymus extract can help strengthen the immune system.
- Selenium (250 mcg per day) may reduce length and frequency.
- Vitamin A (200,000 IU per day for 3 days at onset of outbreak) can help decrease length and severity of symptoms. Pregnant women and those with liver disease should not take these doses of vitamin A.

HERBS
Herbs may be used as dried extracts (capsules, powders, teas), glycerites (glycerine extracts), or tinctures (alcohol extracts). Teas should be made with 1 tsp. herb per cup of hot water. Steep covered 5 to 10 minutes for leaf or flowers, and 10 to 20 minutes for roots.

Topical cream applications of concentrated extracts of lemon balm (*Melissa officinalis*) or glycyrrhizic acid (from licorice root) can provide relief of symptoms and reduce severity and length of outbreak. They may be applied to both oral and genital lesions.

Internal treatment supports antiviral activity and immune function. For acute infection, combine equal parts of the following herbs in a tincture (30 to 60 drops three to four times per day) or a tea (3 to 4 cups per day). Coneflower (*Echinacea purpurea*), licorice root (*Glycyrrhiza glabra*), lemon balm (*Melissa officinalis*), yarrow (*Achillea millefolium*), chamomile (*Matricaria recutita*), and St. John's wort (*Hypericum perforatum*). Do not use licorice if you have high blood pressure. For recurrent infections, substitute lomatium (*Lomatium dissectum*) and astragalus (*Astragalus membranosus*) for yarrow and chamomile, and use the new formula in tincture form, 30 drops three times per day. Lemon balm (*Melissa officianalis*) can be used internally for prevention and treatment.

HOMEOPATHY
Some of the most common remedies used for HSV are listed below. Usually, the dose is 12X to 30C every one to four hours until your symptoms get better.
- *Apis mellifica* when lesions are swollen, stinging, and burning
- *Graphites* for genital herpes on inner thigh with tremendous itching
- *Petroleum* for genital herpes that have spread to anus and thighs

PHYSICAL MEDICINE
Ice packs applied to oral lesions or to the sacral (lower back) area for genital lesions may help reduce pain and inflammation.

ACUPUNCTURE
To boost the immune system and relieve pain.

MASSAGE
Massage helps reduce the effects of stress, which may make HSV worse.

■ FOLLOWING UP
Identifying and avoiding triggers (such as using sunscreen if ultraviolet light activates your symptoms) can help reduce recurrences.

■ SPECIAL CONSIDERATIONS
Getting herpes in the third trimester of pregnancy can be dangerous for both mother and baby. Your health care provider should know that you have had herpes.

■ HERPES ZOSTER (VARICELLA–ZOSTER) VIRUS

Varicella–zoster virus (VZV) is known to cause two diseases: chicken-pox (varicella) and shingles (herpes zoster). Chickenpox is a common contagious disease of children that usually has a benign course. However, chickenpox in adults or people with weakened immune systems can have serious complications. Second attacks of chickenpox are very rare. Shingles is caused by a reactivation of the latent VZV, commonly seen over age 50.

■ SIGNS AND SYMPTOMS

The typical rash of chickenpox is made up of groups of small, itchy blisters surrounded by inflamed skin on the trunk, scalp, face, and extremities, accompanied by low grade fever, fatigue, headache, and loss of appetite. The typical rash of shingles is made up of large blisters that cover a large area of the body, especially the face, trunk, shoulders and neck, and legs. These eruptions follow the path of an infected nerve. Usually only a single nerve is involved, confining the rash to one side of the body. Pain after the rash has disappeared is common because the affected nerve is irritated.

■ WHAT CAUSES IT?

Exposure to an individual with chickenpox at home, at school, or in the hospital is the likely cause of this virus. Later in life, weakening of the immune system from age or disease can make you susceptible to shingles.

■ WHAT TO EXPECT AT YOUR PROVIDER'S OFFICE

Your health care provider will easily be able to diagnose chickenpox because of its characteristic rash. If you have shingles, your provider may order some blood tests. Pain medication, antiviral medication, and symptomatic treatments will likely be prescribed.

■ TREATMENT OPTIONS

The goal is to make the infection last as short a time as possible, and to make you more comfortable while you have it. A vaccine is available for healthy children who have never had chickenpox.

Drug Therapies

- Acetaminophen (Tylenol)—for fever
- Acyclovir—for adolescents and adults with chickenpox in whom symptoms are severe, and for people with shingles
- Valacyclovir—to speed the healing of shingles
- Capsaicin cream (from cayenne pepper), amitriptyline hydrochloride, and fluphenazine hydrochloride—for relief of the pain of shingles
- Prednisone—for relief of the pain of shingles
- Anti-itching drugs—topical agents for chickenpox and shingles

Complementary and Alternative Therapies

Nutritional and herbal support may be helpful.

NUTRITION

- Avoid foods that inhibit immune activity and stimulate inflammation, such as saturated fats, refined foods, sugars, and juice.
- Beta-carotene (50,000 to 100,000 IU per day), zinc (30 to 50 mg per day), vitamin C (1,000 to 1,500 mg three to four times per day), and vitamin E (400 to 800 IU per day) promote healing of lesions.
- Calcium (1,000 to 1,500 mg per day), magnesium (200 mg two to three times per day), and B-complex (50 to 100 mg per day)
- Additional B_{12} (500 to 1,000 mcg) for lingering pain

- Vitamin A (200,000 to 300,000 IU per day for 3 days, then 100,000 to 150,000 IU per day for 3 days, then 50,000 IU per day for three days) helps decrease severity and length of symptoms. Do not take high doses of vitamin A if you are pregnant or have liver disease.

HERBS

Herbs may be used as dried extracts (capsules, powders, teas), glycerites (glycerine extracts), or tinctures (alcohol extracts). Unless otherwise indicated, teas should be made with 1 tsp. herb per cup of hot water. Steep covered 5 to 10 minutes for leaf or flowers, and 10 to 20 minutes for roots.

- Topical cream applications of concentrated extract of glycyrrhizic acid (from licorice root) can provide symptomatic relief. A poultice made from powdered slippery elm *(Ulmus fulva)*, comfrey *(Symphytum officinalis)*, and goldenseal root *(Hydrastis canadensis)* is soothing, aids healing, and reduces the likelihood of secondary infection.
- For acute infection, combine equal parts of the following herbs in a tincture (30 to 60 drops three to four times per day) or a tea (3 to 4 cups per day)and drink. Coneflower *(Echinacea purpurea)*, licorice root *(Glycyrrhiza glabra)*, burdock root *(Arctium lappa)*, lemon balm *(Melissa officinalis)*, chamomile *(Matricaria recutita)*, and St. John's wort *(Hypericum perforatum)*. Do not take licorice if you have high blood pressure.
- Combine equal parts tincture of Jamaican dogwood *(Piscidia erythrina)*, wild lettuce *(Lactuca virosa)*, valerian *(Valeriana officinalis)*, marigold *(Calendula officinalis)*, and St. John's wort *(Hypericum perforatum)* with $1/2$ part yellow jasmine *(Gelsemium sempiverens)*. Take 30 to 60 drops three to four times per day.

HOMEOPATHY

Some of the most common remedies used for VZV are listed below. Usually, the dose is 12X to 30C every one to four hours until your symptoms resolve.

- *Lachesis* for herpes zoster across left side of back with flushes of heat
- *Mezereum* for herpes zoster of the face with headaches and facial pain
- *Petroleum* for herpes zoster with intense itching that is worse at night

PHYSICAL MEDICINE

Tepid oatmeal baths may provide relief from itching and burning. Use Aveeno, as commercially available, or place 1 cup of oats in a sock and let soak in tub. Squeeze the sock to release the soothing oat milk.

Prepare a tea from peppermint leaf *(Mentha piperita)*, cool, and place in a spray bottle. Spray on lesions for temporary pain relief.

ACUPUNCTURE

Immune function may be stimulated with acupuncture treatments.

■ FOLLOWING UP

Your health care provider may want to see you after shingles if you continue to have pain along the course of the affected nerve.

■ SPECIAL CONSIDERATIONS

While chickenpox usually goes away on its own, severe and sometimes fatal infections may occur in newborn infants, in adults, and in people whose immune systems are weakened.

■ HIV AND AIDS

Acquired immune deficiency syndrome, or AIDS, is a worldwide health problem. AIDS is caused by the human immunodeficiency virus (HIV), which attacks white blood cells. About 20 million people throughout the world—heterosexuals and homosexuals alike—are infected with HIV. A massive research effort has produced better treatments, resulting in longer survival and improved quality of life for those with access to the treatments. But there is still no vaccine or cure. The only real defense against AIDS is prevention.

■ SIGNS AND SYMPTOMS

- Fever
- Weight loss
- Night sweats
- Skin lesions or rashes
- Fungus infection in the mouth
- Shortness of breath, cough, or chest pain
- Diarrhea, abdominal pain, or vomiting
- Blurred vision
- Headache
- Depression
- Confusion
- Herpes
- Kaposi's sarcoma
- Malignancies

■ WHAT CAUSES IT?

Infection by the human immunodeficiency virus (HIV) causes AIDS. Seventy percent of HIV transmission occurs through sexual contact. Intravenous drug users transmit HIV by sharing needles. Blood transfusions and blood products caused many infections in the early years of the epidemic, but screening procedures have nearly eliminated this risk in the United States and other developed countries.

■ WHAT TO EXPECT AT YOUR PROVIDER'S OFFICE

If your health care provider suspects HIV infection, he or she will order a blood test to detect the presence of the virus. A stool sample may be requested. You may be sent for a chest X-ray, since a common complication of AIDS is pneumonia. If you have any neurological symptoms, your provider may recommend a computed tomography (CT) scan or analysis of your spinal fluid.

■ TREATMENT OPTIONS

Strong medicines are used to slow the progression of HIV infection to full-blown AIDS, while antibiotics and other therapies are used against complications. At least two antiviral drugs, including a new type called protease inhibitors, are generally taken in combination to fight the infection.

Complementary and Alternative Therapies

These may be effective at slowing the progression from HIV infection to AIDS, and to treat some related infections.

NUTRITION

Avoid megadoses of nutrients unless prescribed by your provider.
- Multivitamin: two to six capsules a day
- Vitamin C (1 to 6 g a day—to bowel tolerance), beta-carotene (150,000 to 300,000 IU a day), and zinc (30 mg a day)
- N-acetyl cysteine (1,500 to 2,000 mg a day): protects the lungs
- Selenium (100 to 400 mcg a day): important antioxidant
- Vitamin E (400 to 800 IU a day): antioxidant
- Vitamin B complex (50 to 100 mg a day): depleted during stress
- Vitamin B$_{12}$ (1000 mcg via intramuscular injection): one injection a month to counter medication side effects

- Magnesium (500 to 750 mg a day): important in protein biosynthesis
- Coenzyme Q10 (10 mg a day): may improve cell ratios
- L-glutamine (30 to 40 g per day in five doses of 6 to 8 g each for at least 7 to 10 days): fuel for cells lining the gastrointestinal tract
- L-carnitine (2,000 mg a day): with wasting or high triglyceride levels

HERBS

Herbs may be used as dried extracts (capsules, powders, teas), glycerites (glycerine extracts), or tinctures (alcohol extracts).
- To stimulate immune function and provide antiviral support: Licorice (*Glycyrrhiza glabra*), $^1/_4$ to $^1/_2$ solid extract twice a day, inhibits HIV reproduction in lab tests; helps regrow liver cells. Do not take licorice if you have high blood pressure. St. John's wort (*Hypericum perforatum*), at 250 mg three times a day, inhibits binding and entry of HIV into host cells and elevates mood. Huang qi (*Astragalus membranaceus*), 250 to 500 mg powdered solid extract, inhibits HIV-1 replication and stimulates the appetite. Use one to two of these.
- To stimulate digestion and prevent diarrhea, take one to three of the following herbs, which stimulate the appetite (15 to 60 drops three times a day with meals): gentian (*Gentiana lutea*) tonic, historically used as an antiparasitic, to be avoided if you have ulcers; dandelion (*Taraxacum officinale*) cholagogue, historically used for liver problems; goldenseal (*Hydrastis canadensis*) as an anti-inflammatory, mild laxative, do not exceed recommended dose for long-term use
- Garlic (*Allium sativum*) is a strong antioxidant, enhances natural killer cell activity in people with AIDS
- Siberian ginseng (*Eleutherococcus sentecosus*) (30 to 60 drops three times a day or 1 cup tea three times a day) increases T-cell, NK cell, and cytotoxic killer cell function
- Milk thistle (*Silybum marianum*): supportive treatment for toxic liver damage, especially important with medications used in HIV/AIDS
- Acidophilus (two to five million organisms three times a day): beneficial gut bacteria that are depleted when you take a lot of antibiotics

HOMEOPATHY

Homeopathy may be useful as a supportive therapy.

PHYSICAL MEDICINE

Weight training may be helpful in maintaining muscle mass.

ACUPUNCTURE

May be very helpful to treat infections and stimulate immune system.

MASSAGE

Massage can enhance the immune system and decrease anxiety.

■ FOLLOWING UP

Complications are common but they can be treated. HIV has a long "dormant" period; the median time for progression to AIDS is 11 years from infection. Patients with AIDS itself generally survive one to two years. Those time spans are beginning to increase as treatments improve.

■ SPECIAL CONSIDERATIONS

If you are HIV-positive and pregnant, taking AZT is the only way to reduce the likelihood of transmitting the virus to your baby. Depending on your own condition, you and your health care provider may decide to postpone treatment until after your first trimester to reduce the risk of birth defects.

■ HYPERCHOLESTEROLEMIA

Hypercholesterolemia, or high cholesterol, occurs when you have abnormally high levels of fats (cholesterol or lipoproteins) in the blood. Lifestyle changes can help reduce cholesterol levels.

■ SIGNS AND SYMPTOMS

High cholesterol has few, if any, symptoms. The key to controlling your cholesterol is to change your lifestyle by exercising regularly, eating a low-fat diet, and losing weight if you need to. When you have your routine physical, get your cholesterol checked.

■ WHAT CAUSES IT?

Risk factors for high cholesterol include the following.
- A diet high in saturated fat
- Cirrhosis
- Poorly controlled diabetes
- Underactive thyroid gland
- Overactive pituitary gland
- Kidney failure
- Porphyria, a disorder caused by deficiencies of certain enzymes
- Heredity
- Alcohol abuse
- Certain drugs

■ WHAT TO EXPECT AT YOUR PROVIDER'S OFFICE

Your health care provider can order a blood test to check for your total cholesterol level at any time. The ideal level is about 120 to 200 milligrams of cholesterol per deciliter of blood (mg/dl) or less. It is important, however, to remember that it is not just the total cholesterol count that matters but the ratio of high-density lipoproteins (HDL, or "good" cholesterol) to low-density lipoproteins (LDL, or "bad" cholesterol).

■ TREATMENT OPTIONS

- Eat a diet low in cholesterol and saturated fat to reduce your LDL level
- Exercise to reduce your LDL level and increase your HDL level
- Drinking a small amount of alcohol may raise your HDL level and lower your LDL level, but more than two drinks could have the opposite effect
- Maintain an appropriate weight
- Stop smoking

Your provider may also prescribe drugs to lower your cholesterol.
- Cholestyramine/cholestipol
- Nicotinic acid
- "Statins," such as Pravastatin, Simvastatin, Atorvastatin, Fluvastatin, and Lovastatin
- Gemfibrozil

Complementary and Alternative Therapies

The digestion, metabolism, and utilization of fats, as well as minimizing the effects of hypercholesterolemia, are areas in which alternative therapies can be very effective.

NUTRITION

- Vegetable proteins have been shown to lower cholesterol levels, while animal and milk proteins have been shown to raise them. Thus a vegetarian or semi-vegetarian diet has been shown to be effective.
- Eat more foods high in omega-3 oils (cold-water fish, nuts, and seeds), which can help decrease cholesterol levels. Include foods that help reduce cholesterol, such as those high in water-soluble fiber (legumes, grains, and pectin-containing fruits, such as apples, grapes, bananas, prunes, lemons, plums, grapefruit, oranges). Reduce consumption of sugar and simple carbohydrates. Eat more foods that support the liver, such as beets, carrots, yams, artichokes, dark bitter greens, and lemons.
- Omega-3 fatty acids (1,000 to 1,500 mg 2 to 3 times per day) lower total cholesterol levels. Found in fish oil capsules and flax seed.
- Selenium (200 mcg per day) for normal processing of fats
- L-taurine (200 mg per day) helps the body excrete extra cholesterol.
- Vitamin C (1,000 mg three times per day) and E (400 to 800 IU per day) are needed for cholesterol metabolism.
- B complex, especially B_{12} (1,000 mcg per day), folic acid (400 to 800 mcg per day), betaine (1,000 mg per day), and B_6 (50 to 100 mg per day) reduce high levels of homocysteine.
- Coenzyme Q10 (50 to 100 mg per day) for your circulatory system
- Chromium (200 mcg one to three times per day) is helpful for people who have high cholesterol as a complication of diabetes.
- Magnesium (200 mg two to three times per day) helps your body function efficiently and lowers blood pressure.
- Panthenine (500 mg three times per day) reduces cholesterol.

HERBS

Herbs may be used as dried extracts (capsules, powders, teas), glycerites (glycerine extracts), or tinctures (alcohol extracts). Unless otherwise indicated, teas should be made with 1 tsp. herb per cup of hot water. Steep covered 5 to 10 minutes for leaf or flowers, and simmer 10 to 20 minutes for roots, barks, and berries. Drink 2 to 4 cups per day.
- Garlic (*Allium sativum*) is most effective when included in the diet in the raw form or taken in capsules.
- Herbs that support the liver may be taken singly or in combination. Herbs to consider include milk thistle (*Silybum marianum*), dandelion root (*Taraxacum*), burdock root (*Arctium lappa*), blue flag (*Iris versicolor*), greater celandine (*Chelidonium majus*), and blue vervain (*Verbena hastata*). Tinctures (15 to 20 drops per dose) or infusions (1 heaping tsp. per dose) are best taken 10 to 20 minutes before meals. Greater celandine should be taken with caution (no more than 2 ml daily), as it can lead to intestinal pain.
- Hawthorn berries (*Crataegus oxyanthoides*) lower high blood pressure and help lower cholesterol levels. Take 200 mg 2 to 3 times per day of dried extract or 30 drops three times per day of tincture.
- Ginger (*Zingiber officinalis*) can lower cholesterol levels.
- Alfalfa (*Medicago sativa*) has been shown to lower cholesterol levels.

HOMEOPATHY

Homeopathy may be useful as a supportive therapy.

ACUPUNCTURE

Acupuncture can assist with improving liver and gallbladder function.

■ FOLLOWING UP

Your provider will check your cholesterol levels regularly.

■ SPECIAL CONSIDERATIONS

It is important that you make a healthy, low-fat diet and regular exercise part of your everyday life to control your cholesterol over the long term.

■ HYPERKALEMIA

Hyperkalemia is an excess of serum potassium. Most potassium in the body (98%) is found within cells; only a small amount usually circulates in the bloodstream. The balance of potassium between the cells and the blood is critical to the body. It affects the way the cell membranes work and governs the action of the heart and the pathways between the brain and the muscles. If you have excess potassium in the blood, it is usually excreted by the kidneys. However, the levels can get too high if your kidneys aren't working right, which is the most common cause of hyperkalemia. Another cause is damaged cells' releasing potassium into the bloodstream faster than even normal kidneys can clear it. Medications or diet may also affect the amount of potassium in the blood. Hyperkalemia is a serious condition that must be treated promptly.

■ SIGNS AND SYMPTOMS

- Fatigue
- Weakness
- Tingling, numbness, or other unusual sensations
- Paralysis
- Palpitations
- Difficulty breathing

■ WHAT CAUSES IT?

Hyperkalemia has many causes, including the following.
- Kidney problems
- Too much acid in the blood, as sometimes seen in diabetes
- Diet high in potassium (bananas, oranges, tomatoes, high protein diets, salt substitutes, potassium supplements)
- Trauma, especially crush injuries or burns
- Addison's disease
- Certain medications

■ WHAT TO EXPECT AT YOUR PROVIDER'S OFFICE

You may not be feeling any effects of your hyperkalemia; your health care provider may discover it during a routine blood test or electrocardiogram. Hyperkalemia can cause life-threatening effects without warning. If you experience the symptoms of hyperkalemia, you should call 911 or get to an emergency room. You should expect to be admitted to the hospital for further tests and so that your condition can be stabilized. You will be given medications to take care of the immediate problem, but more tests may need to be done to determine the underlying cause. If the medications are not successful in lowering the potassium level in your blood, dialysis may be recommended.

■ TREATMENT OPTIONS

The medications that treat hyperkalemia are meant to stabilize cardiac function, promote the movement of potassium from the bloodstream back into the cells, and encourage the excretion of excess potassium.

Drug Therapies

- Insulin—promotes potassium shift from blood to cells
- Sodium bicarbonate—promotes potassium shift from blood to cells
- Beta agonists—promote potassium shift from blood to cells
- Diuretics—cause potassium excretion from kidneys
- Binding resins—promote potassium/sodium exchange in the gastrointestinal system

Complementary and Alternative Therapies

Alternative therapies can provide concurrent support and in treatment of the underlying cause once your condition has been stabilized.

NUTRITION

- Avoid alcohol, caffeine, refined foods, sugar, and saturated fats (meat proteins and dairy products). Eliminate high-potassium foods.
- Drink more water; dehydration can make hyperkalemia worse.
- Eat small amounts of protein and more vegetable proteins and fish than chicken and red meats.
- Small, frequent meals can help prevent hypoglycemia.
- Magnesium (200 mg two to three times per day) helps regulate potassium levels.

HERBS

Herbs may be used as dried extracts (capsules, powders, teas), glycerites (glycerine extracts), or tinctures (alcohol extracts). Teas should be made with 1 tsp. herb per cup of hot water. Steep covered 5 to 10 minutes for leaf or flowers, and 10 to 20 minutes for roots.

Of primary concern is the effect of hyperkalemia on the heart.
- Hawthorn (*Crataegus oxyacantha*) increases cardiac output without increasing cardiac load. It dilates blood vessels, helps stabilize cardiac arrhythmias, and also supports liver function. Compromised liver function and poor fat digestion can make hyperkalemia worse. Drink 3 to 4 cups of tea per day.
- Lily of the valley (*Convalleria majalis*) increases cardiac output and has a regulating effect on heart rhythm. It is a diuretic that relieves swelling and has a neutral to slightly lowering effect on sodium and potassium. This herb has toxic side effects and should not be used without supervision from your health care provider.

HOMEOPATHY

Homeopathy may be useful as a supportive therapy.

PHYSICAL MEDICINE

Contrast hydrotherapy. Alternating hot and cold applications brings nutrients to the site and eases inflammation. Use the applications over the kidneys. Alternate three minutes hot with one minute cold. Repeat three times. This is one set. Do two to three sets per day.

ACUPUNCTURE

Acupuncture may be helpful in supporting normal kidney function.

MASSAGE

Swedish massage may help to stimulate the kidneys.

■ FOLLOWING UP

Your health care provider will probably ask to see you two or three days after you are discharged from the hospital, to repeat the potassium tests and electrocardiogram, and check your kidney function. He or she will review all the medications you are taking, and perhaps advise a change.

■ SPECIAL CONSIDERATIONS

If you are on regular dialysis, make sure you keep strictly to your schedule to avoid hyperkalemia and other serious problems.

For additional information supporting this handout, please refer to our website: www.onemedicine.com/public/products/access

53

■ HYPERTENSION

Hypertension, or high blood pressure, is a very common condition in the U.S. It usually begins after age 20, and up to half of all people over age 65 have high blood pressure. High blood pressure can lead to serious problems such as stroke or heart attack. For this reason, you should try to keep your blood pressure within a normal range, ideally under 140/90 ("140 over 90").

■ SIGNS AND SYMPTOMS

Most people with high blood pressure have primary hypertension, also called essential hypertension. This common form causes no symptoms at all unless the pressure gets extremely high. High blood pressure is often called the "silent killer" because you can feel just fine when you have it—even though damage may be occurring in your body.

Severe hypertension or a hypertensive emergency (usually caused by some other condition) may produce headache, nausea and vomiting, convulsions, visual problems, and other symptoms.

■ WHAT CAUSES IT?

The causes of essential hypertension are unknown. Doctors know only that it is very common and that you are more likely to get it as you get older. Hypertension is more common in African Americans. Factors that increase your risk of high blood pressure include the following.

- Family history
- Lack of exercise
- Alcohol use
- Obesity
- High salt intake
- High sugar intake
- Stress

A rarer kind of hypertension may be caused by other medical conditions, and many medications. Pregnancy also causes blood pressure to rise.

■ WHAT TO EXPECT AT YOUR PROVIDER'S OFFICE

Because blood pressure varies in different circumstances, your health care provider will take your blood pressure at several different times to get an accurate average reading. You may be asked to refrain from smoking, caffeine, and using some medications before coming to the office, because these may raise your blood pressure. You will have a physical examination and may have blood tests or other tests if needed.

■ TREATMENT OPTIONS

Your provider will most likely suggest lifestyle changes, such as eating a low-fat diet, exercising regularly, and losing weight if you need to.

Drug Therapies

A dozen different categories of drugs have been developed to lower blood pressure, with literally hundreds of individual drugs available. Your health care provider will choose the best one for you.

Complementary and Alternative Therapies

Mind/body techniques (such as biofeedback, yoga, and meditation) and nutritional and herbal support may help lower blood pressure.

NUTRITION

- Avoid caffeine and decrease intake of refined foods, sugar, and saturated fats (meats and dairy products). Some kinds of hypertension also respond to a reduction of salt in the diet.
- Eliminate food allergens because these may make hypertension worse.

Increase dietary fiber, vegetables and vegetable proteins, and essential fatty acids (cold-water fish, nuts, and seeds).

- MaxEPA, flax oil, or evening primrose oil (1,000 to 1,500 mg one to two times per day) lowers cholesterol and mildly reduces hypertension. Magnesium (200 mg two to three times per day) mildly dilates blood vessels to decrease blood pressure.
- Zinc (30 mg per day) may help reduce blood pressure associated with high levels of cadmium (usually found in cigarette smokers).
- Coenzyme Q10 (50 to 100 mg one to two times per day) is protective to the cardiovascular system.
- B complex (50 to 100 mg per day) with additional folic acid (800 mcg per day), B_{12} (1,200 mcg per day), and betaine (1,000 mg) may increase resistance to stress and lower blood pressure.
- Vitamin E (400 IU per day) keeps certain types of blood cells from sticking together, improving blood flow.

HERBS

Herbs may be used as dried extracts (capsules, powders, teas), glycerites (glycerine extracts), or tinctures (alcohol extracts). Unless otherwise indicated, teas should be made with 1 tsp. herb per cup of hot water. Steep covered 5 to 10 minutes for leaf or flowers, and 10 to 20 minutes for roots. Drink 2 to 4 cups per day.

- Hawthorn *(Crataegus oxyacantha)*, linden flowers *(Tilia cordata)*, passionflower *(Passiflora incarnata)*, valerian *(Valeriana officinalis)*, and cramp bark *(Viburnum opulus)* may be safely used long-term. These herbs relax and strengthen the cardiovascular system while moderately reducing blood pressure. Combine equal parts in a tincture, 20 to 30 drops three to four times per day.
- Hawthorn as a dried extract, 250 mg three times per day.
- Dandelion leaf *(Taraxecum officinalis)* has a diuretic effect but does not deplete potassium. Drink 3 to 4 cups per day.

Some herbs have a stronger hypotensive (lowering) effect but may also have toxic side effects. These herbs must be used under the supervision of a qualified practitioner: Lily of the valley *(Convallaria majalis)*, night-blooming cereus *(Cactus grandifloris)*, mistletoe *(Viscum album)*, motherwort *(Leonorus cardiaca)*, and Indian tobacco *(Lobelia inflata)*. Combine three to four of these herbs with equal parts of cramp bark and valerian and take 30 to 60 drops three times per day.

HOMEOPATHY

Homeopathy may be useful as a supportive therapy.

ACUPUNCTURE

Acupuncture may help reduce blood pressure and alleviate stress.

MASSAGE

Therapeutic massage may be effective in reducing the effects of stress, helping relaxation, and lowering blood pressure.

■ FOLLOWING UP

Even if you need medication, you will benefit from increased exercise, changes in your diet, and stopping smoking and drinking alcohol.

■ SPECIAL CONSIDERATIONS

Tell your health care provider if you are pregnant, because certain blood pressure medications should not be used in pregnancy.

For additional information supporting this handout, please refer to our website: www.onemedicine.com/public/products/access
Copyright ©2000 Integrative Medicine Communications • 1029 Chestnut St., Newton, MA 02464 • T 877-426-6633 • F 877-426-6630

■ HYPERTHYROIDISM

Hyperthyroidism occurs when your thyroid gland, located at the front of your neck, produces too much thyroid hormone. Hyperthyroidism has three forms that share several symptoms. Hyperthyroidism usually happens between the ages of 20 and 40. It often starts after times of extreme stress or during pregnancy.

■ SIGNS AND SYMPTOMS

- Fast heart rate and palpitations
- High blood pressure
- Swelling at the base of the neck
- Moist skin and increased perspiration
- Shakiness and tremor
- Nervousness and confusion
- Increased appetite accompanied by weight loss
- Difficulty sleeping
- Swollen, reddened, and bulging eyes
- Constant stare (infrequent blinking, lid lag)
- Sensitivity of eyes to light
- Occasionally, raised, thickened skin over the shins, back of feet, back, hands, or even face
- In crisis: fever, very rapid pulse, agitation, and possibly delirium
- Changes in menstrual periods

■ WHAT CAUSES IT?

Researchers suspect that Graves' disease (one form of hyperthyroidism) stems from an antibody that mistakenly stimulates the thyroid to produce too much hormone. Toxic nodular goiter is caused by a noncancerous tumor in nodules that make up the thyroid gland. Secondary hyperthyroidism results when a gland called the pituitary overrides the thyroid's normal instructions, and orders it to make too much thyroid hormone.

■ WHAT TO EXPECT AT YOUR PROVIDER'S OFFICE

Your health care provider will ask you to extend your fingers to see if you have a telltale tremor. Your provider will also examine your thyroid gland while you swallow. You will have blood drawn and may need X rays.

■ TREATMENT OPTIONS
Drug Therapies

Your health care provider will most likely prescribe a single dose of liquid radioactive iodine, which calms down your thyroid gland. Alternatively, your provider may give you thyroid-depressive medication. You may also be prescribed beta-blockers. If drug treatment fails, you may need surgery to remove part of your thyroid.

Complementary and Alternative Therapies

Alternative therapies may be effective at minimizing symptoms of mild thyroid dysfunction.

NUTRITION

Foods that depress the thyroid include broccoli, cabbage, Brussels sprouts, cauliflower, kale, spinach, turnips, soy, beans, and mustard greens. Avoid refined foods, dairy products, wheat, caffeine, and alcohol.

- Essential fatty acids are anti-inflammatory and help your immune system function well. Take 1,000 to 1,500 mg three times per day.
- Bromelain (250 to 500 mg three times per day between meals) reduces swelling.

- Vitamin C (1,000 mg three to four times a day) supports immune function and decreases inflammation.
- Calcium (1,000 mg per day) and magnesium (200 to 600 mg per day) are cofactors for many metabolic processes.
- Vitamin E (400 IU twice a day) can help protect the heart.
- Coenzyme Q10 (50 mg twice a day) can help protect the heart.
- Lithium has antithyroid properties. Doses of as little as 20 mg per day of elemental lithium may augment other antithyroid treatments.

HERBS

Herbs may be used as dried extracts (capsules, powders, teas), glycerites (glycerine extracts), or tinctures (alcohol extracts). Unless otherwise indicated, teas should be made with 1 tsp. herb per cup of hot water. Steep covered 5 to 10 minutes for leaf or flowers, and 10 to 20 minutes for roots. Drink 2 to 4 cups per day. For best results, these herbs should be used under the guidance of an experienced practitioner.

- Bugleweed *(Lycopus virginica)* and lemon balm *(Melissa officinalis)* help to normalize the overactive thyroid. Motherwort *(Leonorus cardiaca)* may relieve heart palpitations and passionflower *(Passiflora incarnata)* reduces anxiety. Combine two parts of bugleweed with one part each of lemon balm, motherwort, and passionflower and take in tincture form, 30 to 60 drops three to four times per day.
- Quercetin (250 to 500 mg three times per day) is an anti-inflammatory.
- Turmeric *(Curcuma longa)* makes the effects of bromelain stronger and should be taken between meals, 500 mg three times per day.
- Milk thistle *(Silibum Marianum)* helps the liver provide proper binding proteins. 300 to 600 mg three times a day.
- Hawthorne berry *(Cratagus oxycantha)* helps protect the heart. Take $\frac{1}{4}$ tsp. of the solid extract, or 1,000 mg of the herb, three times a day.
- Lemon balm *(Melissa officinalis)* inhibits the binding of thyroid-stimulating hormones (TSH) receptors.
- Immune-suppressing herbs such as *Stephania tetranda* and *Hemidesmus indicus* help break the circle of cellular damage.
- Anti-inflammatory herbs such as licorice *(Glycyrrhiza glabra)* and *Rehmania glutinosa* support the adrenals as well.

HOMEOPATHY

Homeopathy may be useful as a supportive therapy.

PHYSICAL MEDICINE

Ice packs to the throat will help decrease inflammation. Castor oil packs to the throat will also reduce inflammation. Apply oil directly to skin, cover with a clean soft cloth and plastic wrap. Place a heat source over the pack and let sit for 30 to 60 minutes. For best results, use for three consecutive days.

ACUPUNCTURE

Acupuncture may be helpful in correcting hormonal imbalances.

MASSAGE

Therapeutic massage may be useful in relieving stress.

■ SPECIAL CONSIDERATIONS

Thyroid problems during pregnancy can cause serious complications.

■ HYPOGLYCEMIA

Hypoglycemia (low blood sugar) is a condition in which there is an abnormally low level of glucose (sugar) in your blood. Normally your body keeps your blood sugar levels within a narrow range through the coordinated work of several glands and their hormones. But factors such as disease or a poor diet can disrupt the mechanisms that regulate your sugar levels. Too much glucose (hyperglycemia) results in diabetes, and too little glucose results in hypoglycemia.

■ SIGNS AND SYMPTOMS

Because glucose (sugar) is the brain's primary fuel, your brain feels the effects of hypoglycemia. The effects include the following.

- Headache
- Excessive sweating
- Blurred vision, dizziness
- Trembling, incoordination
- Depression, anxiety
- Mental confusion, irritability
- Heart palpitations
- Slurred speech
- Seizures
- Fatigue
- Irritability
- Coma

■ WHAT CAUSES IT?

Hypoglycemia can be caused by the following conditions.

- Drugs (such as insulin or alcohol)
- Critical organ failure (kidney, heart, or liver)
- Hormone deficiencies
- Tumors
- Inherited abnormalities
- Lack of an appropriate diet, especially with a critical illness
- With strenuous exercise several hours after eating
- After gastrointestinal surgery

■ WHAT TO EXPECT AT YOUR PROVIDER'S OFFICE

If your symptoms are not severe, your health care provider will order a blood test called a glucose tolerance test (GTT). If your levels are only slightly above normal, your provider may recommend diet and lifestyle changes. If your symptoms are severe, your provider will immediately give you glucose in either an oral or injectable form to bring your blood sugar level back to normal as quickly as possible. Additional tests can determine the cause of your low blood sugar.

■ TREATMENT OPTIONS

It is important to treat low blood sugar immediately to avoid long-term serious effects. Hypoglycemia resulting from exercise several hours after a meal rarely produces serious symptoms. A glass of orange juice and a piece of bread can correct your blood sugar levels within minutes. However, in people with underlying diseases, fluctuating blood sugar levels are more serious and must be treated with oral or injectable forms of glucose. You can take oral glucose if you are able to swallow. If not, your health care provider can give you an injection.

Complementary and Alternative Therapies

Long-term treatment is aimed at the cause of the hypoglycemia, but alternative therapies may also be useful in regulating blood sugar in the short term. Nutritional support should be part of treatment.

NUTRITION

Small frequent meals that are high in protein and complex carbohydrates are best, preferably five or six a day. Cut down on simple carbohydrates including sugar, refined foods, juices, and fruit. Eliminate caffeine, alcohol, and tobacco.

Vitamins and minerals that are important for regulating glucose levels include the following.

- Chromium picolinate: 100 to 200 mcg three times per day with meals
- Magnesium: 200 mg two to three times per day
- Vanadyl sulfate: 10 to 20 mg per day
- Zinc: 15 to 30 mg per day
- B complex: 50 to 100 mg per day
- Niacinamide: 500 mg per day
- Pyridoxine (B_6): 100 mg per day
- Pantothenic acid (B_5): 250 mg per day
- Vitamin C: 1,000 mg two to three times per day
- Vitamin E: 400 IU per day

HERBS

Herbs are generally a safe way to strengthen and tone the body's systems. As with any therapy, it is important to work with your provider on getting your problem diagnosed before you start any treatment. Herbs may be used as dried extracts (capsules, powders, teas), glycerites (glycerine extracts), or tinctures (alcohol extracts). Unless otherwise indicated, teas should be made with 1 tsp. herb per cup of hot water. Steep covered 5 to 10 minutes for leaf or flowers, and 10 to 20 minutes for roots. Drink 2 to 4 cups per day. Tinctures may be used singly or in combination as noted.

- Siberian ginseng *(Eleuthrococcus senticosus)* provides adrenal support. Use tincture 20 drops two times a day or dried extract 100 mg three times a day for two to three weeks with a one week rest before you start taking it again.
- A tincture of equal parts of licorice root *(Glycerrhiza glabra)*, gotu kola *(Centella asiatica)*, Siberian ginseng *(Eleuthrococcus senticosus)*, and ginger root *(Zingiber officinale)* may be used in combination to strengthen the adrenals and help hypoglycemic symptoms. Take 10 to 15 drops three times a day. Do not take licorice if you have high blood pressure.

HOMEOPATHY

Homeopathy may be useful as a supportive therapy.

ACUPUNCTURE

May be beneficial in decreasing stress and increasing coping skills.

■ FOLLOWING UP

Any underlying condition that may be causing your hypoglycemia must be aggressively treated so that your episodes do not recur. If you have hypoglycemia when you exercise, carry healthy snack food with you when you exercise.

■ SPECIAL CONSIDERATIONS

Do not ignore the signs and symptoms of hypoglycemia. Untreated, it can cause irreversible brain damage, coma, or even death.

■ HYPOTHYROIDISM

Hypothyroidism is when your thyroid gland, at the front of your neck, fails to produce enough of a hormone called the thyroid hormone or when your body fails to use thyroid hormone efficiently. There are several different types of hypothyroidism. Perhaps 11 million Americans have hypothyroidism, although only half know it. The disease affects both sexes and all ages. However, middle-aged women are most vulnerable. If you have just developed the disease, you will most likely have muscle aches and often feel cold. Left untreated, hypothyroidism can cause serious health complications.

■ SIGNS AND SYMPTOMS

- Slow pulse
- Lethargy
- Hoarse voice; slowed speech
- Puffy face; drooping eyelids
- Loss of eyebrows from the side
- Intolerance to cold
- Weight gain
- Constipation
- Dry, scaly, thick, coarse hair
- Raised, thickened skin over the shins
- Carpal tunnel syndrome
- Confusion; depression; dementia
- Headaches
- Menstrual cramps or other menstrual disorders
- In children, growth retardation, delayed teething, and mental deficiency

■ WHAT CAUSES IT?

The various forms of hypothyroidism have different causes. In Hashimoto's thyroiditis, antibodies in the blood mistakenly attack the thyroid gland and start to destroy it. Post-therapeutic hypothyroidism occurs when treatment for hyperthyroidism leaves the thyroid unable to produce enough thyroid hormone. And hypothyroidism with goiter results when your diet lacks iodine. The addition of iodine to salt in the U.S. has made this rare.

■ WHAT TO EXPECT AT YOUR PROVIDER'S OFFICE

Your health care provider will test your reflexes. He or she will also examine the palms of your hands and the soles of your feet for evidence of carotene, an orange substance deposited as a result of the disease. Your provider will draw blood and may also want you to take a radioactive iodine uptake test. For this, you drink a liquid containing radioactive iodine. X rays will show whether large amounts of the iodine settle in your thyroid gland.

■ TREATMENT OPTIONS

Drug Therapies

Your health care provider will prescribe drugs that you will take daily. Providers have two alternatives for drug treatment: synthetic thyroid hormone and dried animal thyroid hormone. The provider will want to adjust your dose over a period of several weeks, after regular blood tests to check the amount of thyroid hormone in your blood.

Complementary and Alternative Therapies

Thyroid function can be helped through nutrition and herbs.

NUTRITION

- Avoid foods that suppress thyroid function, including broccoli, cabbage, Brussels sprouts, cauliflower, kale, spinach, turnips, soybeans, peanuts, linseed, pinenuts, millet, cassava, and mustard greens.
- Avoid refined foods, dairy products, wheat, caffeine, and alcohol.
- Essential fatty acids (1,000 to 1,500 mg three times per day) are necessary for hormone production.
- Vitamin C (1,000 mg three to four times per day), vitamin A (10,000 to 25,000 IU per day), B complex [50 to 100 mg/day, augmented with vitamins B_2 (riboflavin, 15 mg), B_3 (niacin, 25 to 50 mg), and B_6 (pyridoxine, 25 to 50 mg)], selenium (200 mcg per day), iodine (300 mcg per day), vitamin E (400 IU per day), and zinc (30 mg per day) are necessary for thyroid hormone production.
- L-tyrosine (500 mg two or three times a day) also supports normal thyroid function. May make high blood pressure worse.
- Calcium (1,000 mg per day) and magnesium (200 to 600 mg per day) help many metabolic processes function normally.

HERBS

Herbs may be used as dried extracts (capsules, powders, teas), glycerites (glycerine extracts), or tinctures (alcohol extracts). Unless otherwise indicated, teas should be made with 1 tsp. herb per cup of hot water. Steep covered 5 to 10 minutes for leaf or flowers, and 10 to 20 minutes for roots. Drink 2 to 4 cups per day.

This combination supports thyroid function: Combine equal parts of the following herbs for a tea (3 to 4 cups per day) or tincture (20 to 30 drops three times per day). Horsetail *(Equisetum arvense)*, oatstraw *(Avena sativa)*, alfalfa *(Medicago sativa)*, and gotu kola *(Centella asiatica)*.

Kelp *(Alaria esculenta)*, bladderwrack *(Fucus vesiculosis)*, and Irish moss *(Chondrus crispus)* may be taken as foods or in capsule form.

Coleus foreskohlii (1 to 2 ml three times a day) stimulates thyroid function with an increase in thyroid hormone production. Also, herbs such as guggul *(Commiphora guggul)* (25 mg of guggulsterones three times a day) and hawthorn *(Crataegus oxyacantha)* (500 mg twice a day) are taken to counteract high cholesterol, which often accompanies hypothyroidism.

HOMEOPATHY

Homeopathy may be useful as a supportive therapy.

PHYSICAL MEDICINE

Contrast hydrotherapy (hot and cold applications) to the neck and throat may stimulate thyroid function. Alternate three minutes hot with one minute cold. Repeat three times for one set. Do two to three sets per day.

ACUPUNCTURE

Acupuncture may be helpful in correcting hormonal imbalances.

MASSAGE

Therapeutic massage can relieve stress and improve circulation.

■ FOLLOWING UP

After you start on thyroid hormone replacement therapy, your provider will want you to have frequent checkups to monitor its effectiveness.

■ INFANTILE COLIC

Colicky babies cry constantly and hard at about the same time each day at least three days a week. About one in five babies, usually a first-born boy, develops colic. Usually seen between 2 weeks and 6 months of age.

■ SIGNS AND SYMPTOMS

- Your baby cries for more than three hours on at least three occasions a week, but is otherwise healthy.
- Your baby kicks a lot, pulls his or her legs up close, and makes tight fists.
- Your baby's tummy seems hard and he or she burps and passes gas often.
- The crying sounds like your baby is in great pain.
- Your baby spits up frequently after feeding.

■ WHAT CAUSES IT?

Providers suspect colic is caused by one or more of the following.

- The baby's nervous or digestive system may be immature
- The baby needs comforting, or is over- or under-stimulated
- If breast-fed, the baby may be reacting to something in the mother's diet
- Antibiotics given at birth, either to the infant or the mother

■ WHAT TO EXPECT AT YOUR PROVIDER'S OFFICE

Your health care provider will ask if the baby is eating well and gaining weight or has diarrhea, fever, or unusual stools. If you are breast-feeding, your health care provider may ask you about foods you have eaten. If your provider decides your baby has colic, you can work together to find ways to relieve your baby's discomfort.

Your provider will also encourage you to take care of yourself, like taking a break or getting help if you are afraid you will harm your baby. Remember that colic usually disappears at 6 months of age. If the treatments you choose do not work, your baby's provider may check for other problems, such as a digestive problem or allergy.

■ TREATMENT OPTIONS

- If breast-feeding, nurse on demand, usually every two to three hours. Avoid caffeine, dairy products, citrus fruits, soy products, and spicy foods. Elevate the infant's head during and after feedings.
- If bottle feeding, ask your health care provider to recommend a formula that is not based on cow's milk and that is not iron-fortified.
- Do not offer your baby solid foods before age 6 months.
- Hold your baby close, offer a pacifier, try rocking or rubbing the back, give your baby a warm bath, take a car ride with the baby, play soft music, or use an infant swing to ease the crying.

Complementary and Alternative Therapies

Eliminating gas-producing foods and using supportive herbal or homeo-pathic therapies can help reduce or eliminate infantile colic. In addition, playing soft music, rocking the infant, or using "white noise" (for example, a dryer) may be helpful in soothing the infant. Reducing stimuli and plac-ing the infant in a dim, quiet room may help calm the baby.

NUTRITION

Acidophilus (especially *Bifidus spp.*) can be given to both the breastfeed-ing mother and infant. Use 1 capsule with meals three times per day for adults; 1 capsule per day for infants (break capsule open and administer powder in divided doses throughout the day).

HERBS

Herbs may be used as dried extracts (capsules, powders, teas), glycerites (glycerine extracts), or tinctures (alcohol extracts). Unless otherwise indi-cated, teas should be made with 1 tsp. herb per cup of hot water. Steep covered 5 to 10 minutes for leaf or flowers, and 10 to 20 minutes for roots. Drink 2 to 4 cups per day.

A tea made from fennel seed *(Foeniculum vulgare)* or anise seed *(Pimpinella anisum)* may be given directly to the infant (1 tsp. before and after feedings) or drunk by the breast-feeding mother (1 cup three to six times per day). Both fennel and anise act as gastrointestinal relaxants and help expel gas.

Other herbs that have relaxing effects and help reduce colic are lemon balm *(Melissa officinalis)*, catnip *(Nepeta cateria)*, peppermint *(Mentha piperita)*, spearmint *(Mentha spicata)*, and linden flower *(Tilia cordata)*. These may be added to the above tea as needed.

HOMEOPATHY

Some of the most common remedies used for colic are listed below. Usually, the dose is 12X to 30C every one to four hours until your symp-toms get better. For infants, dissolve about 5 pellets in 1/4 cup of water and give 1 tsp. every 4 hours.

- *Carbo vegetalis* for flatulent colic and burping
- *Chamomilla* for colic with irritability that is relieved by constant holding and walking
- *Magnesia phosphoricum* for colic that is better when the baby bends at the waist
- Combination remedies for colic are commercially available

PHYSICAL MEDICINE

Warm baths may help relax and soothe colicky infants. Add 3 to 4 drops of essential oil of lavender or lemon balm to enhance the benefit.

MASSAGE

Clockwise abdominal massage may help relieve spasm and expel gas. Use 3 to 5 drops of tincture of catnip *(Nepeta cateria)* in 1 to 2 tsp. of almond or olive oil to enhance effectiveness. Apply warmth.

■ FOLLOWING UP

Use whatever works, and remember that your baby will outgrow the colic in a few weeks or months. Keep in mind, however, that colicky babies often grow up to have other allergy-related health problems, such as ear infec-tions, asthma, and digestive problems.

■ SPECIAL CONSIDERATIONS

Never shake your baby. This can cause serious or fatal brain damage. If you are feeling overwhelmed, try the steps listed below.

- Have someone else watch your baby while you get away for a while.
- Join a support group.
- Call your baby's health care provider.

■ INFLUENZA

Influenza, or "flu," is an infection of the respiratory tract (breathing passages) caused by a virus. Its symptoms are usually more severe than the common cold and are more likely to affect your whole body. While most cases run their course in one to two weeks, life-threatening complications such as pneumonia are possible, especially in the elderly or people with chronic illnesses.

■ SIGNS AND SYMPTOMS

- Fever that comes on suddenly (101 to 104 degrees Fahrenheit)
- Chills
- Headache
- Muscle aches
- Fatigue
- Nonproductive cough
- Sore throat
- Sneezing, runny nose, stuffy nose
- Loss of appetite
- Nausea, vomiting, or diarrhea, especially in children

■ WHAT CAUSES IT?

Influenza is caused by viruses that are spread through the air by sneezes and coughs. Some cause very mild illness, or none at all. Others can suddenly change their form to bypass our bodies' defenses. People most likely to get influenza are those whose immune systems are not working properly, or those whose lifestyle or work often brings them into contact with sick people.

Since there are many types of influenza virus, and because they change over time, a new vaccine is offered every fall. Getting vaccinated reduces your chances of getting the flu, and reduces its severity if you do get it.

■ WHAT TO EXPECT AT YOUR PROVIDER'S OFFICE

Your health care provider will probably be able to diagnose your case of flu from a physical examination and a description of your symptoms. He or she may take a throat swab to identify a particular viral strain, or a chest X ray if there is concern about complications such as pneumonia.

■ TREATMENT OPTIONS

The faster you get to your health care provider after you start feeling the effects of the flu, the better. Specific medicines to fight the flu work best if begun within two days. You also may use over-the-counter medicines and other therapies to relieve your symptoms.

Drug Therapies

Your health care provider may advise you to take acetaminophen (Tylenol) or other non-aspirin pain relievers, a cough suppressant, and a decongestant. Never give aspirin to children or teenagers with a viral illness because of the risk of a life-threatening disease called Reye's syndrome. Antibiotics are not effective against the viruses that cause influenza, but some health care providers prescribe them for patients who are particularly vulnerable to bacterial pneumonia, a common complication of influenza.

Complementary and Alternative Therapies

A combination of herbs and nutrition may be quite effective at relieving symptoms and speeding healing. The basis of treatment is rest and fluids.

NUTRITION

- Vitamin C (1,000 mg three to four times per day), vitamin A (25,000 IU per day), or beta-carotene (200,000 IU per day), and zinc (25 to 90 mg per day) are nutrients that optimize immune system functioning. Women who are or may become pregnant in the next three months should not take high doses of vitamin A. No one should use high doses of vitamin A and zinc for longer than two to six weeks.
- Decrease sugar consumption. Sugar decreases immune system activity.

HERBS

Herbs may be used as dried extracts (capsules, powders, teas), glycerites (glycerine extracts), or tinctures (alcohol extracts). Unless otherwise indicated, teas should be made with 1 tsp. herb per cup of hot water. Steep covered 5 to 10 minutes for leaf or flowers, and 10 to 20 minutes for roots. Drink 2 to 4 cups per day.

- Coneflower (*Echinacea angustifolia*)—helps immune system
- Goldenseal (*Hydrastis canadensis*)—immune modulating, anti microbial, bitter, astringent
- Licorice (*Glycyrrhiza glabra*)—antiviral, anticolic, soothing
- Yarrow (*Achillea millefolium*)—antibacterial, astringent
- Elder (*Sambucus canadensis*)—reduces swelling and irritation
- St. John's wort (*Hypericum perforatum*)—antiviral, pain reliever

Mix a combination of coneflower and goldenseal with two to four of the other herbs listed. Drink 3 to 6 cups tea per day, or take 30 to 60 drops tincture three to six times per day.

Garlic and ginger tea (2 to 3 cloves of garlic and 2 to 3 slices of fresh ginger) keeps the lungs clear and acts as an antimicrobial. May be used in addition to above herbs.

HOMEOPATHY

Some of the most common remedies used for flu are listed below. Usually, the dose is 12X to 30C every one to four hours until your symptoms get better.

- Combination remedy of *Aconite, Gelsemium, Eucalyptus, Ipecacuanha, Phosphorus, Bryonia,* and *Eupatorium perfoliatum* (trade name Oscillococcinum) can be very effective.
- *Gelsemium* for influenza that leaves the patient weak and forgetful
- *Eupatorium perfoliatum* for influenza with deep achiness, especially with sneezing and coughing
- *Nux vomica* for influenza with violent vomiting and irritability

ACUPUNCTURE

May help you generally feel better and speed healing.

■ FOLLOWING UP

In most cases your flu symptoms will ease in one to five days, but they can last as long as two weeks. If you don't start to feel better within a few days, or if you begin having difficulty breathing, contact your health care provider.

■ SPECIAL CONSIDERATIONS

Studies suggest that pregnancy may increase the risk of serious influenza complications due to stresses on the body and changes in the immune system. Therefore the Centers for Disease Control and Prevention (CDC) has recommended vaccination for women who will be in the second or third trimester of pregnancy during the flu season.

For additional information supporting this handout, please refer to our website: www.onemedicine.com/public/products/access

59

■ INSECT BITES AND STINGS

Insect bites can cause an allergic reaction. More people have allergic reactions to stinging insects than to biting insects.

■ SIGNS AND SYMPTOMS
- Red, swollen, warm lump or hives
- Itching, tenderness, pain
- Sores from scratching; can be infected
- Serious allergic reactions when symptoms spread (This is called anaphylaxis). These can include difficulty breathing, dizziness, nausea, diarrhea, fever, muscle spasms, or loss of consciousness. Call for emergency medical help right away.

■ WHAT CAUSES IT?
Stinging insects include bumblebees, yellow jackets, hornets, wasps, and fire and harvester ants. Biting insects include conenose bugs, mosquitoes, horseflies, deerflies, spiders, bedbugs, and black flies.

■ WHAT TO EXPECT AT YOUR PROVIDER'S OFFICE
Your health care provider will determine if you are having, or are at risk of having a serious allergic reaction. If you are having an allergic reaction, your provider will give you drugs to stop it. When you feel better, you may have a series of shots to prevent a strong reaction if you are bitten again.

■ TREATMENT OPTIONS
Large local reactions usually go away in three to seven days with no treatment. For symptom relief, use the following.
- Ice pack or wet compresses
- Antihistamines and analgesics for itching and swelling
- 1 tsp. meat tenderizer mixed with 1 tsp. water applied to bite

For a systemic reaction, your provider may prescribe the following:
- Antibiotics—if infection is suspected
- Epinephrine—repeat every 15 to 20 minutes until you are better
- Intravenous (IV) epinephrine for shock
- Injections of antihistamine (e.g., Benadryl) to decrease itching

Complementary and Alternative Therapies
Anaphylaxis requires immediate medical attention.

High doses of bioflavonoids and vitamins may reduce severity and duration of reaction.

NUTRITION
- B complex (50 to 100 mg a day), especially B_1 (50 to 100 mg one to two times a day) and B_{12} (1,000 mcg a day) can be used in prevention as a mosquito repellent.
- Vitamin C helps reduce histamine release, resulting in a milder reaction. For severe reactions take 1,000 mg every two hours to the limit of your bowel tolerance (i.e., loose stools) which may be more than 10,000 mg a day. After acute episode, take 1,000 mg three to four times a day.
- Bromelain (250 to 500 mg four times a day between meals) is a proteolytic enzyme that has anti-inflammatory effects.

HERBS
Herbs may be used as dried extracts (capsules, powders, teas), glycerites (glycerine extracts), or tinctures (alcohol extracts). Unless otherwise indi-

cated, teas should be made with 1 tsp. herb per cup of hot water. Steep covered 5 to 10 minutes for leaf or flowers, and 10 to 20 minutes for roots. Drink 2 to 4 cups per day.
- Licorice root *(Glycyrrhiza glabra)* reduces inflammation. Take 500 to 1,000 mg every three to four hours during acute reaction. Do not use licorice root if you have high blood pressure.
- Quercetin is a bioflavonoid that has powerful anti-inflammatory effects. Take 500 to 800 mg every two hours for severe reactions.
- Turmeric *(Curcuma longa)* strengthens the effects of bromelain. Take 250 to 500 mg four times a day with bromelain.
- Combine equal parts of coneflower *(Echinacea purpurea)*, cleavers *(Galium aparine)*, oat straw *(Avena sativa)*, red clover *(Trifolium pratense)*, elder *(Sambucus canadensis)*, and marigold *(Calendula officinalis)*. This is best used as a tea, 4 to 6 cups per day, to increase hydration. Tincture may be used as well (30 to 60 drops four times a day).
- Poultice of bentonite clay and goldenseal powder *(Hydrastis canadensis)* with enough water to make a paste. Add several drops of essential oil (4 to 6 drops per tbsp. of paste), such as lavender, peppermint, chamomile, or tea tree. Use this topically with severe inflammation and swelling as it has soothing properties.
- Poultice of raw grated potato or plantain leaves *(Plantago major)*.
- Make a strong tea from peppermint *(Mentha piperita)* using 1 heaping tsp. per cup. Place in spray bottle and chill. Spray on stings and bites to relieve itching.
- Witch hazel mixed with a few drops of lavender oil can be used as a cooling compress.
- Bug repellent herbs include lavender, citronella, eucalyptus, and pennyroyal. Mix 15 drops of each essential oil with one ounce of food-grade oil (for example, almond or olive). May need frequent application, three to four times per day.

HOMEOPATHY
Some of the most common remedies used for insect bites are listed below. Usually, the dose is 12X to 30C every one to four hours until your symptoms get better.
- *Aconite* for acute swelling with anxiety and fear
- *Apis mellifica* for stinging pains with rapid swelling
- *Belladonna* for rapid, intense swelling with redness and heat
- *Ledum* for puncture wounds
- Topical homeopathic preparations containing *Ledum, Arnica, Calendula, Hypericum,* or *Urtica* may provide symptomatic relief. Do not apply over broken skin.

ACUPUNCTURE
May be helpful in reducing inflammation.

■ FOLLOWING UP
Sometimes serious reactions happen again soon after the first reaction stops. Your provider may want to observe you for 8 to 12 hours.

■ SPECIAL CONSIDERATIONS
- If you have had a serious reaction to an insect bite, keep an emergency insect sting kit and wear a medical alert bracelet.
- Keep bites clean and, to prevent infection, don't scratch.
- When outdoors, avoid perfumes and floral-patterned or dark clothing.

■ INSOMNIA

Insomnia is the inability to fall or stay asleep. It often makes daytime functioning more difficult. At some time during the year, about one-third of adults suffer from insomnia.

■ SIGNS AND SYMPTOMS

- Difficulty falling asleep
- Frequent waking
- Early-morning waking
- Sense of unsatisfying sleep
- Daytime drowsiness and impaired functioning

■ WHAT CAUSES IT?

If your health care provider has ruled out physical and mental causes, your insomnia is probably a result of one of the following.

- Idiopathic insomnia—no specific cause (about half of all cases)
- Situational insomnia—caused by work, school, stress, or family stress
- Substance abuse—caffeine, alcohol, drugs, stimulants, decongestants, bronchodilators, or long-term sedative use
- Night work or jet travel across time zones
- Menopause—30 to 40 percent of menopausal women
- Age—as a person grows older, it's normal for sleep to be less deep

■ WHAT TO EXPECT AT YOUR PROVIDER'S OFFICE

Your health care provider will check for possible medical causes for your insomnia. Sleep disorders, such as sleep apnea and narcolepsy, are diagnosed by a test called a polysomnogram.

■ TREATMENT OPTIONS

Sedative drugs are often used. Side effects include daytime sleepiness, loss of muscle coordination, and addiction.

Complementary and Alternative Therapies

Herbs and nutrition can help you treat insomnia. Mind/body treatments, such as yoga, psychotherapy, and relaxation methods may be helpful.

NUTRITION

- Calcium/magnesium: regulate relaxation, especially with muscle tension and physical restlessness, 500/250 Ca/Mg twice a day
- B-complex: B vitamins are depleted under stress; however, they may be stimulating in certain individuals, so take in the morning.
- 5-HTP is a form of tryptophan particularly helpful for difficulty staying asleep. Dose is 50 mg before bed. 5-HTP will help within one week if it will help at all. Dietary sources of tryptophan include turkey, eggs, fish, dairy products, bananas, and walnuts.
- Melatonin: helps prevent jet lag. Dose is one to three mg before bed. Note that a lower dose may be effective when a higher dose is not.
- Niacinamide: muscle relaxant, gentle tranquilizer. Dose is 70 to 280 mg per day, either in divided doses during the day or at bedtime.

HERBS

Herbs may be used as dried extracts (capsules, powders, teas), glycerites (glycerine extracts), or tinctures (alcohol extracts). Unless otherwise indicated, teas should be made with 1 tsp. herb per cup of hot water. Steep covered 5 to 10 minutes for leaf or flowers, and 10 to 20 minutes for roots. Drink 2 to 4 cups per day.

- Chamomile *(Chamomilla recutita):* mild sedative, calms gastric upset. One cup of chamomile tea before bed is often all that is needed for mild insomnia. Causes gastric upset in some people.
- Lemon balm *(Melissa officinalis)* alone, or with catnip *(Nepeta cataria)*: nervous sleeping disorders and mild digestive complaints; one cup tea or 30 to 60 drops tincture one to three times a day.
- Passionflower *(Passiflora incarnata):* the above-ground (aerial) parts, taken 2 to 4 ml one half hour before bedtime.
- Valerian *(Valeriana officinalis):* sedative, soothing, bitter. Side effects of too high a dose may be nausea or grogginess. Traditionally used with passionflower *(Passiflora incarnata)* and hops *(Lupuli strobulus)* to treat acute stress. If you have depression, you should avoid hops. Dose is equal parts herb at 1 cup one to three times a day, or tincture 30 to 60 drops one to three times a day.
- Kava kava *(Piper methisticum):* spasmolytic, anxiolytic, sedative; very effective for short-term management of stress and insomnia. Do not use for more than three months without medical supervision. Dose is 15 to 30 drops ($^1/_2$ to 1 ml) tincture one to three times a day, or $^1/_4$ to $^1/_2$ ml of concentrated liquid extract three times a day.
- St. John's wort *(Hypericum perforatum):* for insomnia with anxious depression; dose is 15 to 60 drops ($^1/_2$ to 2 ml) three times a day, or 250 mg three times a day for depression. Side effects may include skin rash, sensitivity to sunlight, and gastric upset.
- Jamaican dogwood *(Piscidia piscipula):* Jamaican dogwood is a powerful remedy for insomnia, particularly when the sleeplessness is due to nervous tension and pain. Taken 1 to 2 ml just before bedtime. Jamaican dogwood combines well with passionflower, valerian, kava and St. John's wort.
- Essential oils (three to five drops added to a bath): commonly used herbs are lavender *(Lavendula officianalis),* rosemary *(Rosemarinus officinalis),* and chamomile *(Chamomilla recutita).*

HOMEOPATHY

Some of the most common remedies used for insomnia are listed below. Usually, the dose is 12X to 30C every one to four hours until your symptoms get better.

- *Arsenicum alba* for insomnia caused by anxiety
- *Nux vomica* for insomnia from overuse of stimulants, caffeine, drugs
- *Coffea cruda* for insomnia from a racing mind, especially if the stress is caused by adjusting to a positive event
- *Ignatia imara* for insomnia (or excessive sleeping) after grief

ACUPUNCTURE

May be effective at treating both insomnia and some of its underlying causes.

MASSAGE

May be beneficial for its overall relaxing properties.

■ FOLLOWING UP

Often insomnia stops when the stressful events in your life end.

■ SPECIAL CONSIDERATIONS

Establishing good sleep habits is the best method to avoid insomnia. A healthy diet and regular exercise also help. Alcohol disrupts the quality of sleep, so regular use before bed should be avoided.

■ INTESTINAL PARASITES

There are two main types of intestinal parasites: helminths and proto-zoa. Helminths are worms with many cells. Usually, helminths cannot multiply in the human body and will eventually clear up without infecting you again. Protozoa have only one cell. They can multiply inside the human body.

■ SIGNS AND SYMPTOMS

Symptoms include the following.

- Diarrhea
- Nausea or vomiting
- Gas or bloating
- Dysentery (loose stools containing blood and mucus)
- Rash or itching around the rectum or vulva
- Stomach pain or tenderness
- Feeling tired
- Weight loss
- Passing a worm in your stool

■ WHAT CAUSES IT?

The following factors put you at higher risk for getting intestinal parasites.

- Living in or visiting an area known to have parasites
- International travel
- Poor sanitation (for both food and water)
- Poor personal cleanliness
- Age—children are more likely to get infected
- Exposure to child and institutional care centers
- Acquired immune deficiency syndrome (AIDS)

■ WHAT TO EXPECT AT YOUR PROVIDER'S OFFICE

Your health care provider will ask if you have traveled overseas recently and whether you have recently lost weight. Your provider will examine you. If he or she thinks you have an intestinal parasite, you will probably have one or more of the following tests.

- Fecal testing (examination of your stool) can identify both helminths and protozoa. Stool samples must be collected before antidiarrhea drugs or antibiotics are given, or X-rays with barium are taken. Three (five for pinworm) stool samples are needed to find the parasite.
- The string test is used occasionally. For this test, you swallow a string that is then pulled back up. Then samples of your stomach contents on the string are tested.
- The "Scotch tape" test identifies pinworm by placing tape around the anus at night.
- Your health care provider may use X-rays with barium to diagnose more serious problems caused by parasites, although this is usually not required.

■ TREATMENT OPTIONS

Drug Therapies

Your health care provider will choose the drug most effective against your intestinal parasite. Drug treatment may be just one dose or several over a period of weeks. Be careful to take the medicine just as it is prescribed or it may not work.

Complementary and Alternative Therapies

While alternative treatments may be helpful in getting rid of intestinal parasites, your health care provider must find out what kind of organism is causing your problems before you start treatment. The following nutritional guidelines will help keep organisms from growing. It is impor-tant to maintain good bowel habits during treatment.

NUTRITION

- Avoid simple carbohydrates such as are found in refined foods, fruits, juices, dairy products, and all sugars.
- Eliminate caffeine and alcohol.
- Eat more raw garlic, pumpkin seeds, pomegranates, beets, and car-rots, all of which have antiworm properties. Drink a lot of water and get plenty of dietary fiber to promote good bowel elimination.
- Digestive enzymes will help restore your intestinal tract to its normal state, which makes it inhospitable to parasites. Papain taken 30 min-utes before or after meals helps kill worms. Acidophilus supplements help normalize bowel bacteria (one capsule with meals).
- Vitamin C (1,000 mg three to four times a day), zinc (20 to 30 mg per day), and beta-carotene (100,000 IU per day) support the immune system.

HERBS

Herbs are generally a safe way to strengthen and tone the body's systems. As with any therapy, it is important to work with your health care provider on getting your problem diagnosed before you start any treatment. Herbs may be used as dried extracts (capsules, powders, teas), glycerites (glycer-ine extracts), or tinctures (alcohol extracts). Many of the herbs used to treat intestinal parasites have toxic side effects. Use them only under the supervision of a qualified practitioner. He or she will treat you with the most gentle herb that is effective for the type of parasite you have.

HOMEOPATHY

Some of the most common remedies used for intestinal parasites are listed below. Usually, the dose is 12X to 30C every one to four hours until your symptoms get better.

- *Cina* is specific for pinworms; with restless agitation and itching rectum
- *Rumex crispus* for marked itching immediately on undressing
- *Spigellia* for worm infestations with piercing and sharp pains

MASSAGE

May help stimulate bowel function and elimination.

■ FOLLOWING UP

Your health care provider will retest your stool to be sure your parasite is gone, and will give you advice to help you avoid reinfection. Follow these instructions carefully. Getting a parasite a second time can cause more serious health problems.

■ SPECIAL CONSIDERATIONS

The seriousness and length of illness varies with the specific intestinal par-asite. Complications occur more often in older people and in people who already have serious illnesses, such as AIDS.

Intestinal parasites can be more serious if you are pregnant. Your health care provider will tell you which drugs are safe to take during pregnancy. Treatment for intestinal parasites during pregnancy should be closely mon-itored by a qualified practitioner.

■ IRRITABLE BOWEL SYNDROME

Irritable bowel syndrome (IBS) occurs when muscles in your intestines contract faster or slower than normal. This causes pain, cramping, gassiness, sudden bouts of diarrhea, and constipation.

Two types of IBS exist. In spastic colon IBS, you experience constipation, diarrhea, or both, and you often have pain after eating. Painless diarrhea IBS involves the sudden onset of diarrhea during or after meals, or upon waking. Between 10 and 20 percent of the population has IBS at some time. The syndrome often starts in adolescents or young adults. It affects three times as many women as men and is often associated with stress.

■ SIGNS AND SYMPTOMS

- Cramping pain in your lower abdomen
- Bloating and gassiness
- Changes in your bowel habits
- Diarrhea or constipation, or both alternately
- Immediate need to move your bowels when you wake up or during or after meals
- Relief of pain after bowel movements
- Feeling of incomplete emptying after bowel movements
- Mucus in your stool

■ WHAT CAUSES IT?

The underlying cause remains unknown. But the syndrome has no relation to actual disease, and it does not lead to other diseases.

■ WHAT TO EXPECT AT YOUR PROVIDER'S OFFICE

Your health care provider will feel your abdomen to check for signs of pain. He or she will place a gloved finger in your rectum to check its condition. If you're female, you may have a pelvic examination. The provider may use a sigmoidoscope—a flexible instrument inserted into the rectum—to examine your lower colon. You may be asked to provide three days' worth of stool samples. Your provider may also want samples of your blood and urine. The provider may also want an ultrasound or X-rays.

■ TREATMENT OPTIONS

Try to avoid stressful situations that have triggered IBS in the past. Try to establish regular bowel habits.

Drug Therapies

Several "anticholinergic agents," prescribed by your provider, can reduce the pain of spasm. If you have diarrhea, antidiarrheal medications can help.

Complementary and Alternative Therapies

IBS has many underlying causes that can often be successfully treated with alternative therapies. Stress reduction techniques through biofeedback, hypnosis, or counseling can help you deal with stress.

NUTRITION

- Removal of known food allergens or irritants is important. The most common food allergens are dairy products, wheat, corn, peanuts, citrus, soy, eggs, fish, and tomatoes. An elimination/challenge trial may help uncover sensitivities. Eliminate all suspected allergens from the diet for two weeks. Add back one food every three days and wait for reaction to the challenge.
- If you suffer from gassiness, eliminate beans, cabbages, and other "gassy" vegetables from your diet, as well as apple juice, grape juice, bananas, nuts, and raisins.
- Fiber supplementation can help reduce pain, cramping, and gas. Supplements include psyllium, flax meal, slippery elm (*Ulmus rubra*) powder, and marshmallow root (*Althea officinalis*) powder.
- Digestive enzymes taken 20 minutes before meals can help enhance digestion and normalize bowel function.
- One teaspoon of raw bran with each meal, supplemented by extra fluids, provides fiber reliably.
- Pro-flora supplements such as acidophilus and lactobacillus species taken two to three times per day can help to rebalance normal bowel bacteria and reduce gas and bloating.
- Magnesium 200 mg two to three times per day and B-complex (50 to 100 mg per day) with extra B_5 (pantothenic acid; 100 mg per day) may help reduce the effects of stress.
- Low-fat diets may relieve abdominal pain following meals.

HERBS

Herbs may be used as dried extracts (capsules, powders, teas), glycerites (glycerine extracts), or tinctures (alcohol extracts). Unless otherwise indicated, teas should be made with 1 tsp. herb per cup of hot water. Steep covered 5 to 10 minutes for leaf or flowers, and 10 to 20 minutes for roots. Drink 2 to 4 cups per day.

- Enteric-coated peppermint oil: one to two capsules (0.2 ml peppermint oil per capsule) three times a day after meals
- A tea of fennel seed (*Foeniculum vulgare*) or ginger root (*Zingiber officinalis*) taken after meals promotes good digestion.
- A tincture of equal parts of the following before meals (30 drops three times per day): valerian (*Valeriana officinalis*), passionflower (*Passiflora incarnata*), anise seed (*Pimpinella anisum*) extract, meadowsweet (*Filependula ulmaria*), wild yam (*Dioscorea villosa*), and milk thistle (*Silybum marianum*)

HOMEOPATHY

Homeopathy may be useful as a supportive therapy.

PHYSICAL MEDICINE

- Electric heating pads, hot water bottles, and long hot baths can relieve painful spasms and cramping in the abdomen.
- Regular exercise, such as walking, can reduce stress and encourage bowel movements if you are constipated.
- Castor oil pack. Apply oil directly to skin, cover with a clean soft cloth and plastic wrap. Place a heat source over the pack and let sit for 30 to 60 minutes.
- Abdominal breathing helps to induce the relaxation response and may aid normal physiological functioning (such as digestion).

ACUPUNCTURE

Acupuncture can help relieve IBS episodes.

MASSAGE

Therapeutic massage may help in reducing the effects of stress.

■ FOLLOWING UP

Be aware that the syndrome itself may cause you stress.

■ LARYNGITIS

With laryngitis, the voice box and the area around it become irritated and swollen. When you have the condition, you will find your voice changing. You may find yourself unable to speak above a whisper, or even lose your voice entirely for a few days. Laryngitis rarely causes serious trouble in adults. But it can cause complications in children—notably croup, a swelling of the throat that makes it seem as if a child has something caught in his or her throat.

■ SIGNS AND SYMPTOMS

- An unnatural change in your voice
- Hoarseness
- Loss of your voice
- Tickling, scratchiness, and rawness in your throat
- A constant urge to clear your throat
- Fever, general feeling of lethargy and tiredness, and difficulty breathing mark more severe cases

■ WHAT CAUSES IT?

Viruses or bacteria infect the larynx, or voice box, and cause it to swell. That produces irritation and soreness, and changes the voice, making you sound hoarse and unable to speak above a whisper, or even causing you to lose your voice entirely for a few days. Often, the virus comes from another ailment, such as a cold, the flu, or bronchitis. Overuse of your voice, by screaming or shouting for long periods, can worsen the irritation and swelling produced by the infection. Smokers and people who work around fumes to which they are allergic often have chronic laryngitis.

■ WHAT TO EXPECT AT YOUR PROVIDER'S OFFICE

Your health care provider will examine your throat and take a culture if it looks red. Your provider will also use a device that looks like a dentist's mirror to examine your throat and larynx. This procedure, called indirect laryngoscopy, enables him or her to check for swelling.

■ TREATMENT OPTIONS

In most cases you can treat laryngitis yourself. Expect to rest your voice for a week or so. Avoid any irritants that might affect your larynx, such as tobacco smoke and cold air. Stay clear of alcohol. Plenty of rest can also speed your recovery. You can also take a more active role in relieving your symptoms by drinking plenty of warm fluids. Broth, honey, lemon juice, and weak tea can all soothe irritation and scratchiness. Gargle several times a day with 1/2 teaspoon of salt in a glass of warm water. Inhale warm steam (cover your head with a towel and lean over a pan of simmering water). Alternatively, take frequent hot showers, or use a humidifier. If your children have laryngitis, make sure that they rest as much as possible.

Drug Therapies

If you have a bacterial infection, your health care provider will prescribe an antibiotic. Amoxicillin and tetracycline are the most common. Take all the pills prescribed, even if you feel better, to ensure that the infection doesn't return. If your laryngitis is related to allergies, your health care provider may recommend antihistamines and inhaled steroids.

Complementary and Alternative Therapies

Alternative treatments may be effective in cases of acute, chronic, or recurrent laryngitis.

NUTRITION

- Zinc lozenges (as commercially available): boosts the immune system and relieves soreness.
- Vitamin C (1,000 mg three to four times per day): needed for proper immune function and to strengthen mucous membranes.
- B-complex (50 to 100 mg per day): enhances immune function, especially during stress.

HERBS

Herbs are generally a safe way to strengthen and tone the body's systems. As with any therapy, it is important to work with your provider on getting your problem diagnosed before you start any treatment. Herbs may be used as dried extracts (capsules, powders, teas), glycerites (glycerine extracts), or tinctures (alcohol extracts). Unless otherwise indicated, teas should be made with 1 tsp. herb per cup of hot water. Steep covered 5 to 10 minutes for leaf or flowers, and 10 to 20 minutes for roots. Drink 2 to 4 cups per day. Tinctures may be used singly or in combination as noted.

- Slippery elm *(Ulmus rubra)* soothes irritated tissues and promotes healing.
- Licorice *(Glycyrrhiza glabra)* has antiviral properties and is soothing to the throat. Do not take licorice if you have high blood pressure.

Gargles: Use 5 drops of each tincture listed below in $1/4$ cup of water. Gargle and swallow four to six times a day.

- Laryngitis gargle: Coneflower *(Echinacea purpurea)*, sage *(Salvia officinalis)*, and marigold *(Calendula officinalis)* are soothing and anti-inflammatory herbs.
- Antimicrobial gargle: Coneflower, goldenseal *(Hydrastis canadensis)*, and myrrh *(Commiphora molmol)* are antibacterial and immune-stimulating herbs. (Use goldenseal with caution during pregnancy.)
- Pain-relief gargle: Propolis, peppermint *(Mentha piperita)*, and ginger *(Zingiber officinalis)* are antimicrobial and pain-relieving herbs.

HOMEOPATHY

Some of the most common remedies used for laryngitis are listed below. Usually, the dose is 12X to 30C every one to four hours until your symptoms get better.

- *Aconite* for laryngitis that comes on after a shock
- *Spongia tosta* for laryngitis from coughing
- Phosphorus for hoarseness that is painless or with burning pains
- *Arum* for laryngitis from overuse of larynx
- *Causticum* for hoarseness that comes with every cold

ACUPUNCTURE

Acupuncture may be helpful in enhancing immune function.

MASSAGE

Therapeutic massage is helpful in reducing the effects of stress.

■ FOLLOWING UP

Check back with your health care provider if the laryngitis outlasts your other symptoms. If you smoke, stop.

■ SPECIAL CONSIDERATIONS

Call your health care provider if you have problems breathing or swallowing, if your throat bleeds, or if you have a high temperature.

■ LOW BACK PAIN

Low back pain affects 60 to 80 percent of the adult U.S. population at one time or another. Low back problems affect the spine's flexibility, stability, and strength, which can cause pain, discomfort, and stiffness.

■ SIGNS AND SYMPTOMS

- Tenderness, pain, and stiffness in the lower back
- Pain that radiates into the buttocks or legs
- Difficulty standing erect or standing in one position for a long time
- Discomfort while sitting
- Weakness and leg fatigue while walking

■ WHAT CAUSES IT?

Low back pain is usually caused by strain from lifting, twisting, or bending. However, some low back pain can be a symptom of a more serious condition, such as an infection, a rheumatic or arthritic condition, or ovarian cysts. It may be caused by a ruptured or bulging disk, the strong, spongy, gel-filled cushions that lie between each vertebra. Compression fractures of the bones in the spine can also cause low back pain, especially in older women with osteoporosis. In addition, poor overall fitness, smoking, and general life dissatisfaction increase a person's risk for low back problems.

■ WHAT TO EXPECT AT YOUR PROVIDER'S OFFICE

Your health care provider will ask you to stand, sit, and move. He or she will likely check your reflexes and perhaps your response to touch, slight heat, or a pinprick. He or she may also recommend strength testing on a treadmill. You may also need a blood test, X rays, a magnetic resonance imaging scan, or computed tomography scan.

■ TREATMENT OPTIONS

In general, low back pain can be relieved and prevented with lifestyle changes. Exercising to strengthen your muscles, maintaining a healthy weight, and practicing good posture lowers your risk. Learning to bend and lift properly, sleeping on a firm mattress, sitting in supportive chairs, and wearing supportive shoes are important factors. For long-term back pain, your provider may recommend stronger medications or surgery.

Drug Therapies

If you have an episode of low back pain, your health care provider will likely recommend one to two days of bed rest and 10 days of nonsteroidal anti-inflammatory drugs (NSAIDS) such as ibuprofen.

Complementary and Alternative Therapies

Alternative therapies can be effective for easing muscle tension, correcting spinal imbalances, relieving discomfort, and averting long-term back problems by improving muscle strength and joint stability.

NUTRITION

- B-complex: B_1 (50 to 100 mg), B_2 (50 mg), B_3 (25 mg); B_5 (100 mg); B_6 (50 to 100 mg); B_{12} (100 to 1,000 mcg), folate (400 mcg per day) all reduced with stress and pain
- Vitamin E (400 IU per day), vitamin C (1,000 to 3,000 mg per day)
- Calcium (1,500 to 2,000 mg) and magnesium (700 to 1,000 mg) to regulate muscle contraction and ease spasm
- Bromelain (250 to 500 mg three times per day on an empty stomach) anti-inflammatory, works especially well with turmeric

HERBS

Herbs may be used as dried extracts (capsules, powders, teas), glycerites (glycerine extracts), or tinctures (alcohol extracts). Teas should be made with 1 tsp. herb per cup of hot water. Steep covered 5 to 10 minutes for leaf or flowers;10 to 20 minutes for roots. Mix three to six of the following (one cup tea or 30 to 60 drops of tincture three to six times per day).

- Relaxants: Black haw *(Viburnum prunifolium)* relaxant; petasites *(Petasites hybridus),* acute muscle spasm, not for long-term use; valerian *(Valeriana officinalis),* antispasmodic, especially with sleeplessness; wild yam *(Dioscorea villosa),* antispasmodic, especially with joint pains and long-term stress; turmeric anti-inflammatory, especially with digestive problems; Jamaican dogwood *(Piscidea piscipula),* relaxant
- Pain relief: White willow bark *(Salix alba),* anti-inflammatory and analgesic; devil's claw *(Harpagophytum procumbens),* analgesic, anti-inflammatory; St. John's wort *(Hypericum perforatum),* anti-inflammatory
- Circulatory stimulants: rosemary leaves *(Rosemariana officinalis),* especially with digestive problems; gingko *(Ginkgo biloba),* especially with poor circulation
- Topical treatment may be helpful for acute problems. Mix one to two drops of essential oil or 5 to 10 drops of tincture into 1 tbsp. vegetable oil, and rub into the affected area. St. John's wort for nerve pain; leopard's bane *(Arnica montana)* anti-inflammatory, external use only; lobelia *(Lobelia inflata)* antispasmodic

HOMEOPATHY

Some of the most common remedies for this condition are listed below.

- *Aesculus* for dull pain with muscle weakness
- *Arnica montana* especially with pain as a result of trauma
- *Colocynthis* for weakness and cramping in the small of the back
- *Gnaphalium* for sciatica that alternates with numbness
- *Lycopodium* for burning pain, especially with gas or bloating
- *Rhus toxicodendron* for stiffness and pain in the small of the back

PHYSICAL MEDICINE

- Chiropractic or osteopathic manipulation can help relieve pain.
- Contrast hydrotherapy. Alternate hot and cold applications. Alternate three minutes hot with one minute cold. Repeat three times. This is one set. Do two to three sets per day.
- Castor oil pack. Apply oil directly to skin, cover with a clean soft cloth and plastic wrap. Place a heat source over the pack and let sit for 30 to 60 minutes.

ACUPUNCTURE

May help relieve spasm and increase circulation to the affected area.

MASSAGE

Massage may be helpful both acutely and to prevent chronic problems.

■ SPECIAL CONSIDERATIONS

Chronic low back problems can interfere with everyday activities, sleep, and concentration. When symptoms are severe, your mood and sexuality may be affected. While depression is usually not the cause of chronic low back pain, it often complicates treatment.

■ MENOPAUSE

Menopause marks the end of a woman's reproductive years. It is a normal biological event (except with surgery). Women begin menopause at the average age of 51. Although women now live longer, the age at which menopause begins has not changed. This means most women will live a third of their lives after menopause.

■ SIGNS AND SYMPTOMS

- Menstrual bleeding slows and then stops; process takes about four years
- Hot flashes—flushing of face and upper trunk; may occur with heart palpitations, dizziness, headaches
- Night sweats—depression and irritability may result from insomnia
- Cold hands and feet
- Vaginal symptoms—dryness, bleeding after intercourse, itching
- More frequent urination, burning, nighttime urination
- Depression, irritability, tension; usually occurs with sleep disturbances
- Facial hair growth and wrinkles
- Osteoporosis—bone breaks become more likely
- Coronary heart disease (CHD)—twice as many women die from CHD than cancer

■ WHAT CAUSES IT?

Lower estrogen and progesterone production--as the result of fewer functioning follicles (the cell structure that houses the eggs)--leads to the end of menstruation. There may be a genetic link for the age of onset. Smoking lowers the age at which menopause begins.

■ WHAT TO EXPECT AT YOUR PROVIDER'S OFFICE

Your health care provider will give you an examination that includes a Pap smear and will describe the benefits and risks of different treatments.

■ TREATMENT OPTIONS

Drug Therapies

- Estrogen helps relieve hot flashes and vaginal symptoms. Estrogen slows osteoporotic bone loss and fractures. It may prevent CHD and Alzheimer's disease. Estrogen increases your risk of breast cancer, uterine cancer, gallbladder disease, and blood clotting. Side effects include bloating, nausea, adult-onset asthma, and breast tenderness.
- Estradiol is another type of estrogen. It brings the estrogen directly into your bloodstream. Estradiol is available in a patch or gel.
- Vaginal estrogen creams help vaginal and urinary symptoms. It takes four to six weeks for the cream to work. There is a new intravaginal ring that slowly releases estrogen.
- Progesterone prevents uterine cancer that occurs with estrogen therapy.
- Methyltestosterone increases libido and may decrease osteoporosis of the spine. Facial hair growth is a side effect.
- Alendronate is as effective as estrogen in preventing osteoporosis.
- Aspirin is an alternative treatment for CHD.

Complementary and Alternative Therapies

Alternative medicine has much to offer for improving cardiovascular health and preventing osteoporosis. Relaxation techniques, stress management, yoga, and meditation can help with perimenopausal symptoms. Exercise increases endorphin release, which helps relieve pain and elevates mood. Walking, swimming, and biking are less stressful on the joints.

NUTRITION

- Soy (25 to 50 mg soy a day) contains soy isoflavones (phytoestrogens), which may relieve hot flashes and vaginal symptoms and offer increased protection from osteoporosis and breast cancer.
- Vitamin E (400 to 1,600 IU a day) can balance vasomotor instability, decrease hot flashes, and is cardioprotective. High doses are not recommended for women with high blood pressure.
- Take calcium/magnesium (1,000/500 mg a day for women taking estrogen and 1,500/750 mg a day for those who are not) with meals. Citrate or citramate forms may be the most absorbable forms.
- Avoiding smoking, alcohol, caffeine, and spicy foods may help decrease hot flashes.
- A combination of vitamin C (1,200 mg), hesperidin (900 mg), and hesperidin methyl chalcone (900 mg) may relieve hot flashes.
- Gamma-oryzanol (from rice bran oil) 300 mg per day gives partial or total relief of hot flashes in over 80 percent of users.

HERBS

Herbs may be used as dried extracts (capsules, powders, teas), glycerites (glycerine extracts), or tinctures (alcohol extracts). Teas should be made with 1 tsp. herb per cup of hot water. Steep covered 5 to 10 minutes for leaf or flowers; 10 to 20 minutes for roots. Drink 2 to 4 cups per day.

- Black cohosh (*Cimicifuga racemosa*) relieves vasomotor symptoms and depression; Remifemin is the most tested extract of black cohosh. Long-term use is safe; 2 mg a day
- Chaste tree (*Vitex agnes-castus*) for irregular menstrual cycles; may take up to six months for full therapeutic effect
- Angelica (*Angelica archangelica*) relieves vasomotor symptoms.
- Licorice (*Glycyrrhiza glabra*), an estrogen-balancing herb especially for chronic stress; do not use if you have high blood pressure; 250 mg three times a day, 30 to 60 drops tincture three times a day, or 1 cup of tea three times a day
- Ginkgo (*Ginkgo biloba*) improves circulation to cold hands and feet; also used to treat depression; may take up to 12 weeks for full effect; 120 mg two to three times a day

HOMEOPATHY

Some of the most common remedies used are listed below. Usually, the dose is 12X to 30C every one to four hours until your symptoms get better.

- *Mulimen*—German combination remedy (chasteberry, black cohosh, St. John's wort, cuttlefish ink) for hot flashes
- Homeopathic estrogen—by prescription only
- *Ferrum phosphoricum, graphites, lycopodium*—for symptoms occurring during sexual intercourse
- *Amyl nitrosum, lachesis, sulphur*—for hot flashes

PHYSICAL MEDICINE

Kegel exercises increase pelvic muscle tone, helping to prevent incontinence and bladder or uterine prolapse.

ACUPUNCTURE

Acupuncture enhances endorphin release and stimulates kidney function. It may also help to balance hormones and relieve vasomotor symptoms.

MASSAGE

Massage increases circulation. Use water-soluble, nonestrogen lubricants, vegetable oil, or vitamin E oil for vaginal atrophy.

■ MOTION SICKNESS

Motion sickness is nausea and dizziness that occurs when traveling in a moving vehicle such as a car, boat, or airplane.

■ SIGNS AND SYMPTOMS

Motion sickness can produce the following symptoms.

- Dizziness
- Paleness
- Cold sweating
- Excess saliva production
- Nausea
- Vomiting
- Fatigue
- Headache

■ WHAT CAUSES IT?

Motion sickness happens when signals from the balance system of your body conflict with visual cues. For example, your body may sense rolling motions that you cannot see from inside a ship's cabin. Conversely, during a "virtual reality" simulation, your eyes perceive movement that your body does not experience. In addition, the structures of your inner ears can become unbalanced.

It is not known why some people develop motion sickness and others do not. Motion sickness is more likely to be seen in young people, women, and people of Asian ancestry. Those who are fearful and anxious during a trip, or who more frequently experience nausea or vomiting, may also be prone to motion sickness.

■ WHAT TO EXPECT AT YOUR PROVIDER'S OFFICE

Motion sickness generally clears up once you leave the car, boat, or airplane, so you'll rarely find yourself in a health care provider's office during an episode. But your provider may be able to recommend ways to prevent and treat the condition for your next trip.

■ TREATMENT OPTIONS

Antihistamines are effective for both prevention and treatment. These products should not be used if you have breathing problems, glaucoma, or an enlarged prostate that causes difficulty when you urinate. Antihistamines often cause drowsiness and should not be used while driving. The drowsiness effect is more pronounced with some antihistamines than with others; ask your health care provider which one is best for you.

For longer trips, you might want to try a scopolamine patch placed behind an ear six to eight hours before you travel. The effects of it last up to three days. Side effects may include dry mouth, drowsiness, blurred vision, and disorientation.

Complementary and Alternative Therapies

Digestive herbs or homeopathic remedies may be helpful in preventing and relieving motion sickness. As with most therapies, alternative therapies for motion sickness are best used before the onset of symptoms.

NUTRITION

Avoid alcohol and caffeine. If you have respiratory problems, eliminate foods that produce inflammation and mucus, such as dairy products, fruit, and sugar. Ginger root *(Zingiber officinalis)* sliced and chewed may prevent the onset of motion sickness. Encapsulated ginger, crystallized ginger,

or ginger snaps may also help. Ginger has been shown to be more effective than antihistamines if taken one hour before traveling. Sips of lemon water may help relieve nausea during an episode.

HERBS

Herbs are generally a safe way to strengthen and tone the body's systems. As with any therapy, it is important to work with your health care provider on getting your problem diagnosed before you start any treatment. Herbs may be used as dried extracts (capsules, powders, teas), glycerites (glycerine extracts), or tinctures (alcohol extracts). Unless otherwise indicated, teas should be made with 1 tsp. herb per cup of hot water. Steep covered 5 to 10 minutes for leaf or flowers, and 10 to 20 minutes for roots. Drink 2 to 4 cups per day.

- Ginger root *(Zingiber officinalis)* in a tea (frequent small sips) or tincture (30 drops in $1/2$ cup of water as needed). May add peppermint *(Mentha piperita)* or chamomile *(Matricaria recutita)* if there is vomiting.
- Black horehound *(Ballota nigra)* may help relieve nausea secondary to inner ear problems. May be used as tea (1 cup three times per day) or tincture (30 drops three times per day).

HOMEOPATHY

Some of the most common remedies used for motion sickness are listed below. For acute prescribing use 3 to 5 pellets of a 12X to 30C remedy every one to four hours until acute symptoms resolve.

- *Cocculus* for motion sickness from watching moving objects
- *Petroleum* for motion sickness with cold sensation in the abdomen
- *Tabacum* for unrelenting nausea with cold sweat

ACUPUNCTURE

Acupressure may reduce symptoms of sea sickness. Use "Sea Bands" as commercially available.

MASSAGE

Massage or other relaxation techniques may help control motion sickness.

■ FOLLOWING UP

Take steps to prevent motion sickness on your next trip.

- Avoid reading while traveling.
- Focus on the view outside.
- Be the driver; the one in control is less likely to experience motion sickness.
- Get plenty of fresh air.
- Avoid eating or drinking heavily.
- Look for a seat or cabin near the center of the vehicle, where it moves the least.

If you do get sick, don't despair. Motion sickness generally clears up soon after you stop traveling, and has no long-term complications. Report any unusual side effects from motion-sickness medications to your health care provider.

■ SPECIAL CONSIDERATIONS

Pregnant women with nausea from morning sickness are more likely to experience motion sickness. You should not take antihistamines if you are pregnant. Talk with your health care provider before taking any medications or supplements during pregnancy.

For additional information supporting this handout, please refer to our website: www.onemedicine.com/public/products/access   67

Copyright ©2000 Integrative Medicine Communications • 1029 Chestnut St., Newton, MA 02464 • T 877-426-6633 • F 877-426-6630

■ MYOCARDIAL INFARCTION

Myocardial infarction (MI) is also called a heart attack. A heart attack occurs when an artery leading to the heart becomes totally blocked. A heart attack is a medical emergency. Seek immediate medical attention if you or someone else is having the symptoms listed below.

■ SIGNS AND SYMPTOMS

- Pain, heaviness, tightness, burning—in chest, back, left arm, jaw, neck
- Difficulty breathing
- Dizziness, weakness
- Nausea, vomiting
- Irregular heartbeat

■ WHAT CAUSES IT?

Atherosclerosis, the process of plaque buildup in an artery until it becomes closed, is the most frequent cause of heart attacks. Heart attacks can also result from heart-muscle spasms or hereditary heart problems. The following increase your risk of getting a heart attack.

- Smoking
- High-fat diet, excess body weight
- Family history of early MI
- Diabetes
- Oral contraceptives
- Hypertension (high blood pressure)
- Being male, or a female who has gone through menopause
- Cocaine or amphetamine abuse

■ WHAT TO EXPECT AT YOUR PROVIDER'S OFFICE

If you think that you are having a heart attack, call for medical assistance immediately. Treating a heart attack within 90 minutes can save a person's life. In the emergency room, the following three things will happen very quickly to determine if you are having a heart attack.

- You will have an electrocardiogram (EKG).
- A health care provider will ask you about your symptoms and perform a physical examination.
- You will have a blood test to evaluate your cardiac enzyme levels.

■ TREATMENT OPTIONS

Blood must be brought back to the affected area of the heart immediately. Three methods for doing this are drug therapy, angioplasty (using one of several methods to clear the blocked blood vessel, such as inflating a balloon inside it or holding it open with a device called a stent), and surgery.

Drug Therapies

Your health care provider may prescribe one or several drugs to help bring blood back to the blocked artery, keep your heartbeat regular, lower your blood pressure, control pain, and improve blood flow. These drugs may include aspirin, heparin, nitroglycerin, beta blockers, and angotensin-converting enzyme (ACE) inhibitors.

Complementary and Alternative Therapies

Alternative therapies are most appropriate to reduce your risk of a first MI, minimize damage from an MI, and reduce the risk of a subsequent MI. It is important that you first get your condition diagnosed and stabilized by a medical professional.

NUTRITION

- L-carnitine (9 grams per day intravenously for five days, then 6 grams per day by mouth for 12 months) within 24 hours of onset of chest pain decreases left ventricular dilation.
- A diet high in antioxidants (vitamin C, vitamin E, and beta-carotene) and soluble dietary fiber, and low in fat is beneficial.
- Bromelain (400 to 800 mg per day) may help dissolve plaque.

HERBS

Herbs should not be used in place of immediate medical attention. Herbs can be used as general heart tonics and specifically applied to treating conditions associated with MI, such as atherosclerosis, congestive heart failure, high cholesterol levels, high blood pressure, and high fat levels in the blood.

HOMEOPATHY

Homeopathy should never be used instead of immediate medical attention.

PHYSICAL MEDICINE

Beneficial for rehabilitation

ACUPUNCTURE

Useful for pain and rehabilitation

MASSAGE

Beneficial for rehabilitation and prevention

■ FOLLOWING UP

You may reduce your risk of heart attack by avoiding known risk factors. Get aerobic exercise (such as walking, biking, or swimming) for at least 20 minutes three times per week. If you haven't exercised much in the past, walking is a great way to start. Reducing stress can also help lower your risk of MI. Learn stress-reduction techniques such as deep breathing and meditation. Gentle exercise such as yoga and tai chi can also help you reduce your stress level. Eat a low-fat diet and stay at the proper weight.

If you have diabetes or high blood pressure, follow your health care provider's instructions to keep it under control. If you are a woman and have gone through menopause, you may want to consider hormone replacement therapy—it can lower your risk of heart disease. Talk to your provider about your options.

■ OBESITY

Obesity is excess body fat. Approximately 33 percent of Americans 20 to 75 years of age are overweight, and of these, approximately one third are severely obese.

■ SIGNS AND SYMPTOMS

A person whose BMI is greater than 30 (your weight in kilograms divided by the square of your height in meters).

■ WHAT CAUSES IT?

Being overweight usually reflects a poor diet, poor eating habits, and a lack of exercise. Genetics may also play a role. There are a number of rare syndromes that cause obesity. The following factors can put you at risk.

- Other family members are obese
- Overeating or a high-fat diet
- Little or no physical activity
- Some prescription medications
- Psychological factors (such as death of a loved one)

■ WHAT TO EXPECT AT YOUR PROVIDER'S OFFICE

Your health care provider will give you a thorough physical examination and will take blood samples to measure blood sugar and cholesterol levels. He or she will also check your blood pressure.

■ TREATMENT OPTIONS

Lifestyle changes, such as eating better and exercising more, are essential. Your health care provider may suggest drugs to help with your weight loss; however, most cannot be taken over the long term.

Complementary and Alternative Therapies

Alternative therapies can help stabilize blood sugars, promote a customize-tailored exercise plan, and treat emotional well-being. Mind/body techniques can be helpful.

NUTRITION

- Protein: You may do better with a high protein, low carbohydrate diet.
- Fluid: 6 to 8 glasses daily of nonsugared, caffeine-free drinks.
- Fiber: increasing dietary fiber (for example, fruits and vegetables) promotes weight loss.
- Allergies: Many people find that avoiding allergenic foods (wheat, dairy, soy, peanuts, eggs, and citrus) improves digestion.
- Multiple vitamin to address dietary imbalances.
- Chromium picolinate (200 to 500 mcg, once or twice per day): increases insulin sensitivity, and stabilizes blood sugars.
- Vitamin C (3,000 to 6,000 mg per day): speeds up metabolism and is needed for cholesterol metabolism.
- Essential fatty acids (primrose oil, 2 to 4 g per day; flaxseed oil): one study showed reduction in appetite and some weight loss.
- Lecithin, choline, methionine (1 g per day of each): aids proper fat metabolism and decreases fat cravings.
- Thiamine (2.5 mg per day): plays a role in fatty-acid metabolism and may decrease ketone formation; increased ketones may play a role in hunger; to avoid imbalance, supplement with a B-complex: B_1 (50 to 100 mg), B_2 (50 mg), B_3 (25 mg); B_5 (100 mg); B_6 (50 to 100 mg), B_{12} (100 to 1,000 mcg), folate (400 mcg) per day.
- Kelp (1,000 to 2,000 mg per day, equivalent to 250 to 500 mcg of iodine per day): may aid in weight loss because it provides nutrients for thyroid functioning.
- L-glutamine (1,000 mg three times per day): may blunt carbohydrate craving.
- Coenzyme Q10 is important in fatty-acid metabolism, may help break down fat into energy.
- 5-Hydroxytryptophan (5-HTP; 100 to 300 mg per day): reduces food intake by making you feel full. It acts as an anti-depressant.

HERBS

Herbs may be used as dried extracts (capsules, powders, teas), glycerites (glycerine extracts), or tinctures (alcohol extracts). Unless otherwise indicated, teas should be made with 1 tsp. herb per cup of hot water. Steep covered 5 to 10 minutes for leaf or flowers, and 10 to 20 minutes for roots. Drink 2 to 4 cups per day.

A combination of four to six of the following herbs can be taken three times per day before meals (1 cup tea or 30 drops tincture):

- Peppermint *(Mentha piperita)* helps relieve gas, relieves spasms, historically to reduce appetite
- Bladder wrack *(Fucus vesiculosus)* historic use in obesity
- Parsley *(Petroselinum crispum)* diuretic, for gastrointestinal needs
- Dandelion *(Taraxacum officinale)* diuretic, dyspepsia
- Hawthorne *(Cretaegus oxyacantha)* good for blood vessels
- St. John's wort *(Hypericum perforatum)* antidepressant
- Valerian *(Valeriana officinalis)* bitter spasmolytic, sedative
- Milk thistle *(Silybum marianum)* dyspepsia, for liver and gallbladder
- Lavender *(Lavendula officinalis)* reduces gas, relieves spasms
- Gentian *(Gentiana Lutea)* reduces gas, digestive stimulation

HOMEOPATHY

Homeopathy may be useful as a supportive therapy.

PHYSICAL MEDICINE

Exercise is critical. While 20 minutes of aerobic exercise per day is ideal, as little as 10 minutes per day can help stabilize blood sugar and thereby reduce cravings. Gentle exercise (walking, yoga, swimming, biking) can increase cardiovascular health without great stress on joints.

ACUPUNCTURE

Acupuncture can be used to help balance the body's metabolism, stabilize blood sugar, correct digestive disorders, control certain eating disorders, aid in elimination and relieve stress, anxiety, and depression.

MASSAGE

May be beneficial. By decreasing stress, cortisol is decreased, which will help to stabilize blood sugar and prevent or treat diabetes.

■ FOLLOWING UP

Your health care provider may also suggest counseling to help you along as you lose weight.

■ SPECIAL CONSIDERATIONS

If you are obese, you are at risk for diabetes, heart problems, and other conditions. Obesity during pregnancy can put you and your baby at risk.

■ OSTEOARTHRITIS

Osteoarthritis is characterized by degenerative joint changes that cause pain, tenderness, and limited range of motion, The most common form of arthritis, it most frequently affects the hands, feet, knees, shoulders, hips, and spine. Osteoarthritis affects men and women almost equally.

■ SIGNS AND SYMPTOMS
- Morning stiffness or stiffness after inactivity for less than 15 minutes
- Joint pain, worsened by movement and improved with rest
- Soft-tissue swelling
- Bony crepitus (crackling noise with movement)
- Bone deformities (for example, on fingers)
- Limited range of motion
- Subluxation (incomplete or partial dislocation of a joint)

■ WHAT CAUSES IT?
Primary osteoarthritis appears to be caused by overuse of a joint (for example, seen in baseball pitchers, ballet dancers, dock workers), which leads to a destruction of the cartilage. Fractures and other abnormalities may also lead to osteoarthritis. There may be a genetic predisposition to osteoarthritis. Secondary osteoarthritis is associated with an underlying medical condition.

■ WHAT TO EXPECT AT YOUR PROVIDER'S OFFICE
Your health care provider will give you a thorough physical examination to determine the extent of your disability. Your provider will help you manage pain and avoid joint deformation and disability.

■ TREATMENT OPTIONS
The goals of treatment are to reduce pain, minimize disability, and maintain range of motion and mobility.

Drug Therapies
- Acetaminophen—to reduce pain
- Nonsteroidal anti-inflammatory drugs (NSAIDs) such as ibuprofen and naproxen—to reduce pain and inflammation
- Tramadol—for pain control
- Glucocorticoids—for symptomatic relief
- Capsaicin cream—to reduce pain

Complementary and Alternative Therapies
Alternative therapies can help improve joint function and decrease inflammation. Exercise that combines muscle strengthening and aerobic conditioning can help improve joint stability and function.

NUTRITION
- Reduce proinflammatory foods such as refined foods, sugar, saturated fats (meat and dairy products), and omega-6 fatty acids (such as evening primrose or flaxseed oil).
- Omega-3 fatty acids reduce inflammation. Increase intake of cold-water fish, nuts, and seeds or supplement with essential fatty acids (such as fish oil, 1,000 to 1,500 mg twice a day).
- Increase intake of whole grains, vegetables, and legumes.
- Vitamin C (1,000 mg three to four times a day) to support cartilage.
- Vitamin E (400 to 800 IU a day) inhibits breakdown of cartilage.
- Vitamin A (5,000 IU a day) or beta-carotene (50,000 IU a day), zinc

(20 to 30 mg a day), and selenium (200 mcg a day) are antioxidants that protect cartilage and reduce damage secondary to inflammation.
- Boron (3 mg a day) helps slow joint degeneration.
- Essential fatty acids (1,000 to 1,500 mg twice a day) reduce inflammation.
- Glucosamine sulfate (500 mg three times a day) has, in at least some studies, been shown to be more effective than ibuprofen at relieving pain as well as being better tolerated than ibuprofen or other NSAIDs.
- S-adenosylmethionine, or SAM (1,200 mg a day for 21 days, tapering to 200 mg a day). SAM stimulates production of cartilage and is a mild analgesic and anti-inflammatory agent. Do not take if you are manic-depressive.
- Niacinamide (500 to 1,000 mg three times a day) increases joint mobility and reduces pain.

HERBS
Herbs may be used as dried extracts (capsules, powders, teas), glycerites (glycerine extracts), or tinctures (alcohol extracts). Unless otherwise indicated, teas should be made with 1 tsp. herb per cup of hot water. Steep covered 5 to 10 minutes for leaf or flowers, and 10 to 20 minutes for roots. Drink 2 to 4 cups per day.
- Hawthorn *(Crataegus oxyacantha)* and bilberry *(Vaccinium myrtillus)* are high in flavonoids, especially anthocyanidins and proanthocyanidins, which enhance the integrity of connective tissue. Take 100 to 200 mg dried extract two to three times per day.
- Devil's claw *(Harpagophytum procumbens)*, yucca *(Yucca bacata)*, turmeric *(Curcuma longa)*, black cohosh *(Cimicifuga racemosa)*, ginger root *(Zingiber officinalis)*, and meadowsweet *(Filependula ulmaria)* may be combined in equal parts as tea (1 cup three times per day) or tincture (30 to 60 drops three times per day) to reduce inflammation and relieve pain.

HOMEOPATHY
Some of the most common remedies used for osteoarthritis are listed below. Usually, the dose is 12X to 30C every one to four hours until your symptoms get better.
- *Arnica montana* for arthritis with sore, stiff joints
- *Bryonia alba* for arthritic pain that is worse with movement and cold
- *Pulsatilla* for wandering arthritis that is worse with heat and on initiating movement but is relieved by continued movement
- *Rhus toxicodendron* for arthritis that is worse on waking in the morning, in damp and cold weather, and with exertion

ACUPUNCTURE
Acupuncture can relieve pain and reduce inflammation.

■ SPECIAL CONSIDERATIONS
- Manic-depressive people should not take SAM because its antidepressant activity may lead to a manic episode.
- High doses of nicotinamide have been associated with liver damage and glucose intolerance. Since osteoarthritis appears to be made worse by obesity, you should lose weight.
- Many pregnant women are normally too young to have primary osteoarthritis; however, if you have an underlying condition associated with osteoarthritis (secondary osteoarthritis), consult your health care provider concerning the safety of the usual medications.

■ OSTEOMYELITIS

Osteomyelitis is a bone infection, which can occur in practically any bone in the body. Bacteria usually cause the infection, but fungi can occasionally have the same effect. Osteomyelitis is rare in the U.S. and it affects children more than adults.

The disease takes several forms, according the way the infection traveled to the bone and the type of bone infected. Infections can reach the bone via open fractures or surgery on fractures, from body tissues next to the bone, from artificial joints, and from ulcers in the foot. People who inject street drugs and patients who receive kidney dialysis are particularly vulnerable to osteomyelitis.

■ SIGNS AND SYMPTOMS

The symptoms of osteomyelitis include the following.

- Intense pain and a sensation of heat at the site of the affected bone
- Small areas of tenderness and swelling
- Persistent back pain that is not relieved by rest, heat, or pain killers
- Abscesses containing pus in tissue surrounding the painful bone
- Fever, in some cases
- Fatigue

■ WHAT CAUSES IT?

Several different types of bacteria or fungi can infect bones, often after a fracture or other injury, or as the result of a joint replacement. The infection can also spread beyond the bone, creating abscesses in muscles and other tissues outside the bone.

■ WHAT TO EXPECT AT YOUR PROVIDER'S OFFICE

After you describe your symptoms, your health care provider will feel your skin above the affected bone, to check for tenderness. He or she will take blood samples to check for osteomyelitis and the type of bacterium or fungus responsible. Your provider may also want to sample the bone itself. This will involve inserting a needle through the skin and into the bone, and snipping off a small piece of the bone for testing. Your provider may also want you to have a bone scan, which uses a mildly radioactive compound to highlight infected areas in the bones. You may also need a computed tomography scan or magnetic resonance imaging, two types of imaging tests that produce more detailed information than conventional X rays.

■ TREATMENT OPTIONS

Taking medication should clear up an infection that was found early. The type of medication you need depends on the type of bacteria or fungi that caused your osteomyelitis. Your health care provider may recommend bed rest, particularly if the infection affects your back, and he or she may put you in a cast or splint to immobilize the affected bones and joints.

Complementary and Alternative Therapies

Alternative therapies can be used along with medical treatment to strengthen your immune system and help you recover.

NUTRITION

For overall immune support and help with healing, use the following.

- Vitamin C (1,000 mg three or four times a day)
- Zinc (30 to 50 mg per day, then reduce to 25 mg per day)
- Vitamin E (400 to 800 IU per day)
- Vitamin A (10,000 to 15,000 IU per day). Do not use if you are, or may become, pregnant.
- Acidophilus (1 to 3 capsules per day, or 1 to 5 million organisms per day)—to prevent antibiotic-induced diarrhea and yeast infections

HERBS

Herbs are generally a safe way to strengthen and tone the body's systems. As with any therapy, it is important to work with your provider on getting your problem diagnosed before you start any treatment. Herbs may be used as dried extracts (capsules, powders, teas), glycerites (glycerine extracts), or tinctures (alcohol extracts). Unless otherwise indicated, teas should be made with one teaspoon herb per cup of hot water. Steep covered 5 to 10 minutes for leaf or flowers, and 10 to 20 minutes for roots. Drink two to four cups per day.

Use one or more herbs from each category. Make a tincture using equal parts. Take 15 to 60 drops three to four times a day.

- For immune support: coneflower *(Echinacea angustifolia),* lomatium *(Lomatium dissectum),* astragalus *(Astragalus membranaceus)*
- To fight infection: goldenseal *(Hydrastis canadensis),* barberry *(Berberis vulgaris),* garlic *(Allium sativum)*
- To relieve pain: valerian *(Valeriana officianalis),* St. John's wort *(Hypericum perforatum)*
- For improved circulation: *ginkgo biloba* 120 mg twice a day

Herbs called alteratives are traditionally known as blood cleansers. Use an infusion of red clover *(Trifolium pratense),* burdock root *(Arctium lappa),* yellow dock *(Rumex crispus),* yarrow *(Achillea millefolium),* cleavers *(Galium aparine),* and licorice root *(Glycyrrhiza glabra).* Drink two to three cups a day. Do not use licorice if you have hypertension.

To help with the healing of abscesses, make a paste from the powders of goldenseal root *(Hydrastis canadensis)* and slippery elm *(Ulmus fulva).* Apply as needed.

HOMEOPATHY

Some of the most common remedies used for osteomyelitis are listed below. Usually, the dose is 12X to 30C every one to four hours until your symptoms get better.

- *Arnica* for use after trauma or injury, especially with bruising or a bruised, "beat up" feeling
- *Ledum* for puncture wounds that lead to abscesses, especially if they feel better with cold applications
- *Silica* for enlarged glands or abscesses, especially in depleted patients

ACUPUNCTURE

May help stimulate immune response, reducing inflammation, pain, swelling, and fever

MASSAGE

Massage should be avoided because it could spread the infection.

■ FOLLOWING UP

Expect your health care provider to monitor you carefully during your treatment.

■ OSTEOPOROSIS

Osteoporosis is the continual breakdown of bone. It can cause fractures, deformity, and death. Osteoporosis affects over 25 million people each year; 80 percent of them are women.

■ SIGNS AND SYMPTOMS
- Periodontal disease
- Loss of height
- Hunched back
- Back pain

■ WHAT CAUSES IT?
Osteoporosis occurs when bone breaks down faster than it is formed. Lack of estrogen in the body causes 95 percent of all cases of osteoporosis. Other causes include glucocorticoid and heparin use, hyperthyroidism, and calcium deficiency. Osteoporosis may be hereditary. Women approaching or experiencing menopause are at increased risk.

■ WHAT TO EXPECT AT YOUR PROVIDER'S OFFICE
Ask your health care provider about having a bone density test to determine if you have begun to loose bone mass. Your provider will talk to you about preventative treatment options.

■ TREATMENT OPTIONS
Drug Therapies
Hormone replacement therapy is the most common treatment for osteoporosis. It works to slow the speed of bone loss. Your provider may also recommend supplements such as calcium to help slow bone loss.

Complementary and Alternative Therapies
Nutritional and herbal support aid the absorption of essential vitamins and minerals. Include exercise and stress management in any treatment program.

NUTRITION
- Eliminate refined foods, alcohol, caffeine, tobacco, sugar, phosphorous (carbonated drinks and dairy products), aluminum-containing antacids, and high amounts of sodium chloride (table salt) and animal proteins. Sea salt, soy sauce, tamari, or kelp granules are preferable to table salt.
- Increase intake of complex carbohydrates, essential fatty acids (cold-water fish, nuts, and seeds), legumes, and soy. Isoflavones found in soy may slow bone loss and increase bone building activity. Studies suggest 30 to 50 mg per day of soy to maintain bone mass.
- Dark berries (blueberries, blackberries, cherries, and raspberries) contain anthocyanidins, which help stabilize collagen found in bones.
- Mineral-rich foods, especially nondairy sources of calcium, should be increased. Although these are lower in actual calcium content, they provide calcium that is easier for your body to use. Particularly beneficial are almonds, blackstrap molasses, dark leafy greens, sardines, sea vegetables, soy, tahini, prunes, and apricots.
- Calcium citrate or aspartate (1,000 to 1,500 mg per day) are the preferred forms of calcium.
- Magnesium (200 mg two to three times per day) enhances calcium uptake, is necessary for hormone production, and protects the heart. Magnesium may actually increase bone density and may be a more important mineral than calcium for preventing osteoporosis.
- Vitamin K (100 to 500 mcg per day) helps increase calcium uptake. Foods high in vitamin K include dark leafy greens.

- Boron (0.5 to 3 mg per day) helps calcium absorption. Women at high risk for breast cancer should use boron with caution.
- Manganese (5 to 20 mg per day) helps produce the collagen foundation for calcium.
- Zinc (10 to 30 mg per day) aids normal bone growth. Copper (1 to 2 mg per day) is needed with long-term zinc supplementation.
- Chromium (200 to 600 mcg per day) should be used in patients with unstable blood sugars.
- Essential fatty acids (1,000 mg twice a day) aid hormone production.
- B-complex (50 to 100 mg per day) reduces the effects of stress. Elevated cortisol levels from stress increase bone loss. Take folic acid (1 to 5 mg/day), B_6 (100 mg/day), and B_{12} (1,000 mcg per day).

HERBS
Herbs may be used as dried extracts (capsules, powders, teas), glycerites (glycerine extracts), or tinctures (alcohol extracts). Teas should be made with 1 tsp. herb per cup of hot water. Steep covered 5 to 10 minutes for leaf or flowers; 10 to 20 minutes for roots. Drink 2 to 4 cups per day.

Some herbs have phytoestrogen or progesterone properties, and women may choose to take them instead of, or in addition to, conventional hormone replacement therapy. Natural progesterone may be more effective at increasing bone density than synthetic progestins. It is important to note that natural progesterone may not be strong enough to offset the risk of uterine cancer posed by conventional estrogen replacement therapy. The following are examples of herbs that can help treat osteoporosis.
- Black cohosh, licorice *(Glycyrrhiza glabra)*, and squaw vine *(Mitchella repens)* help balance estrogen levels. Do not take licorice if you have high blood pressure.
- Chaste tree, wild yam *(Dioscorea villosa)*, and lady's mantle *(Alchemilla vulgaris)* help balance progesterone levels.
- Kelp *(Nereocystis luetkeana)*, bladderwrack *(Fucus vesiculosis)*, oatstraw *(Avena sativa)*, nettles *(Urtica diocia)*, and horsetail *(Equisetum arvense)* may also help support a sluggish thyroid.
- Milk thistle *(Silybum marianum)*, dandelion root *(Taraxacum officinalis)*, vervain *(Verbena hastata)*, and blue flag *(Iris versicolor)* support the liver and may help restore hormone ratios. Taken together as a tea before meals, they enhance digestion.
- Topical applications of natural progesterone. Your provider should check your progesterone levels periodically.

HOMEOPATHY
Some of the most common remedies used for osteoporosis are listed below. Usually, the dose is 12X to 30C every one to four hours until your symptoms get better. A combination of homeopathic tissue salts such as *Calcarea fluoricum,* and *Silica* may be helpful.

ACUPUNCTURE
Acupuncture can help hormone imbalances and poor blood sugar control.

MASSAGE
Massage may enhance circulation.

■ SPECIAL CONSIDERATIONS
Osteoporosis may take root during the teen years. Adequate calcium and magnesium intake and proper nutrition and exercise are the primary preventative measures for osteoporosis.

■ OTITIS MEDIA

Otitis media is an infection of the middle ear, the area just behind the eardrum. It happens when the eustachian tubes, which drain fluid and bacteria from the middle ear out to the throat, become blocked. Otitis media is common in infants and children, because their immune systems are immature and their eustachian tubes are easily clogged. It is important that children with otitis media be seen by a health care provider, because there can be serious complications if the infection is left untreated.

■ SIGNS AND SYMPTOMS

Acute otitis media causes pain, fever, difficulty in hearing, and general signs of illness such as vomiting and diarrhea. In infants, the clearest sign of otitis media is often incessant crying.

■ WHAT CAUSES IT?

Blockage of the eustachian tubes may be caused by the following.
- Respiratory infection
- Allergies
- Tobacco smoke or other environmental irritants
- Infected or overgrown adenoids
- Sudden increase in pressure (such as during an airplane landing)
- Drinking while lying on the back, such as with a propped bottle
- Excess mucus and saliva produced during teething

Otitis media appears most frequently in the winter. It is not contagious in itself, but a cold may spread among a group of children and cause some of them to get ear infections.

■ WHAT TO EXPECT AT YOUR PROVIDER'S OFFICE

Your health care provider will use an otoscope to examine your child's eardrums, and look for signs of infection.

■ TREATMENT OPTIONS

Antibiotics are generally prescribed to be taken for a week to 10 days, and it is important to follow these instructions to avoid a relapse. You can give your child acetaminophen or ibuprofen to relieve the pain.

If your child repeatedly gets ear infections, you may consider having tympanostomy tubes put in. In this procedure, a tiny tube is inserted into the eardrum, keeping open a small hole through which fluids can drain to the outside. Tympanostomy tube insertion is a 10- to 15-minute procedure done under general anesthesia. Usually the tubes fall out by themselves or are removed in your provider's office.

Complementary and Alternative Therapies

NUTRITION

Eliminate food allergens from the diet. Common allergenic foods are dairy products, soy, citrus, peanuts, wheat, fish, eggs, corn, tomatoes.

Essential fatty acids reduce swelling and help the immune system function. Children should be supplemented with cod liver oil or other fish oils ($^1/_2$ to 1 tsp. per day). Vitamin C (100 to 250 mg two to three times per day) enhances immunity and decreases inflammation. Vitamin C from rose hips or palmitate is citrus-free and hypoallergenic.

HERBS

Herbs may be used as dried extracts (capsules, powders, teas), glycerites (glycerine extracts), or tinctures (alcohol extracts). Unless otherwise indicated, teas should be made with 1 tsp. herb per cup of hot water. Steep covered 5 to 10 minutes for leaf or flowers, and 10 to 20 minutes for roots. Drink 2 to 4 cups per day.

Herbal eardrops may be effective at reducing infection, pain, and fluid accumulation. Do not use eardrops if your provider suspects perforation of the eardrum. An ear oil from mullein *(Verbascum thapsus)* and garlic *(Allium sativum)* can reduce pain and treat the infection. For otitis with pain, include one of the following oils: St. John's wort *(Hypericum perforatum)*, Indian tobacco *(Lobelia inflata)*, or monkshood *(Aconitum napellus)*. Place three to five drops in the ear 2 to 4 times per day. Monkshood is toxic if taken internally.

Coneflower *(Echinacea angustifolia, purpurea,* and *pallida)* may be taken internally as tincture or glycerite, 20 drops three to four times a day. The following herbs also may be taken internally: eyebright *(Euphrasia officinalis),* cleavers *(Galium aparine),* marigold *(Calendula officinalis),* and elderberry *(Sambucus canadensis)* combined in a tea (2 to 4 oz. three times a day), tincture (10 to 20 drops three times a day), or glycerite (20 drops three times a day).

HOMEOPATHY

Some of the most common remedies used for otitis media are listed below. Usually, the dose is 12X to 30C every one to four hours until your symptoms get better.
- *Aconite* for an ear infection that comes on suddenly after exposure to cold or wind; child has bright red ears and high fever
- *Belladonna* for sudden onset of ear infection with great pain
- *Chamomilla* for ear infection with intense irritability, especially if your child is teething

PHYSICAL MEDICINE

A hot pack applied to the ear and side of the neck may relieve pain. Blanch half an onion, wrap in cheesecloth and apply to your child's ear while it is still hot (be sure it has cooled enough to not burn the skin). The sulphur bonds in the onion will be soothing. May also use a hot water bottle or a sock filled with raw rice and heated.

MASSAGE

Gentle massaging of the neck may assist lymph flow, which may speed healing.

■ FOLLOWING UP

Let your health care provider know if your child's ear infection does not improve within 24 to 48 hours.

■ SPECIAL CONSIDERATIONS

You can reduce your child's risk of ear infection by reducing his or her exposure to respiratory infections and tobacco smoke. For children who are old enough to chew gum, xylitol-sweetened gum has been shown to lessen the frequency of ear infections as well as dental cavities.

■ PARKINSON'S DISEASE

Parkinson's disease is a progressive disorder of the central nervous system. It causes tremors (especially in the hands) and rigidity (especially in the face). The disease affects men and women equally, primarily after age 60. However, approximately 10 percent of those with the disease are under age 40. Although no cure for the disease is available at this time, drug therapy can help alleviate the symptoms.

■ SIGNS AND SYMPTOMS

- Shaking
- Poor balance
- Stiffness and rigid limbs
- Walking problems
- Extremely slow movement
- Involuntary eye closure

Secondary symptoms may include the following.

- Memory loss
- Constipation
- Sleep disturbances
- Dementia
- Speech, breathing, swallowing problems
- Stooped posture

■ WHAT CAUSES IT?

Parkinson's disease is caused by the loss of brain cells that produce the neurotransmitter (brain chemical) dopamine, which affects muscle activity. The brain's inability to produce enough of these cells may be due to environmental factors (such as toxins or viruses), heredity, certain other brain chemicals, the aging process, and heroine use.

■ WHAT TO EXPECT AT YOUR PROVIDER'S OFFICE

Since no test can positively identify Parkinson's, your provider will rely largely on interviews with you and your family. He or she may order brain scans to measure dopamine activity. Genetic testing may help identify a specific illness (like Huntington's disease) linked to the disease.

■ TREATMENT OPTIONS

Drug Therapies

Several drugs treat the symptoms of Parkinson's, but they do not cure the disease. It is quite common for your provider to change medications and adjust dosages. Certain drugs used for the treatment of other diseases, especially glaucoma, heart disease, and high blood pressure, can influence the treatment of Parkinson's disease.

Psychotherapy can help you cope with associated conditions such as depression. Speech, physical, and occupational therapy may help.

Complementary and Alternative Therapies

Alternative therapies may provide some relief of symptoms and slow the progression of the disease.

NUTRITION

- Essential fatty acids are anti-inflammatory. A mix of omega-6 (evening primrose, black currant, borage, pumpkin seed) and omega-3 (flax seed and fish oils) may be best (2 tbsp. oil per day or 1,000 to 1,500 mg twice a day).
- Antioxidants vitamin C (1,000 mg three times a day), vitamin E (400 to 800 IU per day), and the trace mineral selenium (200 mcg) may slow progression of Parkinson's. Other antioxidants are alpha-lipoic acid, grape seed extract, and pycnogenol.
- A vitamin B complex is helpful.

- Vitamin B$_6$ (10 to 100 mg per day) may help with symptom control, but should be given with zinc (30 mg per day).
- Manganese: excessive exposure increases the risk of Parkinson's
- Amino acids: Low-protein diets may help control tremors. However, D-tyrosine (100 mg per kg per day) increases dopamine turnover.
- Glutathione: antioxidant, (200 mg twice a day)
- Choline increases brain function; various forms include lecithin, phosphatidyl choline, and DMAE (Dimethylaminoethanol)
- Neurotransmitters made from amino acids such as glutamic acid and GABA (Gamma-aminobutyricacid) are used for Parkinson's

HERBS

Herbs may be used as dried extracts (capsules, powders, teas), glycerites (glycerine extracts), or tinctures (alcohol extracts). Unless otherwise indicated, teas should be made with 1 tsp. herb per cup of hot water. Steep covered 5 to 10 minutes for leaf or flowers, and 10 to 20 minutes for roots. Drink 2 to 4 cups per day.

- Gotu kola *(Centella asiatica)*: historic use in Parkinson's. One cup tea twice a day, or 30 to 60 drops tincture twice a day
- Ginkgo *(Ginkgo biloba)*: circulatory stimulant and an antioxidant (as a supplement 120 mg per day)
- Hawthorn *(Crataegus oxyacantha)*: circulatory stimulant, antioxidant (2 to 5 g per day)
- Milk thistle *(Silybum marianum)*, globe artichoke *(Cynara scolymus)*, and *Bupleurum* species provide liver support.
- St. John's wort *(Hypericum perforatum)*, skullcap *(Scutellaria laterifolia)*, oats *(Avena sativa)*, and lemon balm *(Melissa officinalis)* help support the structure of the nervous system.

HOMEOPATHY

Usually, the dose is 12X to 30C every one to four hours until your symptoms get better.

- *Argentum nitricum* for ataxia (loss of muscle coordination), trembling, awkwardness, painless paralysis
- *Causticum* for Parkinson's with restless legs at night, contractures
- *Mercurius vivus* for Parkinson's that is worse at night, especially with panic attacks
- *Plumbum metallicum* especially with arteriosclerosis
- *Zincum metallicum* for great restlessness, and depression

MASSAGE

May help with increasing circulation and decreasing muscle spasm.

PHYSICAL MEDICINE

Chelation therapy may be effective if the Parkinson's is due to heavy metal toxicity or environmental toxins.

ACUPUNCTURE

May be helpful, particularly for the tremor involved.

■ FOLLOWING UP

Since Parkinson's disease advances with time, you will need to be under constant medical care. Drug treatments often become less effective over time, and you must keep a close eye on your symptoms.

■ SPECIAL CONSIDERATIONS

Exercise will also help you improve mobility.

■ PEPTIC ULCER DISEASE

Peptic ulcers are sores in the lining of either the duodenum (duodenal ulcers) or the stomach (gastric ulcers). The duodenum is located at the beginning of the small intestine. About 10 percent of all people get ulcers, and they often recur.

■ SIGNS AND SYMPTOMS
- Duodenal ulcers often cause pain with burning or gnawing sensations. This pain often occurs after eating and is relieved by antacids and milk. Increased pain, vomiting blood, tarry or red stools, or losing a lot of weight are signs of serious complications.
- Gastric ulcers often cause gnawing or burning pain. One day your pain may be relieved from food or an antacid and the next day these may not help at all. You may have vomiting or nausea.

■ WHAT CAUSES IT?
When the stomach's natural protections from acid stop working, you can get an ulcer. There are a few different ways this happens.
- A kind of bacteria called *Helicobacter pylori* causes 90 percent of duodenal ulcers and 70 to 80 percent of gastric ulcers.
- Drugs like ibuprofen can cause gastric ulcers.
- Zollinger–Ellison syndrome causes diarrhea and ulcers.
- Certain diseases, like alcoholism, can cause ulcers.

■ WHAT TO EXPECT AT YOUR PROVIDER'S OFFICE
Your provider may take an X-ray of your stomach. You will drink a liquid, called barium, which makes your gastointestinal tract show up on the X-ray. Or you may have an endoscopic exam, where a thin tube with a small camera-like device on the end explores your stomach. Your provider will also give you a urea breath test or a blood test for *H. pylori.*

■ TREATMENT OPTIONS
- If you have *H. pylori,* you will probably be given two or three different drugs (antibiotics and stomach acid-reducing drugs).
- Antacids and other medications to reduce acid
- Colloidal bismuth compounds can destroy *H. pylori.*
- If you have a perforated ulcer, an obstruction, or bleeding, or if you do not respond to medical treatments, you may need to have surgery.

Complementary and Alternative Therapies
Nutritional and herbal support help to heal stomach lining, fight infection, and reduce recurrence.

NUTRITION
- Avoid dairy products, caffeine, alcohol, and sugar. Coffee, even decaffeinated, should be eliminated because of irritating oils.
- Eliminate any known food allergens.
- Include sulfur-containing foods such as garlic, onions, broccoli, cabbage, Brussels sprouts, and cauliflower in your diet. Sulfur is the basis of glutathione, which provides antioxidant protection to the stomach lining. N-acetyl cysteine (200 mg twice a day) is also a precursor to glutathione.
- Bananas contain potassium and plantain, both of which yield benefits.
- Acidophilus (one capsule with meals) can help normalize bowel bacteria and inhibit growth of *H. pylori.*
- Essential fatty acids (1,000 to 1,500 mg two to three times per day) reduce inflammation and inhibit the growth of *H. pylori.*

- Vitamin C (1,000 mg three times per day) decreases nitrosamines, which are linked to stomach cancer, and inhibits growth of *H. pylori.*
- Zinc (30 to 50 mg per day) enhances healing.
- Vitamin E (400 IU per day) enhances healing.
- Vitamin A (50,000 IU per day for 2 weeks followed by 10,000 to 25,000 IU per day) for longer term maintenance
- Glutamine (500 mg three times per day) promotes healing of ulcers. Cabbage juice (1 qt. per day) is high in glutamine.

HERBS
Herbs may be used as dried extracts (capsules, powders, teas), glycerites (glycerine extracts), or tinctures (alcohol extracts). Unless otherwise indicated, teas should be made with 1 tsp. herb per cup of hot water. Steep covered 5 to 10 minutes for leaf or flowers, and 10 to 20 minutes for roots. Drink 2 to 4 cups per day.
- DGL (deglycyrrhizinated licorice), 250 mg four times a day 15 to 20 minutes before meals and one to two hours after the last meal of the day, increases local circulation and speeds healing of the stomach lining. Safe for people with high blood pressure.
- Quercetin (250 to 500 mg before meals) or catechin (500 to 1,000 mg before meals) are bioflavonoids that reduce gastric inflammation.
- Powders of slippery elm *(Ulmus rubra)* and marshmallow root *(Althea officinalis)* may be taken singly or together, 1 tsp. two to three times per day to decrease inflammation and encourage healing.
- For a soothing tea, combine equal parts of three to six of the following herbs in a tea and sip before meals. Chamomile *(Matricaria recutita),* lemon balm *(Melissa officinalis),* catnip *(Nepeta cateria),* passionflower *(Passiflora incarnata),* meadowsweet *(Filependula ulmaria),* peppermint *(Mentha piperita),* and valerian *(Valeriana officinalis).*
- Bismuth subcitrate (120 mg four times a day for eight weeks) may be helpful in eradicating *H. pylori* and reducing recurrence of peptic ulcer disease. Combining it with barberry *(Berberis vulgaris),* goldenseal *(Hydrastis canadensis),* or Oregon grape *(Berberis aquifolium)* may make its antimicrobial effects stronger. Take one or more in tincture form, 30 to 60 drops three times a day.

HOMEOPATHY
Some of the most common remedies used for peptic ulcers are listed below. Usually, the dose is 12X to 30C every one to four hours until your symptoms get better.
- *Argentum nitricum* for abdominal bloating with belching and pain
- *Arsenicum album* for ulcers with intense burning pains and nausea; take it if you cannot bear the sight or smell of food and are thirsty.
- *Lycopodium* for bloating after eating with burning that lasts for hours; take it if you feel hungry soon after eating and wake hungry.

ACUPUNCTURE
Acupuncture may improve overall digestive function.

MASSAGE
Therapeutic massage can relieve stress and increase sense of well-being.

■ FOLLOWING UP
If you are not better after a month, return to your provider. If you are pregnant, talk with your health care provider before taking any medications or supplements.

■ PERICARDITIS

Pericarditis is an inflammation of the pericardium, a sac surrounding the heart. The most common form is acute pericarditis, which can usually be treated without hospitalization. Common in adolescents and young adults, acute pericarditis affects males more than females. Pericardial effusion is a form that results when fluid builds up in the pericardium. It is a more serious condition that can require hospitalization and possibly surgery. Constrictive pericarditis is a form that is a chronic condition and worsens gradually over a long period of time. It may ultimately require surgery. Pericardial effusion and constrictive pericarditis can occur together.

■ SIGNS AND SYMPTOMS

The signs and symptoms of pericarditis vary somewhat.
Acute pericarditis:
- Chest pain
- Fever
- Flushed appearance
- Muscle pain
- Pain with swallowing
- Feelings of anxiousness, discomfort, or uneasiness

Pericardial effusion:
- Difficulty breathing
- A bluish skin color

Constrictive pericarditis:
- Difficulty breathing
- Congestion in the lungs
- Fatigue
- Abdominal swelling

■ WHAT CAUSES IT?

Acute pericarditis and pericardial effusion have a large number of possible causes, including viruses, bacteria, fungi, cancer, trauma to the heart (such as chest injury), drug reactions, and radiation exposure. In many cases, however, the actual cause is unknown. Constrictive pericarditis usually results from repeated cases of acute pericarditis.

■ WHAT TO EXPECT AT YOUR PROVIDER'S OFFICE

Your health care provider will listen to your heart and lungs, take your pulse, and probably tap your chest and back. Your provider will probably order a number of tests, which may include blood work, an electrocardiogram, an echocardiogram, chest X-ray, computed tomography (CT) scan, or magnetic resonance imaging (MRI).

■ TREATMENT OPTIONS

Pericarditis is usually treated with aspirin or nonsteroidal anti-inflammatory drugs (NSAIDS, such as ibuprofen), but steroid medications may be prescribed.

Complementary and Alternative Therapies

Alternative therapies may have benefit as supportive treatments for some of the causes of pericarditis. Hawthorn *(Crataegus oxycantha)* is a cardiac tonic with very low toxicity that could be used along with whatever therapy your provider deems most appropriate.

NUTRITION
- Vitamin C (1,000 mg three times per day) may help decrease inflammation. It also aids in fighting infection, and is an antioxidant.
- Coenzyme Q10 (50 mg bid) is an important antioxidant that may help prevent heart muscle damage and speed recovery.
- Your provider may recommend sodium restriction if you have constrictive pericarditis.
- If your pericarditis is of viral origin, your provider may recommend supplementation with vitamin A (300,000 IU/day for 3 days).
- Flaxseed oil (3 g twice per day) helps decrease inflammation.
- Avoid saturated fats, alcohol, and sugars, which can lead to increased inflammation and lowered immune function.
- Consume at least five servings of fruits and vegetables per day. These foods are anti-inflammatory and protect the heart.

HERBS
Herbs may be used as dried extracts (capsules, powders, teas), glycerites (glycerine extracts), or tinctures (alcohol extracts). Unless otherwise indicated, teas should be made with 1 tsp. herb per cup of hot water. Steep covered 5 to 10 minutes for leaf or flowers, and 10 to 20 minutes for roots. Drink 2 to 4 cups per day.
- Hawthorn *(Crataegus oxyanthoides)* can help prevent high blood pressure and hardening of the arteries. Dose is 60 drops tincture three times per day 1 tsp. berries steeped for 10 minutes in hot water, or 100 to 250 mg three times per day as a supplement.
- Linden *(Tilea europea)* is used for high blood pressure with nervous tension, and may be useful adjunctive treatment where there is anxiety. Dose is 1 tsp. dried blossoms per cup hot water three times a day or 60 drops tincture three times a day.
- Blue monkshood *(Aconitum napellus)* has been described as an herbal remedy for pericarditis without significant effusion. CAUTION: As this herb can be highly toxic, even fatal, it is not recommended unless prescribed by an experienced health care provider.

HOMEOPATHY
Some of the most common remedies used for pericarditis are listed below. Usually, the dose is 12X to 30C every one to four hours until your symptoms get better.
- *Aconite* for sudden, sharp pains accompanied by anxiety (especially fear of dying) and restlessness
- *Spongia tosta* for the sensation that the chest will explode, anxiety, light-headedness, sweating; patient may be flushed
- *Cactus grandiflorus* for the feeling that there is a band around the chest or a great weight on the chest; palpitations; feels better in the open air and worse at night

ACUPUNCTURE
Can be very helpful in decreasing inflammation, enhancing immune response, and regulating cardiac function.

■ FOLLOWING UP
Your provider may order a follow-up X-ray or electrocardiogram.

■ PERTUSSIS

Pertussis is a violent cough, sometimes called whooping cough. A vaccine for pertussis was developed in 1948. Before then, children in the United States often died from it. The disease is rising again because fewer people are getting vaccinated.

■ SIGNS AND SYMPTOMS

The three phases of the disease are listed below.
Catarrhal phase (lasts one to two weeks):

- Upper respiratory infection; begins like the common cold
- Low-grade fever (less than 100.4°F)
- Loss of appetite

Paroxysmal phase (lasts one to four weeks):

- Cough increases (2 to 50 times a day) and fever decreases.
- Sudden, forceful breathing in causes the whooping sound.
- A sudden intense bout of coughing (paroxysms) causes bulging and tearing eyes, tongue sticking out, and bluish discoloration.
- Vomiting or choking may follow coughing bouts.

Convalescent phase (lasts two weeks to several months):

- Cough slowly goes away.

■ WHAT CAUSES IT?

A type of bacteria causes pertussis, and it is spread through droplets coughed into the air. It is a highly contagious disease.

■ WHAT TO EXPECT AT YOUR PROVIDER'S OFFICE

Your health care provider will will prescribe an antibiotic, which helps prevent the disease from spreading. Patients with complications, severe coughing bouts, or who are under one year of age are hospitalized.

■ TREATMENT OPTIONS

- Antibiotics and quarantine stop the spread of pertussis (the patient is isolated for seven days).
- Corticosteroids may reduce the severity and length of coughing bouts.
- Albuterol reduces the severity of cough (do not use suppressants).

Complementary and Alternative Therapies

Pertussis can be treated with nutrition, herbs, and homeopathy.

NUTRITION

Note: Doses given are for children. Adults should double the amounts.

- Eliminate dairy, bananas, wheat, and meat products.
- Encourage small, frequent meals of vegetable broths, steamed vegetables, and fresh fruit (especially pineapple and grapes).
- Vitamin C (200 to 500 mg three times per day), zinc (10 to 15 mg per day), and beta-carotene (10,000 to 25,000 IU per day).

HERBS

Herbs may be used as dried extracts (capsules, powders, teas), glycerites (glycerine extracts), or tinctures (alcohol extracts). Teas should be made with 1 tsp. herb per cup of hot water. Steep covered 5 to 10 minutes for leaf or flowers, and 10 to 20 minutes for roots.

Catarrhal stage: Choose two herbs from each of the first three categories. Combine in equal parts in a tea ($1/2$ cup every three to four hours), a tincture or glycerite (30 drops every three to four hours).

Paroxysmal stage: In addition to the above formula, combine 2 parts of catnip with two to four of the other antispasmodic herbs in a tincture or glycerite (20 drops every one to two hours).

Immune-stimulating herbs:

- Coneflower *(Echinacea purpurea)*
- Usnea lichen *(Usnea spp.)*
- Garlic *(Allium sativum)*
- Astragalus *(Astragalus membranaceus)*

Expectorants:

- Licorice root *(Glycyrrhiza glabra)*
- Elecampane *(Inula helenium)*
- Mullein *(Verbascum thapsus)*

Antiseptics:

- Thyme *(Thymus vulgaris)*
- Hyssop *(Hyssopus officinalis)*
- Anise seed *(Pimpinella anisum)*

Antispasmodics:

- Indian tobacco *(Lobelia inflata)* (not more than $1/4$ of combination)
- Catnip *(Nepeta cateria)*
- Chamomile *(Matricaria recutita)*
- Cramp bark *(Viburnum opulus)*
- Valerian *(Valeriana officinalis)*

HOMEOPATHY

Some of the most common remedies for pertussis are listed below.

- *Aconite* for sudden onset of cough and great thirst for cold drinks
- *Belladonna* for sudden onset, high fever with irritability
- *Drosera* for coughing when lying or from tickle in the throat
- *Bryonia alba* for cough that is dry and painful
- *Arnica montana* for painful cough with nosebleed
- *Antimonium tartaricum* for rattling cough and weakness
- *Ipecacuanha* for persistent nausea with cough and gagging

PHYSICAL MEDICINE

- Chest rubs. Use 3 to 6 drops of essential oil (camphor, thyme, eucalyptus, rosemary) with 1 tbsp. food-grade oil (almond, flax, or olive).
- Castor oil pack. Apply oil directly to chest, cover with a clean soft cloth and plastic wrap. Place a heat source over the pack and let sit for 30 to 60 minutes. Use daily.
- Place 3 to 6 drops of essential oil in a humidifier or a warm bath.
- Alternating hot and cold applications to the chest or back. Alternate three minutes hot with one minute cold.
- Warming sock treatment. Before bed, place cold, damp socks on warmed feet and cover with dry wool socks overnight.

ACUPUNCTURE

May enhance immunity and decrease duration and severity of infection.

MASSAGE

Foot massage has a relaxing effect and can help induce sleep.

■ FOLLOWING UP

Complete recovery is expected unless there are complications.

■ SPECIAL CONSIDERATIONS

Vaccinations are 80 to 90 percent effective. They last about 12 years.

For additional information supporting this handout, please refer to our website: www.onemedicine.com/public/products/access

77

■ PHARYNGITIS

With pharyngitis, a virus or bacterium irritates your throat, or pharynx. Both viral and bacterial forms of pharyngitis can make your throat sore and make swallowing difficult. If you have a severe case, you may find it hard to breathe. Most cases of acute pharyngitis last a few days with treatment. If you smoke, face regular exposure to environmental irritants, or have a continuing infection in your sinuses, lungs, or mouth, you may develop chronic pharyngitis, in which your symptoms will come back from time to time. The viral form of pharyngitis usually accompanies a cold, flu, or mononucleosis. Strep throat is the best-known example of a bacterial form of pharyngitis.

■ SIGNS AND SYMPTOMS

The symptoms of pharyngitis include the following.
- Sore throat
- Pain when swallowing
- In rare cases, difficulty breathing
- Inflammation of the membrane lining your throat
- An extra membrane or the appearance of pus in your throat (can appear as white patches on tonsils or back of throat)
- Fever
- Enlarged lymph nodes in your neck

■ WHAT CAUSES IT?

Viruses or bacteria infect the pharynx—your throat—and cause it to swell. That accounts for the soreness and difficulties in swallowing. Viruses that cause pharyngitis usually come into your body with a cold, the flu, or a similar infection. Bacteria that cause the disease can enter the body through open wounds, skin infections, and common routes of sexually transmitted diseases.

■ WHAT TO EXPECT AT YOUR PROVIDER'S OFFICE

Your health care provider will examine your throat and take a swab from it to test whether a virus or bacteria have caused the infection. The provider may also take a blood sample to check your white blood cell count, which can determine the cause of your pharyngitis.

■ TREATMENT OPTIONS

If you have a bacterial form of pharyngitis, your health care provider will prescribe an antibiotic. Penicillin taken by mouth is the most commonly prescribed. If you have an allergy to penicillin, your provider will prescribe erythromycin or another antibiotic.

If you have the viral form of pharyngitis, your health care provider will probably advise you to treat yourself at home. Get plenty of rest. Avoid any irritants that might affect your throat, such as smoke from cigarettes, cigars, or pipes, and cold air. Avoid drinking alcohol. Aspirin or other over-the-counter pain medicines will help relieve the pain and soreness in your throat. However, aspirin should not be given to children under 18. Gargling several times a day with half a teaspoon of salt in a glass of warm water will also help reduce your discomfort, as will throat lozenges.

Complementary and Alternative Therapies

Strep infection should be treated with antibiotics. Alternative treatments can be effective in cases of acute, chronic, or recurrent pharyngitis.

NUTRITION
- Zinc (30 mg per day or lozenges) boosts the immune system and relieves soreness.
- Vitamin C (1,000 mg three to four times per day) is needed, as your bowel tolerates, for proper immune function and to strengthen mucous membranes.
- Beta-carotene (50,000 to 100,000 IU per day) restores the integrity of mucous membranes and supports immune function.

HERBS
Herbs may be used as dried extracts (capsules, powders, teas), glycerites (glycerine extracts), or tinctures (alcohol extracts). Unless otherwise indicated, teas should be made with 1 tsp. herb per cup of hot water. Steep covered 5 to 10 minutes for leaf or flowers, and 10 to 20 minutes for roots. Drink 2 to 4 cups per day.
- Slippery elm *(Ulmus rubra):* Soothes irritated tissues and promotes healing. Use as lozenge or tea.
- Licorice *(Glycyrrhiza glabra):* Antiviral and soothing to the throat. Use as lozenge or tea. Do not take licorice if you have high blood pressure.
- Garlic/ginger tea *(Allium sativum/Zingiber officinalis):* Antimicrobial and warming herbs. Use two cloves of garlic and two to three slices of fresh ginger root. Simmer in 1 cup of water for 10 minutes. Drink warm. May add lemon and honey for flavor.
- Tincture of two parts coneflower *(Echinacea purpurea),* two parts goldenseal *(Hydrastis canadensis),* and one part propolis, should be taken every three to four hours. Place 30 drops in $1/4$ cup water. Gargle and swallow.

HOMEOPATHY
Some of the most common remedies used for pharyngitis are listed below. Usually, the dose is 12X to 30C every one to four hours until your symptoms get better.
- *Apis* for red, swollen throat with burning pains. Patient is thirstless and feels better with cold drinks.
- *Belladonna* for bright red throat and tongue that feels worse on the right side; especially if you are thirsty.
- *Lycopodium* for dryness of throat; pain begins on right side and goes to left. Pain is relieved with hot drinks.

PHYSICAL MEDICINE
Chiropractic treatment may be a helpful adjunct, especially in children.

ACUPUNCTURE
Acupuncture may be helpful in improving immune function.

MASSAGE
Massage can reduce the effects of stress.

■ FOLLOWING UP
Acute pharyngitis usually goes away within a week or two. Check with your health care provider if you still have symptoms after that time.

■ SPECIAL CONSIDERATIONS
Do not use goldenseal during pregnancy.

▪ PREECLAMPSIA

Preeclampsia is a dangerous combination of high blood pressure, fluid retention, and high levels of protein in the urine of women after their 20th week of pregnancy. Sometimes called toxemia, it affects about one in 20 pregnant women. If not treated, preeclampsia can worsen into eclampsia, a potentially fatal condition that involves seizures and coma. Preeclampsia puts unborn children and their mothers at risk.

▪ SIGNS AND SYMPTOMS

Preeclampsia:

- High blood pressure (above 140/90)
- Large increase in your systolic (top number) or diastolic (bottom number) blood pressure
- Excessive weight gain (more than five pounds in a week)
- Sudden weight gain over one or two days
- Retention of fluids, which causes the hands and face to swell, (pregnancy naturally causes the ankles to swell slightly, which is not necessarily a sign of preeclampsia)
- Reduction in the amount of your urine

Eclampsia:

- Pain in the upper right side of your abdomen
- Disturbances to your vision, such as seeing flashing lights

▪ WHAT CAUSES IT?

Nobody knows what causes preeclampsia. However, certain women have a higher risk of developing it in pregnancy. They include women in their first pregnancy; teenagers and women over 40 who are pregnant; women carrying multiple fetuses; women who have already suffered preeclampsia; African-American women; and women who have had high blood pressure, diabetes, or kidney disease.

▪ WHAT TO EXPECT AT YOUR PROVIDER'S OFFICE

Once you have described your symptoms, your health care provider will take your blood pressure and examine your face and hands for evidence of fluid retention. He or she will want samples of your blood and urine, for tests to differentiate between preeclampsia and other diseases. Your provider will probably want you to collect all the urine you produce during a full day.

▪ TREATMENT OPTIONS

If you have a mild case of preeclampsia, your health care provider may recommend that you rest in bed. You should lie on your left side, to prevent the weight of your uterus from pressing against important blood vessels. You should drink a lot of water to help you urinate and get rid of excess fluids. Your provider will want to monitor your blood pressure and urine every couple of days.

If your pregnancy is far along (28 weeks or more) and you have severe preeclampsia, your provider may admit you to the hospital, where you will receive drugs to induce labor or a Cesarean section.

Your practitioner may prescribe the following drugs, which are given intravenously.

- Magnesium sulfate or hydralazine to reduce your blood pressure
- Calcium gluconate intravenously if your blood pressure falls too low
- Furosemide to encourage you to urinate more

Complementary and Alternative Therapies

If you have preeclampsia, you should be under the care of an obstetrician. Complementary and alternative therapies can be used with medical treatment. Some of the most common ones are described below.

NUTRITION

- Omega-3 oils (1,000 mg three times a day) are highly beneficial in pregnancy, and help reduce swelling.
- Increasing protein intake may help minimize preeclampsia.
- Magnesium (200 mg two to three times per day) helps reduce high blood pressure.

HERBS

Herbs are generally a safe way to strengthen and tone the body's systems. As with any therapy, it is important to determine a diagnosis before pursuing treatment. Herbs may be used as dried extracts (capsules, powders, teas), glycerites (glycerine extracts), or tinctures (alcohol extracts). Unless otherwise indicated, teas should be made with 1 tsp. herb per cup of hot water. Steep covered 5 to 10 minutes for leaf or flowers, and 10 to 20 minutes for roots. Drink 2 to 4 cups per day. Tinctures may be used singly or in combination as noted.

Herbs that can be used to treat mild hypertension in pregnancy include the following: Passion flower *(Passiflora incarnata),* hawthorn berries *(Crataegus oxyanthoides),* cramp bark *(Viburnum opulus),* milk thistle *(Silybum marianum),* and Indian tobacco *(Lobelia inflata).* Use equal parts of each in a tincture, 20 drops three to four times a day.

ACUPUNCTURE

May be helpful in lowering blood pressure and generally increasing circulation.

▪ FOLLOWING UP

Your health care provider will monitor you carefully for the first few days after you have delivered your child. He or she will keep you in the hospital for several days to several weeks after you have delivered your baby, depending on the severity of the preeclampsia. You should have checkups at least every two weeks for the first several months after leaving the hospital.

▪ SPECIAL CONSIDERATIONS

If you wear rings, remove them as soon as you start having symptoms. Swollen fingers can make it difficult (or even impossible) to remove rings, and they may begin to cut off circulation in your fingers.

The symptoms of preeclampsia can appear gradually and suddenly get worse. See your health care provider regularly for checkups during your pregnancy, which you should do regardless of your risk of preeclampsia. He or she can recognize the early signs of preeclampsia and get treatment for you immediately.

■ PRIMARY PULMONARY HYPERTENSION

Pulmonary hypertension occurs when blood circulation through your lungs is restricted by narrowed blood vessels. To maintain blood flow through these narrowed blood vessels, pulmonary artery pressure increases. Pulmonary hypertension can occur by itself, but is often caused by an existing disease. It is a rare condition that mostly affects women in their 30s or 40s.

■ SIGNS AND SYMPTOMS

The most common symptom is shortness of breath with exercise, progressing to shortness of breath while at rest. Other symptoms are:

- Getting tired easily
- Fainting
- Cough
- Chest pain
- Swelling of the lower extremities
- Coughing up blood

■ WHAT CAUSES IT?

Many cases have no known cause. Some conditions that are associated with pulmonary hypertension include the following.

- Congenital heart disease
- Mitral stenosis or regurgitation
- Certain kinds of lung disease
- Obesity, especially with sleep apnea
- Chronic obstructive pulmonary disease (COPD)
- Cocaine abuse
- Use of dexfenfluramine and other diet drugs

■ WHAT TO EXPECT AT YOUR PROVIDER'S OFFICE

Your health care provider will give you a thorough examination and order laboratory tests to diagnose your condition.

■ TREATMENT OPTIONS

If your pulmonary hypertension is the result of an underlying disease, that disease must be treated. You must avoid excessive physical stress or exercise. If your disease has progressed, you may be advised to have lung or heart–lung transplantation.

Drug Therapies

Some treatments your health care provider may use include the following.

- Supplemental oxygen
- Vasodilator therapy for those with no underlying disease
- Anticoagulant therapy is used if the primary disease is thromboembolic pulmonary disease.
- Diuretics for right ventricular failure

Complementary and Alternative Therapies

NUTRITION

- Coenzyme Q10 (100 mg twice a day) supports cardiac function, is an antioxidant, and oxygenates tissues.
- L-Carnitine (500 mg three times per day) improves endurance and is needed for efficient cardiac function.
- Magnesium aspartate (200 mg two to three times per day) increases efficiency of cardiac muscle and decreases vascular resistance.
- Potassium aspartate (20 mg per day) improves the ability of the heart muscle to contract.
- Vitamin E (400 IU per day) is an antioxidant and protects the heart.
- Vitamin C (1,000 to 1,500 mg three times per day) is an antioxidant, improves vascular integrity, and stimulates immune function.

- Taurine (500 mg twice a day) enhances cardiac function.
- Selenium (200 mcg per day) is a cardioprotective antioxidant.
- Choline (250 to 500 mg per day) and inositol (150 to 200 mg per day) positively affect heart and lung activity.

HERBS

Herbs may be used as dried extracts (capsules, powders, teas), glycerites (glycerine extracts), or tinctures (alcohol extracts). Combine the following herbs in equal parts in tincture form and take 30 drops three to four times per day.

- Hawthorn (*Crataegus oxyacantha*) helps your heart work more efficiently without making it work harder. Strengthens the integrity of and mildly dilates blood vessels.
- Garlic (*Allium sativum*) helps you cough up mucus, lowers blood pressure, stimulates your immune system, and helps prevent hardening of the arteries.
- Rosemary (*Rosemarinus officinalis*) strengthens cardiac function, prevents hardening of the arteries, prevents spasms, and improves circulation to the lungs.
- Linden flowers (*Tilia cordata*) prevents spasms, lowers blood pressure, prevents hardening of the arteries, relaxes your respiratory system, and helps you cough up mucus. Also stimulates immune function.
- Ginkgo (*Ginkgo biloba*) improves peripheral blood flow and decreases platelet aggregation.
- Indian tobacco (*Lobelia inflata*) stimulates respiratory function, reduces spasms, and lowers blood pressure. Used in high doses this herb can have toxic side effects. Using small amounts in a formula (one fourth or less) will minimize the risk of toxicity.

HOMEOPATHY

Homeopathy may be useful as a supportive therapy.

PHYSICAL MEDICINE

Caster oil pack. Apply oil directly to chest, cover with a clean soft cloth and plastic wrap. Place a heat source over the pack and let sit for 30 to 60 minutes.

Contrast hydrotherapy. Alternate hot and cold applications to the chest. Alternate three minutes hot with one minute cold and repeat three times. This is one set. Do two to three sets per day. For very sick patients use cool and warm applications to decrease the contrast.

Steams. Using three to six drops of essential oils in a humidifier, vaporizer, atomizer, or warm bath will stimulate respiration and circulation. Consider eucalyptus, rosemary, thyme, or lavender.

ACUPUNCTURE

May support treatment of symptoms through an increase in circulation.

■ FOLLOWING UP

The prognosis for pulmonary hypertension is generally poor.

■ SPECIAL CONSIDERATIONS

For the most part, women who have primary pulmonary hypertension should not get pregnant because the condition is dangerous for both mother and baby.

■ PROSTATITIS

Prostatitis is usually caused by bacteria, but a nonbacterial form of the disease also exists. Prostatitis is the most common genitourinary ailment in men younger than age 50, but the bacterial form occurs most often in men age 70 and older. If left untreated, infection can spread to the testicles and epididymis (tubules in back of the testis) and, in severe cases, destroy the prostate gland.

■ SIGNS AND SYMPTOMS

- Recurrent urinary tract infections (UTIs)
- Frequent and urgent urination
- Difficult or painful urination
- Urinating at night
- Fever; chills
- Generalized sense of ill health
- Painful ejaculation
- Bloody semen
- Sexual dysfunction
- Pain in the lower back, pelvis, or perineum (lining of the pelvic area)

■ WHAT CAUSES IT?

Risk factors for prostatitis include the following.
- Recent urinary tract infection
- Prior sexually transmitted diseases, such as gonorrhea or chlamydia
- Smoking
- Excess alcohol consumption

■ WHAT TO EXPECT AT YOUR PROVIDER'S OFFICE

Your health care provider will do a physical examination of the prostate and use laboratory tests, such as urine analysis or blood cultures.

■ TREATMENT OPTIONS

Drug Therapies

Several antibiotics and other drugs are used to treat prostatitis. They are usually given orally, except in cases of sudden and severe prostatitis, which may require intravenous administration. The treatments may last 4 to 12 weeks, depending on how severe the infection is. Stool softeners, anti-inflammatory agents (such as ibuprofen), and hot sitz baths may also relieve symptoms.

Surgical Procedures

If fever and pain persist, you may need surgery.

Complementary and Alternative Therapies

NUTRITION

- Vitamin C (1,000 mg three to four times a day)
- Zinc (60 mg a day) has been shown to reduce the size of the prostate.
- Selenium (200 mcg a day) is an antioxidant concentrated in the prostate.
- Essential fatty acids (1,000 to 1,500 mg one to two times a day) are anti-inflammatory for optimum prostaglandin concentrations.
- Pumpkin seeds have been used historically for a healthy prostate.
- Avoid simple sugars, alcohol (especially beer), and coffee; drink plenty of water (48 oz. a day).

HERBS

Herbs may be used as dried extracts (capsules, powders, teas), glycerites (glycerine extracts), or tinctures (alcohol extracts). Teas should be made

with 1 tsp. herb per 1 cup of hot water. Steep covered 5 to 10 minutes for leaf or flowers, or 10 to 20 minutes for roots.

Studies show saw palmetto *(Serenoa ripens)* may be as effective as Proscar (a common prostate medication). Dose of 160 mg twice a day is difficult to achieve in tea or tincture; extract standardized for 85 to 95 percent of fatty acids and sterols is recommended.

Cernilton, a flower pollen extract (500 to 1,000 mg two to three times a day), has been used extensively in Europe to treat prostatitis caused by inflammation or infection. It also has a contractile effect on the bladder and relaxes the urethra.
- Bearberry *(Arctostaphylos uva-ursi):* diuretic, urinary antiseptic
- Goldenseal *(Hydrastis canadensis):* diuretic, antiseptic, antimicrobial
- Coneflower *(Echinacea purpurea):* improves immune function
- Corn silk *(Zea mays):* diuretic, soothing demulcent

Take a combination of the above herbs (1 cup tea or 60 drops tincture three times a day).

HOMEOPATHY

Some of the most common remedies used for prostatitis are listed below. Usually, the dose is 12X to 30C every one to four hours until your symptoms get better.
- *Chimaphila umbellata* for retention of urine with an enlarged prostate
- *Pulsatilla* for pain after urination, especially involuntary urination
- *Pareira* for painful urination, especially with painful urging
- *Lycopodium* for painful urination with reddish sediment in the urine, especially with impotence
- *Thuja* specifically if there is a forked stream of urine

PHYSICAL MEDICINE

Kegel exercises increase pelvic circulation and improve muscle tone.

Contrast sitz baths: You will need two basins that you can comfortably sit in. Fill one basin with hot water, one with cold water. Sit in hot water for three minutes, then in cold water for one minute. Repeat this three times to complete one set. Do one to two sets a day, three to four days a week.

ACUPUNCTURE

May improve urinary flow and decrease swelling and inflammation.

MASSAGE

May help reduce symptoms. Focus may be on the lower abdominal area, lower back, and around the sacrum.

■ FOLLOWING UP

Be sure you follow your health care provider's instructions for treatment and keep using the treatment as directed even if you start to feel better.

■ SPECIAL CONSIDERATIONS

Men should have a yearly prostate examination after age 40, even if they have no symptoms of prostate problems. In recurring cases, you may need ongoing treatment with periodic checkups.

■ PSORIASIS

Psoriasis is a skin disorder that appears as raised, reddish-pink areas covered with silvery scales and red borders. Psoriasis most commonly appears on the scalp, elbows, knees, groin, and lower back. It "comes and goes," and may appear as a few spots or involve large areas. It is not contagious, either to other body parts or other people. More than 6 million people in the United States have psoriasis, which is seen in both sexes and all age groups. It can be triggered by emotional stress and can run in families. Severe cases can be physically painful and emotionally traumatic due to its unsightly appearance. Approximately 10 percent of psoriasis sufferers develop psoriatic arthritis, a painful arthritic condition.

■ SIGNS AND SYMPTOMS

The following are symptoms of psoriasis.
- Raised skin lesions, deep pink with red borders and silvery surface scales; may be cracked and painful
- Blisters oozing with pus (usually occurs on the palms or soles)
- Pitted, discolored, and possibly thickened fingernails or toenails
- Itchy skin in some people
- Joint pain (psoriatic arthritis) in some people

■ WHAT CAUSES IT?

The cause of psoriasis is uncertain, but researchers do know that it involves a higher-than-normal rate of skin-cell production. Dead skin cells accumulate and form thick patches. Several underlying factors may trigger the disorder or flare-ups, including the following.
- Faulty immune system
- Genetics (hereditary)
- Emotional stress
- Obesity
- Skin injuries or sunburn
- Streptococcal (strep) infection (symptoms sometimes first appear two weeks after strep throat)
- Certain drugs (gold, lithium, beta-blockers)
- Acidic foods
- Alcohol

■ WHAT TO EXPECT AT YOUR PROVIDER'S OFFICE

Your health care provider will examine your skin and ask questions about your physical and emotional health. You may need a blood test to check levels of calcium, zinc, and certain other elements.

■ TREATMENT OPTIONS

Your provider may suggest one or several different treatment options.
- Topical creams and lotions
- Medications
- Light therapy
- Changes in your diet
- Vitamin or mineral supplements
- Exercise
- Elimination therapy (in which you discontinue taking certain medications or eating certain foods)

Drugs used to treat psoriasis include corticosteroids, cancer-treatment medications, vitamin A derivatives, and nonsteroidal anti-inflammatory drugs (NSAIDs, such as ibuprofen) for pain or inflammation. Topical creams and lotions for psoriasis may include corticosteroids, petroleum jelly, vitamin D_3, coal tar ointments or shampoos, ultraviolet light therapy (short exposures to sunlight), liquid nitrogen (to freeze moderate-sized lesions to reduce chance that they'll grow larger).

Complementary and Alternative Therapies

You may benefit from mind/body therapies and stress management. Exercise can help too, as can drinking plenty of water.

NUTRITION

- Eliminate alcohol, simple sugars, inflammatory fats (meat, dairy). Avoid acidic foods (pineapple, oranges, coffee, tomato) and any allergic foods (wheat, citrus, milk, corn, eggs).
- Essential fatty acids: omega-3 and omega-6 (oily fish, flaxseed oil, 1,000 mg two times per day)
- Vitamins: B_{12} (100 to 1,000 mcg) may need to be intramuscular injections, folate (400 mcg per day), vitamin E (400 to 800 IU per day)
- Minerals: zinc (30 mg per day), selenium (200 mcg per day)
- Quercetin: 500 mg three times per day before meals
- Digestive enzymes help with proper protein digestion

HERBS

Herbs may be used as dried extracts (capsules, powders, teas), glycerites (glycerine extracts), or tinctures (alcohol extracts). Teas should be made with 1 tsp. herb per cup of hot water. Steep covered 5 to 10 minutes for leaf or flowers, and 10 to 20 minutes for roots.
- Milk thistle *(Silybum marianum)* stops breakdown of substances that contribute to psoriasis, protects the liver
- Yellow dock *(Rumex crispus)*, red clover *(Trifolium pratense)*, and burdock *(Arctium lappa)* are alternatives.
- Sarsaparilla *(Smilax sarsaparilla)* can be effective in psoriasis
- Coleus *(Coleus forskohlii)* has been historically used for psoriasis

Mix equal parts of the above herbs and use 1 cup tea three times per day or 30 to 60 drops tincture three times per day. This is especially effective if sipped. Take 5 to 15 minutes before meals to stimulate digestion. Coleus *(Coleus forskohlii)* (tincture, 1 ml three times a day) has been used historically for psoriasis.

Topical creams may relieve discomfort. Chickweed *(Stellaria media)* relieves itching and marigold *(Calendula officinalis)* speeds healing of open lesions.

HOMEOPATHY

Be aware that homeopathic treatment of skin problems can result in an initial worsening before resolution.

■ FOLLOWING UP

See your provider regularly until your psoriasis is under control.

■ SPECIAL CONSIDERATIONS

In pregnancy, oral medications can be damaging to a fetus and topical creams can be absorbed into the bloodstream.

■ PULMONARY EDEMA

Pulmonary edema occurs when too much fluid accumulates in the lungs, often due to heart attacks, heart disease, or acute severe asthma. It requires immediate medical attention.

■ SIGNS AND SYMPTOMS

Symptoms often begin suddenly and get worse quickly. They include:

- Extreme shortness of breath and difficulty breathing
- Tightness and pain in the chest
- Wheezing, coughing
- Paleness
- Sweating
- Bluish nails and lips
- Pink, frothy mucus coming from nose and mouth

■ WHAT CAUSES IT?

Some risk factors for pulmonary edema include the following.

- High blood pressure
- Diabetes
- Coronary or valvular heart disease
- Obesity
- Smoking
- Exposure to high altitude
- Heroin overdose
- Central nervous system injury
- Infection
- Pregnancy
- Hyperthyroidism
- Hanta virus
- Inhaled toxins
- Stress
- Blood transfusion

■ WHAT TO EXPECT AT YOUR PROVIDER'S OFFICE

Immediate treatment is required because an attack is life-threatening. Once the initial attack is under control, your provider will order blood tests and a urine test to look for what may have caused the attack. You will also undergo a chest X-ray and electrocardiogram.

■ TREATMENT OPTIONS

Medications include diuretics to remove excess fluid from the lungs and morphine to relieve congestion. In rare cases, surgery may be needed.

Complementary and Alternative Therapies

Alternative therapies can strengthen the cardiopulmonary system.

NUTRITION

- Increase dietary potassium and magnesium when using diuretics (for example, bananas, apricots, nuts, seeds, and green leafy vegetables).
- Coenzyme Q10 (100 mg twice a day) supports cardiac function.
- L-carnitine (500 mg three times per day) improves endurance.
- Magnesium aspartate (200 mg two to three times per day) increases efficiency of cardiac muscle. Magnesium and calcium (1,000 mg per day) improve fluid exchange in the body.
- Potassium aspartate (20 mg per day) improves ability of heart muscle to contract and should be supplemented with diuretic use.
- Vitamin E (400 IU per day) is an antioxidant and protects your heart.
- Vitamin C (1,000 to 1,500 mg three times per day) is an antioxidant.
- Taurine (500 mg twice a day) enhances cardiac function.
- Raw heart concentrate (100 to 200 mg per day) provides essential nutrients to the heart.
- Selenium (200 mcg per day) protects heart and lung tissues.
- Choline (250 to 500 mg per day) and inositol (150 to 200 mg per day) positively affect heart and lung activity.

HERBS

Herbs may be used as dried extracts (capsules, powders, teas), glycerites (glycerine extracts), or tinctures (alcohol extracts). Teas should be made with 1 tsp. herb per cup of hot water. Steep covered 5 to 10 minutes for leaf or flowers, and 10 to 20 minutes for roots.

The following are best administered in a tea (4 to 6 cups per day), although a tincture may be used (30 to 60 drops four times per day). Combine three of the these herbs with equal parts of two to three additional herbs from the following categories, according to the underlying cause. Cleavers (*Gallium aparine*), yarrow (*Achillea millefolium*), oatstraw (*Avena sativa*), elder (*Sambucus canadensis*), red clover (*Trifolium pratense*), fresh parsley (*Petroselenium crispus*), and dandelion leaf (*Taraxacum officinalis*).

For pulmonary edema that does not originate with the heart:

- Garlic (*Allium sativum*) helps you cough up mucus, lowers blood pressure, and stimulates your immune system. (Garlic can also be taken as capsules, 1,000 to 4,000 mg per day.)
- Rosemary (*Rosemarianus officinalis*) strengthens cardiac function.
- Linden flowers (*Tilia cordata*) reduce spasms, lower blood pressure, prevent hardening of the arteries, relax your respiratory system.
- Indian tobacco (*Lobelia inflata*) stimulates respiratory function, reduces spasms, and lowers blood pressure.
- Thyme leaf (*Thymus vulgaris*) helps you cough up mucus, tones the respiratory system, and increases circulation.

For pulmonary edema originating with the heart:

- Hawthorn (*Crataegus oxyacantha*) helps your heart work better.
- Motherwort (*Leonorus cardiaca*) has antispasmodic properties, relieves heart palpitations, and enhances cardiac function.
- Rosemary strengthens blood vessels and is a heart tonic.

HOMEOPATHY

Homeopathy may be useful as a supportive therapy.

PHYSICAL MEDICINE

Alternating hot and cold applications with hand or foot baths may help circulation. Alternate three minutes hot with one minute cold. Repeat three times. This is one set. Do two to three sets per day.

Castor oil pack. Apply oil directly to the chest, cover with a clean soft cloth and plastic wrap. Place a heat source over the pack and let sit for 30 to 60 minutes.

ACUPUNCTURE

Acupuncture may improve cardiopulmonary function.

MASSAGE

Massage can assist with increasing circulation and lymphatic drainage.

■ FOLLOWING UP

Continued medication and surveillance may be required.

■ SPECIAL CONSIDERATIONS

Pregnant women who are obese and have high blood pressure are at increased risk for pulmonary edema.

■ RAYNAUD'S PHENOMENON

Raynaud's phenomenon is a condition where blood vessels in the fingers and toes (and sometimes in the earlobes, nose, and lips) constrict. It is usually triggered by cold or by emotional stress. Episodes are intermittent and may last minutes or hours. Approximately 5 to 10 percent of the U.S. population is affected, and women are affected five times more often than men. It usually occurs between the ages of 20 and 40 in women and later in life in men.

■ SIGNS AND SYMPTOMS

- Changes in skin color in the fingers or toes and sometimes in the nose, legs, or earlobes (may occur in three phases: white, blue, then red)
- Throbbing, tingling, numbness, and pain
- Deterioration of the pads on fingertips or toes
- Gangrenous ulcers near fingertips

■ WHAT CAUSES IT?

Risk factors for Raynaud's phenomenon include the following.

- Cigarette smoking
- Age in women (onset primarily between the ages of 20 and 40)
- Occupation (for example, using vibrating tools such as chain saws and jackhammers)
- Drug use, including some cancer drugs, narcotics, and over-the-counter cold medications
- Electric shock injury
- Previous frostbite
- Repetitive physical stress (for example, typing or playing the piano)
- Primary pulmonary hypertension
- Exposure to cold
- Psychological stress
- General medical conditions such as rheumatoid arthritis, scleroderma, systemic lupus erythematosus, and carpal tunnel syndrome

■ WHAT TO EXPECT AT YOUR PROVIDER'S OFFICE

Your health care provider may conduct several laboratory tests, such as the antinuclear antibody test, to look for antibodies associated with connective tissue disease or other autoimmune disorders. If you have Raynaud's phenomenon, your provider will most likely begin with a conservative approach involving non-drug and self-help measures (for example, dressing warmly, avoiding the cold, controlling stress).

■ TREATMENT OPTIONS

One of the most important preventive measures you can take is to stop smoking because nicotine shrinks arteries and decreases blood flow. Other preventive measures include the following.

- Protecting yourself from cold, especially outdoors in the winter
- Guarding against cuts and other injuries to affected areas
- Exercising, such as raising your arms above your head and then whirling them vigorously, to increase circulation

Drug Therapies

Several types of drugs are used to treat Raynaud's phenomenon. Calcium-channel blockers can reduce the frequency and severity of attacks. Vasodilators (drugs that open up blood vessels) are also recommended.

Surgical Procedures

If attacks become extremely frequent and severe and interfere with your well-being and ability to work or function, a surgical procedure called sympathectomy may be used. This surgery becomes less effective as the disease advances.

Complementary and Alternative Therapies

NUTRITION

- Vitamin E (400 to 800 IU per day) improves circulation and helps certain blood cells function well.
- Vitamin C (1,000 mg two to three times per day) supports connective tissue and reduces swelling.
- B-complex (50 to 100 mg per day) reduces stress.
- Coenzyme Q10 (100 mg two times per day) promotes healthy tissues.
- Calcium (1,500 mg per day) and Magnesium (200 mg 3 times per day) relieves spasm.
- Omega-3 oils (1,500 mg two to three times per day) reduce swelling and help certain blood cells function well.
- Zinc (30 to 50 mg per day) boosts your immune system.

HERBS

Herbs are generally a safe way to strengthen and tone the body's systems. As with any therapy, it is important to work with your provider on getting your problem diagnosed before you start any treatment. Herbs may be used as dried extracts (capsules, powders, teas), glycerites (glycerine extracts), or tinctures (alcohol extracts). Unless otherwise indicated, teas should be made with 1 tsp. herb per cup of hot water. Steep covered 5 to 10 minutes for leaf or flowers, and 10 to 20 minutes for roots. Drink 2 to 4 cups per day. Tinctures may be used singly or in combination as noted. The following herbs are circulatory stimulants with other properties as well. Use one or more tinctures in combination. Take 20 to 30 drops two times per day.

- Hawthorn berries (*Crataegus oxyanthoids*) strengthens and mildly dilates blood vessels
- Ginkgo (*Ginkgo biloba*) (120 to 160 mg per day for dried extracts) keeps blood cells from sticking together
- Rosemary (*Rosemariana officianalis*) is a gentle relaxant
- Ginger root (*Zingiber officinale*) is a mild soothing agent
- Prickly ash bark (*Xanthoxylum clava-herculis*) enhances lymph activity and integrity of blood vessels

HOMEOPATHY

Homeopathy may be useful as a supportive therapy.

ACUPUNCTURE

Acupuncture may be useful as an adjunct therapy.

■ FOLLOWING UP

Most milder cases can be brought under control through self-help measures.

■ SPECIAL CONSIDERATIONS

Many drugs used to treat Raynaud's phenomenon can affect a growing fetus and should not be used by pregnant women.

■ REITER'S SYNDROME

Reiter's syndrome has many possible symptoms, with arthritis (joint inflammation) being an important one. There is no cure for Reiter's syndrome, but you can control the symptoms.

■ SIGNS AND SYMPTOMS
- Arthritis—includes pain, swelling, stiffness, and redness of joints. Usually occurs on one side of the body and usually involves joints of the spine, pelvis, legs, fingers, toes, wrists, feet, or ankles.
- Conjuctivitis (inflammation under eyelids)—usually brief and mild
- Iritis (inflammation of the iris)—affects 5 percent of people with Reiter's and needs immediate medical treatment to avoid eye damage
- Urinary tract infection—burning during urination may or may not occur; may have pus drainage from penis
- Painless, shallow ulcers on the penis
- Pus-filled sores on soles, palms, and penis; mouth sores
- Weight loss, malaise, morning stiffness, fever
- Heart problems (rarely)

■ WHAT CAUSES IT?
Reiter's is a reactive arthritis, which means that another illness triggers it. Scientists do not know what actually causes Reiter's. But they know that the following factors often precede Reiter's.
- HLA-B27 gene—20 percent of people who have this gene get Reiter's; about 80 percent of people with Reiter's have the HLA-B27 gene.
- Bacterial triggers, such as salmonella, shigella, campylobacter
- Sexually transmitted disease triggers, such as chlamydia
- White males ages 20 to 40 are at higher risk.

■ WHAT TO EXPECT AT YOUR PROVIDER'S OFFICE
Tell your health care provider about any intestinal conditions or sexually transmitted diseases you have had recently. You may have a blood test to exclude other diseases and to see if you have the HLA-B27 gene.

■ TREATMENT OPTIONS
Drug Therapies
- Nonsteroidal anti-inflammatory drugs (NSAIDs)
- Corticosteroids
- Sulfasalazine—a promising experimental drug for arthritis
- Methotrexate—an experimental drug taken orally or by injection for chronic arthritis; frequent blood and liver tests are needed

Your provider may also prescribe drugs to treat specific symptoms.

Complementary and Alternative Therapies
Alternative therapies may be effective with fewer side effects than drugs.

NUTRITION
- Glucosamine sulfate (500 mg three times a day): stimulates cartilage growth and may be as effective for pain relief as NSAIDs without the side effects.
- Avoid nightshade family (tomatoes, potatoes, eggplant, peppers, tobacco); decrease saturated fats and alcohol (which can cause inflammation); increase oily fish, nuts, and flaxseed (which can decrease inflammation); increase fruits and vegetables (bioflavonoids).
- Vitamin C (1,000 to 3,000 mg a day), vitamin E (400 to 800 IU a day), beta-carotene (25,000 IU per day), selenium (200 mcg a day)
- Essential fatty acids (2 tbsps. oil a day or 1,000 to 1,500 mg twice a day): mix of omega-6 (evening primrose) and omega-3 (flaxseed)
- Minerals: zinc (45 mg a day), copper (1 mg a day), bromelain (500 mg three times a day) to reduce inflammation

HERBS
Herbs may be used as dried extracts (capsules, powders, teas), glycerites (glycerine extracts), or tinctures (alcohol extracts). Unless otherwise indicated, teas should be made with 1 tsp. herb per cup of hot water. Steep covered 5 to 10 minutes for leaf or flowers, and 10 to 20 minutes for roots. Drink 2 to 4 cups per day.

Turmeric *(Curcuma longa),* 400 mg three times a day: helps with morning stiffness and joint instability, works well when taken with bromelain

For urethritis: Mix three to four of these herbs in equal amounts and use 1 tsp. of mixture. Drink 1 cup tea three times a day or 30 drops tincture three times a day. Take daily during an acute flare-up and two weeks of the month as a preventative.
- Juniper *(Juniperus communis):* a diuretic, for inflammatory conditions of the urinary tract; avoid if you have kidney disease.
- Uva ursi *(Arctostaphylos uva-ursi):* used as an antibacterial and anti-inflammatory for lower urinary tract; for acute cases of Reiter's only
- Horsetail *(Equisetum arvense):* soothing diuretic
- Licorice *(Glycyrrhiza glabra):* soothing, anti-inflammatory, do not take if you have high blood pressure.
- Meadowsweet *(Filipendula ulmaria):* anti-inflammatory

For iritis:
- Horsetail, licorice, meadowsweet (see dosage directions above)
- Eyebright *(Euphrasia officinalis)* and bilberry *(Vaccinium myrtillus)* have been historically used for inflammation of the eyes. Drink 30 to 60 drops tincture three times a day, or 1 cup tea three times per day, or use tea to make compresses for acute relief: soak a cotton ball or cloth in a cooled tea and place over the eyes.

ACUPUNCTURE
As with other forms of arthritis, acupuncture may be effective at stimulating the immune system and reducing inflammation.

■ FOLLOWING UP
The initial attack usually lasts three to six months. Most people maintain near-normal lifestyles with physical and occupational adjustments.

■ RHEUMATOID ARTHRITIS

Rheumatoid arthritis (RA) occurs when your body's immune system attacks and destroys the tissues that make up your joints. The joints become swollen, stiff, and painful. In later stages, the joints can become deformed. Other areas of your body can also be affected, including your lungs, heart, blood vessels, and eyes. About 1 percent of the U.S. population suffers from RA. Typically, it strikes between the ages of 30 and 60, but it can occur at any age.

■ SIGNS AND SYMPTOMS

- Stiffness, swelling, and pain in and around certain joints, especially after not moving for a while (for example, when waking)
- Affected joints typically include hands, fingers, wrists, ankles, feet, elbows, and knees.
- Generally, if a joint on the right side of your body is affected, the same joint on the left side is also affected.
- Feeling tired and run-down with swollen lymph glands, a low fever, little or no appetite, and weight loss
- Appearance of small bumps under the skin near the affected joints

■ WHAT CAUSES IT?

Medical researchers do not know why RA develops. Genes may play some as yet unknown role. It also is possible that a change in the body, such as an infection or hormonal shift, can trigger its development.

■ WHAT TO EXPECT AT YOUR PROVIDER'S OFFICE

Your health care provider will assess the swelling and pain in each joint and will likely ask you to demonstrate how well you can use that joint. During the physical examination, your provider will take your temperature and check your lymph nodes and spleen for swelling. Your provider may order X-rays and blood and urine tests. In some cases, a small amount of fluid may be taken from the affected joint for examination. These tests help rule out other causes of your symptoms and confirm a diagnosis of RA.

■ TREATMENT OPTIONS
Drug Therapies

The following drugs are used to treat RA.
- Nonsteroidal anti-inflammatory drugs (NSAIDs) such as ibuprofen
- Disease-modifying antirheumatoid drugs (DMARDs) such as gold salts, antimalarials, methotrexate, cyclophosphamide, and others
- Corticosteroids (glucocorticoids) such as prednisone
- Combination therapy uses two or more DMARDs together.
- Experimental therapy uses newly developed drugs. Several of these attack cells in your immune system that destroy joint tissues.

Complementary and Alternative Therapies

The goal of therapy is to decrease inflammation and preserve joint function. Treatment is long term.

NUTRITION
- The most common allergic foods are wheat, corn, and dairy. An elimination diet may identify whether these foods constitute a problem: avoid allergenic foods completely for two weeks, then reintroduce the foods one at a time, every three days, and note if your RA symptoms get worse. Citrus, chocolate, alcohol, red meat, spices, and carbonated drinks may also aggravate RA.
- A vegetarian diet high in antioxidants and flavonoids (green tea, blueberry, elderberry) and low in saturated fats

- A small percentage of people respond dramatically to a diet free of nightshades. These include peppers, eggplant, tomatoes, and white potatoes. A month-long trial is recommended.
- One clinical study demonstrated that selenium combined with vitamin E reduces RA symptoms. Dose is 50 to 75 mcg per day of selenium and 400 to 800 IU of vitamin E.
- Zinc (45 mg per day) and manganese (45 mg per day)
- Omega-3 fatty acids keep white blood cells from producing substances that cause swelling. Dose is 1,000 to 1,500 IU per day.
- Bromelain: anti-inflammatory when taken between meals. Dose is 2,000 to 2,500 mg twice a day.
- Quercetin: stabilizes mast cells, found in increased numbers in the synovial membranes of affected joints. Dose is 250 to 500 mg three times per day, on an empty stomach.

HERBS
Herbs may be used as dried extracts (capsules, powders, teas), glycerites (glycerine extracts), or tinctures (alcohol extracts). Teas should be made with 1 tsp. herb per cup of hot water. Steep covered 5 to 10 minutes for leaf or flowers, and 10 to 20 minutes for roots.
- Devil's claw (*Harpagophytum procumbens*): analgesic, anti-inflammatory
- Ginseng (*Panax ginseng*): adaptogen (tonic for long-term stress), specific for chronic disease and the effects of suppressive medications
- Ginger (*Zingiber officinale*): antispasmodic, digestive stimulant
- Valerian (*Valariana officinalis*): relaxant, reduces spasms
- Blue flag (*Iris versicolor*): stimulates liver to process effects of inflammation
- Wild yam (*Dioscorea villosa*): specific for RA, helps reduce spasms
- Horsetail (*Equisitum arvense*): diuretic, stabilizes connective tissue

Devil's claw and three to five of the above herbs can be mixed as either tincture 30 to 60 drops three times per day, or 1 cup tea three times per day.

HOMEOPATHY
Some of the most common remedies used for rheumatoid arthritis are listed below. Usually, the dose is 12X to 30C every one to four hours until your symptoms get better.
- *Rhus toxicodendron* for arthritis that feels worse in the morning, in damp, cold weather, or before a storm
- *Bryonia alba* for arthritis that feels better with pressure, feels worse with any movement, or cold weather
- *Ruta graveolens* for arthritic pains that feel worse after exertion, feel better after resting, especially with a history of strains or sprains
- *Calcarea carbonica* for arthritis that is associated with weakness

ACUPUNCTURE
May decrease pain and joint inflammation, and slow progress of RA

MASSAGE
May be helpful in relieving symptoms and increasing mobility

■ FOLLOWING UP
Make regular visits to your health care provider to monitor the progress of the disease and side effects of drugs you may be taking.

■ ROSEOLA

Roseola is mainly a childhood disease. Almost all of the cases of roseola occur in the first two or three years of life. Roseola begins with a high fever, usually followed by a rash. About 30 percent of all children in the United States get roseola. There is also a type of roseola that occurs in adults who have a serious illness.

■ SIGNS AND SYMPTOMS

- Sudden high fever (103° to 106° F), which usually lasts three to four days. Your child will most likely remain alert in spite of the fever.
- Rash appears as the fever goes away and lasts three to four days. It may look like measles or rubella. There are rose-colored bumps two to three millimeters in diameter. The rash usually appears first on the trunk of the body. It may spread to the neck, arms, and legs but rarely to the face.
- Seizures happen in 5 to 35 percent of all cases of roseola. They will not cause brain damage, and they usually go away when the fever goes down. Seizures may also occur without the rash.
- Breathing problems, ear infections, and diarrhea occur in about half the cases.

■ WHAT CAUSES IT?

Roseola is caused by the human herpes virus 6 (HHV-6). It is still unknown how the disease is spread but it may be present in saliva. The incubation period is 5 to 15 days.

■ WHAT TO EXPECT AT YOUR PROVIDER'S OFFICE

Your child's health care provider may take blood to check for other conditions and complications. He or she will take your child's temperature and talk to you about how to take care of your child's roseola at home.

■ TREATMENT OPTIONS

- Drugs such as acetaminophen (Tylenol) lower the fever. They also can reduce the discomforts and aches of the fever. Acetaminophen can cause liver damage if you take it for long periods or in high doses. Do not use aspirin because it may cause a very serious illness called Reye's syndrome.
- Make sure your child drinks a lot of fluids to prevent dehydration.
- Sedatives may reduce the chance of seizure.
- Phenobarbital is sometimes given for seizures.

Complementary and Alternative Therapies

Herbal teas are anti-fever, and calming. Adult doses are listed, unless otherwise specified. The formula to determine the child's dose is (age of child divided by 20) x adult dose. Adult doses may given to the mother to treat breastfeeding babies.

NUTRITION

Immune stimulating: vitamin C (1,000 mg three times a day), zinc (30 to 60 mg per day), and beta-carotene (250,000 IU/day).

HERBS

Herbs may be used as dried extracts (capsules, powders, teas), glycerites (glycerine extracts), or tinctures (alcohol extracts). Unless otherwise indicated, teas should be made with 1 tsp. herb per cup of hot water. Steep covered 5 to 10 minutes for leaf or flowers, and 10 to 20 minutes for roots.

- Catnip (*Nepeta cataria*) lowers fever and reduces spasms
- Peppermint (*Mentha piperita*) reduces gas, has been historically used for colds and fevers
- Elder (*Sambuccus nigra*) calms your child and reduces fever
- Fennel (*Foeniculum vulgare*) for an upset stomach and upper respiratory irritation; calming
- Yarrow (*Achillea millifolium*) reduces fever, helps appetite loss
- Chamomile (*Matricaria recutita*) stimulates immune system, is a relaxant (to allow for sleep)

Mix four to six of the above and drink as a tea, 1cup three to four times per day or as a tincture, 60 drops three to four times per day. In addition, a strong tea (2 tbsp. herb) can be added to a bath to keep fever down.

Garlic (*Allium Sativum*)/ginger (*Zingiber officinale*) tea (one to three cloves garlic and one to three slices of fresh ginger) may be drunk to stimulate the immune system and prevent upper respiratory infections. Lemon and a sweetener may be added for flavor. Do not give honey to children under 2 years old.

HOMEOPATHY

Some of the most common remedies used for roseola are listed below. Usually, the dose is 12X to 30C every one to four hours until your symptoms get better.

- *Aconitum nappellus* for rapid onset of high fever
- *Belladonna* for high fever where the face or body are burning hot to the touch, especially with irritability and sensitivity to noise or light
- *Chamomilla* for fever with one cheek red and the other pale, with hypersensitivity and irritability
- *Pulsatilla* for fever, child is thirstless, clingy, and wants to be held

PHYSICAL MEDICINE

Warming socks. Wet cotton socks with cold water, wring them out, and put on the feet. Put on dry wool socks over the cotton socks and go to bed. This treatment, while uncomfortable at first, will help disperse a fever and allow for a good night's sleep.

Wet sheet wrap. Wrap the child in a cotton sheet that is wet with cold water and wrung out. Then wrap the child in another blanket. Especially in infants, this will disperse a fever and allow a restful sleep.

ACUPUNCTURE

Acupressure for children may be quite calming and help reduce the fever.

MASSAGE

Gentle massage may relieve discomfort. A foot massage may help relax the child. Some children will not want to be touched, however.

■ FOLLOWING UP

Most children get well within about a week with no problems. If your child has a seizure, call your provider or emergency room immediately.

■ SPECIAL CONSIDERATIONS

Avoiding infected children is the only prevention. There is no vaccine for roseola.

■ SEIZURE DISORDERS

Seizures occur when nerve cells in your body misfire. Types of seizures vary. Recurrent seizures from one of many chronic processes are considered epilepsy. However, seizures are not considered to be epilepsy if they occur only once or are correctable.

■ SIGNS AND SYMPTOMS

- Aura (before generalized seizures), including lethargy, depression, irritability, involuntary jerks of limbs, abdominal pains, pale complexion, headache, constipation, or diarrhea
- Loss of consciousness
- Total body muscle spasms
- Temporary cessation of breathing
- Bluish color of skin and mucous membranes
- Dilated pupils that do not react to light
- Bowel or bladder incontinence
- Increased pulse and blood pressure
- Increased salivation and sweating
- Deep coma, post-seizure confusion, and deep sleep

■ WHAT CAUSES IT?

Seizures are caused by hyperexcitable nerve cells in the brain (cerebral cortex) that fire abnormally. No one knows why this happens.. The conditions listed below are associated with seizure activity.

- Central nervous system infection (bacterial meningitis, encephalitis)
- Drug toxicity or withdrawal (for example, alcohol or illicit drug use)
- Genetic mutations
- Head trauma
- Electrolyte or metabolic abnormalities
- Drugs that lower the seizure threshold
- High fevers
- Brain abnormalities (for example, tumors, stroke)
- Low sugar and low calcium levels in the blood

■ WHAT TO EXPECT AT YOUR PROVIDER'S OFFICE

Precipitating events (for example, head trauma) and risk factors (for example, family or personal history of seizures) are important factors to be discussed with your provider. It is also important to note how you felt before and after the seizure. Your provider will do blood tests for baseline values and an electroencephalogram (EEG) to help in your diagnosis.

■ TREATMENT OPTIONS

The goal of therapy is to stop the seizures, to minimize adverse drug effects, to prevent recurrences, and to help you readjust to your home life and work environment after a seizure.

Drug Therapies

Your health care provider will most likely prescribe medication to help control your seizures (approximately 30 to 70 percent of people who have a seizure will have a second seizure within one year). You may need to try several medications before you find one that works for you.

Complementary and Alternative Therapies

Some mild seizures may be controlled by alternative therapies.

NUTRITION

- Diet: a high-fat, low-protein, low-carbohydrate (ketogenic) diet may help control the frequency of seizures. Some studies have shown a connection with food allergies and seizures in children. Avoid alcohol, caffeine, and aspartame.
- Taurine (500 mg three times per day): amino acid that has been shown in studies to inhibit seizures
- Folic acid (400 mcg per day): depleted during seizures and in some people with seizures, although higher doses than 400 mcg may actually precipitate some seizures. Should be taken with B_{12}
- B_{12} (100 to 200 mcg per day)
- B_6 (20 to 50 mg per kilogram of body weight): especially in children may help control seizures.
- Magnesium: 500 to 750 mg per day (should be in a 1:1 ratio in people taking calcium) for normal muscle and nervous system function
- Manganese: (5 to 15 mg per day) depleted in people with epilepsy
- Zinc (30 mg per day) may be depleted by some medications
- Dimethyl glycine (100 mg twice a day): may decrease medication requirements

HERBS

Herbs may be used as dried extracts (capsules, powders, teas), glycerites (glycerine extracts), or tinctures (alcohol extracts). Teas should be made with 1 tsp. of herb per cup of hot water. Steep covered 5 to 10 minutes for leaf or flowers; 10 to 20 minutes for roots. Drink 2 to 4 cups per day.

- Passionflower *(Passiflora incarnata):* to both prevent and treat seizures, may be effective without side effects, especially where stress is a precipitating factor. Dose is 30 drops three to four times per day.
- Skullcap *(Scutellaria lateriflora):* antispasmodic and calmative herb
- Valerian *(Valeriana officinalis):* spasmolytic, sedative

The above herbs may be used singly or in combination as 1 cup tea three times per day or 30 to 60 drops tincture three times per day. In addition, use milk thistle *(Silybum marianum)* to protect the liver from effects of medications (70 to 210 mg three times per day).

HOMEOPATHY

Some of the most common remedies used for seizure disorders are listed below. Usually the dose is 12X to 30C every one to four hours until your symptoms get better.

- *Artemesia vulgaris* for convulsions after exertion or visual stimulation
- *Oenanthe* for violent seizures, especially when they are worse during a woman's menstrual period or after a head injury
- *Bufo* for convulsions accompanied by delayed development in children
- *Cicuta* for violent seizures with arching of the back
- *Cuprum metallicum* for seizures with mental dullness and/or difficulty breathing
- *Causticum* for seizures during menstrual periods or after a fright
- *Belladonna,* especially for convulsions followed by nausea

PHYSICAL MEDICINE

Chiropractic, osteopathic, or naturopathic manipulation may be helpful, especially in children or for seizures after head trauma.

ACUPUNCTURE

Acupuncture may be helpful with specific acupressure points that have been used to stop seizures.

■ FOLLOWING UP

Determining the best dosage or drug combinations is an inexact science; your provider will monitor you until your seizures are under control.

■ SEXUAL DYSFUNCTION

Sexual dysfunctions cover a wide variety of disorders, including male impotence, premature ejaculation in males, spasms of the vagina, pain with sexual intercourse, and problems with sexual desire (libido) and response. Men over age 65 are at increased risk for impotence. Impotence, however, is not a normal part of aging. The causes of sexual disorders vary, and include psychological causes and some medical conditions, such as illness or injury.

■ SIGNS AND SYMPTOMS

- Premature or abnormal ejaculation in men
- Inability to achieve or maintain an erection (impotency)
- Pain during intercourse
- Lack or loss of sexual desire
- Difficulty achieving orgasm
- Inadequate vaginal lubrication in women

■ WHAT CAUSES IT?

- Age 65 and over in men
- Depression or anxiety
- Stressful life events
- Certain medical conditions

■ WHAT TO EXPECT AT YOUR PROVIDER'S OFFICE

Your health care provider will do a physical examination. He or she may ask about your ethnic, cultural, religious, and social background, which can influence your sexual desires, expectations, and attitudes. Blood tests can help distinguish between psychological and physical causes for sexual dysfunctions. Other tests for men may include penile tumescence measurements, which are done while you are sleeping to determine whether an impotence problem is psychological or physical.

■ TREATMENT OPTIONS

Antidepressants can be taken by men and women whose sexual dysfunction is related to depression. Vasodilators administered by injection are sometimes used for impotence. Viagra (sildenafil citrate), a relatively new drug for treating impotence, can have serious side effects in some men. Over-the-counter products are available as creams or gels for women whose bodies produce inadequate lubrication.

A variety of psychological, behavioral, and interpersonal therapies are also available for many sexual disorders.

Surgery on the veins in the penis can be performed in severe cases, but this treatment is still considered experimental. An implant in the penis may help impotence if the problem does not respond to other treatment.

Complementary and Alternative Therapies

Sexual dysfunction secondary to decreased circulation, hormonal imbalance, depression, or anxiety may be reduced with alternative therapies.

NUTRITION

- Vitamin C (1,000 mg three times per day) supports vascular integrity.
- Vitamin E (400 IU per day), B6 (50 to 100 mg per day), and zinc (30 mg per day) to support hormone production.
- Magnesium (200 mg twice a day) supports hormone production.
- B-complex (50 to 100 mg per day) helps reduce stress.

HERBS

Herbs may be used as dried extracts (capsules, powders, teas), glycerites (glycerine extracts), or tinctures (alcohol extracts). Unless otherwise indicated, teas should be made with 1 tsp. herb per cup of hot water. Steep covered 5 to 10 minutes for leaf or flowers, and 10 to 20 minutes for roots.

For sexual dysfunction related to poor circulation:
- Ginkgo *(Ginkgo biloba,* 50 to 100 mg per day) increases peripheral circulation and may improve sexual function.
- Hawthorn *(Crataegus oxyacantha),* rosemary *(Rosemarinus officinalis),* ginger root *(Zingiber officinale),* and prickly ash bark *(Xanthoxylum clava-herculis)* are circulatory stimulants. Use singly or in combination, 3 cups of tea per day or 20 to 30 drops tincture three times per day.
- Yohimbe bark *(Pausinystalia yohimbe)* can be used for sexual dysfunction, under the supervision of your provider.

For sexual dysfunction secondary to hormonal imbalance:
- Chaste tree *(Vitex agnus-cactus)* helps normalize pituitary function but must be taken long-term (12 to 18 months) for effectiveness.
- Saw palmetto *(Serenoa repens)* may help hormone balance.
- Damiana *(Turnera diffusa)* may support testosterone levels. It also tones the central nervous system and may help relieve anxiety.
- Milk thistle *(Silybum marianum),* dandelion root *(Taraxacum officinale),* and vervain *(Verbena hastata)* support the liver and may help restore hormone ratios. Use equal parts in a tea (1 cup before meals), or tincture (15 to 20 drops before meals).

For sexual dysfunction associated with depression or anxiety:
St. John's wort *(Hypericum perforatum),* kava kava *(Piper methysticum),* skullcap *(Scutellaria laterifolia),* lemon balm *(Melissa officinalis),* passionflower *(Passiflora incarnata),* and gotu kola *(Centella asiatica).* Combine equal parts in a tea (1 cup twice a day) or tincture (20 to 30 drops twice a day). May take six weeks for results.

HOMEOPATHY

Homeopathy may be useful as a supportive therapy.

PHYSICAL MEDICINE

Contrast sitz baths promote circulation. You will need two basins that you can comfortably sit in. Sit in hot water for three minutes, then in cold water for one minute. Repeat this three times to complete one set. Do one to two sets per day three to four days per week.

MASSAGE

Therapeutic massage can reduce the effects of stress.

■ FOLLOWING UP

Most sexual dysfunctions are long-term and require professional care.

■ SPECIAL CONSIDERATION

Certain drugs and herbs used for treating these psychological or physical disorders may have serious side effects. Marital counseling and other forms of interpersonal therapy are also important.

■ SINUSITIS

Sinusitis is a swelling and infection of the sinuses near the nose. About 31 million adults and children in the United States have sinusitis each year. Sinusitis usually begins with an acute sinus infection that lasts for two to four weeks. A chronic sinus infection is one that continues for four weeks or longer.

■ SIGNS AND SYMPTOMS

- Nasal discharge (yellow or green), postnasal drip
- Headache, pain, sinus tenderness, or toothache
- Cough or sore throat
- Fever, in half of patients
- Loss of smell
- General tiredness

■ WHAT CAUSES IT?

The sinuses cannot drain properly and become infected. Some common causes for this include the following.

- Common cold (upper respiratory tract infection)
- Allergies (hay fever, tobacco smoke, dry air, pollutants)
- Infected tooth
- Swimming
- Disease or an abnormal structure in the sinus area
- Physical injury to the sinuses

■ WHAT TO EXPECT AT YOUR PROVIDER'S OFFICE

Your health care provider will give you a physical examination and will prescribe an antibiotic. You may need to have special tests to determine the cause of your sinusitis if it does not go away.

■ TREATMENT OPTIONS

Drug Therapies

The first time you get sinusitis you will probably be prescribed an antibiotic called amoxicillin. Sinus infections often come back. If yours does, you may be given a stronger broad-spectrum antibiotic. Decongestants can help with uncomfortable symptoms. Do not take decongestants if you have problems with urinating or have a heart condition. Use nasal sprays only for the prescribed amount of time. Your provider may also prescribe a nasal steroid spray.

Complementary and Alternative Therapies

A combination of physical medicine and herbal or homeopathic treatment is often effective for treating both acute and chronic sinusitis.

NUTRITION

- Vitamin C (1,000 mg three times a day), zinc (30 to 60 mg per day), beta-carotene (15,000 IU per day) to support immunity.
- Bromelain (500 mg three times a day between meals) and quercetin (500 mg three times a day between meals) are anti-inflammatory
- Avoid mucus-producing foods, such as dairy products, bananas, and any known food allergens.
- Drink plenty of fluids. Decrease sugar intake.

HERBS

Herbs may be used as dried extracts (capsules, powders, teas), glycerites (glycerine extracts), or tinctures (alcohol extracts). Unless otherwise indicated, teas should be made with 1 tsp. herb per cup of hot water. Steep covered 5 to 10 minutes for leaf or flowers, and 10 to 20 minutes for roots.

- Wild indigo *(Baptesia tinctoria)*—specific for sinus infections
- Eyebright *(Euphrasia officinalis)*—reduces inflammation, specifically for sinus problems
- Licorice *(Glycyrrhiza glabra)*—antiviral, soothing, especially with exhaustion or heartburn. Do not use if you have high blood pressure.
- Coneflower *(Echinacea purpurea)*—stimulates the immune system
- Goldenseal *(Hydrastis canadensis)*—antiviral, antibacterial

A combination of all of the above herbs, equal parts, may be very effective. 1 cup tea or 30 to 60 drops tincture every two to four hours. May add:

- Jamaican dogwood *(Piscidia piscipula)* or St. John's wort *(Hypericum perforatum)*, in equal parts, may be added for pain relief.
- Garlic/ginger tea—two to three cloves of garlic and two to three slices of fresh ginger. Steep 5 to 15 minutes and drink, breathing in the steam. Stimulates immune system and drainage.
- Essential oils may be used for bath or steam. For a steam, place two to five drops in a pot, bring to a simmer, and hold your head over the pot. For a bath, add 5 to 10 drops of oil to the bath. Eucalyptus, lavender, and thyme are specific for upper respiratory infections. Lavender and rosemary are also very calming.

HOMEOPATHY

Some of the most common remedies used for sinusitis are listed below. Usually, the dose is 12X to 30C every one to four hours until your symptoms get better.

- *Arsenicum album* for sinusitis with watery discharge
- *Kali bichromicum* for sinusitis with thick "gluey" discharge
- *Pulsatilla* for thick, bland, greenish discharge
- *Nux vomica* for sinusitis with a "stopped up" feeling

PHYSICAL MEDICINE

- Contrast hydrotherapy. Alternate hot and cold applications. Apply wet washcloths over the sinus area. Alternate three minutes hot with one minute cold. Repeat three times. This is one set. Do two to three sets per day.
- Nasal wash. Mix salt and water to taste like tears. Rinse each nostril by holding your head sideways over the sink and letting water run from the upper nostril to the lower nostril. Keep nostrils lower than throat to prevent salt water from draining into the back of the throat.

ACUPUNCTURE

May be helpful for both acute and chronic sinusitis.

■ FOLLOWING UP

If you are not better in a few weeks, you may be sent to an ear, nose, and throat specialist for tests to find the cause of your sinus infection.

■ SPECIAL CONSIDERATIONS

Some serious diseases are caused by sinusitis or can have similar symptoms. Be sure to see your health care provider if you are not feeling better or have new symptoms. Tell your provider if you may be pregnant.

■ SLEEP APNEA

People with sleep apnea stop breathing for short periods of time while they are asleep. You generally don't wake up fully when this happens, but in the morning you don't feel rested, and you feel sleepy during the day. Sleep apnea can be caused by a blocked upper airway (called obstructive apnea), by your brain not signaling your lungs to breathe (central apnea), or by a combination of these two problems.

■ SIGNS AND SYMPTOMS

The symptoms of sleep apnea include the following.
- Loud, irregular snoring, then quiet periods of at least 10 seconds when breathing stops; these episodes can happen up to 100 times or more each hour
- Daytime sleepiness, always feeling tired
- Morning headaches, sore throat, dry mouth, cough
- Feeling depressed, moody, irritable
- Unable to concentrate or remember
- Possible impotence or high blood pressure

■ WHAT CAUSES IT?

Apnea is caused by many physical conditions (such as obesity, or large tonsils and adenoids). The typical person with sleep apnea is an overweight, middle-aged man who has allergies, but apnea can occur at any age and in women as well as men. Sometimes drugs such as alcohol, sleeping pills, or heart medications can trigger apnea. It can also be inherited.

■ WHAT TO EXPECT AT YOUR PROVIDER'S OFFICE

People who have sleep apnea often seek medical help because they feel tired all the time or because their partner complains of loud snoring. Your health care provider will check your weight and blood pressure and ask about allergies. He or she may send you home with a device to check your oxygen levels while you sleep. Your provider may also refer you to a sleep clinic for overnight testing.

■ TREATMENT OPTIONS

- A few drugs hold promise, but most have some undesirable side effects.
- Several mask and ventilator devices are available, as well as dental appliances worn in your mouth. These may be uncomfortable at first.
- Sometimes surgery is needed, but your provider will most likely recommend that you try devices or drugs first.

Making the following lifestyle changes can help obstructive apnea.
- Lose weight.
- Minimize your use of alcohol, antihistamines, or tranquilizers.
- Get treatment for allergies and colds or sinus problems.
- Gargle with salt water (without swallowing) to shrink your tonsils.
- Develop regular sleep habits, and especially make sure you get enough sleep at night.
- Sleep on your side or sitting up rather than on your back. You may want to sew a couple of tennis balls to the back of your sleepwear or put pillows behind you so you stay on your side.
- Use an air humidifier at night.
- Don't smoke or expose yourself to other irritants (such as dust or perfumes).
- Raise the head of your bed by placing bricks under the headboard.

Complementary and Alternative Therapies

Alternative therapies may be useful in treating sleep apnea caused by allergies. Homeopathy and nutrition are most likely to have a positive effect. While many supplements are touted as good for weight loss, none have proven to be as effective as eating less and exercising more.

NUTRITION

- Diet: Try eliminating mucus-producing foods (dairy and bananas) for two weeks, reintroducing them and noticing any difference.
- Essential fatty acids (EFAs) moderate inflammatory response, decrease allergic response; EFAs are found to be low in obese people.
- Chromium helps regulate insulin and decrease insulin resistance; Chromium may not be effective at burning fat, but effective at stabilizing blood sugar and decreasing sugar cravings.

HOMEOPATHY

Some of the most common remedies used for sleep apnea are listed below. Usually, the dose is 12X to 30C every one to four hours until your symptoms get better.
- *Grindelia* is recommended if you also have advanced heart or lung illness, and if you wake suddenly with the feeling that you are suffocating.
- *Lachesis* is recommended if you also have frequent nightmares, are unable to sleep on your right side, and talk in your sleep.
- *Sambucus* nigra is recommended if you have trouble breathing at night, and if you wake suddenly with the feeling that you are suffocating, especially if you have asthma or a nasal blockage.
- *Spongia* is recommended if you wake with a feeling of suffocation, you have a harsh, dry cough, and your throat feels tight, ticklish, or dry.
- *Digitalis* can help if you have a slow heartbeat that may be accompanied by palpitations.
- *Opium* can help if you snore loudly and your sleep is very deep and hard to disturb, especially if you have a condition called narcolepsy (inability to control falling asleep).
- *Sulfur* is recommended if you have trouble falling asleep and have nightmares, especially if you also have skin rashes that become worse with heat.

ACUPUNCTURE

May be helpful in treating sleep apnea.

■ FOLLOWING UP

Sleep apnea is a serious condition that can cause fatal heart problems, so it's crucial to stick with your treatment plan. If you are using a mask and ventilator equipment, be sure to take care of them. Keep in contact with your health care provider or sleep clinic to make sure your treatment is working.

■ SPECIAL CONSIDERATIONS

If you are pregnant, you may have nasal congestion that makes you snore in a way that people with apnea do, but this is not apnea. If you have apnea and become pregnant, be sure to continue your treatment so that your condition will not affect your baby.

■ SPRAINS AND STRAINS

Sprains and strains often result from sports or exercise, but can easily result from any physical activity. Sprains result from an injury to a ligament (the connective tissue that links bones together at joints), most often in the ankle, knee, elbow, or wrist. Strains are tears in muscle tissue, commonly occurring in the muscles that support the neck, thigh, groin, and ankle.

■ SIGNS AND SYMPTOMS

Sprains and strains cause pain and swelling. You may have joint instability or disability if the injury is serious, involving a muscle or ligament tear.

■ WHAT CAUSES IT?

Sprains generally result from a twisting force applied to a joint while it is bearing weight, which causes the ligament to stretch beyond its natural limit. Muscle strains occur when the weight load on a muscle is greater than what the weakest part of the muscle can bear. Strains usually occur during activities that require a muscle to be stretched and bear weight at the same time. You are at risk for a sprain or strain if you do the following.

- Exercise without warming up properly
- Use athletic equipment that does not fit properly
- Participate in sports and activities that you are not conditioned for

■ WHAT TO EXPECT AT YOUR PROVIDER'S OFFICE

Your health care provider may take an X ray. If your injury is severe, he or she may also order an MRI. You may need to have the injured limb wrapped in an elastic bandage or put in a soft cast.

■ TREATMENT OPTIONS

You may want to take a mild pain reliever such as aspirin, acetaminophen, ibuprofen, or naproxen to reduce swelling. Limit activity that involves the injured area for at least seven days. Your health care provider will recommend that you treat the injury with RICE: rest, ice (wrapped in a cloth or a towel—do not apply ice directly to the skin), compression, and elevation of the affected area. Apply RICE as needed over the first several days following the injury.

Complementary and Alternative Therapies

Specific nutrients and herbs may help restore the integrity of connective tissue, reduce swelling, and provide pain relief.

NUTRITION

- Vitamin C (1,000 to 1,500 mg three times a day) to reduce swelling and support connective tissue.
- Bromelain (250 to 500 mg three times a day between meals) helps reduce swelling.
- Beta carotene (50,000 IU per day) is needed to make collagen.
- Zinc (15 to 30 mg per day) helps you heal faster.
- Vitamin E (400 IU/day) has antioxidant effects.
- Adequate protein intake is important.

HERBS

Herbs may be used as dried extracts (capsules, powders, teas), glycerites (glycerine extracts), or tinctures (alcohol extracts). Unless otherwise indicated, teas should be made with 1 tsp. herb per cup of hot water. Steep covered 5 to 10 minutes for leaf or flowers, and 10 to 20 minutes for roots. Drink 2 to 4 cups per day.

Bioflavanoids are found in dark berries and some plants. They help reduce swelling and strengthen the tissues that are affected by sprains and strains. The following may be taken in dried extract form as noted.

- Quercetin: 250 to 500 mg three times a day
- Hawthorn (*Crataegus oxyacantha*): 500 mg three times a day
- Turmeric (*Curcuma longa*) makes the effect of bromelain stronger. Take 250 to 500 mg each of turmeric and bromelain, three times a day between meals.

The following combination of herbs reduces spasm and stimulates cirulation. Black cohosh (*Cimicifuga racemosa*), cramp bark (*Viburnum opulus*), Jamaican dogwood (*Piscidia erythrina*), feverfew (*Tanacetum parthenium*), poke root (*Phytolacca americana*), and valerian (*Valeriana officinalis*). Combine equal parts in a tea (1 cup three to four times per day), or tincture (15 drops every 15 minutes until you feel better, up to eight doses; or 20 to 30 drops four times per day).

HOMEOPATHY

Some of the most common remedies used for this condition are listed below. Usually, the dose is 12X to 30C every one to four hours until your symptoms get better.

- *Arnica montana* for acute injury with bruised sensation and sensitivity to pressure
- *Rhus toxicodendron* for sprains and strains with great restlessness
- *Ruta graveolens* for stiffness and pain from injury or chronic overuse
- Topical homeopathic creams containing leopard's bane (*Arnica montana*) or St. John's wort (*Hypericum perforatum*) may provide pain relief. Do not apply over broken skin.
- *Arnica* oil may be applied topically for pain relief, provided the skin is not broken.

PHYSICAL MEDICINE

Castor oil pack. Apply oil directly to skin, cover with a clean soft cloth and plastic wrap. Place a heat source over the pack and let sit for 30 to 60 minutes. For best results, use for three consecutive days.

ACUPUNCTURE

Acupuncture may provide pain relief and increase local circulation.

MASSAGE

Therapeutic massage is effective at increasing circulation and may relieve spasm in surrounding muscle groups.

■ FOLLOWING UP

Your health care provider probably won't need to see you again unless your injury was severe or you have complications.

■ SPECIAL CONSIDERATIONS

Be careful of recurring sprains and strains. Once a muscle or tendon is injured, it is susceptible to reinjury, especially if you return to full activity too soon. Sprains and strains are easy to prevent. Basic physical fitness and strength training with proper warm-up and cool-down reduce the stress to muscles and joints.

■ TENDINITIS

Tendinitis is the painful inflammation of a tendon and its ligaments, which attach it to the bone. It often results from the stress of repetitive movements. Acute tendinitis may become chronic if it is not treated. The areas most commonly affected by tendinitis are the shoulder (rotator cuff tendinitis or impingement syndrome), elbow (tennis elbow or golfer's elbow), wrist and thumb (de Quervain's disease), knee (jumper's knee), and ankle (Achilles tendinitis). Calcific tendinitis, which occurs when calcium deposits build up in a joint, often appears in people with a chronic disease, such as diabetes.

■ SIGNS AND SYMPTOMS
- Minor edema (swelling)
- Tenderness in affected limb
- Pain that worsens when you move the affected limb
- Warmth and redness
- Crepitus (crackling)

■ WHAT CAUSES IT?
Although the exact cause of tendinitis is unknown, it can result from overuse, undertraining, or poor technique in sports, repetitive movement in certain occupations, falling, lifting or carrying heavy objects, and extreme or repeated trauma. It may also be seen with certain inflammatory conditions (for example, Reiter's syndrome, ankylosing spondylitis), autoimmune disorders (for example, diabetes mellitus), and some infections.

■ WHAT TO EXPECT AT YOUR PROVIDER'S OFFICE
Your health care provider will give you a thorough physical examination. X-rays may be taken and other diagnostic tests may be performed.

■ TREATMENT OPTIONS
Treatment can include applying ice, taking painkillers, getting rest, temporary immobilization, massage, steroid injections, phonophoresis (use of ultrasound with a drug applied to the skin over the affected joint), light exercise, physical therapy, and surgery in some cases.

Drug Therapies
- Nonsteroidal anti-inflammatory drugs (NSAIDs)
- Injections of lidocaine and corticosteroids
- Colchicine (for calcific tendinitis only)

Complementary and Alternative Therapies
- Ice, especially after the initial injury
- Rest
- Massage
- Temporary immobilization of the affected limb (slings, splints)
- Flexibility and strengthening exercises after acute phase has passed
- Physical therapy (such as range-of-motion exercises)
- Ultrasonography (phonophoresis)—high-frequency sound to heat an area and increase the blood supply
- Transcutaneous electrical nerve stimulation (TENS)—electricity used to control pain

NUTRITION
- Vitamin C (500 to 1,000 mg three times a day) to aid in healing, increase immune function, and reduce inflammation
- Calcium (1,500 mg a day) and magnesium (750 mg a day) to aid healing of connective tissues and muscles

- Vitamin A (15,000 IU a day) for immune function and healing
- Vitamin E (400 to 800 mg a day) to reduce inflammation
- Bromelain (250 to 750 mg three times a day between meals) to reduce swelling
- Essential fatty acids (1,000 to 15,000 IU one to three times a day): anti-inflammatory

HERBS
Herbs may be used as dried extracts (capsules, powders, teas), glycerites (glycerine extracts), or tinctures (alcohol extracts). Unless otherwise indicated, teas should be made with 1 tsp. herb per cup of hot water. Steep covered 5 to 10 minutes for leaf or flowers, and 10 to 20 minutes for roots. Drink 2 to 4 cups per day.
- Bioflavonoids (500 to 1,000 mg three times a day) to reduce inflammation and maintain healthy collagen (protein found in connective tissue, skin, cartilage, and other tissue)
- Curcumin (*Curcuma longa*), yellow pigment of tumeric, (200 to 400 mg three times a day between meals) to reduce inflammation
- Willow (*Salix alba*) bark tea (2 to 3 tsps. in 1 cup of boiling water three times a day) for pain relief (Caution: if you are allergic to aspirin, do not take aspirinlike herbs.)
- Licorice (*Glycyrrhiza glabra*) (3 cups tea a day) to reduce inflammation (Do not use if you have high blood pressure.)
- Comfrey (*Symphytum officinale*) (1 tsp. in 1 cup boiling water four times a day) to aid healing and for pain relief

HOMEOPATHY
Homeopathic remedies for tendinitis include creams or gels. *Arnica* cream by itself or in combination with *Calendula officinalis, Hamamelis virgineana, Aconitum napellus,* and *Belladonna,* applied three to six times a day, speeds healing and decreases discomfort. For acute injuries, always start with *Arnica.*

Internally, the dose is usually 12X to 30C every one to four hours until the symptoms get better.
- *Bryonia* for pains that are worse with the slightest motion or when jarred. The pain feels worse with cold and better with heat.
- *Phytolacca* for tendinitis where the pain is focused at the insertion of the tendons and feels worse with heat
- *Rhus toxicodendron* for tendinitis that is worse in the morning
- *Rhododendron* for tendinitis that gets worse with barometric changes

PHYSICAL MEDICINE
- Orthotics or heel lift and shoe correction (Achilles tendinitis)
- Elbow strap and small (2 lb.) weights (tennis elbow)
- Contrast hydrotherapy. Alternate hot and cold applications. After the first 24 to 48 hours, soak affected part for three minutes in hot water, then 30 seconds in cold water.

■ FOLLOWING UP
Tendinitis often has three stages: Stage 1 is characterized by a dull ache following activity, which improves with rest; stage 2, by pain with minor movements (for example, dressing); and stage 3, by constant pain.

■ SPECIAL CONSIDERATIONS
Recurrences are common, particularly for athletes and people whose work requires repetitive motions.

■ THYROIDITIS

Thyroiditis is an inflammation of the thyroid gland. There are several types of thyroiditis, but each of them generally produce three phases: overactive thyroid (hyperthyroidism), underactive thyroid (hypothyroidism), and return to normal. It usually takes one year to complete this cycle. Young to middle-aged women seem most at risk, although some forms of thyroiditis are seen in both men and women of all ages. With some forms, hypothyroidism may develop years later even if the thyroiditis has resolved.

■ SIGNS AND SYMPTOMS

Depending on the type of thyroiditis, the thyroid gland can have one of the following characteristics.

- Firm and enlarged, but not tender
- Enlarged and painful, with pain extending to the jaw or ears
- Enlarged but not painful; or enlarged on only one side, hard like a stone, and sticking to other neck structures

You may also have one or more of the following symptoms.

- Cool, dry skin, slow pulse rate (less than 60 beats per minute), swelling around the eyes, hoarseness, or slow reflexes
- No desire to eat, feeling tired and unenergetic, and a slight fever
- A rapid heartbeat, slight nervousness, anxiety, weight loss of 5 to 10 pounds, and increased sweating

■ WHAT CAUSES IT?

Thyroiditis can be caused by immune disorders, viruses, and fever disorders. Sometimes thyroiditis develops if you have Graves' disease (a thyroid disorder). In some cases, there is no identifiable cause.

■ WHAT TO EXPECT AT YOUR PROVIDER'S OFFICE

Your health care provider will feel your neck to see what the thyroid gland feels like and may order blood tests to check the levels of thyroid hormones and other factors. You may be given pain medication or something to help you feel more normal.

■ TREATMENT OPTIONS

For moderate pain, your health care provider may suggest aspirin or another pain reliever. If the pain is severe, you may be given steroids.

Complementary and Alternative Therapies

Alternative therapies can help when used along with the medications your provider prescribes.

NUTRITION

- Foods that depress thyroid activity are broccoli, cabbage, Brussels sprouts, cauliflower, kale, spinach, turnips, soy, beans, and mustard greens. These foods should be included in the diet for hyperthyroid conditions and avoided for hypothyroid conditions.
- Avoid refined foods, sugar, dairy products, wheat, caffeine, alcohol.
- Essential fatty acids are anti-inflammatory and necessary for hormone production. Take 1,000-1,500 flaxseed oil mg three times per day.
- Calcium (1,000 mg per day) and magnesium (200 to 600 mg per day) help many metabolic processes function correctly.

Your health care provider may also recommend specific nutritional supplements for a hyperthyroid or hypothyroid condition.

HERBS

Herbs may be used as dried extracts (capsules, powders, teas), glycerites (glycerine extracts), or tinctures (alcohol extracts). Unless otherwise indicated, teas should be made with 1 tsp. herb per cup of hot water. Steep covered 5 to 10 minutes for leaf or flowers, and 10 to 20 minutes for roots. Drink 2 to 4 cups per day.

For hyperthyroid conditions:

- Bugleweed *(Lycopus virginica)* and lemon balm *(Melissa officinalis)* help normalize the overactive thyroid.
- Motherwort *(Leonorus cardiaca)* relieves heart palpitations and passionflower *(Passiflora incarnata)* reduces anxiety. Combine two parts of bugleweed with one part each of lemon balm, motherwort, and passionflower in a tincture, 30 to 60 drops three to four times per day.
- Quercetin (250 to 500 mg three times per day) is an anti-inflammatory.
- Turmeric *(Curcuma longa)* makes the effect of bromelain stronger and should be taken between meals, 500 mg three times per day.
- Ginkgo biloba *(Ginkgo folium)* 80 to 120 mg two times per day.

For hypothyroid conditions:

- A combination that supports thyroid function includes herbs rich in minerals. Combine the following for a tea (3 to 4 cups per day) or tincture (20 to 30 drops three times a day): horsetail *(Equisetum arvense)*, oatstraw *(Avena sativa)*, alfalfa *(Medicago sativa)*, gotu kola *(Centella asiatica)*, and bladderwrack *(Fucus vesiculosis)*.

HOMEOPATHY

Homeopathy may be useful as a supportive therapy for both "hyper" and "hypo" conditions of the thyroid.

PHYSICAL MEDICINE

For hyperthyroid conditions:

- Ice packs to the throat will help decrease inflammation.

For hypothyroid conditions:

- Contrast hydrotherapy. Alternate hot and cold applications. Alternate three minutes hot with one minute cold. Repeat three times. This is one set. Do two to three sets per day.
- Exercise helps improve thyroid function.

ACUPUNCTURE

Acupuncture may be helpful in correcting hormonal imbalances and addressing underlying deficiencies and excesses involved in thyroiditis.

MASSAGE

Therapeutic massage may relieve stress and increase the sense of well-being.

■ FOLLOWING UP

Your health care provider may need to check you each year.

■ SPECIAL CONSIDERATIONS

If you are pregnant or just had a baby, you may develop Hashimoto's thyroiditis.

For additional information supporting this handout, please refer to our website: www.onemedicine.com/public/products/access
Copyright ©2000 Integrative Medicine Communications • 1029 Chestnut St., Newton, MA 02464 • T 877-426-6633 • F 877-426-6630

■ ULCERATIVE COLITIS

Ulcerative colitis (UC) is a disease in which the lining of your large intestine (colon) becomes inflamed. This inflammation leads to the formation of raw sores, or ulcers, causing pain and bloody diarrhea. UC can begin at any age, but most people who get it are in their early twenties. For most, UC comes and goes for the rest of their lives. Most people can control attacks by taking medicine and adjusting their diet. But in about one-quarter of people with UC, surgery becomes necessary.

■ SIGNS AND SYMPTOMS

UC usually begins gradually with bloody diarrhea, rectal bleeding, cramping or pain in the belly, and growing urgency to move your bowels. Depending on which area of the colon is affected, the stool may be normal or hard and dry. Other symptoms might be fever, fatigue, weight loss, loss of appetite, anemia from loss of blood, pus in stools, malnutrition, and slow growth in children. UC can also affect parts of the body outside the colon, causing skin sores, mouth sores, joint pain, and inflammation of the eyes, liver, kidneys, or gallbladder.

■ WHAT CAUSES IT?

Nobody knows what causes UC. It might start with an infection. Ten to 20 percent of people with UC have at least one family member with an intestinal disorder called inflammatory bowel disease (IBD).

■ WHAT TO EXPECT AT YOUR PROVIDER'S OFFICE

Your health care provider will take stool and blood samples, and will look inside your rectum through a flexible tube called an endoscope. You may also have an X ray, with or without barium (a chalky liquid that makes organs and structures easier to see on an X-ray image).

■ TREATMENT OPTIONS

Support groups such as the Crohn's-Colitis Foundation of America (CCFA) may be helpful.

Drug Therapies

Most people who have UC use more than one medication. Your provider may prescribe drugs such as sulfasalazine or corticosteroids.

Complementary and Alternative Therapies

NUTRITION

- Decrease refined foods, sugars, and saturated fats.
- Eliminate all food allergens from the diet. Common allergenic foods are dairy, soy, citrus, peanuts, wheat, fish, eggs, corn, tomatoes.
- A rotation diet, in which the same food is not eaten more than once every four days, may help reduce symptoms.
- Dairy products, Brassica vegetables (cabbage, Brussels sprouts, broccoli, cauliflower, and kale) and gluten-containing grains (wheat, oats, barley, triticale, rye) may make UC worse.
- Fiber supplementation can help reduce abdominal pain, cramping, and gas: psyllium, flax meal, slippery elm (*Ulmus fulva*) powder, and marshmallow root (*Althea officinalis*) powder.
- Proflora supplements taken two to three times a day.

- Essential fatty acids may protect intestinal lining. Max-EPA or fish oil (3 to 4 g, up to 18 g per day).
- Bromelain (250 to 500 mg between meals) for inflammation.

Inflammatory bowel disease which may be associated with UC is associated with low levels of many vitamins and nutrients. Ask you provider about taking supplements.

HERBS

Herbs may be used as dried extracts (capsules, powders, teas), glycerites (glycerine extracts), or tinctures (alcohol extracts). Teas should be made with 1 tsp. herb per cup of hot water. Steep covered 5 to 10 minutes for leaf or flowers, and 10 to 20 minutes for roots.

- Enteric-coated peppermint oil: one to two capsules (0.2 ml peppermint oil per capsule) three times per day after meals. Peppermint oil (*Mentha piperita*) is a potent relaxant that reduces bowel irritability.
- A tincture of equal parts of the following herbs may be taken before meals (20 to 30 drops three times per day): cramp bark (*Viburnum opulus*), passionflower (*Passiflora incarnata*), meadowsweet (*Filependula ulmaria*), wild yam (*Dioscorea villosa*), valerian (*Valeriana officinalis*), and lemon balm (*Melissa officinalis*).
- Use equal parts of the following in a tincture (30 drops four times per day): coneflower (*Echinacea purpurea*), goldenseal (*Hydrastis canadensis*), and geranium (*Geranium maculatum*)
- Licorice root (*Glycyrrhiza glabra*) and marshmallow root (*Althea officinalis*) promote healing of the gastrointestinal lining. Make a tea of licorice root by steeping one tsp. in one cup of hot water for 20 minutes. Drink three cups per day. (Contraindicated in hypertension.) For marshmallow root tea, soak one heaping tbsp. of root in one quart of cold water overnight. Strain and drink throughout the day. Do not take licorice if you have high blood pressure.
- Quercetin (250 to 500 mg before meals) for food sensitivities.

HOMEOPATHY

Some of the most common remedies for this condition are listed below.

- *Arsenicum album* for intense cramping and burning, with scanty dark blood in stool. Patient is restless, chilly, and anxious.
- *China* for extreme bloating and gurgling in abdomen
- *Phosphorus* for painless diarrhea with prostration and thirst
- *Sulfur* for morning diarrhea that drives patient out of bed
- *Mercurius vivus* for IBD with canker sores and metallic taste

PHYSICAL MEDICINE

Castor oil pack. Apply oil directly to skin, cover with a clean soft cloth and plastic wrap. Cover with a heat source and let sit for 30 to 60 minutes.

ACUPUNCTURE

Acupuncture can help relieve spasm and normalize digestive function.

■ FOLLOWING UP

People who have UC for a long time are more likely to get colon cancer than other people, and must be checked for it regularly.

■ URETHRITIS

Urethritis is infection and inflammation of the lining of the urethra, the narrow tube that carries urine out of the body and which, in men, also carries semen. Urethritis is caused by bacteria and may involve the bladder, prostate, and reproductive organs. It can affect males and females of all ages; females are at higher risk.

■ SIGNS AND SYMPTOMS

In both sexes, but particularly in women, the disease may not show symptoms. When it does, symptoms include the following.
In men:
- Burning during urination
- Pus or whitish mucous discharge from the penis
- Burning or itching around the penile opening

In women:
- Painful urination
- Unusual vaginal discharge

■ WHAT CAUSES IT?

- Bacteria and other organisms entering the urethra
- Bruising during sexual intercourse (in women)
- Infection reaching the urethra from the prostate gland or through the penis opening (in men)
- Bacterial infection after you have taken a course of antibiotics
- Reiter's syndrome
- Sexually transmitted diseases (STDs), such as chlamydia, syphilis, or HIV/AIDS

■ WHAT TO EXPECT AT YOUR PROVIDER'S OFFICE

A physical examination of your genitals will be necessary, and laboratory tests will be done on a urine sample and a specimen of mucus taken from inside the urethra and, in women, the vagina.

■ TREATMENT OPTIONS

Treatment consists of antibiotic medications to kill the disease-causing bacteria. All sex partners should be treated. Abstaining from sexual activity is recommended until the treatment is completed, because disease can remain active even after symptoms have disappeared.

Complementary and Alternative Therapies

Nutrition, herbs, and homeopathic remedies are useful in fighting infection, relieving pain, and stengthening the urinary system.

NUTRITION

You can make the following changes in your diet to help treat urethritis.
- Eliminate any known food allergens.
- Eliminate refined foods, sweetened fruit juices, caffeine, alcohol, and sugar, which may compromise immunity and irritate the urinary tract.
- Cranberries and blueberries are helpful because they contain substances that stop bacteria from adhering to the urinary tract.
- Vitamin C (1,000 mg three times per day) makes your urine more acidic, which keeps bacteria from growing.
- Beta-carotene (25,000 to 50,000 IU per day) is necessary for immune function and healthy mucous membranes.
- Zinc (30 to 50 mg per day) helps your immune system.

HERBS

Herbs may be used as dried extracts (capsules, powders, teas), glycerites (glycerine extracts), or tinctures (alcohol extracts). Teas should be made with 1 tsp. herb per cup of hot water. Steep covered 5 to 10 minutes for leaf or flowers, and 10 to 20 minutes for roots.

Herbal therapy should begin at the first sign of symptoms and continue for three days after the symptoms go away. Teas provide the best treatment for infectious urethritis because the additional fluid intake helps the "flushing action." Combine two herbs from each of the following categories and drink 4 to 6 cups per day.
Urinary antiseptics fight bacteria and include the following.
- Uva ursi (*Arctostaphylos uva ursi*)
- Buchu (*Agathosma betulina*)
- Thyme leaf (*Thymus vulgaris*)
- Pipsissewa (*Chimaphila umbellata*)

Urinary astringents tone and heal the urinary tract and include the following.
- Horsetail (*Equisetum arvense*)
- Plantain (*Plantago major*)
- Cleavers (*Galium aparine*)

Urinary demulcents soothe the urinary tract and include the following.
- Corn silk (*Zea mays*)
- Couch grass (*Agropyron repens*)
- Marshmallow root (*Althea officinalis*) is best used alone in a cold infusion. Soak 1 heaping tbsp. of marshmallow root in 1 qt. of cold water overnight. Strain and drink during the day in addition to any other urinary tea.

For advanced or recurrent infections, prepare a tincture of equal parts goldenseal (*Hydrastis canadensis*) and coneflower (*Echinacea purpurea*). Take 30 drops four to six times per day in addition to the urinary tea.

For noninfectious urethritis or for urethritis with severe pain and spasm, add kava kava (*Piper methysticum*) to any of the above formulas.

A periwash may be helpful in reducing pain with urination. Place 1 tsp. of the coneflower/goldenseal tincture in an 8-oz. peri bottle. Fill with water. Rinse off after each time you urinate.

HOMEOPATHY

Some of the most common remedies used for urethritis are listed below. Usually, the dose is 12X to 30C every one to four hours until your symptoms get better.
- *Staphysagria* for urinary infections associated with sexual intercourse
- *Apis mellifica* for stinging pains that are made worse by warmth
- *Cantharis* for intolerable urging with "scalding" urine
- *Sarsaparilla* for burning after urination

ACUPUNCTURE

Acupuncture may be helpful in enhancing your body's immune function.

■ FOLLOWING UP

If your urethritis was caused by a sexually transmitted disease, your sexual partners may need to be treated as well.

■ SPECIAL CONSIDERATIONS

STDs can cause permanent damage to reproductive organs and infertility in both sexes. They also can cause difficulties during pregnancy; premature delivery; low birth weight; and infections in newborns.

■ URINARY INCONTINENCE

Urinary incontinence is the inability to control urination. It affects more than 13 million people of all ages in the United States. It is more common in the elderly and women.

Incontinence is classified as either stress incontinence (caused by coughing, laughing, sneezing), urge incontinence (losing urine when suddenly feeling the urge to urinate), overflow incontinence (continually leaking urine), functional incontinence (in people with a brain injury), or transient incontinence (temporary incontinence). Treatment is highly effective in more than 80 percent of cases. Exercise and behavioral therapies are most successful.

■ SIGNS AND SYMPTOMS
- Not being able to hold your urine until you get to a bathroom
- Frequent and unusual urges to urinate

■ WHAT CAUSES IT?
- Stretched pelvic muscles from pregnancy and childbirth
- Low estrogen levels in women
- Enlarged prostate in men
- Side effects of certain medications
- Urinary tract infections (UTIs)
- Frequent constipation
- Damage to or diseases of the brain or spinal cord (for example, dementia, spinal cord injury, multiple sclerosis, stroke)
- Weakened muscles that control urination (urethral sphincter and pelvic-floor muscles)

■ WHAT TO EXPECT AT YOUR PROVIDER'S OFFICE

Your health care provider will give you a physical examination and may ask you some questions about your past prostate problems, pregnancy, hysterectomy, your pattern of urinating, when your urine leakage occurs, and whether you strain or experience discomfort when you urinate. You may be asked to cough vigorously to see if it causes urine loss, a sign of stress incontinence.

Your provider may suggest urine tests to detect infection, urinary stones, diabetes, and other underlying causes. A pelvic ultrasound may be performed to examine your bladder, kidneys, and urethra.

■ TREATMENT OPTIONS
- Exercises: Kegel exercises strengthen muscles that control urination. While increased muscle tone requires long-term exercise, squeezing the muscles just before coughing or sneezing provides initial relief.
- Biofeedback: Electronic devices inserted into the vagina or rectum aid in muscle identification for exercise therapy.
- Relaxation techniques may help you go longer without urinating.
- Habit training helps establish regularity of urination.

Several types of drugs are available to help muscle control. Surgery is also helpful, particularly in women with stress incontinence and for men with an enlarged prostate. Various other options exist as well, such as catheters, urethral plugs, condom catheters, and absorbent pads or underwear.

Complementary and Alternative Therapies
Alternative therapies mainly involve Kegel exercises, biofeedback, and preventing any conditions that worsen incontinence. Yoga may help as well.

NUTRITION
- Eliminate caffeine, alcohol, sweetener substitutes, simple sugars.
- Cranberries and blueberries contain substances that keep bacteria from adhering to the bladder. This may help prevent infections that can make incontinence worse, and helps deodorize urine.
- Vitamin C (1,000 mg three times a day) keeps bacteria from growing in urine.
- Beta-carotene (25,000 to 50,000 IU per day) helps your immune system function properly and keeps mucous membranes healthy.
- Zinc (30 mg per day) supports immune function.
- Calcium (1,000 mg per day) and magnesium (500 mg per day) taken together may improve control of the muscles used in urination.

HERBS
Herbs may be used as dried extracts (capsules, powders, teas), glycerites (glycerine extracts), or tinctures (alcohol extracts). Teas should be made with 1 tsp. herb per cup of hot water. Steep covered 5 to 10 minutes for leaf or flowers; 10 to 20 minutes for roots. Drink 2 to 4 cups per day.

Urinary astringents tone and heal the urinary tract and can be taken long-term at 1 cup per day or 30 drops tincture per day.
- Horsetail (Equisetum arvense) helps connective tissue integrity.
- Plantain (Plantago major) is an astringent and demulcent.

Marshmallow root (Althea officinalis) is a urinary demulcent, best used alone in a cold infusion. Soak 1 heaping tbsp. of marshmallow root in 1 qt. of cold water overnight. Strain and drink during the day in addition to other teas.

HOMEOPATHY
Some of the most common remedies used for urinary incontinence are listed below. Usually, the dose is 12X to 30C every one to four hours until your symptoms get better.
- *Causticum* for stress incontinence, especially with retention from holding the urine and frequent urges to urinate
- *Natrum muriaticum* for stress incontinence, vaginal dryness and pain during sex, especially with a history of grief
- *Pareira* for retention of urine from an enlarged prostate
- *Sepia* for stress incontinence with sudden urge to urinate, especially with prolapsed uterus and vaginitis
- *Zincum* for stress incontinence, urinary retention from prostate problems, unable to urinate standing

ACUPUNCTURE
May help, depending on cause of the incontinence

■ FOLLOWING UP
Exercise and behavioral therapy are highly successful when closely adhered to. You may need close monitoring by your health care provider and support from someone close to you to stay committed to these lifestyle changes.

■ SPECIAL CONSIDERATIONS
If you are pregnant, consult with your provider before taking any medication. For men, regular prostate examinations can detect problems early.

■ URINARY TRACT INFECTION IN WOMEN

Urinary tract infections (UTIs) are caused by bacteria and are 10 times more common among women than men. About 30 percent of UTIs go away and do not recur. When UTIs do recur, it is often because the treatments used to suppress bacteria seem to work at first, but do not produce a lasting cure. UTIs can also recur when a woman is infected again by a different kind of bacterium.

■ SIGNS AND SYMPTOMS

- Pain or burning when urinating
- The need to urinate more often than usual
- A feeling of urgency when you urinate
- Blood or pus in the urine
- Cramps or pain in the lower abdomen
- Chills or fever (fever may be the only symptom in infants and children)
- Strong-smelling urine
- Pain during sexual intercourse

■ WHAT CAUSES IT?

Some risk factors include the following.

- A new sex partner or multiple partners
- More frequent or intense intercourse
- Diabetes
- Pregnancy
- Use of irritating products such as harsh skin cleansers
- Use of irritating contraceptives such as diaphragms and spermicides
- Use of birth control pills
- Heavy use of antibiotics
- A blockage in the urinary tract (benign masses or tumors)
- A history of UTIs, especially if the infections were less than six months apart

■ WHAT TO EXPECT AT YOUR PROVIDER'S OFFICE

Your health care provider will feel your abdomen and kidneys for changes and use laboratory tests, such as a urine culture, to find out if you have a UTI. If the usual treatments do not work, your provider will explore the possibility that you have some other condition. Other illnesses can cause symptoms that mimic a UTI, such as sexually transmitted diseases.

■ TREATMENT OPTIONS

Drug Therapies

Several antibiotics and other drugs are used to treat UTIs. The most effective antibiotics are usually taken for 7 to 10 days. Shorter courses of treatment are available, and your health care provider may prescribe an antibiotic that you take for one to three days.

Complementary and Alternative Therapies

NUTRITION

- Drink a lot of fluids, such as herb teas and water. Avoid sweetened fruit juices and other sweetened drinks.
- Eliminate refined foods, fruit juices, caffeine, alcohol, and sugar.
- Cranberries and blueberries contain substances that inhibit the binding of bacteria to bladder tissue. Drinking unsweetened cranberry juice regularly seems to help lower the risk of UTIs and can help cure one if you drink it when you first feel symptoms.
- Vitamin C (1,000 mg three times per day) makes urine acidic, which inhibits bacterial growth.
- Beta-carotene (25,000 to 50,000 IU per day) is necessary for immune function and mucous membrane integrity.
- Zinc (30 to 50 mg per day) supports immune function.

HERBS

Herbs may be used as dried extracts (capsules, powders, teas), glycerites (glycerine extracts), or tinctures (alcohol extracts). Teas should be made with 1 tsp. herb per cup of hot water. Steep covered 5 to 10 minutes for leaf or flowers, and 10 to 20 minutes for roots.

Start herbal therapy at the first sign of symptoms and continue for three days after you start feeling better. Teas work best for treating UTIs because the additional fluid intake helps the "flushing action." Combine two herbs from each of the following categories and drink 4 to 6 cups per day.

- Urinary antiseptics are antimicrobial: uva ursi (*Arctostaphylos uva ursi*), buchu (*Agathosma betulina*), thyme leaf (*Thymus vulgaris*), pipsissewa (*Chimaphila umbellata*)
- Urinary astringents tone and heal the urinary tract: horsetail (*Equisetum arvense*), plantain (*Plantago major*)
- Urinary demulcents soothe the inflamed urinary tract: corn silk (*Zea mays*), couch grass (*Agropyron repens*)

Marshmallow root (*Althea officinalis*) is best used alone in a cold infusion. Soak 1 heaping tbsp. of marshmallow root in 1 qt. of cold water overnight. Strain and drink during the day in addition to any other urinary tea.

For advanced or recurrent infections prepare a tincture of equal parts of goldenseal (*Hydrastis canadensis*) and coneflower (*Echinacea purpurea*). Take 30 drops four to six times per day.

HOMEOPATHY

Some of the most common remedies used for UTI are listed below. Usually, the dose is 12X to 30C every one to four hours until your symptoms get better.

- *Staphysagria* for UTI's associated with sexual intercourse. The number one homeopathic UTI remedy.
- *Apis mellifica* for stinging pains that are exacerbated by warmth
- *Cantharis* for intolerable urging with "scalding" urine
- *Sarsaparilla* for burning after urination

■ FOLLOWING UP

Preventive measures you can follow:

- Urinate both before and after intercourse.
- Have your health care provider recheck the fit of your diaphragm if you use one.
- Avoid sex while you are being treated for a UTI.

■ SPECIAL CONSIDERATIONS

If you are pregnant, you are more at risk for developing a UTI.

■ UROLITHIASIS

Commonly called kidney stones, urolithiasis means stones in the urinary tract. These stones occur four times more often in men than women, with 240,000 to 720,000 Americans affected yearly. The pain of having a stone has been compared to that of childbirth. The stones can be made of calcium, uric acid, oxalate, struvite, or cystine.

■ SIGNS AND SYMPTOMS

You may have no symptoms if the stone is noted on an X-ray for an unrelated condition. Or you may have some or all of the following.

- Sudden onset of excruciating pain in the buttocks area
- Abdominal pain
- Nausea and vomiting
- You are constantly moving to relieve the pain
- Pain in the genital area as the stone moves
- Fever and chills

■ WHAT CAUSES IT?

Kidney stones occur because the small bowel absorbs too much calcium, your diet is too high in calcium or another mineral, you have intestinal problems, a urinary tract infection, or an inherited disorder. You may not be drinking enough fluids (especially in the summer) or exercising enough.

■ WHAT TO EXPECT AT YOUR PROVIDER'S OFFICE

If you are in extreme pain, your health care provider may give you a strong pain reliever. Then your health care provider will need a urine sample to check for infection and to see if your urine is acid or alkaline, which indicates the type of stone. You may need to collect your urine for 24 hours if this is not your first stone. Your provider will also take a blood sample.

With time, the stone generally passes out of the body by itself. If it doesn't or if you have severe pain, bleeding, fever, nausea, or can't urinate, your provider can shatter the stone with shock waves, and the smaller pieces can pass with much less pain. Only rarely is surgery needed.

■ TREATMENT OPTIONS

Usually taking pain relievers and drinking at least six to eight glasses of water a day, plus one at bedtime and another during the night, enables the stone to pass more easily. You may need to urinate through a strainer to collect the stone and give it to your health care provider for analysis.

You may need pain medication while the stone is moving through your system. After it passes, you may need other drugs so that you don't form stones again.

Complementary and Alternative Therapies

Symptomatic urolithiasis requires medical attention. Alternative therapies aid in reducing the risk of recurrent episodes and increasing the overall vitality of the urogenital system. Start with nutritional guidelines for prevention of recurrence. Herbs and homeopathic remedies can be used for acute pain relief and long-term toning of the urinary tract.

NUTRITION
- Reduce your intake of sugar, refined foods, animal products (meats and dairy), caffeine, alcohol, soda, and salt.

- Drink more water and eat more fiber, vegetables, whole grains, and vegetable proteins.
- Cut down on oxalate-containing foods such as spinach, rhubarb, beets, nuts, chocolate, black tea, wheat bran, strawberries, and beans.
- Include foods rich in magnesium and low in calcium, such as barley, bran, corn, rye, oats, soy, brown rice, avocado, banana, and potato.
- Magnesium citrate (200 to 400 mg per day) may increase the solubility of calcium oxalate and calcium phosphate.
- Pyridoxine (B_6, 10 to 100 mg per day) is essential for the metabolism of oxalic acid, a component of some stones.
- Folic acid (5 mg per day) helps break down uric acid stones.

HERBS
Herbs are generally a safe way to strengthen and tone the body's systems. As with any therapy, it is important to work with your health care provider on getting your problem diagnosed before you start any treatment. Herbs may be used as dried extracts (capsules, powders, teas), glycerites (glycerine extracts), or tinctures (alcohol extracts). Unless otherwise indicated, teas should be made with 1 tsp. herb per cup of hot water. Steep covered 5 to 10 minutes for leaf or flowers, and 10 to 20 minutes for roots. Drink 2 to 4 cups per day. Tinctures may be used singly or in combination as noted.

- For acute pain relief, combine tinctures of wild yam *(Dioscorea villosa)*, cramp bark *(Viburnum opulus)*, kava *(Piper methysticum)*, and Jamaican dogwood *(Piscidia erythrina)*. Take 15 drops every 15 minutes for up to 8 doses.
- Drink an infusion of equal parts of gravel root *(Eupratorium purpureum)*, corn silk *(Zea mays)*, pipsissewa *(Chimaphila umbellata)*, and kava *(Piper methysticum)*. Use 1 tsp. of herb mixture per 1 cup water. Drink 3 to 4 cups per day.

HOMEOPATHY
Some of the most common remedies used for urolithiasis are listed below. Usually, the dose is 12X to 30C every one to four hours until your symptoms get better.

- *Berberis* for sharp sticking pains that radiate to your groin.
- *Colocynthis* for restlessness and pain that feels better when you bend forward.
- *Ocimum* for nausea and vomiting from the pain.

PHYSICAL MEDICINE
Castor oil pack. Used externally, castor oil is a powerful anti-inflammatory. Apply oil directly to skin, cover with a clean soft cloth (for example, flannel) and plastic wrap. Place a heat source (hot water bottle or heating pad) over the pack and let sit for 30 to 60 minutes. For best results, use for three consecutive days.

■ FOLLOWING UP

Fifty percent of patients pass the stone in 48 hours. If there are complications, your health care provider may refer you to a urologist or admit you to the hospital. After you pass the stone, keep drinking fluids and change your diet to reduce the chance of forming more stones in the future.

■ SPECIAL CONSIDERATIONS

Shock-wave therapy is not appropriate for women of childbearing age. If you think you might be pregnant, tell your health care provider. He or she will also want to rule out ectopic pregnancy or a ruptured ovarian cyst.

■ VAGINITIS

There are many types of vaginitis of which 40 percent are caused by candida, a yeast-like fungus. When it multiplies in the vaginal tract, the disorder is called vulvovaginitis. Women often refer to it as a "yeast infection." About 75 percent of women get candida vaginitis at some time in their lives.

■ SIGNS AND SYMPTOMS

- Itching in the vagina and vulva
- Vaginal discharge (small amounts are normal, however)
- Red, swollen, painful vaginal mucous membranes and external genitalia
- Satellite lesions (tender, red, pus-filled bumps, which can spread to thighs and anus)

■ WHAT CAUSES IT?

Candida is a yeast-like fungus that grows in the vagina. When there is too much of it, it causes infection. The following increase your chance of getting a yeast infection.

- Antibiotics—especially broad-spectrum types
- Pregnancy—from increased heat and moisture and hormonal shifts
- Diabetes
- Corticosteroid use
- Human immunodeficiency virus (HIV) infection
- Taking birth control pills
- Being overweight
- High sugar intake
- Wearing panty hose, tight clothing, or non-cotton underwear

■ WHAT TO EXPECT AT YOUR PROVIDER'S OFFICE

Your health care provider will give you a pelvic examination and swab your vagina to check for candida. You probably will also have a Pap smear. Some women have chronic yeast infections. If this happens, your provider may want to do additional tests.

■ TREATMENT OPTIONS

Topical therapies (70 percent to 90 percent effective):
- Insert cream or vaginal suppository in the vagina.
- Some brands may also be used externally for lesions

Oral therapies (75 percent to 92 percent effective).
- Do not take if pregnant or think you may be.

Complementary and Alternative Therapies

Alternative therapies may help to treat acute and chronic vaginitis.

Use only one of the following douches at one time. Do not douche during menstrual periods. For first time or acute infection try the vinegar douche or boric acid capsules. For chronic vaginitis, use the herbal combination douche. For recurrent vaginitis, use the Betadine douche. Stop douching if you are in pain or your symptoms get worse.

- White vinegar: 1 to 2 tbsp. to 1 pint of water. Douche daily for 10 to 14 days.
- Boric acid: One capsule (600 mg) inserted daily for 10 to 14 days. May cause irritation or problems from systemic absorption.
- Herbal combination: Mix equal parts of oregano leaf (*Origanum vulgare*), goldenseal root (*Hydrastic canadensis*), and coneflower

(*Echinacea purpurea*). Steep 1 heaping tbsp. of herbal mixture in 1 pint of water. Cool and douche daily for 10 to 14 days.
- Povidone iodine (Betadine): Douche with one part iodine to 100 parts water twice daily for 10 to 14 days. Prolonged use can suppress thyroid function.

NUTRITION

- Avoid simple and refined sugars (breads, pasta, baked goods, sweets), dairy products, alcohol, peanuts, fresh or dried fruit, fruit juice, and food allergens. Eat plenty of protein, vegetables, and grains.
- Lactobacillus acidophilus re-establishes normal bacteria in the body and prevents the overgrowth of candida. Take one capsule orally two to three times per day. Insert one capsule into the vagina nightly during treatment (not to exceed 14 nights).
- Vitamin A (10,000 IU per day) or beta-carotene (50,000 IU per day) enhances the integrity of the vaginal lining. Remember to avoid high doses of vitamin A in pregnancy or if you may become pregnant within the next three months.
- Zinc (30 mg per day) and vitamin E (400 to 800 IU per day) are essential for immune function.
- Vitamin C (1,000 mg three to four times per day) enhances immunity and helps restore the integrity of vaginal lining.

HERBS

Herbs may be used as dried extracts (capsules, powders, teas), glycerites (glycerine extracts), or tinctures (alcohol extracts). Unless otherwise indicated, teas should be made with 1 tsp. herb per cup of hot water. Steep covered 5 to 10 minutes for leaf or flowers, and 10 to 20 minutes for roots. Drink 2 to 4 cups per day.

- Pau d'arco tea has antifungal effects.
- Garlic (*Allium sativum*) has antimicrobial, antifungal, and immune-stimulating properties. Prepare a tea with two cloves of garlic. May add fresh lemon and honey for flavor.

HOMEOPATHY

Some of the most common rededies for vaginitis are listed below. Usually the right dose is 12X to 30C every one to one to four hours until your symptoms get better.

- *Calcarea carbonica* for intense itching with thick white or yellowish discharge that is worse before you start your period.
- Borax for burning pains with egg-white colored discharge.
- *Sepia* for burning pains with milky white discharge and pressure in vaginal area, especially if you feel depressed and irritable.
- *Graphites* for backache with thin white discharge that is worse in the morning and when walking.
- *Arsenicum album* for when you have burning, discharge.
- Homeopathic combinations are available as creams to apply vaginally.

ACUPUNCTURE

Acupuncture may be helpful in improving immune function.

■ FOLLOWING UP

To keep infections away, use unscented soap, take showers instead of baths, and cleanse after bowel movements by wiping from front to back.

■ SPECIAL CONSIDERATIONS

Yeast infections occur twice as often during pregnancy.

■ WARTS

Warts are small, generally harmless, and usually painless growths on the skin. Warts can be disfiguring and embarrassing, however, and occasionally they will hurt or itch. The different types of warts include the following.

- *Common warts: usually on the hands, but can appear anywhere*
- *Flat warts: generally found on the face and back of the hands*
- *Genital warts: normally found on the external genitalia, in the pubic area, and in the area between the thighs, but can appear inside the vagina and in the anal canal*
- *Plantar warts: found on the soles of the feet*

Warts affect all age groups. Genital warts are quite contagious, while common, flat, and plantar warts are much less likely to spread from person to person. All warts can spread from one part of the body to another. Some warts will disappear without treatment, although it can take as long as six months to two years. Whether treated or not, warts that disappear often reappear.

■ SIGNS AND SYMPTOMS

- Common warts: usually begin as tiny, smooth, flesh-colored eruptions and grow into rough growths perhaps $1/4$ inch across or in clusters
- Flat warts: small flesh-colored or pink growths with flat tops
- Genital warts: tiny eruptions that grow to resemble common warts
- Plantar warts: rough, flattened, callus-like growths, often with tiny black dots in the center; frequently tender; can disrupt your posture, resulting in leg or back pain

■ WHAT CAUSES IT?

Warts are caused by a common virus in humans, the human papillomavirus (HPV). Your risk of getting warts is increased by direct contact with warts or the fluid in warts (notably genital warts), using communal facilities (such as locker rooms), skin trauma, and diseases or drugs that weaken your immune system.

■ WHAT TO EXPECT AT YOUR PROVIDER'S OFFICE

Warts can generally be diagnosed by location and appearance. Your health care provider may want to cut into a wart to confirm that it is not a corn, callus, or other similar-appearing growth, but rarely will your provider have to order laboratory tests. If you have genital warts, your provider will want to check inside your anus and (in women) vagina.

■ TREATMENT OPTIONS

Medical treatments include drug therapy (usually the first-line treatment), cryosurgery ("freezing" the wart to destroy tissue), electrosurgery, lasers, and cutting out the wart. Unless your wart is causing significant problems, you should avoid treatments that have risks or could result in scarring.

Drug Therapies

Common, flat, and plantar warts: nonprescription preparations using salicylic acid are available over the counter.

Genital warts: in most cases, your health care provider will either apply podophyllin weekly or prescribe a podofilox for you to apply.

Complementary and Alternative Therapies

Nutritional and herbal support may enhance immune function and minimize recurrence of HPV, the virus that causes warts.

NUTRITION

Some changes you can make in your diet include the following.

- Eliminate caffeine, alcohol, refined foods, and sugar.
- Avoid saturated fats (animal protein and dairy products).
- Increase whole grains, fresh vegetables, fruits, legumes, and essential fatty acids (nuts, seeds, and cold-water fish).
- Vitamin C (1,000 to 1,500 mg three times per day), beta-carotene (100,000 IU per day), vitamin E (400 IU per day), and zinc (15 to 30 mg per day) support immune function and healing. Vitamin E may also be put directly on a wart to treat it.
- B complex (50 to 100 mg per day) helps reduce the effects of stress, which can weaken your immune system.
- Folic acid (800 mcg per day) is recommended for genital warts.
- Selenium (200 mcg per day) supports immune function.

HERBS

Herbs may be used as dried extracts (capsules, powders, teas), glycerites (glycerine extracts), or tinctures (alcohol extracts). Unless otherwise indicated, teas should be made with 1 tsp. of herb per cup of hot water. Steep covered 5 to 10 minutes for leaf or flowers, and 10 to 20 minutes for roots. Drink 2 to 4 cups per day.

Combine tinctures of one part goldenseal *(Hydrastis canadensis)* with two parts each of the following herbs: lomatium *(Lomatium dissectum),* licorice root *(Glycyrrhiza glabra),* coneflower *(Echinacea purpurea),* osha *(Ligusticum porteri),* and thuja leaf *(Thuja occidentalis).* Take 30 drops twice a day. Do not take licorice if you have high blood pressure.

Topical applications are most effective for treating warts. Stop any topical application if irritation should develop in the surrounding skin. For plantar, flat, and common warts use the following applications.

- Banana peel patch. Cut a piece of banana peel and place it over the wart before going to bed. Tape in place.
- Raw garlic patch. Cover the wart and surrounding skin with a thin layer of castor oil or olive oil. Apply a thin slice of fresh garlic and tape in place.

To maximize benefit, place two to four drops of tincture of thuja or greater celandine *(Chelidonium majus)* on the wart before covering with peel or garlic. This application may need to be repeated nightly for up to three weeks. The wart will turn black as it begins to die.

For external genital warts, paint the warts with vitamin A or beta-carotene once or twice daily. Add 3 to 4 drops each of thuja, echinacea, and lomatium for best results.

HOMEOPATHY

Homeopathy may be useful as a supportive therapy.

ACUPUNCTURE

Acupuncture may be helpful in stimulating your immune system.

■ SPECIAL CONSIDERATIONS

Do not use podophyllin if you are pregnant.

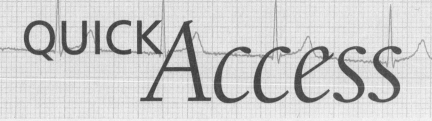

QUICK Access

HERBS

Aloe
Barberry
Bilberry
Black Cohosh
Burdock
Cat's Claw
Cayenne
Celery Seed
Chamomile, German
Chamomile, Roman
Comfrey
Devil's Claw
Echinacea
Eucalyptus
Evening Primrose
Feverfew
Flaxseed
Garlic
Ginger
Ginkgo Biloba
Ginseng, American
Ginseng, Asian
Ginseng, Siberian
Goldenseal
Grape Seed Extract
Green Tea
Hawthorn
Kava Kava
Lemon Balm
Licorice
Milk Thistle
Pau D'Arco
Peppermint
Saw Palmetto
St. John's Wort
Stinging Nettle
Valerian

■ ALOE

Aloe vera has a long history of use as a medicinal plant, with written records of its use going back to 1750 BC. Today it is grown in most subtropical and tropical locations, including the Caribbean, southern United States, Latin America, and the Middle East. Many people also grow a small potted version indoors for use in healing minor burns and cuts.

■ PLANT DESCRIPTION

Aloe vera is a perennial plant with yellow flowers. Its tough, fleshy, spearlike leaves can grow up to 20 inches long, and the whole plant up to 4 feet high. Only the leaves are used for medicine, but different parts of the leaves are used for different purposes. The clear, thick gel that is most commonly associated with aloe vera comes from the inner part of the leaf. Between this gel and the outer skin of the leaf are some special cells that contain a bitter yellow juice. When this juice is dried, it forms aloe latex.

■ WHAT'S IT MADE OF?

Aloe gel contains glycoproteins, which stop pain and inflammation and speed the healing process, and polysaccharides, which stimulate skin growth and repair. The anthraquinones in aloe latex work as powerful laxatives, and in smaller amounts, these chemicals can help stop kidney stone formation.

Aloe gel can be used to heal both internal and external wounds. It greatly speeds the healing of many skin injuries, including ulcerations, burns, and frostbite. Aloe latex is a powerful laxative, but because it can cause painful cramping, it is not used frequently. In smaller doses, aloe latex can help prevent kidney stones or reduce their size. It is also useful as a stool softener, particularly in people who have painful hemorrhoids.

Aloe juice is a liquid form of aloe gel that you can take internally. Because it has antibacterial properties, aloe juice can be used to treat bacterial infections in the gastro-intestinal tract. It is also effective for healing peptic ulcers because it reduces the stomach acids that aggravate ulcers.

Recent studies have shown that acetylated mannose, an antiviral component of aloe, has important HIV-fighting properties. Acetylated mannose attacks the virus itself, but more important, it greatly enhances the action of AZT, a powerful drug used to treat HIV infection. If taken in conjunction with aloe, the amount of AZT taken for HIV could be reduced by 90 percent, which would greatly reduce the expense and side effects associated with AZT.

■ AVAILABLE FORMS

Aloe gel is best fresh from an aloe plant, but it is also available commercially in a stabilized gel form. Aloe latex is available in a powdered form or in 500-mg capsules for use as a laxative. Aloe juice is a liquid form of the gel.

■ HOW TO TAKE IT

Aloe gel is best when taken fresh from the plant. Many people keep an aloe plant in their kitchen to treat minor burns or cuts. It can also be effective for treating hives and poison ivy. To use the gel, slit a leaf lengthwise and remove the gel inside. Apply liberally to affected area.

Aloe latex has been used traditionally as a laxative, but it is used infrequently in the US. Because it can produce painful cramping, other gentler herbal laxatives such as cascara and senna are recommended first.

For kidney stones and as a stool softener, take 0.05 to 0.2 grams of dry aloe extract (latex).

For HIV, take 800 to 1600 mg of acetylated mannose per day. This is equivalent to .5 to 1 liter of aloe vera juice, although amounts of acetylated mannose may vary in different products.

■ PRECAUTIONS

Aloe gel is safe for external use, unless it causes a rare allergic reaction. Discontinue use if it irritates the skin. Aloe gel is not useful for treatment of deep wounds. Aloe latex may cause severe intestinal cramps or diarrhea. Pregnant or nursing women should not take aloe latex because it may cause uterine contractions and trigger miscarriage. Aloe latex is not recommended for gastrointestinal illness, intestinal obstruction, appendicitis, or stomach pain of unknown cause. It may aggravate ulcers, hemorrhoids, diverticulosis, diverticulitis, colitis, or irritable bowel syndrome. If it's taken over a long period of time, aloe latex can cause dependence or disturb the electrolyte balance. It may also cause urine to turn a harmless red color. Children under 12 should not use aloe latex.

■ POSSIBLE INTERACTIONS

Chronic use of aloe latex could cause potassium deficiency, which could interfere with certain heart medications. The potential for potassium deficiency is greater if you use aloe latex with thiazide diuretics, licorice, or corticosteroids.

■ BARBERRY

Medicinal use of barberry goes as far back as ancient Egypt, where pharaohs and queens took it with fenel seed to ward off the plague. Today, it is said to ease the pain of arthritis and rheumatism, and the flare-ups of psoriasis. The types of infections that barberry can help fight involve the throat, urinary tract, gastrointestinal tract, and lungs, as well as yeast infections and diarrhea.

The bark of the root and stem are used for medicine. Both are yellow, and Native Americans and Europeans used them for dyeing cloth. But the ingredients in the bark are also what make barberry a useful medicine. The bark contains alkaloids that are considered antibiotic by some people, and which cause, according to herbalists, infection-fighting stimulation of your body's mucous membranes.

In order to understand what this means, if you place a drop of barberry on your tongue, you will probably feel your mouth water. This is not because it tastes good; it's actually somewhat bitter. But as your mouth waters, according to herbalists, it is helping the body to fight infections. It does this by stimulating parts of your body's immune system.

■ PLANT DESCRIPTION

Barberry is a shrub that can grow to about nine feet and has gray, thorny branches. Its leaves have spiny teeth. Between April and June, bright yellow flowers bloom. These become dark red berries in the fall, which grow in drooping bunches. You can use the ripe berries for jam, or in ways similar to cranberries. Barberries are a little more sour and less bitter than cranberries.

■ WHAT'S IT MADE OF?

Barberry bark and root bark contain many types of chemicals called isoquinoline alkaloids. Scientists and researchers have studied these constituents for many years, and have found that they do indeed have antibiotic actions. Some of them lower fevers, reduce swelling, lower blood pressure, and help normalize heart rate and the contractions of the heart muscle.

■ AVAILABLE FORMS

Barberry comes as tea, powdered in capsules, in fluid extracts or tinctures, and as a topical ointment. Extracts are standardized to 8 to 12 percent isoquinoline alkaloid content.

■ HOW TO TAKE IT

If you have been taking antibiotics frequently because you get the same infections over and over again, your health care provider may discuss herbal alternatives to prescription drugs. There are many reasons for this. Barberry may help you feel better and give you a break from other treatments. Also, resistance to antibiotics is rising. In order to avoid this, many providers are looking into other ways to treat illnesses. Another reason is that your body changes in response to antibiotics, and these changes are not always good. The normal bacteria that we all have inside us, which actually helps us to fight against infection, can get wiped out with regular antibiotics. Your provider may want to help you restore this "good" bacteria by letting you have a little time off from antibiotics.

Barberry may also be recommended to you as an ointment for arthritis or psoriasis for similar reasons: medicines used regularly to treat these conditions can upset your body's balance. Often, the side effects caused by strong medications trigger reactions in the body that can seem like an entirely new illness.

Whatever the reason, once you and your health care provider have decided that discontinuing medications will pose no risk to your health, barberry may be recommended. It may also be recommended as a preventive method.

You should never take barberry longer than five to seven days. If your stomach is sensitive, three to five days is probably long enough. For sore throats, bladder infections, diarrhea, bronchitis, or yeast infections, choose from the following.

- Tea: 2 to 4 g steeped dried root three times daily
- Tincture (a 1:5 solution made from herb and alcohol, or herb, alcohol, and water): 3 to 6 ml ($1/2$ to $1 1/2$ tsp. three times daily)
- Dry extracts: 250 to 500 mg three times daily
- For arthritis/psoriasis/skin disorders: 10 percent extract of barberry in ointment, applied to the skin three times daily

It is important to remember that some infections can be very dangerous if regular antibiotics are not taken for them. Never try to take an herb like barberry in place of a stronger antibiotic if a stronger antibiotic is needed. Make sure to follow your health care provider's instructions.

■ PRECAUTIONS

Barberry is safe with appropriate use, but do not use it if you are pregnant.

■ POSSIBLE INTERACTIONS

Large doses for a prolonged period of time may irritate your stomach and intestines, and may make it difficult for your body to get enough B vitamins.

■ BILBERRY

Bilberry berries and leaves are used for herbal medicines. The berries contain compounds called anthocyanosides, which are known to strengthen blood vessels and improve circulation, and can be useful in treating eye disorders, such as diabetic retinopathy, cataracts, and glaucoma, and circulation disorders, such as varicose veins and hemorrhoids. These same compounds also strengthen the retina, the part of the eye that controls night vision and helps the eye adapt to light changes. During World War II, British fighter pilots ate bilberries before going on nightly bombing raids because their night vision improved as a result.

Bilberry leaves have been used to control blood sugar levels in people with diabetes, but there is no documented evidence of how successful this treatment is. While bilberries are safe in any amount, bilberry leaves taken in large amounts over a long period of time can become toxic, and limited use is recommended.

Dried bilberries have been used for many years to treat diarrhea. The dried berry is high in tannin, which helps control and reduce the intestinal inflammation that can cause diarrhea.

Bilberry extract can also help protect the stomach against ulcers. It stimulates production of stomach mucus, which protects against digestive acids. And because it relaxes muscles, it can help relieve menstrual cramps.

■ PLANT DESCRIPTION

Bilberry is a shrub that grows to about 16 inches high. It has oval, pointed leaves and small pink and white flowers, which bloom from April through June. In the late summer, its dark purple berries are ripe to pick. Bilberry is a botanical relative of blueberry, cranberry, and huckleberry, and its fruit looks and tastes much like the American blueberry. The fruit can be eaten fresh or dried, or used in jams and preserves.

■ WHAT'S IT MADE OF?

The most important compounds in bilberry fruit and extract are the anthocyanosides. These compounds help build stronger capillaries and improve circulation to all areas of the body. They also reduce the stickiness of blood platelets, keeping them from causing blood clots. These compounds also help increase production of rhodopsin, a pigment that improves night vision and helps the eye adapt to light changes. Bilberry leaves are high in chromium, which may be why they seem to help control blood sugar levels

in people with diabetes. Dried bilberries are high in tannin and pectin, which have an astringent action that controls the inflammation that causes diarrhea.

■ AVAILABLE FORMS

Bilberries may be eaten fresh or dried. Bilberry tea may also be made from fresh or dried berries, or from the leaves. Bilberry extract comes powdered as capsules and should be standardized to 25 percent anthocyanidins. The extract contains the highest percentage of anthocyanidins, making it the most effective form of bilberry.

■ HOW TO TAKE IT

Because bilberry contains compounds that strengthen and build the body's circulation system, you can take it as a preventive measure if you have a family history of circulatory problems, such as varicose veins, hemorrhoids, or atherosclerosis. Bilberry also supports healthy eye function and can be taken to help prevent and treat eye disorders that come with aging or diabetes, such as cataracts, glaucoma, macular degeneration, and diabetic retinopathy. You can also take bilberry to improve night vision. Bilberry is an effective treatment for diarrhea, but if diarrhea continues for more than three to four days, you should consult your health care provider.

- For eye conditions and circulation: standardized bilberry extract (with 25 percent anthocyanidin) in encapsulated form, dosage of 480 mg a day in two to three divided doses. After improvement, maintenance dosage of 240 mg daily. Maintenance dosage used for prevention.
- For menstrual cramps and ulcer prevention: 20 to 40 mg bilberry extract three times a day, 2 to 4 ml tincture (1:5) three times a day, or eat a half cup of fresh bilberries.
- For diarrhea: 5 to 10 crushed dried bilberries in cold water, brought to a boil for 10 minutes, then strained.
- For diabetes: Pour boiling water over 1 g (approximately $1^1/_2$ teaspoons) bilberry leaf and strain after 10 to 15 minutes. Use long-term only under the supervision of your health care provider.

■ PRECAUTIONS

Bilberry fruit and extract are safe, with no known side effects. They are considered safe for use during pregnancy and nursing. Bilberry leaf is safe with appropriate usage, but should not be taken in large quantities over an extended period of time because it may become toxic.

■ POSSIBLE INTERACTIONS

None known

■ BLACK COHOSH

More than two centuries ago, Native Americans discovered that the root of the black cohosh plant (Cimicifuga racemosa) helped relieve many female problems, including menstrual cramps and hot flashes, headaches, irritability, and other signs of menopause. Because it was used mostly to treat women, they called black cohosh "squawroot."

The discomfort caused by menopause is typically treated with a synthetic form of the female sex hormone estrogen. Estrogen has eased millions of women through this life change, yet it often causes side effects. The most serious is an increased risk of breast cancer. Many women fear breast cancer so much that they suffer through menopause without treatment. A small but growing number of women who want relief without estrogen's side effects are discovering the benefits of black cohosh. The herbal therapy provides the same relief estrogen does, with no known serious side effects.

■ PLANT DESCRIPTION

Black cohosh is made from the roots of a member of the buttercup family. The tall, flowering plant grows in forests of the United States and Canada. Black cohosh also is called black snakeroot, bugbane, bugwort, and squawroot.

■ WHAT'S IT MADE OF?

The compound in black cohosh that acts like estrogen is called cimicifugin (macrotin). Black cohosh contains several other substances including starch and sugars.

■ AVAILABLE FORMS

Black cohosh is available in several forms. The most familiar are capsules and tablets. Black cohosh is also available as a liquid tincture that can be mixed in water and as a dried root that's simmered in water to make a drink similar to tea.

■ HOW TO TAKE IT

Although black cohosh's comeback in the United States is relatively new, European women have used it for more than 40 years. Scientists in Europe and the United States have conducted several studies that prove the botanical treatment helps women while producing few side effects. The evidence was strong enough to convince the German government to approve black cohosh as a nonprescription drug. The U.S. Food and Drug Administration (FDA) regulates it as a dietary supplement along with vitamins, minerals, and other botanicals.

Black cohosh has been proven effective in treating the following conditions.
- Premenstrual discomfort
- Painful menstruation
- Hot flashes
- Headache associated with menopause
- Heart palpitations associated with menopause
- Nervousness and irritability associated with menopause

Native Americans used black cohosh to treat other symptoms unrelated to menstruation or menopause. Scientists today see promise in black cohosh's ability to treat a variety of ailments. But they haven't studied its use in treating these problems as thoroughly as they have in treating symptoms of menstruation and menopause. Other conditions that may improve with black cohosh include the following.
- Inflammation, such as arthritis and rheumatism
- Mild high blood pressure
- Respiratory congestion from colds

The recommended daily dose is 40 mg. If you're using black cohosh tincture, that equals 2 ml three times a day in water or tea. You may prefer capsules or tablets. Two will likely give you the recommended daily dose. To make a black cohosh drink, put 20 g of dried root in 34 oz. of water. Bring to a boil, then simmer 20 to 30 minutes until the liquid is reduced by a third. Strain, cover, and store in the refrigerator or a cool, dry place. The liquid keeps up to 48 hours.

If the dosage for your brand of black cohosh differs, follow the recommendation of the manufacturer or your health care provider. As with most drugs and supplements, tell your provider about your interest in taking black cohosh. You should feel relief within six to eight weeks. Continue taking the treatment for up to six months.

■ PRECAUTIONS

Studies in Germany have found no serious side effects with black cohosh. The botanical treatment does not appear to increase women's cancer risk, although you should talk to your provider before taking black cohosh if you've had breast cancer or are in a high-risk group. Avoid black cohosh if you're breastfeeding or pregnant. It can stimulate contractions and lead to premature labor.

Some patients taking high doses of black cohosh have reported side effects, including the following.
- Abdominal pain
- Diarrhea
- Dizziness
- Headaches
- Joint pains
- Nausea
- Slow heart rate
- Tremors
- Visual dimness
- Vomiting

Do not confuse black cohosh with blue cohosh, which is a botanical used to treat some of the same problems black cohosh helps. But scientists have not studied blue cohosh thoroughly and its safety is uncertain.

■ POSSIBLE INTERACTIONS

Because black cohosh acts like estrogen, side effects may be more bothersome if it's taken with hormonal drugs. Avoid black cohosh if you're taking birth control pills or hormone-replacement therapy (HRT).

■ BURDOCK

During the Middle Ages, English herbalists preferred burdock root over sarsaparilla in treating boils, scurvy, and rheumatism. Native American healers were quite fond of burdock as a medicinal plant. American herbalists have used the roots and seeds as a blood purifier and pain reliever for more than two centuries.

Both the root and leaves are used in herbal remedies, but most recipes call for the root. Burdock is valued mainly as a treatment for arthritis, gout, and other inflammatory conditions. It is thought to help gout and rheumatism by stimulating the liver. Burdock is used as a diuretic, and it promotes perspiration, which make it effective in treating gout.

Burdock has been used by herbalists worldwide to treat a variety of ill-nesses, including pneumonia, abscesses, acne, fever, dandruff, and throat infections, as well as inflammation. However, the evidence that burdock is effective in treating gout, arthritis, and skin diseases is mostly anecdotal.

■ PLANT DESCRIPTION

Burdock originally grew in Europe and northern Asia. A member of the thistle family, this biennial is now widespread throughout the United States. It is a stout, common weed with many spreading branches, and grows to a height of three to four feet. Its purple flowers bloom between June and October. Burdock has alternate, wavy, heart-shaped leaves that are green on the top and whitish on the bottom. The deep roots are brownish-green, or nearly black on the outside. The roots are the most important part of the plant used for medicinal purposes.

Burdock grows well in the wild. It thrives in light, well-drained soil. Herbalists usually collect burdock leaves during the first year of growth, and harvest the roots in the fall of the first year after planting (or during the following spring before the flowers bloom).

■ WHAT'S IT MADE OF?

Burdock contains active compounds called sesquiterpene lactones. It contains a high percentage of a carbohydrate called inulin (or fructosan). It also contains a volatile oil, plant sterols, tannins, and fatty oil. Herbalists have traditionally used burdock root and leaves in treatments for arthritis, rheumatism, gout, skin disorders, scurvy, venereal diseases, psoriasis, and other skin disorders. But experts don't know for sure which active ingredients in burdock root are responsible for its healing properties.

■ AVAILABLE FORMS

Burdock products are made from fresh or dried roots or leaves. You can usually buy it as dried root powder, a decoction (liquid made by boiling down the herb in water), a tincture (a solution of the herb in alcohol, or water and alcohol), or a fluid extract.

■ HOW TO TAKE IT

Burdock root is a favorite among traditional herbalists for treating rheuma-tism, gout, skin eruptions, and cystitis. Burdock stimulates the appetite, so modern experts recommend it for anorexia nervosa. It is also used as a diuretic, for gastrointestinal symptoms, or externally to heal rough, scaly skin and psoriasis.

Scientific research done nearly 50 years ago showed that burdock root has some antibiotic properties. There's also evidence that it is effective in treating boils. Some people even claim that burdock root is helpful for diabetes. But the research on diabetes is not clear-cut. In one study, burdock lowered blood sugar; in another study, burdock actually made the symptoms of diabetes worse in animals.

A recent study showed that burdock blocked dangerous chemicals from causing damage to cells, suggesting to the possibility that burdock may help decrease the risk of developing cancer from toxic chemicals.

You can take burdock in the following forms as a daily supplement.
- Dried root: 2 to 6 g in decoction three times a day
- Tincture (1:5): 8 to 12 ml three times a day
- Fluid extract (1:1): 2 to 6 ml three times a day
- Tea: 2 to 6 g in 500 ml water

■ PRECAUTIONS

There are no known risks associated with using burdock. But be careful if you touch it because there is a slight chance of getting skin irritation from handling burdock. If you're pregnant or nursing, don't take burdock because it might stimulate your uterus to abort the fetus. In any case, at this point it's best to avoid taking excessive amounts of burdock (especially burdock root) because experts haven't studied the toxic effects of this plant in-depth yet.

■ POSSIBLE INTERACTIONS

If you're taking medication for diabetes, don't take large amounts of bur-dock because it can interfere with the action of these medications. If you have diabetes, talk with your health care provider before taking this or any other supplement.

■ CAT'S CLAW

Tribal people in the regions where cat's claw grows have used medi- cines prepared from the root bark for at least 2,000 years. They've used it to treat so many illnesses that it sounds like an amazing superdrug. For example, sexually transmitted diseases, arthritis, ulcer, and cancer are all reported to be cured by cat's claw.

After these claims got the attention of scientists in Europe, tests were able to show that ingredients in cat's claw do have some potentially powerful qualities. These ingredients together are able to reduce inflammation, destroy certain viruses, and stop the spread of some cancer cells. Much more research needs to be done on this plant and its medicinal properties. Still, cat's claw ranked among the top 10 herbs sold in American natural food stores by 1997.

■ PLANT DESCRIPTION

Cat's claw is a climbing shrub with thick vines growing as long as 100 feet. It is found in the Amazon rainforest and in tropical countries in South America and Central America. Much of the cat's claw available in the United States, as well as information about it, comes from Peru.

Curved, claw-like thorns grow on the stem—that's how cat's claw got its name. Bitter, water-like liquid collects inside the stem. People in South and Central America reportedly drink this on occasion to stop hunger, thirst, and fatigue.

■ WHAT'S IT MADE OF?

Cat's claw preparations are made by scraping the bark off the root of the vine. The root contains many types of plant chemicals. Some tannins also occur in the root (tannins are also found in tea). Quinovic acid glycosides help reduce inflammation and fight against some types of viruses.

Because collecting the root to get the bark kills the plant, herbalists look for other sources of these important ingredients. Right now, the inner bark of the vine seems to be a good alternative.

■ AVAILABLE FORMS

Both standardized and crude bark cat's claw are available. Crude bark is crushed and used to make tea. Standardized liquid or dried products are usually preferable: standardization is the quality control of herb manufacture.

■ HOW TO TAKE IT

Cat's claw reportedly has immune stimulant and anti-inflammatory actions. Most likely, if you or your provider have decided to add cat's claw to your daily therapy, it is probably because your immune system could use a little push or because your digestive tract is a little off kilter. You may have fre- quent colds or other viruses, or you may be trying to relieve irritable bowel syndrome, diverticulitis, or even Crohn's disease.

If you've decided to take cat's claw, choose between one of the prepara- tions listed below and take as directed by your health care provider or the product packaging.

Remember that because cat's claw has not been extensively researched, it is extremely important to get it from a reputable manufacturer.

Conventional Use
For treating mild stomach pains, sore throats, and colds; immune function; and minor injuries.
- Tea: 1 g root bark to 250 ml water, boil 10 to 5 minutes, cool, and strain. Drink 1 cup, three times daily
- Tincture (solution made from herb and alcohol, or herb, alcohol, and water): 1 to 2 ml two to three times daily
- Dry, encapsulated standardized extract: 20 to 60 mg daily

■ PRECAUTIONS

The people who live where cat's claw grows say that it is very safe and nontoxic. However, until science has proven this, there are some precau- tions to keep in mind.

The American Herbal Products Association (AHPA) gives cat's claw a class 4 safety rating. This means that the AHPA doesn't have enough evidence to base a clear rating on. AHPA does, however, believe that the tannin content of cat's claw taken in high doses might cause some abdominal pain or gas- trointestinal problems. Some researchers say that cat's claw should not be used in skin grafts or patients receiving organ transplants, or in patients with HIV, AIDS, or tuberculosis.

It is not to be used in children who are under three years of age. Breastfeeding and pregnant women also should not take cat's claw.

You might notice loose stools or diarrhea while taking cat's claw. This side effect is mild and tends to go away with continued use of cat's claw.

■ POSSIBLE INTERACTIONS

Do not use cat's claw if you receive immunizations, fresh or frozen blood plasma, or drugs that use animal protein or peptide hormones, such as animal sera, intravenous hyperimmunoglobulin therapy, intravenous thymic extracts, or bovine or porcine insulin.

■ CAYENNE

Cayenne, also known as red pepper, was first introduced to the world outside the Americas by the Caribbean Indians, who gave it to Columbus. Since then its popularity has spread, and it has become an important spice, particularly in Cajun and Creole cooking, and in the cuisines of southeast Asia, China, southern Italy, and Mexico. Capsaicin is the ingredient in cayenne that makes it hot. Even though cayenne tastes hot, capsaicin actually helps lower body temperature, which is one of the reasons that people in hot climates like to eat so much of it. Capsaicin also contributes to many of cayenne's other medicinal properties to stimulate the cardiovascular system, relieve pain on the surface of the skin or in joints, improve digestion, act as an expectorant, and fight bacteria.

Cayenne lowers levels of cholesterol in the blood, which helps lower blood pressure. It also prevents blood in your arteries from clotting. These properties help prevent heart disease, such as atherosclerosis (hardening of the arteries).

Even though cayenne can sting your tongue, it is actually a powerful pain reliever. It initially stimulates, but then decreases the intensity of pain signals in the body. This makes it particularly effective for people with chronic pain, since it takes several days to see significant results. Those who suffer from shingles, pain from diabetes, postmastectomy pain, and other postsurgical pain, may especially benefit from several different cayenne or capsaicin creams that are available. The capsaicin in cayenne not only relieves the pain of osteoarthritis and rheumatoid arthritis, but it also helps reduce the swelling from these conditions when used as a rub.

Cayenne improves digestion by stimulating production of digestive juices in the stomach and by fighting bacteria that could cause infection. Its antibacterial power also fights diarrhea caused by infection. As an expectorant, it thins mucus and helps move it out of the lungs. Because it also strengthens lung tissue, it is helpful for those with emphysema.

■ PLANT DESCRIPTION

Cayenne is a shrub that grows in subtropical and tropical climates. Its fruit grows into long pods that turn red, orange, or yellow when they are ripe. The fruit is eaten raw or cooked, or is dried and powdered into the spice that has been used for centuries in food and medicines.

■ WHAT'S IT MADE OF?

Studies have shown that capsaicin, the most active ingredient in cayenne, lowers blood cholesterol levels and decreases the intensity of pain signals in the body. It is also an antioxidant (which helps protect your cells from damage) and an antibacterial.

■ AVAILABLE FORMS

Cayenne may be taken by eating raw or cooked red pepper. Dried red pepper is available powdered, which may be added to food, stirred into juice, tea, or milk, or taken in capsule form. It also comes in creams for external use (should contain at least 0.025 percent capsaicin).

■ HOW TO TAKE IT

Because cayenne is so good for your heart, adding it regularly to food or taking it in capsule form can help prevent heart disease. Although it is spicy, it actually aids digestion and is not irritating to most ulcers. It is powerful even in small doses, so it is best not to take more than you would eat with food.

As a pain reliever, cayenne powder or cream can help relieve toothache, shingles, arthritis, psoriasis, and other kinds of chronic pain. Although it may cause some initial burning or itching, this should go away quickly. Because cayenne works by first stimulating and then decreasing the intensity of pain signals in the body, the pain may increase slightly but then should diminish greatly over the first few days.

As an external pain reliever (that is, when applied to the skin), capsaicin cream (0.025 to 0.075 percent capsaicin) may be applied directly to the affected area up to four times a day (brand names include Zostrix, Axsain, Capzasin-P).

For improved digestion and prevention of heart disease, capsaicin may be taken in capsules (30 to 120 mg, three times daily). You can make an infusion by adding $1/4$ to $1/2$ tsp. of powder to a cup of boiling water and drinking it.

■ PRECAUTIONS

Keep cayenne away from your eyes, and wash your hands thoroughly after use. Because cayenne does not dissolve easily in water, use vinegar to remove it. Capsaicin cream may cause skin irritation in some people. Test it on a small area of your skin before extended use. If it causes irritation, discontinue use. It may cause stomach irritation, but does not worsen duodenal ulcers. Do not use it for children under age 2. It is safe for use during pregnancy. It is not known if the spicy compounds are transferred through breast-feeding.

■ POSSIBLE INTERACTIONS

Do not take cayenne if you have high blood pressure or are being treated for high blood pressure.

■ CELERY SEED

Celery seed, whose sharp, refreshing flavor you may have tasted in pickles or sauerkraut, is also a useful herbal medicine. Celery seed has had varied uses around the world for thousands of years. Recent scientific studies have shown that certain chemicals in celery seed may actually help problems such as high blood pressure, arthritis, and anxiety. Celery seed may also help prevent cancer.

Celery seed has long been used to treat both arthritis and muscle spasm. Several chemicals in celery seed block inflammation or relieve pain. Others chemicals relax muscles that are in spasm. Celery seed contains calcium, which can help relax muscle cramps.

Certain chemicals in celery seed are anti-bacterial, while others are diuretic, meaning that they help remove water from the body in the form of urine. This helps wash away bacteria and the minerals that cause kidney and bladder stones.

Several chemicals in celery seed are hypotensive, meaning that they help lower blood pressure. Celery seeds are also rich in calcium, which may also lower blood pressure.

Celery seed has long been used in traditional medicine to treat gout and kidney stones. It lowers the levels of uric acid in the body.

Studies in lab animals show that celery seed prevents liver damage caused by toxic chemicals. It has been used for centuries as a liver tonic.

Celery seed strengthens muscles in the uterus, which helps increase menstrual flow.

A compound in celery seed called limonene acts as a mild tranquilizer. The calcium in celery seed helps calm tense nerves.

Celery seed may also help prevent cancer. A number of chemicals in celery seed prevented tumors in lab animals exposed to cancer-causing substances.

■ PLANT DESCRIPTION

Celery seeds come from the same plant whose stalks we've all eaten and cooked with. If you've never seen the stalks in their natural habitat, the celery plant is slender and stands about two to three feet tall. It has three to five segmented leaves, and flowers with small white petals. The seeds come from the flowers, are very small, are tan to dark brown, and have a strong, pleasant smell.

■ WHAT'S IT MADE OF?

Volatile oils (including apiol), flavonoids, boron, calcium, iron, limonene, sodium, zinc, 3-N-butyl-phthalide, alpha-linolenic-acid, beta-eudesmol, guaiacol, isoimperatorin, isoquercitrin, limonene, p-cymene, terpinen-4-ol, umbelliferone.

■ AVAILABLE FORMS

- Fresh or dried seeds
- Tablets
- Capsules filled with celery seed oil
- Celery seed extract, in which the active ingredients of celery seed have been extracted by alcohol or glycerin

■ HOW TO TAKE IT

- Celery seed oil capsules or tablets: Take one to two capsules or tablets three times a day, as directed by your health care provider.
- Celery seed extract: Take $1/4$ to $1/2$ tsp. three times a day, or as directed by your health care provider. (Always take with plenty of juice or with water at mealtime, unless instructed otherwise.)
- Whole celery seeds: Prepare a tea by pouring boiling water over one teaspoon (1 to 3 g) of freshly crushed seeds. Let it steep for 10 to 20 minutes before drinking. Drink this tea three times a day.

■ PRECAUTIONS

- Do not use celery seed if you are, or could be, pregnant.
- Celery seed is a safe herb. One word of caution, though. If you use it as a diuretic, consult your doctor first. Diuretics can deplete your body of potassium, which is an essential nutrient.
- Also, don't use celery seeds from a garden packet. Most seeds sold for planting have been treated with chemicals and shouldn't be taken internally.

■ POSSIBLE INTERACTIONS

None that are known

■ CHAMOMILE, GERMAN

Peter Rabbit's mother gave him a cup of chamomile tea after he returned from his day of danger in Mr. MacGregor's garden to settle his stomach, calm him down, and make him sleepy. But the medicinal use of chamomile starts way before the story of Peter Rabbit. Ancient Egyptians, Romans, and Greeks used chamomile flowers to relieve sunstroke, fevers, and colic. Germans use a phrase to describe chamomile, "alles zutraut," which means that chamomile can cure anything.

If you take German chamomile as a tea or liquid extract, it can help stop pains from gas, heartburn, and ulcers. If you use it as a cream or ointment on your skin, it can help reduce symptoms of psoriasis, eczema, or radiation burns from cancer therapies. As an ointment, chamomile may also help heal wounds that have taken a long time to get better. You can put steeped chamomile flowers, or tinctures (solutions made from herb and alcohol, or herb, alcohol, and water), into bathwater and soak in it; this can help heal a number of skin problems, including hemorrhoids. Inhale the steam from a pot of chamomile tea or a few drops of chamomile oil in boiling water when you have a cold. When the tea cools, you can use it as a mouthwash or gargle to help reduce pain from gum disease or mouth sores.

■ PLANT DESCRIPTION

The tiny daisy-like flowers of German chamomile can soothe irritated stomachs, lungs, and skin. The flowers have white collars circling raised, cone-shaped, yellow centers and are less than an inch wide, growing on long, thin, light green stems. Sometimes chamomile grows wild and close to the ground, but you can also find it bordering herb gardens. It can reach up to three feet high. Chamomile can mean either German chamomile or Roman (English) chamomile.

■ WHAT'S IT MADE OF?

The flowers are put into tea bags for tea, or crushed and steamed so that the oil they contain, which is blue, can be taken out and packaged separately. The oil contains ingredients that stop swelling and help reduce the growth of bacteria, viruses, and even fungi, which can contribute to or cause swelling and pain.

■ AVAILABLE FORMS

German chamomile is available as dried flower heads, tea, liquid extract, and topical ointment.

■ HOW TO TAKE IT

There are many uses for chamomile. Irritation from chest colds, slow-healing wounds, abscesses, gum inflammation, psoriasis, eczema, children's conditions such as chickenpox, diaper rash, and colic are common reasons for taking chamomile tea, baths, or tinctures. Usually, chamomile is used when symptoms arise. If you are using it for ulcer, heartburn, or another potentially serious condition, and your symptoms are not going away or are getting worse, see your health care provider as soon as you can.

- To relieve colic, ulcer, stomach pain, heartburn, and gas, make a tea of 2 to 3 g of the herb, steeped in hot water, three to four times daily between meals, or take 5 ml of 1:5 chamomile tincture three times daily.
- To use as a gargle or mouthwash for mouth sores or gum disease, make a tea of 2 to 3 g of the herb, steeped in hot water, then let it cool, and gargle as often as desired.
- For soothing the lungs during a cold or to calm a cough, pour a few drops of essential oil into steaming water and inhale the steam, or prepare tea and inhale the steam.
- To soothe hemorrhoids, cuts, eczema, or insect bites, use $1/4$ lb. of dried flowers per bath, or use alcohol extracts of chamomile flowers in the tub.
- To use as a douche, use 3 to 10 percent infusion (herb steeped in water; also called a "tea").
- For poultices applied to inflamed skin, use a 3 to 10 percent infusion (herb steeped in water; also called a "tea").
- For psoriasis, eczema, or dry and flaky skin, apply cream with a 3 to 10 percent crude drug chamomile content.

■ PRECAUTIONS

Chamomile is generally safe to use. Highly concentrated tea may cause vomiting, however. If you're allergic to ragweed, you should avoid chamomile, because they are both in the same family.

Chamomile should not be used in large amounts during pregnancy or while breastfeeding. If you are pregnant discuss with your doctor whether or not you should take chamomile.

■ POSSIBLE INTERACTIONS

There have been no reports of drug interactions with chamomile. However, it is probably safer to avoid chamomile while taking anticoagulant (blood-thinning) medications.

■ CHAMOMILE, ROMAN

Most likely it was Roman chamomile, which is also called English chamomile, that Peter Rabbit was sent to bed with in order to calm him down in Beatrix Potter's The Tale of Peter Rabbit. *The story was written at the start of the 20th century, but chamomile is still used in Europe today as a calming medicine. It is also used for heartburn and excess gas that may be due to nervousness. You might also find it in face creams, drinks, hair dyes, shampoos, and perfume.*

Roman chamomile may reduce nausea, vomiting, and the formation of gas in your intestines. It may also help to calm you down, lessen the swelling from cuts, or hemorrhoids, and make conditions such as eczema and gingivitis (swollen gums) less uncomfortable. Its uses are practically identical to the uses for German chamomile, and for good reason: they share the same active ingredients.

Roman chamomile has not been used in human studies as much as German chamomile, so claims on its use for specific health conditions will have to be verified through future research. Unfortunately, this means that many people assume Roman chamomile is not worth taking, without realizing that Roman chamomile is already added to many teas, ointments, and other types of medicinal preparations.

■ PLANT DESCRIPTION

Roman chamomile originates from northwestern Europe and Northern Ireland, where it creeps close to the ground but can also reach up to one foot in height. Gray-green leaves grow from the stems, and the flowers have yellow centers surrounded by white petals, like miniature daisies. The flowers smell like apples.

■ WHAT'S IT MADE OF?

Chamomile teas, ointments, and extracts all start with the white and yellow flower head. If these heads are not made into tea, they are crushed and steamed to produce a blue oil, which has medicinal benefits. Ingredients in the oil stop swelling and help reduce the growth of bacteria, viruses, and fungi that can contribute to pain.

■ AVAILABLE FORMS

Roman chamomile is available as dried flowers in bulk, tea, tinctures, and in creams and ointments.

■ HOW TO TAKE IT

Roman chamomile can be taken a number of ways. One easy way is to drink a cup of hot chamomile tea if your stomach is bothering you or if you are having trouble sleeping. In general, the dosages listed below will probably help relieve your stomachaches and may improve your appetite. Chamomile is also good for reducing pain during your menstrual period, and the swelling of your gums if you have gingivitis.

- Dried flowers, as tea, 1 to 4 g three times daily, or 70 percent alcohol extract, 1 to 4 ml three times daily.
- For hemorrhoids or skin problems, add a couple of tea bags to your bathwater or a few drops of Roman chamomile tincture. If you want to use an ointment, choose products that contain 3 percent to 10 percent dried chamomile flower heads.

■ PRECAUTIONS

Roman chamomile is generally safe to use, but you shouldn't take it as medicine during pregnancy or while breastfeeding. It is considered safe in tea, however.

Roman chamomile contains an ingredient, called anthemic acid, which could cause vomiting if taken in high doses.

There is a report that an individual had a severe allergic reaction after drinking Roman chamomile tea. That person was allergic to ragweed, which is in the same plant family as Roman chamomile. If you are allergic to ragweed, you should not use Roman chamomile. If you don't know whether you are allergic to ragweed, ask your health care provider about your risk for this allergy. Most likely, you can take any form of chamomile safely.

■ POSSIBLE INTERACTIONS

Interactions with other drugs or herbs haven't been reported, but it is safer to avoid chamomile if you are taking blood thinners.

■ COMFREY

Comfrey is traditionally used for superficial wounds, and to reduce the inflammation of sprains and broken bones. Allantoin, which is good for healing wounds, is a key active ingredient in the roots and leaves of comfrey. Comfrey herb and leaf also contain rosmarinic acid, which helps decrease inflammation and helps heal blood-vessel injuries in the lungs.

■ PLANT DESCRIPTION

Comfrey is a herbaceous perennial that originated in Europe and temperate parts of Asia.

■ WHAT'S IT MADE OF?

Comfrey products are made from the leaves or other parts of the plant grown above the ground. They can also be made from the roots, but root preparations are more likely to cause poisoning. Comfrey contains allantoin, rosmarinic acid, and pyrrolizidine-type alkaloids.

Some think that comfrey is a beneficial herb, but scientific studies show that this herb can be very toxic. If you drink comfrey preparations or take it internally in other forms you run the risk of being poisoned. Some people have even died from eating or drinking comfrey remedies.

Many comfrey plants contain poisonous compounds called pyrrolizidine alkaloids (PA), which are very toxic to the liver. Echimidine is the most poisonous pyrrolizidine alkaloid found in comfrey. Common comfrey *(Symphytum officinale)* doesn't usually contain dangerous pyrrolizidine alkaloids, but it sometimes does. Some comfrey products are made from other comfrey species that have dangerously high levels of echimidine, such as prickly comfrey *(S. asperum)* and Russian comfrey *(S. uplandicum)*.

The roots of all comfrey plants contain 10 times as much poisonous compound as the leaves. Do not use comfrey root unless you are being closely supervised by a qualified practitioner.

■ AVAILABLE FORMS

Comfrey ointments (containing 5 to 20 percent comfrey), creams, poultices, and liniments are made from the fresh or dried herb, fresh or dried leaf, or root of comfrey species. Use only products made from leaves of common comfrey *(S. officinale)*. PA-free comfrey preparations are also available. Do not use products made from the root of the comfrey plant and those made from *S. asperum* and *S. uplandicum*.

■ HOW TO TAKE IT

Scientific studies in animals show that comfrey has healing and pain-relieving properties. You can apply comfrey herb and leaf preparations to your skin to relieve pain from fractures, sprains, minor wounds, bruises, pulled muscles and ligaments, sprains, blunt injuries, and broken bones.

Recommended dosage:
Stick to herb and leaf ointments, creams, and other topical preparations. Use only the amount recommended on the label and never more than this amount. You shouldn't use comfrey remedies for more than four to six weeks in any given year.

■ PRECAUTIONS

Comfrey is basically safe if you follow the recommended dosages and use it only externally. Never use any comfrey preparation on broken skin.

If you take comfrey internally as a beverage or in another form for a long period of time, you risk getting a liver disorder (hepatic veno-occlusive disease). There have also been cases of atropine poisoning from taking comfrey remedies by mouth. Plant collectors sometimes unknowingly mix together raw plant material from comfrey and belladonna, and the atropine poisoning is actually caused by elements in the belladonna plant. Always make sure you're using reputable commercial brands that have good quality manufacturing practices. And read the label carefully.

- Don't use products made from comfrey root at all.
- Limit your use of comfrey leaf and herb preparations to four to six weeks per year.
- If you're pregnant or nursing, do not use comfrey products.

■ POSSIBLE INTERACTIONS

If you follow the dosage and safety guidelines for taking comfrey, there should not be any negative interactions.

■ DEVIL'S CLAW

Devil's claw is the common name for Harpagophytum procumbens *and* Harpagophytum zeyheri, *which belong to the sesame family. Originally from southern Africa and Madagascar, they are now found in the savannas and on the outskirts of the Kalahari Desert in South Africa and Namibia. Both plants are used to make the devil's claw root, or* Harpagophytum radix. *Medical researchers have found that devil's claw root can reduce inflammation and reduce pain.*

For thousands of years the Khoisan peoples of the Kalahari Desert have used devil's claw root, in remedies for treating pain and complications of pregnancy and in topical ointments for treating skin problems. Today, devil's claw is sold as a digestive aid and appetite stimulant. It also has mild pain-relieving action.

■ PLANT DESCRIPTION

Devil's claw doesn't have an odor, but it contains substances that make it taste bitter. It is a leafy perennial with branching roots and shoots. It has secondary roots, or tubers, that grow out of the main and lateral roots.

■ WHAT'S IT MADE OF?

Devil's claw herbal preparations are made from sliced or pulverized dried tubers. You can make teas (infusions) from commercially available dried devil's claw root. The tubers contain active compounds called monoterpenes, of which harpagoside is the most important active compound.

■ AVAILABLE FORMS

Devil's claw is available as whole or ground root tubers. You can make teas (infusions) from dried devil's claw root.

■ HOW TO TAKE IT

Health care providers use devil's claw root to treat loss of appetite, rheumatism, arthritis, fever, myalgia, tendinitis, gastrointestinal problems, and liver and gallbladder problems. Devil's claw is also an effective therapy for degenerative musculoskeletal conditions (disorders of locomotive system). It is also used as a pain reliever (analgesic), sedative, and diuretic.

Studies in animals have shown that devil's claw reduces the inflammation associated with arthritis. However, other studies have not demonstrated any anti-inflammatory properties. Devil's claw seems to work differently from most nonsteroidal anti-inflammatory drugs (NSAIDs). Its active compound, harpagoside (or a related compound called harpagide) is changed into another substance inside the body. The new substance, harpagogenin, may be the active ingredient that actually decreases the inflammation associated with arthritis.

You can take devil's claw as a dried root, a liquid extract, or a tincture (solution made from herb and alcohol, or herb, alcohol, and water). If you are taking it for a serious medical condition such as rheumatism, always first consult with your health care provider.

Recommended dosages for general use:
- Dried tuber: Take 0.1 to 0.25 g 3 times a day, encapsulated or made as decoction (liquid prepared by boiling down herb in water)
- Liquid extract (1:1 in 25 percent alcohol): Take 0.1 to 0.25 ml 3 times a day
- Tincture (1:5 in 25 percent alcohol): Take 0.5 to 1.0 ml 3 times a day

■ PRECAUTIONS

Devil's claw is nontoxic and safe, with virtually no side effects if taken in the recommended therapeutic doses. However, no one yet knows for sure whether devil's claw may be toxic if you take it long-term. And if you've been diagnosed with gastric ulcers, duodenal ulcers, or gallstones, you shouldn't take devil's claw unless your health care provider recommends it.

Devil's claw is cardioactive, which means it can act on the heart. If you have a serious medical condition, you should not use this herb without the advice of a qualified health care provider.

Some people think that devil's claw can cause miscarriage, but there is no scientific evidence that this is true. If you are pregnant, you should check with your health care provider before taking devil's claw or any other herbal supplement.

■ POSSIBLE INTERACTIONS

None known.

For additional information supporting this handout, please refer to our website: www.onemedicine.com/public/products/access

115

■ ECHINACEA

Native Americans used echinacea since at least the 1600s. They used the plant to treat snakebite, gum and mouth disease, colds, coughs, blood poisoning, sore throat, stomach and intestinal pain. It was also historically used for scarlet fever, syphilis, malaria, blood poisoning, and diphtheria. Through the 1800s, it was the most widely used plant drug in the United States, dispensed by both traditional doctors and the "nature doctors" (who were also called Eclectic physicians). It remained on the national list of official plant drugs in the United States until the 1940s and was most likely taken off this list because the conditions it had been used for were by then being treated with antibiotics.

In the 1980s, experiments with echinacea demonstrated that it still had possible therapeutic applications. Today, some people note that echinacea reduces the amount of time it takes for a cold or flu to run its course. It is also used for nasal, sinus, and bronchial illnesses, and echinacea ointments can speed the healing of wounds that are slow to heal.

■ PLANT DESCRIPTION

Echinacea has tall stems and bears single flowers that look similar to black-eyed Susans, except that echinacea flowers are pink or purple, and the cone in the middle is usually a purplish brown. The cone (the "eye" in black-eyed Susan) is actually a seed head and is very large on echinacea flowers. It has sharp spines that look like a stiff comb or an angry hedgehog. This is actually where echinacea got its name: *echinos* is Greek for hedgehog. Of nine species, three are used medicinally, which vary in appearance from the intensity of petal color to the stiff or drooping way the petals encircle the seed head.

■ WHAT'S IT MADE OF?

Many plant chemicals are involved in echinacea's effects: polysaccharides, flavonoids, caffeic acid derivatives, essential oils, polyacetylenes, alkylamides, and alkaloids. Polysaccharides are known to trigger cells in the body that fight infection.

■ AVAILABLE FORMS

Extracts, tinctures, tablets, capsules, ointments, and stabilized fresh extracts are available.

■ HOW TO TAKE IT

Echinacea's immune stimulant actions reduce inflammation and help the body fight bacteria and viruses. Tests show that echinacea stimulates immune system cells into action. When these cells are activated, white blood cells are more ready to wrap themselves around illness-causing invaders and to move viruses or bacteria out of your system, prevent them from reproducing themselves, or simply stop their activity.

While many individuals choose to take echinacea on a daily basis during the winter to help prevent colds and flu, studies have not consistently shown that this type of use is effective. On the other hand, echinacea can reduce the length of time that you have a cold or the flu. And, if you have rheumatoid arthritis and have trouble with steroid-based anti-inflammatory drugs, echinacea may provide you with very mild relief and no side effects.

For general immune system stimulation, during colds, flu, upper respiratory tract infection, or bladder infection, choose from the following forms and take three times a day.
- 1 to 2 g dried root, as tea
- 2 to 3 ml of 22 percent ethanol extract standardized to contain 2.4 percent beta-1,2-fructofuranosides
- 200 mg of powdered extract containing 6.5:1, or 3.5 percent, echinacoside
- Fluid extract (1:1): .5 ml to 1 ml
- Tincture (1:5): 1 to 3 ml
- Stabilized fresh extract: .75 ml

For arthritis, take 15 drops daily of a standardized extract produced by a reputable manufacturer.

For slow-healing wounds, apply creams or ointments as desired.

■ PRECAUTIONS

The American Herbal Products Association gives echinacea a class 1 safety rating, so it's safe as long as you use it as recommended by your health care provider or as instructed on the product label. In Germany, continual use of echinacea is restricted to eight weeks. Discuss long-term use with your health care provider.

Echinacea is a member of the *Compositae* family and as such may rarely cause an allergic reaction.

When you take echinacea orally, you will notice a strong numbing and tingling sensation on your tongue. This is normal and goes away quickly.

Some cases of skin rash and itching have been reported, but these are rare. Do not use echinacea if you have tuberculosis, leukoses, diabetes, collagenosis, multiple sclerosis, AIDS, HIV infection, or an autoimmune disease. If you are pregnant, consult with your health care provider before taking echinacea.

■ POSSIBLE INTERACTIONS

Do not use if you are currently taking immunosuppressant therapy.

■ EUCALYPTUS

The Aborigines—native Australians—used the leaves of eucalyptus to help heal wounds and reduce fevers. They also knew that if they were stuck without water in the desert area of Australia known as the Outback, they could dig up some eucalyptus roots, which are filled with water, to have a drink.

Eucalyptus leaves and the oil they produce kill bacteria, and ease breathing difficulties in people with croup, asthma, and bronchitis. It is also used externally for chest congestion, to ease aches and pains, and as a deodorant. If you've ever used Vicks VapoRub, then you probably remember the cool yet burning sensation that the balm left on your skin, and the way the minty, spicy smell cleared your sinuses to help you breathe. That's how eucalyptus essential oil works.

Eucalyptus is added to perfume, soap, and some foods and drinks. Its also used as an insect repellent and is added to wax candles and insect sprays. If you have dust mite allergies, you might want to consider adding a few drops of eucalyptus essential oil to your washer the next time you do laundry. Recent research suggests that this greatly reduces the numbers of dust mites, and that will help you breathe easier.

If you have cockroaches in your home, try putting a couple drops of eucalyptus essential oil on a few rags and leaving them overnight in your cupboards (be careful not to let the rags touch food or dishes). But remember that eucalyptus oil is highly toxic to humans and should be used with care. If you have children, make sure you store essential oils well out of their reach.

■ PLANT DESCRIPTION

Eucalyptus is native to Australia, where it is the primary food in the diet of koala bears. Today it is grown all over the world, including the United States. There are many species of eucalyptus. Some are the size of an ornamental shrub, and some grow to be giant trees. The type of eucalyptus that is most often used medicinally is called blue gum or Australian fever tree. It can grow as high as 230 feet. Its 4- to 12-inch leaves are dark green and shiny. Its blue-gray bark peels, and under it is a cream-colored bark.

■ WHAT'S IT MADE OF?

Eucalypus extracts and teas are made from soaking leaf material in an alcohol solution that draws out active components. Some of these active components are called tannins and flavonoids. Leaf essential oil, prepared from steam distillation, is mostly made up of an active component called cineole. It also contains other plant chemicals.

■ AVAILABLE FORMS

Eucalyptus is available as liquid essential oil, essential oil in ointment form, leaf tincture (solution made from herb and alcohol, or herb, alcohol, and water), crude leaf, and tea. Commercial cough drops, syrups, vaporizer fluid, liniments, toothpaste, and mouthwash may contain eucalyptus oil or its main ingredient, cineole.

■ HOW TO TAKE IT

Eucalyptus is used to treat inflammation of the chest, lungs, nose, and throat. It can kill a number of strains of bacteria, as well as some types of fungus. When applied to your skin, it can help to relieve rheumatic pain. Before using the following or any dosages, talk to your health care provider and follow his/her instructions.

- Eucalyptus leaf as infusion (tea): 1 to 2 g per cup three times a day
- Eucalyptus leaf tincture (for congestion): $^{1}/_{2}$ to 1 ml a day
- Oil for topical application (sore joints or chest rub for congestion): 30 ml oil to 500 ml lukewarm water
- Eucalyptol: 0.05 to 0.2 ml (1 to 2 drops per cup boiling water) daily
- Eucalyptus oil (for topical application): add $^{1}/_{2}$ to 1 ml (15 to 30 drops) of oil to $^{1}/_{2}$ cup of carrier oil (sesame, olive, etc.). For inhalation, add 5 to 10 drops of oil to 2 cups boiling water; place towel over head and inhale steam.

■ PRECAUTIONS

Do not use eucalyptus if you are pregnant or breast-feeding.

Eucalyptus oil is not toxic when used outside of the body. It should not be taken internally.

The American Herbal Products Association gives eucalyptus leaf a class 2d safety rating. Class 2d means that there are restrictions to an herb's use. In the case of eucalyptus leaf extracts, people with inflammation of the gastrointestinal tract or bile duct inflammatory disease should not use eucalyptus leaf extract. You also shouldn't use it if you have liver disease. Ask your health care provider if either of these conditions apply to you. You also should avoid taking too much leaf extract. The tannins in it could cause stomachaches or damage your liver or kidneys if taken in large amounts.

Never apply eucalyptus oil to the face or nose of a child under age 2.

■ POSSIBLE INTERACTIONS

Eucalyptus extract and oil may change the effects of drugs that you may be taking for hypoglycemia (low blood sugar). If you have hypoglycemia, make sure you talk to your health care provider before proceeding with eucalyptus treatments.

■ EVENING PRIMROSE

Evening primrose is native to North America where it was used for both food and medicine. Native Americans boiled and ate the peppery, nutty-flavored root, and used leaf poultices from the plant for bruises and hemorrhoids. European settlers took the root back to England and Germany, where it was planted for food.

Today, evening primrose is mostly grown for its seed oil. The oil, usually called EPO, is used in England to relieve the itchiness of atopic dermatitis, and to ease breast pain and tenderness associated with premenstrual syndrome and other causes. But further research may show its usefulness to extend beyond the treatment of these conditions. Eczema, diabetes, cardiovascular disease, high cholesterol, chronic fatigue syndrome, and even cancer may one day be reasons to use EPO.

■ PLANT DESCRIPTION

A circle of leaves grows close to the ground around evening primrose stems after the first year it is planted. In the second year, flowers grow. The flowers bloom with creamy yellow or bright yellow blossoms from June to September, but only after sunset or on cloudy days.

■ WHAT'S IT MADE OF?

Using a chemical called hexane, oil is taken from the seeds and prepared as medicine. The seeds contain essential fatty acids, or EFAs, which are a necessary part of our diets. The EFAs in evening primrose seeds are linoleic acid (LA) and gamma-linolenic acid (GLA). Because GLA is known to affect systems in the body that cause or reduce inflammation, it may have a major role in treating many illnesses, especially those that cause pain and inflammation.

■ AVAILABLE FORMS

You can get EPO as an oil or in capsules. Usually the capsules are preferred. Keep the product out of direct sunlight—better yet, in the refrigerator, which will prevent the oil from becoming rancid.

EPO is usually standardized to an 8 percent gamma-linolenic acid.

■ HOW TO TAKE IT

Many drugs, such as aspirin, have similar anti-inflammatory and pain relieving effects as EPO. However, these drugs do not supply any kind of dietary fatty acid and they can have side effects. In contrast, EPO gives your body something it may need, with little or no side effects.

If you and your health care provider have decided to try EPO, make sure you keep track of your dosages as well as how the treatment is working for you. Stick with the program that you and your provider have chosen for at least three months. In clinical studies, it has taken that long for effects to be seen, and in many cases, the effects were significant. For example, 60 percent of rheumatoid arthritis patients who took EPO were able to stop or reduce the amount of pain killers they normally took.

Skin rash, mastalgia (breast pain), and premenstrual syndrome (PMS) are the three conditions for which dosages have been recommended. For skin rash, the recommended daily dosage is 6 to 8 g for adults and 2 to 4 g for children. For mastalgia, the recommended dosage is 3 to 4 g daily. For PMS, the recommended dosage is 3 g daily. EPO is available as capsules and as oil. Follow package directions and your health care provider's instructions.

If you are taking EPO for arthritis, dry and scaly skin, or most other conditions, a dosage of about 3 g per day is considered safe. Be sure to discuss this with your health care provider before taking EPO.

■ PRECAUTIONS

The American Herbal Products Association (AHPA) gives EPO a class 1 safety rating, which means it's safe with appropriate use. There have been rare reports of nausea and headaches from using it. Stomach pain and loose stools may be indications that your dosage is too high. Talk to your health care provider about it, and lower your dosage based on his/her instructions.

Taking EPO while breastfeeding is believed to be safe. Breast milk actually contains both LA and GLA, and it may be a necessary part of a newborn's diet. Safety during pregnancy has not been determined—talk with your health care provider.

■ POSSIBLE INTERACTIONS

If you are taking drugs to treat schizophrenia, talk with your health care provider before taking EPO. It can interact with certain types of schizophrenia drugs and could put you at risk for epilepsy.

■ FEVERFEW

Feverfew has been used for centuries in European folk medicine for headache, arthritis, and fever. Feverfew comes from the Latin word, febrifuge, which means fever-reducing. This herb was traditionally used for insect bites, irregular menstruation, stomachaches, and toothache, although modern herbalists do not usually use it for these conditions. Herbalists today use feverfew to treat migraine, arthritis in its early stages, rheumatic diseases, and other conditions.

■ PLANT DESCRIPTION

Feverfew originally came from southeastern Europe. Today, it is widespread throughout Europe, North America and Australia. It is a short perennial that blooms between July and October. In the past, it could be seen in nearly every hedgerow throughout the gardens of England and Germany. People planted feverfew around their homes because they believed it would purify the atmosphere and ward off disease.

The small, daisy-like yellow flowers of this plant show that it belongs to the daisy family. Feverfew looks a little like chamomile, but it has some differences. The yellow-green leaves are alternate, and turn downward with short hairs. The leaves are the most important part for herbal medicine. Feverfew is an aromatic herb with a strong and bitter smell.

■ WHAT'S IT MADE OF?

Feverfew products are usually made from the leaves. Sometimes they are made from the aerial parts (all the parts of the plant that grow above the ground). The migraine-relieving activity of feverfew comes from an active compound called parthenolide. Parthenolide affects smooth muscle in the walls of blood vessels in the brain to block the action of vasoconstrictors like serotonin, prostaglandins, and norepinephrine. Vasoconstrictors narrow blood vessels and are one of the main causes of migraines.

■ AVAILABLE FORMS

Feverfew capsules are usually made from dried leaves. Always look for standardized products that contain at least 0.2 percent parthenolide. If the product is not standardized, you cannot be sure that you are actually getting enough parthenolide. And without parthenolide, you might not reap optimal health benefits.

It is important that you read the label carefully on feverfew products because the amount of parthenolide varies depending upon where the feverfew was grown. Feverfew from some regions of the world has very little or even no parthenolide.

You can also chew leaves from feverfew that you plant yourself or buy from an herbal market. However, be cautious in eating the leaves. About 10 percent of people who chew feverfew leaves get mouth ulcerations, loss of taste, and swelling of their lips, tongue, and mouth.

■ HOW TO TAKE IT

Today, nearly 10 percent of Americans suffer from migraines. Feverfew can provide effective relief for many of these people. It is used to treat migraines in progress and stop migraines before they start. It is most beneficial for migraine sufferers who have not had much success with other medications. (This includes prescription drugs and over-the-counter pain medications.) Feverfew is safe when used according to your health care provider's instructions.

In the 1980s, British researchers found that 70 percent of migraine sufferers who ate two to three fresh feverfew leaves every day got serious relief from their headaches. The British scientists were so amazed by this high success rate that they expanded their research. They discovered that feverfew was much more effective than placebo in reducing migraine severity. And feverfew also decreased symptoms of nausea and vomiting associated with migraine.

In 1997, feverfew ranked number 19 on a list of top-selling herbs at health food stores in the United States. Medical experts are not sure if feverfew reduces the inflammation of arthritis. The evidence so far is conflicting. But some people who have arthritis claim that feverfew helps decrease their pain and stiff joints.

Recommended dosage:
- To treat and prevent migraine, take standardized feverfew extract (minimum 250 mcg parthenolide) two times daily.
- To treat an acute migraine attack, take 1 to 2 g parthenolide daily. For other conditions, take 1 to 2 ml twice a day of 1:1 fluid extract; or 2 to 4 ml twice a day of 1:5 tincture (solution made from herb and alcohol, or herb, alcohol, and water).

■ PRECAUTIONS

Feverfew works best for migraine sufferers who have not responded well to conventional treatment. Sometimes people experience side effects such as abdominal pain, indigestion, flatulence, diarrhea, nausea, vomiting, and nervousness. Because feverfew can alter the menstrual cycle, menstruating women should use it with caution. Pregnant women, nursing women, and children under 2 years old should not take feverfew.

■ POSSIBLE INTERACTIONS

You should not take feverfew if you are taking aspirin, warfarin, or another "blood-thinning" (antithrombotic) drug. If you are taking any of these medications, you should consult your physician or another qualified health care provider before you start taking feverfew.

■ FLAXSEED

Flaxseed has been used throughout the world for food, medicine, and fiber to make clothes, fishnets, and other products. The ancient Egyptians grew flax thousands of years ago, and it is now found throughout the world.

Flax is a rich source of dietary fiber that can help lower cholesterol levels. And flaxseed oil helps improve cardiovascular health. Long before people knew about the health benefits of flaxseed oil, they used whole and milled flax seeds as a laxative. The laxative effect comes from mucilage.

Flaxseed oil contains both omega-3 fatty acids and omega-6 fatty acids. Flaxseed oil is nature's richest storehouse of omega-3 fatty acids. Flaxseed oil contains more than twice as much omega-3 oil as fish oils, and it costs less than fish oils, ounce for ounce. Omega-3 oil has been shown to reduce the risk of arteriosclerosis. Flaxseed oil also contains plant nutrients like phytoestrogens. These are natural estrogen-like substances that can lessen the discomfort of menopause.

■ PLANT DESCRIPTION

Flax is an annual plant that thrives in deep moist soils rich in sand, silt, and clay. The seeds in the flax plant are filled with flaxseed oil, sometimes called linseed oil. (Note: Commercial-grade linseed oil commonly used in furniture restoration is not meant for human consumption.) The husks of the seeds are rich in mucilage. Both the seed oil and mucilage have many nutritional and therapeutic properties.

■ WHAT'S IT MADE OF?

Flax products are made from the seeds found inside the fruits. The seeds contain fatty oils called alpha-linolenic acid (ALA) and linoleic acid. ALA is the omega-3 oil in flaxseed. Flax also contains other important substances like lignans, which may protect you against some types of cancer.

■ AVAILABLE FORMS

You can buy several types of products made from flaxseed. Ripe seeds, linseed cakes, and flaxseed oil are all available at health food or grocery stores. Flaxseed oil can be purchased in liquid form (to use in preparing food) or as softgels that you can take as a dietary supplement.

■ HOW TO TAKE IT

You can benefit from adding flaxseed oil to your diet if you have elevated cholesterol, angina, high blood pressure, psoriasis, eczema, rheumatoid arthritis, or multiple sclerosis.

Flaxseed oil reduces LDL (low-density lipoprotein) cholesterol (the body's "bad cholesterol") and lowers triglyceride levels. Research shows that flaxseed oil gives much better protection against heart attacks than canola oil or olive oil.

Taking flaxseed oil can reduce cancer risk. This is because flaxseed contains the richest sources of lignan building blocks, which play a major role in preventing cardiovascular diseases and cancer. New research indicates that the lignans in flaxseed have both short-term and long-term protective effects against colon cancer.

To make sure that you are getting both essential fatty acids and lignans in your diet, look for flaxseed oil that is rich in lignans. The best way to take flaxseed oil is to add it to foods like salad dressings. But you shouldn't use flaxseed oil for cooking because heat destroys the healthful fatty acids in flaxseed oil.

If you suffer from constipation, gastritis (stomach inflammation), or enteritis (inflammation of the small intestine), try adding flax-seed products to various dishes. Flaxseed is an excellent source of mucilage, which acts as a laxative. And be sure to always drink enough liquid, especially water, if you eat bruised, milled, or whole flaxseed.

Recommended dose:
- Flaxseed: 1 tbsp. whole or bruised (but not ground) seed with 150 ml liquid two to three times a day for gastritis and enteritis. 2 to 3 tbsp. bulk seeds taken with 10 times the amount of water as a bulk laxative
- Poultice: 100 g soaked in boiling water for 10 to 15 minutes, strained, placed in cheesecloth and applied
- Decoction (liquid prepared by boiling down herb in water): 15 g of whole seed simmered in 1 cup water for 10 to 15 minutes
- Flaxseed oil: 1 tbsp. oil daily, added to foods such as salad dressing

■ PRECAUTIONS

You shouldn't have any side effects if you take the recommended doses of flaxseed or linseed oil. But if you eat a large quantity of flaxseed and don't drink enough water, you might get intestinal upset. If you're pregnant or nursing, you can add flaxseed and flaxseed oil to your diet. But be sure to not take more than the recommended dose and discuss with your health care provider first.

■ POSSIBLE INTERACTIONS

Try to avoid taking flaxseed at the same time that you are taking medications or other nutrients. The flaxseed can slow down the absorption of other drugs, vitamins, and minerals. Talk to your health care provider before taking flaxseed if you take any drugs (either prescription or over-the-counter) regularly.

GARLIC

The pungent odor of garlic, which is offensive to some people, is noticeable on your breath and even your skin after you eat it. Despite this, herbalists worldwide consider garlic one of the most important herbal medicines. It has been used as both food and medicine in many cultures for thousands of years. The construction workers who built the Egyptian pyramids ate large amounts of garlic to protect themselves from diseases. Gravediggers in early eighteenth-century France drank a concoction of crushed garlic in wine to keep them from getting a plague that killed many people in Europe. During both World War I and II, soldiers were given garlic to prevent gangrene.

PLANT DESCRIPTION

Garlic originally came from central Asia, and is now found throughout the world. Garlic is a perennial that can grow two feet high or more. The most important part of this plant for medicinal purposes is the compound bulb. Each bulb is made up of 4 to 20 cloves, and each clove weighs about 1 gram.

WHAT'S IT MADE OF?

The main active ingredient in garlic is alliin. Alliin is an odorless chemical relative of the sulfur-containing amino acid cysteine. When garlic bulbs are crushed, alliin is converted into another compound called allicin. Allicin is the active compound that gives garlic its characteristic odor and many of its healing benefits.

Fresh garlic contains about 0.25 to 1.15 percent of allicin. The total amount of sulfur-containing substances in garlic is about 25 to 35 percent after the bulbs have been crushed. Allicin gives garlic its antibiotic effects. Allicin also helps lower cholesterol by blocking cells from making more cholesterol. Ajoene is another important active compound in garlic that helps prevent hardening of the arteries and stroke.

AVAILABLE FORMS

Garlic products are made from whole fresh garlic, fresh or dried garlic cloves, or oil of garlic. But the amount of allicin in commercial products can vary, depending on how the product was prepared, or on the percentage of active compounds in fresh garlic cloves. Not all garlic starts with the same amount of active ingredients.

Aged garlic products are made by fermenting garlic. These products are odor-free, but they don't have many health benefits. Fermentation inactivates most of the active ingredients, so it's important that you carefully read the label on all garlic products. It is best to use standardized garlic products to be sure you're getting a specified concentration of allicin and other active substances.

HOW TO TAKE IT

For years, people have taken garlic to help prevent atherosclerosis (hardening of the arteries) and high blood pressure, colds, coughs, bronchitis, gastrointestinal problems, and menstrual pain. Medical research shows that garlic can kill many types of bacteria, some viruses and fungal infections, and even intestinal parasites. Garlic is also an antioxidant and it can boost your immune system. Garlic may even help prevent cancer. But garlic is best known for its favorable effects on cardiovascular health. Garlic is effective in treating and preventing high cholesterol and triglyceride levels, atherosclerosis, and respiratory infections such as colds and cough.

You can take garlic in the following forms to help prevent cardiovascular problems and the common cold.

- Capsules: 1,000 to 3,000 mg daily (lower doses for prevention, higher for treatment)
- Oil: 0.03 to 0.12 ml, three times a day

PRECAUTIONS

Avoid eating too much garlic because it might give you a stomachache. Also, if you handle too much fresh or dried garlic, you might get burn-like skin lesions or other skin irritations. If you know that your blood clots slowly, don't take large therapeutic doses of garlic. This is especially important if you're going to have surgery. Too much garlic can increase your risk for bleeding during or after the operation. If you're pregnant or nursing, talk to your health care provider before taking or eating large amounts of garlic. In small amounts, it's fine, but extremely large doses can stimulate the uterus and may even cause a miscarriage.

POSSIBLE INTERACTIONS

If you are taking anticoagulant drugs such as aspirin, don't consume large amounts of garlic, either fresh or commercially processed.

■ GINGER

Ginger originally came from China and India, where it has been used in cooking for more than 4,000 years. Because people liked its sharp and spicy flavor so much and found it to be warming and good for stomach pains, it was transplanted worldwide by explorers in warm, tropical places. Ginger root helps relieve the dizziness, sweating, nausea, and vomiting that comes from motion sickness or seasickness. It can also ease sore throats, headaches, some types of menstrual and arthritis pain, and fevers and aches caused by colds and flu.

■ PLANT DESCRIPTION

Ginger rhizome is the knotted, thick, beige tuber you find at your local market. Because it grows underground, it is often called ginger root. Technically, a rhizome is part of a stem that just happens to be underground. The actual root sprawls out from knots on the rhizome. Above the ground are 12-inch long stems with long, narrow, ribbed, green leaves, and white or yellowish-green flowers.

■ WHAT'S IT MADE OF?

Ginger products are made from fresh or dried ginger root or from steam distillation of the oil.

■ AVAILABLE FORMS

Once the rhizome is cut, the active chemicals in the plant, such as zingiberene, bisabolene, gingerol, and shogoal, begin to lose potency. Herbal product companies market ginger as extract, tinctures, capsules, or oils, in order to prevent the loss of these chemicals. Use products that clearly state on the label the amount of ginger you will be getting per dose.

You can also buy fresh ginger root and prepare your own tea by steeping half a handful sliced, or half a teaspoon grated, washed, and unpeeled tuber in hot water; or pour a pint of boiling water over an ounce of sliced rhizome. Let the tea steep for 15 minutes or so, and drink 2 cups of this a day. Another good source of ginger is crystallized ginger. Don't be fooled by the sugar coating; crystallized ginger delivers a sharp bite.

■ HOW TO TAKE IT

How you take it depends on personal preference and what ails you. In general, you should not take more than 2 to 4 grams of ginger a day, in addition to the ginger you may already get from your diet (from items such as ginger ale, ginger snaps, gingerbread, or stir-fried foods). If you are using fresh ginger, make sure you weigh the piece so that you will know approximately how large a chunk equals 2 to 4 grams.

For nausea, gas, or indigestion, take 2 to 4 grams of fresh root daily (0.25 to 1.0 gram of powdered root) or 1.5 to 3.0 ml tincture daily. To prevent vomiting, take 1 gram powdered ginger ($1/2$ tsp.) or its equivalent every four hours as needed, or 2 ginger capsules (1 gram) three times daily. You may also chew a $1/4$-oz. piece of fresh ginger.

For cold symptoms, fever associated with flu, sore throat, menstrual cramps, or headache, steep 2 tbsp. of freshly shredded ginger in boiled water, two to three times daily, or place a drop of ginger oil or a few slices of fresh rhizome in steaming water and inhale.

To relieve arthritis pain, take fresh ginger juice, extract, or tea, 2 to 4 grams daily; rub ginger oil into painful joint; or place fresh root in a warm poultice or compress and apply to painful areas.

■ PRECAUTIONS

The American Herbal Products Association (AHPA) gives fresh ginger root a class 1 safety rating, so it is a safe herb with a wide dosage range. Still, it is always wise to follow recommended dosages. The AHPA gives dried ginger root a class 2b rating, advising that it not be used during pregnancy.

Some women do use ginger to calm symptoms of morning sickness, but this use of ginger is controversial. For safety, do not take more than normal dietary amounts. Ginger eaten as a normal part of the diet is not considered risky.

Do not use ginger if you have gallstones. While ginger use is normally not associated with side effects, too much ginger may cause mild heartburn.

■ POSSIBLE INTERACTIONS

If you are taking cardiac drugs, anticoagulant medication such as warfarin, or drugs for diabetes, and you are considering taking ginger as a preventive-type medicine for motion sickness, vertigo, migraine, uterine cramps, or arthritis, talk to your health care provider first. While no studies have proven the interaction, there is a risk that ginger can either block or increase the effects of some of these drugs.

◾ GINKGO BILOBA

More than 400 published studies have been done on Ginkgo Biloba extract (GBE), making it one of the best researched of all herbal medicines. In Germany and France it is the most frequently prescribed herbal medicine and is in the top five of all prescriptions written in those countries. GBE is a powerful aid to circulatory problems, particularly a lack of blood to the brain, which causes memory loss, vertigo, tinnitus, disorientation, headaches, and depression, especially in the elderly. It has strong antioxidant properties as well, protecting both the central nervous system and the cardiovascular system from damage and the effects of aging.

GBE improves blood circulation by strengthening blood vessels and reducing the stickiness of blood platelets, which can help blood circulate more easily, even when atherosclerosis (hardening of the arteries) is present. This not only helps improve blood flow to the brain, but it also increases blood flow to the limbs and can help prevent or treat heart disease and stroke. It is also used effectively to help prevent mental deterioration for those approaching old age. In a few small studies, GBE seemed to slow and even stop the progress of Alzheimer's disease, particularly in the early stages.

Recent studies have also shown that GBE may reduce impotence caused by impaired blood flow. It also may help reduce certain premenstrual symptoms, specifically fluid retention.

◾ PLANT DESCRIPTION

Ginkgo biloba is the oldest living tree species. It is amazingly adaptable, surviving even the Ice Age and the atomic bomb that destroyed Hiroshima. A single tree can live as long as 1,000 years and grow to a height of 120 feet. It has short branches with fan-shaped leaves and produces inedible fruit that has a strong odor. The fruit contains an edible inner seed. Although Chinese herbal medicine has used both the ginkgo leaf and seed for centuries, modern research has focused on the standardized *Ginkgo biloba* extract (GBE), which is produced from the leaves. This extract is highly concentrated and much more effective than any other product made from the leaves.

◾ WHAT'S IT MADE OF?

Ginkgo biloba is made up of ginkgo flavone glycosides, several terpene molecules unique to ginkgo (ginkgolides and bilobalide), and organic acids. The special terpene molecules are thought to give *Ginkgo biloba* its ability to fight many of the effects of aging. This includes improving blood circulation, reducing inflammation, and protecting brain cells from damage caused by lack of oxygen.

◾ AVAILABLE FORMS

Ginkgo biloba extract standardized to contain 24 percent ginkgo flavone glycosides (50:1 extract) and 6 percent terpene lactones. (There are several different brands of GBE available in the U.S.) Capsules and tincture are also available.

◾ HOW TO TAKE IT

GBE repairs much of the damage that aging inflicts, particularly on the circulatory and nervous systems. It can also strengthen blood vessels. As a result, GBE is most often recommended for older people suffering from signs of dementia, such as disorientation, memory loss, headaches, depression, vertigo, and tinnitus. Your health care provider will determine that these conditions are related to lack of blood flow to the brain and not another condition before recommending GBE. Patients suffering from leg cramps resulting from poor circulation have also seen good results with GBE.

Because GBE strengthens and protects the circulatory and nervous systems, it can be also taken to help prevent heart disease, stroke, and the onset of dementia.

Initial results often take four to six weeks, but should continue to accumulate beyond that period. You may not see any dramatic changes for six months.

- Take 120 mg daily in two or three divided doses of 50:1 extract standardized to 24 percent flavone glycosides. If you have more serious dementia or Alzheimer's disease, you may need to work up to 240 mg daily in two or three divided doses.
- Capsules of dried herb with 10 mg standardized extract (1 to 3 capsules three times a day)
- Tincture (1:5): 2 to 4 ml three times a day
- Fluid extract (1:1): 1 to 3 ml three times a day

◾ PRECAUTIONS

GBE is very safe and side effects are rare. In a few cases, gastrointestinal upset, headaches, and dizziness were reported. GBE does not appear to alter heart rate and blood pressure or to change cholesterol and triglyceride levels. Because it decreases platelet aggregation (stickiness), there is some concern that ginkgo may increase risk of intracranial (brain) hemorrhage. Use with caution in conjunction with other blood-thinning agents (for example, Coumadin). Do not handle or ingest the fruit of *Ginkgo biloba*. The German Commission E reports that a hypersensitivity to *Ginkgo biloba* preparations is the only known reason not to take GBE.

If you are pregnant, you should exercise caution since there is a lack of data concerning showing GBE's effect during pregnancy. Do not give GBE to infants or children.

◾ POSSIBLE INTERACTIONS

None known

■ GINSENG, AMERICAN

Asians consider ginseng the king of all herbs. American ginseng is similar enough to Asian ginseng to chemically have the same effects. American ginseng root is light tan and looks a bit like a human body. Herbalists hundreds of years ago took this likeness to mean that ginseng could cure all human ills. It has been used as a cure-all by many different cultures.

Ginseng is difficult to grow. This difficulty made it a good export crop early on in American history, because it was plentiful in North America. In 1718, American ginseng brought five dollars a pound in Canton, China. In 1773, 55 tons of American ginseng were sold to the Chinese. In 1824, 380 tons were exported. Even Daniel Boone traded ginseng.

According to alternative medicine practitioners, American and Asian ginsengs are best to alleviate stress, fatigue, convalescence, and diabetes, and Siberian ginseng for stress, fatigue, atherosclerosis, and impaired kidney function. Confusion regarding which ginseng (American, Asian, or Siberian) to use for stress, fatigue, and convalescence stems from the suggestion that active components in one type are superior to those in another type. Such superiority has not been demonstrated. Early Russian studies indicated that Siberian ginseng's positive effects exceed those of Asian ginseng's. These results are supported by empirical reports, but have been challenged by investigators who question the validity of the studies and the quality of the Siberian ginseng preparation. At this time, all three ginsengs are regarded as adaptogens, all three have the same side effects, and despite qualitative differences, each is used for similar treatments. Cost, standardization, and the reputation of the manufacturer may be the deciding points in determining which product to use.

■ PLANT DESCRIPTION

The plant has leaves that grow in a circle around a straight stem. Yellowish-green umbrella-shaped flowers grow in the center and produce red berries. Wrinkles around the neck of the root tell how old the plant is. This is important because ginseng is not ready for use until it has grown for four to six years.

■ WHAT'S IT MADE OF?

Ginseng products are made from ginseng root and the long, thin offshoots called root hairs. The main chemical ingredients of American ginseng are ginsenosides and polysaccharide glycans (quinquefolans A, B, and C).

■ AVAILABLE FORMS

White ginseng (dried, peeled) is available in water, water-and-alcohol, or alcohol liquid extracts, and in powders or capsules.

■ HOW TO TAKE IT

Ginseng increases stamina, strength, and well-being. These actions make it sound like a stimulant, such as coffee, but stimulants often affect the action of important parts of the body, so irritability, heart palpitations, addiction, and anxiety are some of the side effects that may result from stimulant use. Ginseng, on the other hand, acts without any of these negative effects.

Your doctor may recommend ginseng if you have just had an illness. If you are elderly, ginseng may shorten the time that it takes you to bounce back from illness or surgery. It may also help you to focus your thoughts.

If you are someone who tends to get a lot of colds or sore throats you may find that taking ginseng reduces the number of these conditions. Ginseng may help if you have difficulty concentrating. Athletes take ginseng to increase both endurance and strength.

In each of these functions, ginseng acts as an adaptogen, which help the body fight against the effects of just about any kind of stress, be it viral, bacterial, emotional, intellectual, or physical. The effects of stress may be as simple as headaches or colds, but they can also be more serious, such as accelerated aging, memory loss, heart disease, cancer, and arthritis.

When taking American ginseng, look for standardized products. Standardization is the only way we have of assuring quality in herbal products. Choose white American ginseng, standardized to 0.03 percent ginsenosides, designated as Rb1.

The recommended dose is 1 to 2 g fresh root, 0.6 to 2 g dried root, or 200 to 600 mg liquid extract daily.

If you are healthy and are using ginseng to increase your physical or mental performance, to prevent illness, or to improve resistance to stress, you should take ginseng at the recommended dosage in cycles. For example, take 1 to 2 g fresh root, 0.6 to 2 g dried root, or 200 to 600 mg liquid extract daily for 15 to 20 days, followed by two weeks without taking ginseng.

For help recovering after an illness, the elderly should take 0.5 g twice a day for three months and then stop. Or take 0.5 g twice a day for a month, followed by a two-month break. Repeat if desired.

■ PRECAUTIONS

The American Herbal Products Association (AHPA) rates American ginseng as a class 2d herb, which indicates that specific restrictions apply. In this case, hypertension (high blood pressure) is the specific restriction, so people with hypertension should not take ginseng products.

People with heart disease, diabetes, and low blood pressure should use caution when taking American ginseng. Do not take ginseng during any acute illness. Do not use ginseng if you are pregnant because its safety during pregnancy has not been determined.

■ POSSIBLE INTERACTIONS

Ginseng may increase the effects of caffeine or other stimulants, making you feel anxious or nervous, or causing sweating, insomnia, or irregular heartbeat.

Ginseng may increase the effects of phenelzine sulfate (Nardil) or other antipsychotics, or medications for blood pressure or diabetes. It may interfere with steroids. Do not take ginseng if you are using these kinds of drugs without consulting your provider first.

■ GINSENG, ASIAN

Ginseng is a light tan, gnarled root, regarded by people in Asian countries to be the king of all herbs. Sometimes the main part of the root looks like a human body, with stringy shoots that look like arms and legs. Herbalists hundreds of years ago took this appearance to mean that ginseng could cure all human ills, and it has been used as a cure-all by many different cultures. The Chinese, however, view ginseng not only as a cure-all, but also as a plant that brings longevity, strength, and wisdom to its users.

American and Asian ginsengs are best to alleviate stress, fatigue, convalescence, and diabetes, and Siberian ginseng for stress, fatigue, atherosclerosis, and impaired kidney function. Confusion regarding which ginseng (American, Asian, or Siberian) to use for stress, fatigue, and convalescence stems from the suggestion that active components in one type are superior to those in another type. Such superiority has not been demonstrated. Early Russian studies indicated that Siberian ginseng's positive effects exceed those of Asian ginseng's. These results are supported by empirical reports, but have been challenged by investigators who question the validity of the studies and the quality of the Siberian ginseng preparation. At this time, all three ginsengs are regarded as adaptogens, all three have the same side effects, and despite qualitative differences, each is used for similar treatments. Cost, standardization, and the reputation of the manufacturer may be the deciding points in determining which product to use.

■ PLANT DESCRIPTION

The ginseng plant has leaves that grow in a circle around a straight stem. Yellowish-green umbrella-shaped flowers grow in the center and produce red berries. Wrinkles around the neck of the root tell how old the plant is. This is important because ginseng is not ready for use until it has grown for four to six years.

■ WHAT'S IT MADE OF?

Ginseng products are made from the ginseng root, and the long, thin off-shoots, called root hairs. The main chemical ingredients in Asian ginseng are the ginsenosides (Rg1 as marker); glycans (panaxans); polysaccharide fraction DPG-3-2; peptides; maltol; and volatile oil.

■ AVAILABLE FORMS

White ginseng (dried, peeled) or red ginseng (unpeeled root, steamed before drying) is available in water, water-and-alcohol, or alcohol liquid extracts, and in powders or capsules.

■ HOW TO TAKE IT

Ginseng increases stamina, strength, and well-being. These actions make it sound like a stimulant, such as coffee. But stimulant drugs often compromise the actions of important parts of the body, and irritability, heart palpitations, addiction, and anxiety are some of the side effects that may result. Ginseng, on the other hand, acts without any of these negative effects, and it has been used safely for at least 2,000 years.

Your doctor may recommend ginseng if you have just had an illness. If you are elderly, ginseng may shorten the time that it takes you to bounce back from illness or surgery. It may also help you to focus your thoughts.

If you are someone who tends to get a lot of colds or sore throats you may find that taking ginseng reduces the number of these conditions. Ginseng may help if you have difficulty concentrating. Athletes take ginseng to increase both endurance and strength. Ginseng may also help reduce the discomforts of menopause.

In each of these functions, ginseng acts as an adaptogen, which help the body fight against the effects of just about any kind of stress, be it viral, bacterial, emotional, intellectual, or physical. The effects of stress may be as simple as headaches or colds, but they can also be more serious, such as accelerated aging, memory loss, heart disease, cancer, and arthritis.

When taking ginseng, look for standardized products. Standardization is the only way we have of assuring quality in herbal products. Choose white or red ginseng, standardized to 1.5 percent ginsenosides, designated as Rg1.

The recommended dose is 1 to 2 g fresh root, 0.6 to 2 g dried root, or 200 to 600 mg liquid extract daily.

If you are healthy and are using ginseng to increase your physical or mental performance, to prevent illness, or to improve resistance to stress, you should take ginseng at the recommended dosage in cycles. For example, take 1 to 2 g fresh root, 0.6 to 2 g dried root, or 200 to 600 mg liquid extract daily for 15 to 20 days, followed by two weeks without taking ginseng.

For help recovering after an illness, the elderly should take 0.5 g twice a day for three months and then stop. Or take 0.5 g twice a day for a month, followed by a two-month break. Repeat if desired.

■ PRECAUTIONS

The American Herbal Products Association (AHPA) rates ginseng as a class 2d herb, which indicates that specific restrictions apply. In this case, hypertension (high blood pressure) is the specific restriction, so people with hypertension should not take ginseng products.

People with heart disease, diabetes, and low blood pressure should use caution when taking ginseng. Do not take ginseng during any acute illness. Do not use ginseng if you are pregnant because its safety during pregnancy has not been determined.

■ POSSIBLE INTERACTIONS

Red ginseng may increase the effects of caffeine or other stimulants, making you feel anxious or nervous and increase your heart rate and blood pressure. You may sweat more, have trouble sleeping, or have irregular heartbeats.

Ginseng may increase the effects of phenelzine (Nardil) or other antipsychotics, or medications for blood pressure or diabetes. It may also interfere with steroids. Do not take ginseng if you are using any of these kinds of drugs without consulting your provider first.

■ GINSENG, SIBERIAN

A Chinese poem describes the thorny branches covering this shrub as looking like a bony jackal's leg. While that doesn't sound very attractive, the poem goes on to say that daily use will "keep your virgin face younger, and prolong your life for ever and ever." The author claims that Siberian ginseng is worth much more than gold and jewels, and for centuries the Chinese have prized Siberian ginseng to prolong life, enhance health, and stimulate both a healthy appetite and a good memory. But it wasn't until the Soviet Union began testing it in the 1950s that published studies began to support some of these uses.

American and Asian ginsengs are best to alleviate stress, fatigue, convalescence, and diabetes, and Siberian ginseng for stress, fatigue, atherosclerosis, and impaired kidney function. Confusion regarding which ginseng (American, Asian, or Siberian) to use for stress, fatigue, and convalescence stems from the suggestion that active components in one type are superior to those in another type. Such superiority has not been demonstrated. Early Russian studies indicated that Siberian ginseng's positive effects exceed those of Asian ginseng's. These results are supported by empirical reports, but have been challenged by investigators who question the validity of the studies and the quality of the Siberian ginseng preparation. At this time, all three ginsengs are regarded as adaptogens, all three have the same side effects, and despite qualitative differences, each is used for similar treatments. Cost, standardization, and the reputation of the manufacturer may be the deciding points in determining which product to use.

■ PLANT DESCRIPTION

Siberian ginseng is a shrub that grows 3 to 10 feet high. Its leaves are attached to a main stem by long branches. Both the branches and the stem are covered with thorns. Flowers, yellow or violet, grow in umbrella-shaped clusters, and turn into round, black berries in late summer. The root itself is brownish, wrinkled, and twisted.

■ WHAT'S IT MADE OF?

Siberian ginseng products are made from the root. The root contains a mixture of components, common to many plants but occurring together in Siberian ginseng, called eleutherosides. Among the other ingredients are chemicals called polysaccharides, which have been found to boost the immune system and lower blood sugar levels in laboratory studies using animals.

■ AVAILABLE FORMS

Siberian ginseng is available in liquid extracts, solid extracts, powders, capsules, and tablets, and as dried or cut root for tea.

■ HOW TO TAKE IT

One of the many actions of Siberian ginseng is to increase your body's resistance to stress. Not only can it help your body cope with daily stresses, but it may also prevent you from becoming ill. Viruses, bacteria, chemicals, extreme working conditions, noise, and pollution are some of the many types of stressors each of us are exposed to every day. Siberian ginseng may help your body get back to normal after experiencing these. It may also help your body get back to normal after you've been ill.

Siberian ginseng also increases mental and physical performance. If you've been having difficulty concentrating at work, Siberian ginseng may help you stay on task. And if your job requires repeated physical labor, it may help with that, too.

Siberian ginseng has these effects because it is an adaptogen, substances that help the body fight against the effects of just about any kind of stress. Although currently unproven, the effects of stress may be as simple as headaches or colds, or they may also be more serious, such as memory loss, heart disease, cancer, arthritis, and accelerated aging. Do not be surprised if one day your provider recommends Siberian ginseng to you for any of these conditions, or for chronic fatigue syndrome or atherosclerosis. These conditions may be someday be scientifically proven to benefit from Siberian ginseng supplementation.

The recommended dose is 2 to 3 g dried root daily (tea, or in capsules). You can also take a tincture (solution made from herb and alcohol, or herb, alcohol, and water), 5 ml three times daily, or a 33 percent alcohol extract, 2 to 4 ml, one to three times daily. Extracts are considered a little more potent than tinctures. In making tincture, 1 part Siberian ginseng may be used in 5 parts liquid; in making an extract, 1 part herb is used in 1 part liquid. Solid extracts, made from dried, powdered root, are also available. Look for products that contain at least 1 percent eleutheroside F, and take 100 to 200 mg three times daily.

If you are taking Siberian ginseng to increase stamina or resistance to stress, you should take one of the forms recommended above for one month, and then wait two months before taking it again for another month. If you are taking it to help beat a chronic condition, such as fatigue, you can take it for three months, followed by 2-to-3 weeks without taking it. (Be sure to take your dosages before 3 P.M. to avoid insomnia.) You can repeat these cycles if you feel you need to, but you should consult with your health care provider first.

■ PRECAUTIONS

The American Herbal Products Association (AHPA) rates Siberian ginseng as a class 1, which means that it is safe when used as directed. However, if you have high blood pressure or are pregnant, you should not use Siberian ginseng.

■ POSSIBLE INTERACTIONS

Siberian ginseng may increase the effects of caffeine or other stimulants, making you feel anxious or nervous, or causing sweating, insomnia, or irregular heartbeat. It should not be used with antipsychotic medications, steroids, or hormones.

■ GOLDENSEAL

Goldenseal was originally introduced to early American settlers by Native American tribes, who used it as a yellow dye, as well as a wash for skin diseases, sore eyes, and various forms of "catarrh" (colds and flu, for example).

Goldenseal may help the symptoms of sore mouth, sore throat, canker sores, gingivitis (infected gums); stomachache, diarrhea, indigestion, constipation, and ulcers; colds and flu; vaginal irritation; earaches; mild conjunctivitis ("pink eye") or other eye irritations. (See your health care provider if eye irritation continues for more than a few days, or if it is severe.)

Goldenseal may also be useful for disinfecting cuts, scrapes, boils, and acne; and for lowering high blood sugar levels (hyperglycemia), which may lead to diabetes.

■ PLANT DESCRIPTION

Goldenseal is a small plant with a single hairy stem. It has two five-lobed, jagged leaves, small flowers, and raspberry-like fruit. The bitter-tasting rhizome, or root, is a bright yellow-brown in color, twisted, and wrinkled. Goldenseal can be found growing wild in rich, shady soil in the northern U.S., but is now grown mostly on farms.

■ WHAT'S IT MADE OF?

Goldenseal contains a compound called berberine that kills many of the bacteria that cause diarrhea. Berberine has also been shown to kill a wide range of other types of germs, such as those that cause yeast infections, as well as various parasites such as tapeworms and giardia. Berberine may also activate your white blood cells, making them more effective at fighting infection. For these reasons, it is used as an all-around disinfectant, both externally and internally. Goldenseal also stimulates the production of bile, a fluid produced by your liver that helps digest fats. Goldenseal is used as a healing tonic for the digestive tract, and is considered helpful for easing chronic constipation, and hemorrhoids.

■ AVAILABLE FORMS

Goldenseal is available as tablets (various concentrations), powdered root in capsules (various concentrations), alcoholic tinctures, and low-alcohol extracts.

■ HOW TO TAKE IT

- Goldenseal in capsules or tablets: 500 to 2,000 mg up to three times a day.
- Goldenseal extract (more concentrated): 0.03 to 0.12 g, up to three times a day.
- For disinfecting cuts, scrapes, boils, and acne, place goldenseal extract or tincture on a clean cloth, and press the cloth gently on the affected area.
- For earaches, mix with olive oil and use as eardrops.
- For sore throat, gums, or mouth, make a mouthwash as follows: In 1 cup of warm water, mix $1/4$ tsp. salt and $1/2$ tsp., or the contents of 1 capsule, of goldenseal powder. (It will not dissolve completely.) Rinse and spit out.
- For cases of vaginal irritation, make a goldenseal douche as follows: Mix $1/4$ tsp. salt and $1/2$ tsp., or the contents of 1 capsule, of goldenseal powder in 1 cup of warm water. Let the mixture settle, and strain out any suspended particles before using it. (Keep the mixture as clean as you can.) Over-douching can make you more susceptible to certain kinds of vaginal infections. See your health care provider if your symptoms do not improve after a few days.
- An eyewash made from goldenseal is good for eye infections and irritations. Use 1 cup of sterile water with $1/4$ tsp. salt and $1/2$ tsp. goldenseal (or the contents of one capsule), and strain out all particles. Discard if the solution becomes cloudy, which indicates bacterial growth.

■ PRECAUTIONS

- Do not use goldenseal if you are pregnant or have high blood pressure.
- If used for long periods of time, goldenseal can irritate the skin, mouth, throat, and vagina. It can also reduce the number of good bacteria in your digestive system, which can cause nausea and diarrhea.
- Large doses may also interfere with your body's ability to absorb B vitamins.

■ POSSIBLE INTERACTIONS

None known

■ GRAPE SEED EXTRACT

Grapes have been used by humans for thousands of years. They were around during the Bronze age. The Greek poet, Homer, who lived about 700 BC, talked of wine made from grapes. The fruit is mentioned in the Bible, and Egyptian tombs and relics have representations of grapes on them.

People have used grapes for purposes other than eating or making into wine or juice. European folk healers, hundreds of years ago, made an ointment from the sap in the stems to cure skin and eye diseases. Leaves were astringent and hemostatic, that is, they were used to stop bleeding, inflammation, and pain, such as the kind brought on by hemorrhoids. Unripe grapes treated sore throats; dried grapes, or raisins, treated consumption, constipation, and thirst. The round, ripe, sweet grapes, however, had the most uses of all, used to treat cancer, cholera, smallpox, nausea, eye infections, and skin, kidney, and liver diseases.

■ PLANT DESCRIPTION

Grapes are native to Asia near the Caspian Sea, but were brought to North America and Europe: European settlers brought grapes to North America in the 1600s. This plant's climbing vine has large, jagged leaves, and its stem bark tends to peel. The grapes themselves may be green, red, or purple.

■ WHAT'S IT MADE OF?

Today we eat grapes or raisins because we like them, and we drink wine and grape juice for the same reason. But in 1970, a biochemist in France isolated from grape seed a material that improves blood circulation—oligomeric proanthocyandin (OPC). It also reduces swelling, and may even prevent heart disease. OPC is one of the substances in red grape juice and red wine that has been shown to have some protective properties against heart disease. Because of its OPCs, grapes are now harvested not only for the food and drink products we are familiar with, but also as a source of these therapeutically active ingredients.

First and foremost, OPCs are antioxidants, which help the body to handle assaults that could eventually cause disease, such as cigarette smoke and environmental chemicals. They are different from a broader category of stress protectors called adaptogens, which also protect you from chemical or physical substances. Antioxidants or adaptogens also protect you from physical and mental exhaustion and help you recover after an illness. Both antioxidants and adaptogens may help us avoid at least two of the big killers today: cardiovascular disease and cancer.

OPC's antioxidant actions may help prevent cardiovascular disease. Some studies suggest that it might reduce the formation of plaques in the arteries, and may help regenerate damaged tissue lining the arteries. If you have a family history of cardiovascular disease, you may want to look into taking OPCs. Chronic venous insufficiency is another reason to take OPCs, as is vision disturbance from diabetic nephropathy or macular degeneration, for example. These uses of OPC have been supported in clinical studies.

Future uses may include the treatment of premenstrual syndrome (PMS), and to stop swelling in the face after plastic surgery. OPC has helped reduce the breast discomfort and aching joints and legs that sometimes occur with PMS, and has decreased recovery time from plastic surgery. Antitumor actions have also been shown.

■ AVAILABLE FORMS

Grape seed extracts are available in fluid extract form or in capsules and tablets. Look for products that are standardized to 95 percent OPC content.

■ HOW TO TAKE IT

Results from clinical trials suggest that grape seed OPCs may help vision difficulty as well as chronic venous insufficiency and its symptoms. Lymphedema, varicose veins, cancer, premenstrual syndrome, dental caries, and circulatory disorders are some of the many other types of conditions that OPC treatment might help with.

As a preventative for arterial plaques, vision disorders, or other conditions, take 50 mg standardized extract per day. For specific illness, 150 to 300 mg per day is recommended, but consult your health care provider and don't self-prescribe.

■ PRECAUTIONS

There are currently no precautions for grape seed OPC use. It is considered very safe.

■ POSSIBLE INTERACTIONS

None have been reported, however, because OPCs are new, and affect blood vessels, circulation, and evidently a significant range of illnesses, drug-herb interactions may crop up. Keep in touch with your health care provider and with developments in grape extract research, particularly if you have diabetes or other serious conditions such as macular degeneration or lymphedema.

■ GREEN TEA

Green tea is not usually prescribed as a remedy for diseases. But people all over the world have noticed that drinking green tea daily has many health benefits. Green tea is an important preventative against cancer, elevated blood fats, hardening of the arteries, and dental cavities. It also protects against bacterial dysentery. Green tea can help ward off a number of fungal, bacterial, and even viral infections (like the common cold) as well.

The difference between green and black teas is in their processing. The fresh leaves are slightly steamed and then quickly dried in green tea. This prevents enzymes in the tea from breaking down nutritious substances called polyphenols, which are the cancer-fighting compounds in green tea. Green tea polyphenols (GTP) are even better antioxidants than vitamins C and E.

Green tea is good for your digestive system. It helps you think more clearly, and even improves your eyesight. Green tea strengthens arteries and reduces excess fats in the blood. It clears phlegm from sore throats, and neutralizes poisons. The tannins in green tea can stop diarrhea. If you want to increase the tannin levels in your tea, let it brew longer.

■ PLANT DESCRIPTION

The tea plant is a large shrub with evergreen leaves. It originally came from China, where it has been used for more than 5,000 years. Today, tea is grown throughout Asia and parts of the Middle East and Africa. Black tea is more common in the United States. But black tea is fermented and not as healthy as green tea. Green tea is unfermented. (Oolong tea is semi-fermented.)

■ WHAT'S IT MADE OF?

The leaf buds and young leaves make the best green tea. Tea contains the purine alkaloids caffeine, theophylline, and theobromine. But the most important active ingredients are polyphenols, which are responsible for many of the therapeutic and preventive actions of green tea.

■ AVAILABLE FORMS

Most green tea products are sold as dried leaf tea. There are also extracts made from the leaves and leaf buds. Green tea has 300 to 400 polyphenols and 50 to 100 mg caffeine per cup. Decaffeinated green tea products contain concentrated polyphenols (60 to 89 percent total polyphenols).

■ HOW TO TAKE IT

One of the active compounds in green tea is as effective as aspirin in keeping blood platelets from clumping together, which improves circulation. And green tea helps stop hardening of the arteries. Population studies show that there's less cancer in countries where people drink green tea every day, but no cause and effect has been established. Black tea does not have the same effect. In fact, if you drink a lot of black tea, you increase your risk for getting cancers of the rectum, gallbladder, and endometrium. Green tea's cancer-fighting effects work best against gastrointestinal cancer, lung cancer, and breast cancer. Green tea is highly recommended as an alternative to coffee and black tea.

Three cups of green tea per day (3 g soluble components, or 240 to 320 g polyphenols) or 300 to 400 mg per day of standardized green tea extract (extracts should contain 80 percent total polyphenols and 55 percent epigallocatechin) is the recommended dosage. Capsules and liquid preparations are also available.

■ PRECAUTIONS

Limit your intake of green tea if you have a sensitive stomach, cardiovascular complications, kidney disorder, overactive thyroid, or tendency toward spasm. If you're prone to anxiety attacks, be careful drinking tea or any caffeinated beverage.

If you're pregnant, don't ingest any products that contain caffeine, including tea. If you must have tea, try to limit yourself to no more than 3 cups of green tea per day. This is a maximum of 200 mg of caffeine per day. And drink your tea over the course of the entire day (but not too late at night). Don't drink it all in a short period of time. You should also avoid tea if you're nursing. Even a small amount of caffeine might give your baby a sleeping disorder.

If you take more than 1.5 grams of tea every day over a long period of time, you might develop serious symptoms. This much caffeine can cause irritability, insomnia, heart palpitation, and dizziness. You may experience vomiting, diarrhea, and headaches, and you might lose your appetite. If you're drinking a lot of tea and start to vomit or have abdominal spasms, you may have caffeine poisoning. Lower your caffeine intake and see your health care provider if your symptoms are severe. The side effects of drinking too much tea are usually not fatal.

■ POSSIBLE INTERACTIONS

If you're taking alkaline drugs (prescription or over-the-counter) it's best to avoid tea. The tannins in tea bind with alkaline drugs, which can make the drugs less effective.

■ HAWTHORN

Hawthorn is used in Europe, particularly in Germany, for patients with deteriorating heart function. It may also be helpful for angina, arteriosclerosis, and some mild types of arrhythmia. If your health care provider has advised you to try hawthorn, you probably have a very mild form of heart disease, and studies indicate that hawthorn may help you manage your condition.

■ PLANT DESCRIPTION

Hawthorn is a common thorny shrub that grows up to five feet tall on hillsides and in sunny wooded areas throughout the world. In May its flowers bloom, but although hawthorn is in the same botanical family as roses, the flowers are not fragrant. They grow in small clusters, and are white, red, or pink. Small berries, called haws, sprout after the flowers. They are usually red when ripe, but they may also be black. Hawthorn leaves are shiny and grow in a variety of shapes and sizes.

■ WHAT'S IT MADE OF?

Hawthorn medicines start with the leaves, the berries, and sometimes, the flowers (only the white flowers are medicinal). These parts are dried and then made into powder. The powder is put into capsules, or added to alcohol or glycerite (a sweet, non-alcohol liquid), along with water, so you can take it in a liquid form. In liquid forms of botanicals, the alcohol and water create a more digestible form.

■ AVAILABLE FORMS

Hawthorn comes in capsules, tinctures, standardized fluid extracts, or solid extracts. You can also make a bitter-tasting tea from dried cut hawthorn leaves, flowers, and berries.

■ HOW TO TAKE IT

Look for standardized hawthorn products. Look for a label that says the product is standardized to contain either 4 to 20 mg flavonoids/30 to 160 mg oligomeric procyanidins, or 1.8 percent vitexin rhamnoside/10 percent procyanidins.

If you are taking hawthorn for heart failure or angina, you will need to take it for at least six weeks, three times a day, before you notice an effect.

■ PRECAUTIONS

The American Herbal Products Association (AHPA) gives hawthorn a class 1 safety rating, which indicates that it is a very safe herb with a wide dosage range. Even so, it is always wise to follow recommended dosage. If you are pregnant, do not use hawthorn.

It is extremely important for you to note any changes you feel while you are taking hawthorn. More pain, more angina attacks, more exhaustion while walking or exercising—these are all good reasons to stop taking hawthorn and see your health care provider right away. Even if you don't experience any of these symptoms, see your health care provider if your condition hasn't improved after six weeks of hawthorn treatment. Your progress should be monitored even if you do feel better, so see your health care provider in either case.

■ POSSIBLE INTERACTIONS

Hawthorn can make the effects of digitalis stronger, so don't use hawthorn if you are taking digitalis. Hawthorn may work with other supplements (such as magnesium or vitamin B_6) or herbs (such as garlic or reishi mushroom) to help your cardiovascular system work better.

■ KAVA KAVA

People in the Pacific Islands, where kava comes from, have probably used kava for thousands of years. First knowledge of it in the West came with one of the expeditions led by Captain James Cook in the 1700s. Natives to the islands used kava as part of important rituals and rites, and it was the focus of many social gatherings. The drink prepared from the roots numbs the mouth. In the 20th century, kava has been given to many important visitors to the Pacific Islands. Hillary Rodham Clinton and Pope John Paul II were given kava during welcoming ceremonies, as were President and Mrs. Lyndon B. Johnson in 1966.

Kava root can reduce stress-related anxiety and the effects of anxiety disorders. At lower dosages, kava helps you be more aware and active, but not tense. At higher dosages, the chemicals in kava root can make you sleepy. But usually, kava is simply calming, as opposed to the heavier sedation of alcohol or antianxiety prescription drugs. Health care providers prescribe kava for pain and stiffness, anxiety, insomnia, menopausal anxiety, uncontrolled epilepsy, pain, and jet lag.

■ PLANT DESCRIPTION

The root comes from a tall shrub that grows in the islands of the Pacific Ocean, including Hawaii. This shrub produces large, green, heart-shaped leaves that grow thickly on the branches, off thick stalks. Long, slender flowers that look like Chinese baby corn grow where the branches meet the stems. The roots look like bundles of woody, hairy branches.

■ WHAT'S IT MADE OF?

Kava root contains chemicals called kavapyrones, which reduce convulsions and cause muscles to relax in laboratory tests using animals. The kavalactones also cause reactions in the brain that are believed to be like those caused by pharmaceutical drugs used for depression and anxiety. Kavalactones are what numbs your tongue if you put liquid kava in your mouth or on your gums.

■ AVAILABLE FORMS

In some cultures, kava is prepared by chewing the root and spitting it into a bowl. The saliva mixes with the root and activates the plant medicine. Today, manufacturers use alcohol or acetate instead. You can find kava in liquid form, as tinctures or extracts, and in capsules or tablets. It's also available powdered or crushed.

■ HOW TO TAKE IT

If your health care provider has recommended kava, make sure you read the label to look for kava products that are standardized to contain a 70 percent kavalactone content. A standardized product is one with a listing of specific amounts of active plant material per dosage.

For the relief of anxiety and insomnia, and to reduce stress, the recommended kava dose is 2.0 to 4.0 g as decoction (a preparation made by boiling down the herb in water) up to three times daily. Take 60 to 600 mg kavalactones daily of standardized formulas or follow your provider's instructions.

Length of treatment varies. It may take four weeks before you notice improvement. Recommendations are not to take kava for longer than three months.

■ PRECAUTIONS

Kava's side effects are mild. It can numb the mouth and may have an unpleasant taste. A very small percentage of people report nausea, headache, dizziness, or skin rash when they take kava. If any of these happen to you, make sure you tell your health care provider. Don't drive if you are taking Kava.

The American Herbal Products Association (AHPA) advises pregnant and breast-feeding women not to take kava. It also advises against taking more than the recommended dosage, using kava for longer than three months at a time, and driving while using kava.

Missionaries to the Pacific islands during the 19th century noticed that people who took kava all the time had yellowish, scaly skin. In a more recent study, people who took 100 times the recommended dose experienced this same yellowing, developed a rash, lost hair, and had trouble with vision, appetite, and breathing. These changes go away when you stop taking kava.

■ POSSIBLE INTERACTIONS

Do not use kava if you are taking barbiturates or while using alcohol. Kava may increase the effect of these drugs.

■ LEMON BALM

Just as mint is known for its soothing effects on the stomach, lemon balm is also used to ease pain and discomfort associated with digestion, including gas and bloating. Lemon balm also calms and relaxes, easing away stress and nervous anxiety, and can help you get to sleep, and has been used for this purpose as far back as the Middle Ages. Today, it is often combined with other calming, soothing herbs, such as valerian, to enhance the overall relaxing effect.

Even before the Middle Ages, lemon balm was used to lift the spirits, and to help heal wounds and reduce the swelling and pain of insect bites. European ointments for cold sores and herpes sores contain high concentrations of lemon balm. Patients say these ointments work better than some prescription medications in easing pain and preventing sores from coming back, and their health care providers confirm this.

■ PLANT DESCRIPTION

Lemon balm comes from Europe and is now grown all over the world. It is grown not only in herb gardens, but also in crops for medicine, cosmetics, and furniture polish manufacturing. The plant grows up to two feet high, sometimes higher if left untended. In the spring and summer, clusters of small, light yellow flowers grow where the leaves meet the stem. The leaves are very deeply wrinkled and range from dark green to yellowish green in color, depending on the soil and climate. If you rub your fingers on them, your fingers will smell tart and sweet, like lemons. The leaves are similar in shape to mint leaves, and in fact, come from the same plant family.

■ WHAT'S IT MADE OF?

Lemon balm preparations are made from the leaves of the plant. Essential oils made from lemon balm leaves contain plant chemicals called terpenes, which cause at least some of the herb's sedative and antiviral effects. Lemon balm also contains ingredients called tannins, which are thought to cause many of the herb's antiviral effects. It also contains eugenol, which calms muscle spasms, numbs tissues, and kills bacteria.

Lemon balm is also used to treat headaches, menarche (delayed menstruation), and chronic fatigue syndrome. It also seems to help in the treatment of a thyroid disorder called Graves' disease. While clinical trials are lack-

ing, the tests that have been done tend to support the herb's many uses. For example, lemon balm essential oil was seen to relax laboratory animals, and smooth muscles that line the digestive tract in these same animals. Studies also suggest that lemon balm extracts affect the thyroid hormones in a way that benefits people with Graves' disease. Research also supports its use for cold sores, or lesions due to herpes viruses.

■ AVAILABLE FORMS

Lemon balm is available as dried leaf that can be bought in bulk. It is also sold as tea, and in capsules, extracts, tinctures, and oil. The creams used in Europe, which contain high levels of lemon balm, are not currently available in the United States, but teas can be used on the skin by applying it with cotton balls.

■ HOW TO TAKE IT

In general, you should read the manufacturer's suggestions for use when taking any herbal product, and consult with your health care provider for brands and dosages that he or she recommends.

For difficulty sleeping, or to reduce stomach complaints, flatulence, or bloating, choose from the following.
- Tea, using 1.5 to 4.5 g herb, several times daily
- 2 to 3 ml tincture three times daily, or the equivalent in fluid extract or encapsulated form

For cold sores or herpes sores, steep 2 to 4 tsp. of crushed leaf in 1 cup boiling water for 10 to 15 minutes. Cool. Apply with cotton balls to the sores throughout the day.

■ PRECAUTIONS

No side effects or symptoms of toxicity have been reported with lemon balm use, but because it is used to bring on menstruation, do not use it if you are pregnant.

■ POSSIBLE INTERACTIONS

Lemon balm may interfere with thyroid medications or other treatments for Graves' disease.

■ LICORICE

Licorice is traditionally used for coughs and as a soothing remedy for the skin. People also take it for spasms and inflammation, for bronchitis, rheumatism, and arthritis. You can also take licorice as a laxative. Many health care providers prescribe licorice root products for peptic ulcer and chronic gastritis. Some providers recommend licorice root to treat primary adrenocortical insufficiency.

■ PLANT DESCRIPTION

Spanish licorice (*Glycyrrhiza glabra*) grows wild in some parts of Europe and Asia. A perennial that grows 3 to 7 feet high, licorice has an extensive branching root system. The roots are straight pieces of wrinkled, fibrous wood, which are long and cylindrical and grow horizontally underground. Licorice roots are brown on the outside and yellow on the inside.

Glycyrrhizin, an active ingredient in licorice root, is 50 times sweeter than sugar. Glycyrrhizin contains a compound called glycyrrhizic acid mixed with potassium and calcium salts. Glycyrrhizin and glycyrrhizic acid are beneficial for peptic ulcers. Licorice must always be used with caution because glycyrrhizin and glycyrrhetic acid can harm the adrenal glands.

■ WHAT'S IT MADE OF?

Licorice products are made from the roots and underground stems of the plant. Glycyrrhizin and glycyrrhetic acid are the most important substances in licorice. The roots also contain coumarins, flavonoids, volatile oils, and plant sterols.

■ AVAILABLE FORMS

Licorice products are made from peeled and unpeeled dried root. There are powdered root and finely cut root preparations, dry extracts, and liquid extracts. Some licorice root extracts have had the harmful compounds removed. These extracts are known as deglycyrrhizinated licorice (DGL), and do not harm the adrenal glands. You may want to use DGL if you have gastric or duodenal ulcers.

■ HOW TO TAKE IT

Licorice root extracts kill staph and strep infections, and acts against viruses such as HIV, hepatitis A, and herpes. Licorice root destroys the yeast that causes Candida infections. Scientific studies show that DGL reduces inflammation and is as effective as some prescription drugs for gastric ulcers.

You can take licorice in the following forms.
- Dried root: 1 to 5 g as an infusion or decoction three times a day
- Licorice tincture: 2 to 5 ml three times a day
- DGL extract: 0.4 to 1.6 g three times a day for peptic ulcer
- DGL extract 4:1: in chewable tablet form 300 to 400 mg 20 minutes before meals for peptic ulcer

■ PRECAUTIONS

You should be very careful if you're taking large amounts of licorice products or if you chew licorice-flavored tobacco or use other licorice-flavored products. If so, you're at risk for licorice poisoning.

If you take more than 20 g of licorice a day, you might have a bad reaction. Too much glycyrrhizin causes a condition called pseudoaldosteronism, which makes you overly sensitive to a hormone in the adrenal cortex. This condition can give you headaches and make you feel tired. It can also make you retain water. An overdose of glycyrrhizin can lead to harmful conditions such as high blood pressure and even heart attack. These symptoms can show up within one week if you're taking more than 100 g of glycyrrhizin every day.

People don't usually die from taking too much licorice or glycyrrhizin, but you can have side effects even if you're taking just an average amount of licorice. Some people get muscle pain, and others get numbness in their arms and legs. Too much licorice can also cause weight gain.

You can avoid these problems if you keep your dosages within the recommended guidelines. If you have any medical problems or concerns, check with your health care provider.

Don't use licorice if you've been told you have high blood pressure, or a kidney, heart, or liver condition. If you're pregnant, do not take licorice products. If you're nursing, don't take licorice. No matter how healthy you are, don't use any licorice product for longer than four to six weeks.

■ POSSIBLE INTERACTIONS

If you're taking thiazide diuretics, don't take licorice products because they can interact with licorice and cause you to lose too much potassium.

■ MILK THISTLE

Milk thistle helps relieve the symptoms of hepatitis, cirrhosis, and inflammatory liver conditions. It is one of the most effective herbs known for treating liver disorders. Even the ancient Greeks knew the virtues of milk thistle for jaundice. Physicians of the Middle Ages used it for liver problems and other conditions, and nursing mothers took milk thistle leaf to increase their milk for breast-feeding.

Milk thistle fruit contains an active ingredient called silymarin. Silymarin is the liver-protecting compound inside milk thistle. Silymarin repairs liver cells damaged by alcohol and other toxic substances. Silymarin also keeps new liver cells from being destroyed by these same substances.

■ PLANT DESCRIPTION

Milk thistle originally came from the Mediterranean. It is now widespread throughout the world, from Europe to Asia, and from Africa to North America. This stout thistle usually grows in dry, sunny areas. The stem branches at the top, and it reaches a height of 4 to 10 feet. The leaves are wide, with white blotches or veins. The flowers are red-purple. The small, hard-skinned fruit is brown, spotted, and shiny. Milk thistle is easy to grow, and it matures quickly, in less than a year.

■ WHAT'S IT MADE OF?

Milk thistle products are made from the seeds inside the fruit. The seeds contain 1.5 percent to 3 percent silymarin. Silymarin is actually made up of a group of compounds called flavonolignands. The most important flavonolignan is silybarin (sometimes called silybin). Other flavonolignans in silymarin are isosilybin, dehydrosilybin, silydianin, and silychristin.

■ AVAILABLE FORMS

- Capsules of standardized dried herb (each capsule contains about 120 to 140 mg silymarin)
- Several teas contain the standardized extract.
- Liquid extract
- Tincture

■ HOW TO TAKE IT

Milk thistle protects the liver from harmful chemicals and alcohol. Silymarin is a more powerful antioxidant than vitamin C and vitamin E. Standardized extracts of milk thistle are beneficial for cirrhosis of the liver, chronic hepatitis B, chronic alcoholic liver diseases, and liver damage from toxins.

Silymarin is the most effective antidote to deathcap mushroom poisoning. Milk thistle standardized extract can stop deadly mushroom poisoning if you take it 10 minutes after you ingest deathcap *(Amanita phalloides)* mushrooms. Always get immediate medical attention if you eat poisonous mushrooms or any other toxic substance.

If you have a liver problem, or if you drink much alcohol (or drank too much in the past), your health care provider may recommend milk thistle for you. This herb can also help protect your liver if you take a lot of acetaminophen (nonaspirin pain reliever). Milk thistle is also beneficial if you need to increase your bile flow, and helps reduce the symptoms of psoriasis.

You should always use standardized capsules whenever possible. This is because the silymarin in milk thistle seeds is hard to absorb. Silymarin can get into your system faster if it is concentrated, and it is most concentrated in standardized capsules. Try to avoid alcohol extracts.

The recommended dose of milk thistle is 12 to 15 g dried herb (200 to 400 mg silymarin) per day.

If you are taking milk thistle to protect your liver, you can take 120 mg silymarin (about 2 capsules) two times a day.

If you are taking milk thistle because your liver is damaged (from alcohol, drugs, or chemicals), the recommended dosage is 120 mg (about 3 capsules) three times a day.

There is a new form of milk thistle called silymarin-phosphatidylcholine complex. This is absorbed better than regular standardized milk thistle. In clinical trials, the silymarin-phosphatidylcholine complex worked better than silymarin by itself for treating liver disorders. A key element in cell membranes, phosphatidylcholine helps the silymarin attach easily to the cell membranes. This keeps toxins from getting inside liver cells.

The recommended dosage for silymarin-phosphatidylcholine complex is 100 to 200 mg two times per day.

■ PRECAUTIONS

The U.S. Food and Drug Administration labels milk thistle a dietary supplement so there are no restrictions on using it. Milk thistle is safe when you follow the recommended dosage. Sometimes this herb has a mild laxative effect. If this happens, take some fiber such as guar gum, psyllium, oat bran, or pectin. The fiber should stop loose stools and any stomach discomfort.

■ POSSIBLE INTERACTIONS

You can take milk thistle with other herbs, nutritional supplements, and drugs. You should ask your health care provider how much milk thistle to take if you have a liver disorder or any other serious medical condition.

■ PAU D'ARCO

Brazilian herbalists use pau d'arco to treat ulcers, diabetes, rheumatism, cancer, and ringworm. It's a very popular tea for Candida fungal infections, inflammation, and other infections. And some traditional healers claim that this tea can even help cure cancer. Pau d'arco has become so popular a remedy in the United States that the trees are in danger of becoming extinct.

■ PLANT DESCRIPTION

Pau d'arco is an herbal tea made from the inner bark of *Tabebuia* evergreen trees. These trees grow in the warm parts of Central and South America. Most pau d'arco comes from a tree in the Amazon rain forest called *Tabebuia avellanedae*. It is a broad-leaf evergreen that grows to a height of 125 feet. The wood of this tree is so hard that it doesn't decay easily.

■ WHAT'S IT MADE OF?

Pau d'arco products are made from the inner bark of *Tabebuia* trees. The bark contains important chemical compounds called naphthoquinones. Some naphthoquinones are beneficial for fighting infection and reducing inflammation. But because most pau d'arco products are not standardized, they may or may not have a significant amount of the important active substances.

Some herbal teas that are labeled pau d'arco aren't really made from *Tabebuia* trees. Always read the label to make sure that you're getting authentic pau d'arco. Look for *Tabebuia avellanedae* as an ingredient.

■ AVAILABLE FORMS

Pau d'arco is sold as dried bark tea, alcohol extract, and nonalcohol (usually glycerin) extract. Most of the chemical research on pau d'arco has been done on the wood and not the bark. The heartwood of *Tabebuia avellanedae* contains naphthoquinones. But it's not easy to tell how much naphthoquinones are in pau d'arco products because they're not standardized. So it is best to buy commercial brands that have a good reputation for quality.

■ HOW TO TAKE IT

Pau d'arco seems to be helpful for treating yeast infections. It is beneficial for vaginal candidiasis and oral thrush candidiasis. Pau d'arco also has some antibiotic and antifungal properties, and it sometimes reduces the inflammation of arthritis. Scientists have found that lapachol, the active ingredient in pau d'arco, can block fungal infections and destroy intestinal parasites. It can kill bacteria and viruses that cause infections such as herpes simplex, influenza, and polio.

You can take pau d'arco as an herbal supplement if you have any of these conditions. But if you have a serious health problem, whether it is an infection or cancer, first check with your health care provider.

Recommended dosage:
If you're making a tea from loose bark, boil 1 tsp. of pau d'arco in 1 cup water (8 oz.) for 5 to 15 minutes.
- Drink 1 cup of this tea two to eight times a day.
- If you're using an extract, follow the manufacturer's directions on the label.
- For tinctures (1:5)—solutions made from herb and alcohol, or herb, alcohol, and water—take 1 ml two or three times per day.
- For capsules, take 1,000 mg three times per day.

■ PRECAUTIONS

It is safe to drink pau d'arco tea and take pau d'arco extract at the recommended dosages. If you drink too much, you might become nauseated. If you have problems with blood clots, don't take pau d'arco unless you've talked to your health care provider first.

■ POSSIBLE INTERACTIONS

You can take pau d'arco with other herbs and medications.

■ PEPPERMINT

Peppermint is helpful for many stomach ailments and promotes good digestion. Because it has a calming and numbing effect, it is useful for headaches and skin irritations. It also relieves many symptoms of colds and flu.

■ PLANT DESCRIPTION

Peppermint plants have square stems, and can grow up to two feet tall. They bloom from July through August, sprouting tiny purple flowers in whorls and terminal spikes. Simple, toothed, and fragrant leaves grow opposite the flowers. Peppermint is native to Europe and Asia, and some varieties are indigenous to South Africa, South America, and Australia. It is naturalized in North America and cultivated in Oregon, Washington, and Wisconsin.

■ WHAT'S IT MADE OF?

Peppermint preparations start with the leaves and flowering tops of the plant. These contain a volatile oil, where you find peppermint's primary active component, menthol.

■ AVAILABLE FORMS

Peppermint may be dried from fresh peppermint leaves, and is also widely available as tea.

Tinctures—Peppermint spirit is an alcoholic solution containing 10 percent peppermint oil and 1 percent peppermint leaf extract. To make your own tincture, add 1 part peppermint oil to 9 parts pure grain alcohol.

Enteric-coated capsules, which are specially coated to allow the capsule to pass through the stomach and into the intestine (0.2 ml of peppermint oil per capsule)

Creams or ointments (should contain 1 to 16 percent menthol)

■ HOW TO TAKE IT

Peppermint is helpful for nausea, diarrhea, indigestion, morning sickness, and flatulence. It calms the muscles of the stomach and improves the flow of bile, which the body uses to digest fats. As a result, food passes through the stomach more quickly, which helps many digestive problems. Peppermint also relaxes the muscles that allow the body to rid itself of painful digestive gas. You can make peppermint tea (infusion) with 1 to 2 tsp. of dried leaves per 8 oz. of hot water. To aid digestion or to soothe an upset stomach, drink 3 to 4 cups of peppermint tea daily. For vomiting, take 3 to 6 g of leaf, or 5 to 15 drops of tincture.

This is a partial list of some other conditions that can be improved by peppermint.

- Menstrual cramps—Because peppermint is so effective for relaxing muscles, it is very helpful for painful cramps.
- Irritable bowel syndrome—Research has shown that enteric-coated peppermint capsules are able to calm and soothe intestinal muscles. This provides pain relief and healing for this common stress-related syndrome. Take 1 to 2 coated capsules three times daily between meals.
- Gallstones—Peppermint oil can help the body break down gallstones, providing a safe alternative to surgery. Take 1 to 2 enteric-coated capsules three times daily between meals.
- Viruses—Peppermint oil has strong antiviral properties, which can fight and kill viruses that cause some flus, mumps, yeast infections, sinusitis, sore throats, cold sores, and genital sores caused by herpes.
- Itching and skin irritations—Peppermint has a soothing and cooling effect on skin irritations caused by hives, poison ivy, or poison oak. Apply menthol in a cream or ointment form no more than three to four times daily.
- Tension headaches and migraines—Research has shown that peppermint oil's ability to relax muscles and relieve pain has made it particularly effective against headache pain. Several studies have proved that applying a tincture of peppermint oil to your forehead can be as effective as taking two acetaminophen tablets. Lightly coat the area and allow to evaporate.
- Colds and flu—Peppermint and its main active agent, menthol, are effective decongestants. Because menthol thins mucus, it is also a good expectorant. It is soothing and calming for sore throats and dry coughs as well.

■ PRECAUTIONS

Peppermint tea is generally safe, but pregnant or nursing mothers should drink only small amounts of peppermint tea. Those with a history of miscarriage should not use peppermint while pregnant.

Rare negative reactions to enteric-coated peppermint oil capsules may include skin rash, heartburn, slow heart rate, and muscle tremors.

Menthol or peppermint oil applied to the skin could cause contact dermatitis or rash. Peppermint oil should be diluted and taken in small amounts, since large doses could cause kidney damage. Pure menthol is poisonous and should never be taken internally. Peppermint oil and menthol should not be applied to the faces of infants and small children. Be careful not to confuse oil and tincture preparations.

■ POSSIBLE INTERACTIONS

None known

■ SAW PALMETTO

There are about 40 published studies on saw palmetto berries, which reduce levels of substances that our bodies use to make hormones such as testosterone and estrogen. While we associate testosterone with men and estrogen with women, both men and women have testosterone and estrogen in their bodies, just in different levels.

For men, too much of a substance called dihydrotestosterone (DHT) has been blamed for a disorder called benign prostatic hyperplasia (BPH). Estrogen may also have something to do with it. In BPH, cells in the prostate gland (a tiny gland that lies behind the urethra) grow too quickly. The gland swells and presses on the urethra, so that it feels as if you constantly need to urinate. A common prescription drug for BPH, Proscar, reduces DHT in order to slow or stop BPH.

Recently, researchers concluded that saw palmetto can be as effective as Proscar in relieving certain symptoms of BPH such as urine flow, which is reduced in BPH, and the constant feeling that you have to urinate. One difference between the two therapies, however, is that Proscar can shrink the size of the prostate, and saw palmetto can't. For this reason, if you have chosen to try saw palmetto for your BPH symptoms, it is very important to do so under the guidance of a health care provider, and to keep regular appointments with him or her so that your progress can be monitored.

Saw palmetto berries were not always used for BPH; Native Americans ate them as part of their diet, and they were also used to increase libido.

■ PLANT DESCRIPTION

Saw palmetto is a fan palm that can reach heights of 10 feet in warm climates. In the United States, it grows in the warm climates of the southeast, from South Carolina to Mississippi and throughout Florida. Lush, green leaves fan out from thorny stems. The plant bears white flowers, which develop yellow olive-like berries. The berries, when ripe, turn bluish-black and are dried for medicinal use.

■ WHAT'S IT MADE OF?

Saw palmetto's active ingredients are fatty acids and plant sterols. However, most likely the fatty acids and sterols are not the only part of the berries that affect hormone production, and it will take more scientific study before we know exactly how saw palmetto works.

The berries also contain high-molecular-weight polysaccharides, which are usually associated with either anti-inflammatory or immune-stimulant effects.

■ AVAILABLE FORMS

You can buy saw palmetto as crude dried berries, tea, powdered capsules, tablets, liquid tinctures, and liposterolic extracts. Look for products that say on the labels that they are standardized and contain 85 to 95 percent fatty acids and sterols.

■ HOW TO TAKE IT

Saw palmetto relieves symptoms of Stage I and II BPH. Common symptoms include frequent need to urinate, a delay before you are able to urinate, dripping after urinating, and having to get up numerous times throughout the night to urinate. The majority of men over 60 are considered to have urinary symptoms attributable to BPH, which can disturb sleep, affect self-confidence, cause constant low-grade anxiety or even pain, and may progress to infections in the bladder or kidneys. If you think you have BPH and your health care provider has suggested that you try saw palmetto, try to keep track of how it affects you. It shouldn't take long for you to notice whether it's helping you.

The recommended dosages for Stages I and II BPH is 160 mg, two times a day, of a fat-soluble saw palmetto extract, which has been standardized to contain 85 to 95 percent fatty acids and sterols.

■ PRECAUTIONS

Saw palmetto is a very mild herb. Side effects are very rare and mild stomach complaints are the only recorded reactions. The American Herbal Products Association gives saw palmetto a class 1 safety rating, which means that it is safe when used as directed.

You should not try to self-diagnose, or self-medicate, BPH. Saw palmetto only relieves the symptoms of BPH, despite the fact that it alters DHT production and testosterone levels. It will not shrink the prostate. Your health care provider should monitor the course of BPH.

Saw palmetto should not be used during pregnancy or breast-feeding.

■ POSSIBLE INTERACTIONS

Saw palmetto may change the effects of contraceptive pills and patches and hormone replacement therapy because it can affect hormone levels.

■ ST. JOHN'S WORT

St. John's wort once was thought to rid the body of evil spirits, but more recently it has been used to treat problems such as depression, anxiety, and sleeplessness. When steeped in oil and applied to the skin, it helps heal wounds and burns. Research suggests it may also be useful in treating infections caused by viruses.

Here are some illnesses and conditions that St. John's wort has been used to treat:

- *Depression. St. John's wort reduces symptoms of depression in people with mild to moderate forms of the condition.*
- *Seasonal affective disorder. Used alone, St. John's wort improves mood. Effects are even greater when the herb is used in combination with light therapy.*
- *Other mood problems. St. John's wort helps reduce anxiety, listlessness, and feelings of worthlessness.*
- *Sleep problems. The herb relieves sleeplessness (insomnia) and the tendency to sleep too long (hypersomnia).*
- *HIV infection and AIDS. Research and patients' experiences suggest St. John's wort may improve the health of people infected with human immunodeficiency virus (HIV), the virus that causes AIDS.*
- *Wounds and burns. In forms that can be applied to the skin, St. John's wort reduces pain and inflammation and promotes healing.*
- *Hemorrhoids. "Red oil," a preparation made by steeping St. John's wort flowers in oil, eases discomfort when applied to hemorrhoids.*

■ PLANT DESCRIPTION

St. John's wort is a shrubby plant with clusters of yellow flowers. The plant is often in full bloom around June 24, the day traditionally celebrated as the birthday of John the Baptist. Both the flowers and leaves are used as medicine.

■ WHAT'S IT MADE OF?

The best-studied active components are hypericin and pseudohypericin, found in both the leaves and flowers. There has been recent research to suggest that these best-studied components may not be the most active in the plant, with significant debate ensuing within the industry. It also includes other components such as essential oils and flavonoids.

■ AVAILABLE FORMS

You can buy St. John's wort in many forms: capsules, liquids, oil-based skin lotions, and teas. You can also buy chopped or powdered forms of the dried herb. Look for products that are standardized to contain 0.3% hypericin.

■ HOW TO TAKE IT

When taken by mouth for depression and other mood problems, the usual dose is 300 to 500 mg at 0.3 percent, three times a day, with meals, for a minimum of four to six weeks. You can also make a tea by steeping 1 to 2 tsp. of dried St. John's wort in a cup of boiling water for 10 minutes. Drink 1 to 2 cups a day for four to six weeks. But keep in mind that the dose you get when you make St. John's wort tea may not be as consistent as what you get in capsules or other products.

For treating wounds, burns or hemorrhoids, use an oil-based preparation of St. John's wort that you can rub onto your skin.

■ PRECAUTIONS

- Depression is a serious condition. If your depression is severe or if you feel like hurting yourself or someone else, see a health care professional before using St. John's wort. There are some conditions that you should not try to treat yourself with herbs or other over-the-counter medicines. A health care professional can help you decide whether St. John's wort is right for you.
- Do not take St. John's wort if you are pregnant or breast-feeding.
- St. John's wort may make your skin unusually sensitive to sunlight. Although this reaction is rare, you should be careful about sun exposure if you have fair skin or if you are taking St. John's wort in large doses or over a long time. Use a sunscreen with a skin protection factor (SPF) of at least 15, and do not use sunlamps, tanning booths or tanning beds.

Side effects of St. John's wort are usually mild and may include:
- Abdominal pain, bloating, constipation
- Nausea, vomiting
- Dizziness
- Dry mouth
- Itching, hives, skin rash
- Sleep problems
- Elevated blood pressure
- Unusual tiredness

■ POSSIBLE INTERACTIONS

St. John's wort is thought to work something like the antidepressants known as monoamine oxidase (MAO) inhibitors. If you are taking a MAO inhibitor, such as Nardil or Parnate, check with your health care provider before using St. John's wort.

Check with your health care provider if you are using a selective serotonin reuptake inhibitor (SSRI), such as Prozac, Paxil, or Zoloft, or any other antidepressant medicine.

If you are taking L-dopa or 5-hydroxytryptophan, check with your health care provider before taking St. John's wort.

Always be careful about taking more than one herb or any combination of drugs and herbs. Check with your provider or pharmacist to make sure the combination is safe.

■ STINGING NETTLE

During medieval times, diuretics and remedies for joint problems were made from stinging nettle. Native American healers used to strike the arms or legs of paralyzed patients with branches of stinging nettle to activate the muscles. This whipping technique, also called flagellation, can also stimulate the organs and relieve the pain of sore muscles and other parts of the body. Stinging nettle has been used in this way for centuries.

The stinging hairs on nettle are like tiny glands that have inside them chemicals that irritate the skin. The hairs are very painful to the touch, but if they irritate an area of the body that is already in pain, the chemicals can actually decrease the original pain. This is why stinging nettle is called a counterirritant. If you get stung with nettle, you can actually relieve the painful nettle stings by applying nettle juice to your skin.

Stinging nettle has been used for hundreds of years to treat rheumatism, eczema, arthritis, gout, and anemia. Today many people use it to treat urinary problems during the early stages of enlarged prostate (benign prostatic hyperplasia, or BPH).

■ PLANT DESCRIPTION

Stinging nettle is the name given to common nettle, garden nettle, and hybrids of these two plants. Originally from the colder northern regions of Europe and Asia, today this herbaceous shrub grows all over the world. Stinging nettle grows well in nitrogen-rich soil, blooms between June and September, and reaches nearly 3 feet high.

The branching stems underground multiply by themselves and have multiple shoots. The leaves are heart-shaped, finely toothed, and tapered at the ends. The entire plant is covered with tiny stinging hairs, mostly on the leaves and stem.

■ WHAT'S IT MADE OF?

Stinging nettle products are usually made from the roots or leaves. In some cases, all the plant parts that grow above the ground are used in herbal preparations. Leaf remedies are useful in treating kidney and urinary tract conditions. The flavonoids and potassium in nettle leaves are most likely responsible for their diuretic action.

Root preparations are used to treat enlarged prostate. They can help reduce some symptoms of BPH (benign prostatic hyperplasia), but they do not make the prostate grow smaller.

■ AVAILABLE FORMS

Stinging nettle is available as dried leaf and as root tincture (a tincture is a solution of the herb in alcohol).

■ HOW TO TAKE IT

You can take nettle herb and leaf remedies to treat lower urinary tract inflammation and to prevent and treat kidney stones. Nettle works as a diuretic if you take enough water with it. If you have difficult urination from an enlarged prostate, nettle root preparation may be helpful.

For lower urinary tract inflammation and kidney stones, take 8 to 12 g leaf tea and ample liquid (at least 2 liters a day). For enlarged prostate, use root tincture (1:10), 4 to 6 g per day. Talk with your health care provider before taking nettle root for BPH.

■ PRECAUTIONS

Stinging nettle is safe when used as directed. But always be careful if you are handling the nettle plant. If your skin touches it, you can get contact urticaria (hives), which will make your skin sting. If you are taking nettle root, you may have some mild side effects, such as mild gastrointestinal irritation, excess fluid, or decreased urine flow.

If you're pregnant, do not take any nettle product. Don't use nettle if you are nursing. Nettle can also alter the menstrual cycle. Always check with your health care provider if you have questions or concerns.

■ POSSIBLE INTERACTIONS

Don't take large amounts of stinging nettle if you're taking central nervous system-depressant medication, or drugs for diabetes, high blood sugar, or low blood sugar.

For additional information supporting this handout, please refer to our website: www.onemedicine.com/public/products/access

139

■ VALERIAN

Valerian eases insomnia, stress-related anxiety, and nervous restlessness. It may also ease menstrual and stomach cramps, and some types of headache. Its main use, however, is to help people sleep.

Doctors, researchers, and herbalists recommend valerian for the treatment of sleep problems because it is both safe and gentle. Unlike sleeping aids you may have already tried, valerian will not cause you to feel tired when you wake up, and it has few, if any, side effects.

■ PLANT DESCRIPTION

Valerian products are made from the root of a tall, wispy plant, which is grown to decorate gardens but also grows wild in damp grasslands. Its umbrella-like heads top grooved, erect, and hollow stems. Its dark green leaves are pointed at the tip and hairy underneath. Small, sweet-smelling white, light purple, or pink flowers bloom in June. The root is light grayish brown and smells like dirty socks.

■ WHAT'S IT MADE OF?

The manufacture of medicinal valerian products begins with pressed fresh root or powdered freeze-dried root (frozen below 400°C). Valerian pressed-root juice added to alcohol or glycerite (sweet, nonalcohol liquid) bases become fluid extracts or tinctures; powdered root goes into capsules and tablets. While we don't know all the plant chemicals that cause valerian's activity, valerenic acid and bornyl in its plant essential oils have important roles.

■ AVAILABLE FORMS

Valerian fluid extracts and tinctures are sold in alcohol or alcohol-free (glycerite) bases. Powdered valerian capsules or tablets are also available, and you can also find valerian tea.

Valerian products are commonly added to formulas that contain other calming herbs, such as passionflower *(Passiflora incarnata),* hops *(Humulus lupulus),* lemon balm *(Melissa officinalis),* and, more recently, kava *(Piper methysticum).* If you are new to herbal therapy, it's a good idea to use valerian without any other herbs. If your provider has recommended valerian to you, it is most likely because he or she feels valerian is the most specific remedy for your condition.

■ HOW TO TAKE IT

When you buy valerian, look for labels that say the product is standardized to contain 0.8 percent valerenic, or valeric, acid. Standardization is the only way to guarantee any level of quality control in an herbal product.

To reduce nervousness, anxiety, or headache or menstrual pain, you may use any of the following. Dosages repeated three times a day will also help you sleep better.

- 2 to 3 g dried root in tea, up to several times daily
- $\frac{1}{4}$ to $\frac{1}{2}$ tsp. (1 to 3 ml) tincture up to several times daily
- $\frac{1}{4}$ tsp. (1 to 2 ml) fluid extract (1:1)
- 150 to 300 mg valerian extract, dried or liquid, standardized to contain 0.8 percent valerenic acid, 1 percent to 1.5 percent valtrate

To get to sleep quicker, take one of the dosages at least 30 to 45 minutes before bedtime. If your insomnia has been long-term, it may take two weeks before you notice an effect. When you notice a change, continue to take valerian for two to four more weeks. A total of four to six weeks is usually the length of treatment advised by herbalists.

After six weeks, take a two-week break to see how you sleep without valerian. If you still have difficulty sleeping, start another four-to-six week course of treatment, or talk with your health care provider about other herbal medicines that may be helpful.

■ PRECAUTIONS

The American Herbal Products Association (AHPA) gives valerian a class 1 safety rating, which indicates that it is a very safe herb with a wide dosage range. Even so, it is always wise to follow the recommended dosage exactly.

If you are pregnant, you should consult with your physician before taking any medication, including herbs.

Some people have a "paradoxical reaction" to valerian. This means that instead of feeling calm or sleepy, they suddenly feel nervous and anxious after they take valerian. If this happens to you, stop taking valerian, and tell your health care provider. This reaction is rare and not life-threatening.

■ POSSIBLE INTERACTIONS

Valerian is a sedative herb and may increase the effects of other anti-anxiety medications or prescription painkillers. It may also interact with antiepileptic drugs in a way that could harm people with epilepsy. Make sure you do not take valerian with any of these kinds of pharmaceuticals. If you are not sure whether a medication you're taking might interact with valerian or any herb, consult your health care provider. And while valerian does not seem to increase the effects of alcohol in the same way that some prescription drugs do, it is not a good idea to consume alcohol while taking valerian.

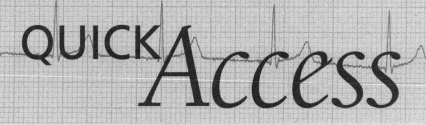

SUPPLEMENTS

5-Hydroxytryptophan (5-HTP)
Alpha-Linolenic Acid (ALA)
Alpha-Lipoic Acid
Brewer's Yeast
Bromelain
Calcium
Cartilage
Chromium
Copper
Creatine
Dehydroepiandrosterone (DHEA)
Ethylenediaminetetraacetic Acid (EDTA)
Flaxseed Oil
Gamma-Linolenic Acid (GLA)
Glutamine
Iron
Lipase
Lysine
Magnesium
Manganese
Melatonin
Phenylalanine
Phosphorus
Potassium
Psyllium
Selenium
Spirulina
Sulfur
Tyrosine
Vanadium
Vitamin A (Retinol)
Vitamin B_1 (Thiamine)
Vitamin B_2 (Riboflavin)
Vitamin B_3 (Niacin)
Vitamin B_5 (Pantothenic Acid)
Vitamin B_6 (Pyridoxine)
Vitamin B_9 (Folic Acid)
Vitamin B_{12} (Cobalamin)
Vitamin C (Ascorbic Acid)
Vitamin D
Vitamin E
Vitamin H (Biotin)
Vitamin K
Zinc

■ 5-HYDROXYTRYPTOPHAN

5-hydroxytryptophan (5-HTP) is an amino acid. The body makes 5-HTP from tryptophan (an essential amino acid) and converts it to serotonin, an important neurotransmitter (brain chemical). 5-HTP dietary supplements help raise serotonin levels in the brain, which may have a positive effect on the following functions and processes: sleep, mood, anxiety, aggression, appetite, temperature, sexual behavior, and pain sensation.

■ USES

5-HTP may be helpful in treating a wide variety of conditions related to low serotonin levels, such as the following.

Depression. Scientists believe that some forms of depression are caused by low levels of serotonin in the brain. Therefore, many of the anti-depressant drugs prescribed for depression increase serotonin levels. 5-HTP is as effective as some antidepressant drugs in treating some individuals with mild to moderate depression, and people treated with 5-HTP have shown improvements in mood, anxiety, insomnia, and physical symptoms.

Fibromyalgia. This is a disorder that causes achy and stiff muscles, tender joints, and ongoing pain at various sites in the body. Although many factors can affect the severity of the disorder, the primary cause of the pain of fibromyalgia is low serotonin levels. 5-HTP has been shown to increase pain tolerance, improve sleep quality, and reduce anxiety and depression in patients with fibromyalgia.

Insomnia. 5-HTP has been shown to reduce the time required to fall asleep and to improve sleep quality.

Migraine. 5-HTP reduces the frequency and severity of migraine headaches with fewer side effects than migraine headache drugs.

Obesity. 5-HTP can decrease carbohydrate intake by promoting a feeling of satiety (fullness), and may result in weight loss in overweight individuals.

Headaches in children. Children with headaches associated with sleep disorders can respond favorably to 5-HTP treatment.

■ DIETARY SOURCES

5-HTP is extracted from the seed of the African plant *Griffonia simplicifolia*. It is purified, and concentrated in dietary supplements.

■ OTHER FORMS

5-HTP is an ingredient in multivitamin and herbal preparations. It is also available as a single ingredient in tablets and capsules. You will find it in doses that include 25 mg, 50 mg, and 100 mg capsules and tablets.

■ HOW TO TAKE IT

Follow the directions indicated on product packages. Some experts recommend taking 50 to 100 mg of 5-HTP per day for most conditions. Higher doses of 5-HTP are necessary to produce beneficial results in certain conditions. Seek the advice of your health care provider before taking more than 100 mg of 5-HTP per day.

■ PRECAUTIONS

5-HTP causes mild gastrointestinal disturbances in some people. These side effects include mild nausea, heartburn, flatulence, feelings of fullness, and rumbling sensations.

Check with your health care provider before taking 5-HTP if any of the following applies to you.
- You have high blood pressure.
- You are pregnant or nursing.
- You have diabetes.
- You are taking antidepressant drugs, such as monoamine oxidase inhibitors (MAOIs) or selective serotonin reuptake inhibitors (SSRIs), or any other prescription medications.

Seek the advice of your health care provider before giving 5-HTP to children or adolescents.

■ POSSIBLE INTERACTIONS

5-HTP may add to the effects of St. John's wort.

Vitamin B_6, niacin, and magnesium help convert 5-HTP to serotonin.

■ ALPHA-LINOLENIC ACID (ALA)

Alpha-linolenic acid (ALA) is an essential fatty acid that comes from plants. It is considered an essential nutrient, which means that your body requires it.

ALA is used as a source of energy by the body. It also serves as the parent substance to omega-3 fatty acids, compounds that regulate blood pressure, blood clotting, heart rate, blood vessel dilation, the immune response, and breakdown of fats. Essential fatty acids are also used to make brain and nervous tissue. Only certain plant products provide ALA. Primarily, they are canola (rapeseed), flaxseed (linseed), and soybean oil. Some fish (for example, mackerel and salmon) contain omega-3 fatty acids. Corn, safflower, cottonseed, sesame, and sunflower oils are rich in fats called omega-6 fatty acids. These two families of fats have very important, but different, roles in the body. It is important to have a balance of omega-6 and omega-3 fatty acids in the diet. Excessive intake of either type of fat can cause health problems.

American diets are typically high in omega-6 fatty acids and low in omega-3 fatty acids. Americans' high consumption of omega-6 oils (corn, safflower, sunflower oils), low intake of fish, and focus on decreasing overall fat in the diet are the primary reasons for inadequate or imbalanced levels of omega-3 fatty acids in the diet. Taking in more omega-6 than omega-3 fatty acids may encourage your body to produce substances that cause inflammation and negatively affect your body's response to disease. These imbalances may make you more susceptible to heart disease, inflammatory conditions such as arthritis and psoriasis, and infections, and can lower your immunity. You may gain significant health benefits by increasing the level of omega-3 fatty acids in your diet. This is especially true if you take in large amounts of omega-6 fatty acids.

■ USES

Omega-3 fatty acids have several proven benefits. They are especially good for your heart, they can provide relief from rheumatoid arthritis, they may be helpful in treating multiple sclerosis and some cases of diabetes, and they may help prevent cancer. Recently, omega-3 fatty acids were shown to help treat migraines and depression. ALA may be useful in treating skin cancer.

ALA and other omega-3 oils are used to help treat the following.
- Heart disease: ALA may reduce the risk of heart disease by improving the arteries that carry blood throughout the body and to the brain, and by lowering cholesterol and triglyceride levels.
- Hypertension (high blood pressure)
- Allergic and inflammatory conditions such as psoriasis and eczema
- Autoimmune diseases, such as multiple sclerosis, lupus, and cancer

■ DIETARY SOURCES

The following foods are good sources of ALA: flax seeds, flaxseed oil, canola (rapeseed) oil, soybean oil, margarine, if made from canola or soybean oil, pumpkin, and walnuts.

■ OTHER FORMS

There are two types of commercial preparations. Cooking oils (canola oil, soybean oil, margarines made from these oils), and medicinal oils (flaxseed oil, gelatin capsules of flaxseed oil).

Several manufacturing methods can destroy the nutrient value of products that contain ALA. Preferred methods are "modified atmospheric packing methods." Generally, high-quality oil will be certified as organic by a reputable company, bottled in light-resistant containers, refrigerated, and marked with an expiration date.

■ HOW TO TAKE IT

There is no recommended dietary allowance (RDA) for ALA.

A healthy diet should include less saturated fats and more polyunsaturated essential fatty acids. Discuss your total fat intake with your health care provider if you are thinking about taking ALA supplements.

■ PRECAUTIONS

You should talk with your health care provider about your regular diet. Your health care provider can help you decide if you should take supplements, and what kind of supplements may be best for you. Remember that ALA supplements are fats, and are high in calories. Avoid products containing hydrogenated fats.

■ POSSIBLE INTERACTIONS

Flaxseed oil, a source of ALA, may increase your body's need for vitamin E. For more information, talk with your health care provider.

■ ALPHA-LIPOIC ACID

Alpha-lipoic acid is an antioxidant, which is a powerful substance that may help slow the aging process and fight disease. More commonly known antioxidants are vitamins A, C, and E. Antioxidants work by attacking "free radicals," waste products created when our bodies turn food into energy. Free radicals cause harmful chemical reactions that can damage cells, making it harder to fight off infections and lowering defenses against cancer and heart disease. In fact, free radical damage may be the basis for the aging process.

Antioxidants work by attaching to free radicals and neutralizing them. Free radicals are useful in small amounts, but when there are too many of them in our bodies, they can cause problems. Today there are more and more sources of free radicals in our environment—for example, ultraviolet rays, radiation, and toxic chemicals in cigarette smoke, car exhaust, and pesticides.

■ USES

Alpha-lipoic acid (also called thioctic acid) works together with other antioxidants such as vitamins C and E. It is important for growth, helps the body produce energy, and aids the liver in removing harmful substances from the body. Alpha-lipoic acid (ALA) also prevents cell damage, controls blood sugar, and removes toxic metals from the blood. In animal studies, alpha-lipoic acid improved brain function as well. Because it is both water- and fat-soluble, ALA can function in almost any part of the body, including the brain.

Alpha-lipoic acid has been used to treat chronic hepatitis because it relieves stress on the liver and helps it rid the body of toxins. It is the standard treatment for Amanita poisoning (Amanita is a highly poisonous mushroom). Alpha-lipoic acid can help lessen the toxic effects of drugs used during surgery and for pain control afterwards. A recommended dose for this purpose is two 100-mg capsules three times daily, with meals, one week before surgery and for two weeks after the operation.

Unlike other substances, alpha-lipoic acid can pass easily into the brain, and studies have shown that ALA has protective effects on brain and nerve tissue. ALA is promising as a treatment for stroke and other brain disorders involving free-radical damage. Animals treated with alpha-lipoic acid had a four times greater survival rate after a stroke.

In more than one study, treatment with ALA helped reduce pain, burning, itching, tingling, and numbness in people who had nerve damage caused by diabetes. Other studies have shown that alpha-lipoic acid speeds the removal of glucose (sugar) from the blood of people with diabetes, and leads to improved heart function.

■ DIETARY SOURCES

Good food sources of alpha-lipoic acid include spinach, broccoli, beef, yeast, kidney, and heart.

■ OTHER FORMS

Alpha-lipoic acid is available in capsule form.

■ HOW TO TAKE IT

Alpha-lipoic acid is made by the body and is available in foods. It can be purchased in various dosages—from 30-mg to 100-mg tablets. Currently there are no established recommended doses. ALA manufacturers suggest one or two 50-mg capsules daily as a dietary supplement.

■ PRECAUTIONS

People with diabetes should consult with their health care provider before taking alpha-lipoic acid because it has been associated with hypoglycemia (low blood sugar). If you are pregnant or nursing, consult your health care provider before taking any supplement.

■ POSSIBLE INTERACTIONS

Alpha-lipoic acid improves the antioxidant function of vitamins C and E, and glutathione, which also is produced by the body.

■ BREWER'S YEAST

Brewer's yeast, which is often called nutritional yeast, was originally a by-product of the brewing of beer. While still used for brewing, it is also now grown as a plant product for its nutritional value. Nutritional yeast is not exactly the same as brewer's yeast. Brewer's yeast was originally used as a nutritional supplement, then other yeasts were made available for this purpose. Brewer's yeast differs from live baker's yeast in that its live yeast cells have been destroyed, leaving the nutrients behind. Live yeast cells can actually deplete the body of B vitamins and other nutrients.

Nutritional yeast contains high levels of many important nutrients, including all of the B vitamins (except for B_{12}), 16 out of 20 amino acids, and 14 different minerals. The amino acids (proteins) in yeast help the body repair tissue and fight disease. Brewer's yeast has a very high protein content, with one tbsp. providing 4.6 g, making it a rich source of protein for vegetarians. It is also high in phosphorus.

■ USES

Because yeast is such a rich source of B vitamins, it enhances the roles these vitamins play in the body. The B-complex vitamins help your body metabolize carbohydrates, fats, and proteins. They also support the nervous system and help maintain the muscles used for digestion.

Different B vitamins play different roles, particularly in their support of the nervous system. They relieve stress, depression, irritability, and fatigue, and also help reduce some effects of aging. When under the pressures of stress or infection, the body needs greater supplies of B vitamins. The body does not store excess B vitamins, so they must be regularly consumed. B vitamins can also help relieve morning sickness.

Biotin, one of the B vitamins that brewer's yeast supplies, has been shown to strengthen brittle nails and improve the health of hair. It also is used to treat infant cradle cap. Biotin helps people with diabetes use insulin more efficiently and is useful for treating diabetic neuropathy.

Brewer's yeast is also an important source of chromium. The U.S. FDA recommends 120 mcg of chromium daily, but 90 percent of Americans are deficient in this important mineral. Chromium has the ability to significantly lower blood cholesterol levels.

Chromium is also an important supplement for those with type 2 (adult onset) diabetes because it can significantly lower blood sugar levels. Without chromium, insulin is not able to work properly and blood sugar levels rise. Researchers have been able to lower some diabetic glucose levels to almost normal levels with daily chromium doses of 1,000 mcg.

Several studies have tested the use of chromium for the treatment of acne, with good results. Chromium's ability to increase the effectiveness of insulin's activity in the body has also led to its consideration as an aid to weight loss. Chromium can be difficult for the body to absorb, but is more easily absorbed when taken with brewer's yeast.

As a source of chromium, brewer's yeast can reduce blood sugar levels in people with type 2 diabetes, lower blood cholesterol levels, help with weight loss, and aid in the treatment of acne.

As a source of B vitamins, brewer's yeast can relieve stress, depression, irritability, and fatigue.

As a source of biotin, brewer's yeast can strengthen hair and nails, and treat cradle cap and diabetes.

■ DIETARY SOURCES

N/A

■ OTHER FORMS

Brewer's yeast comes in flake, powder, tablet, and liquid form.

■ HOW TO TAKE IT

You can dissolve brewer's yeast in juice or water. Four tbsp. per day are recommended. If your diet is low in B vitamins, this amount may cause gas, so it's best to begin with 1 tsp. in a glass of juice and work slowly up to 4 tbsp.

■ PRECAUTIONS

There are no known side effects. However, you should avoid yeast products if you have frequent yeast infections. People who have osteoporosis should avoid yeast because of its high levels of phosphorus. If you take a yeast supplement, also take extra calcium.

■ POSSIBLE INTERACTIONS

None noted

■ BROMELAIN

Bromelain is a digestive enzyme found in the stem and fruit of the pineapple plant (Ananas comosus). It is best known as a digestive aid and for its anti-inflammatory effects in traumatic injuries and after surgery. Bromelain has also been used successfully to treat a number of disorders, including heart disease, arthritis, upper respiratory tract infection, and Peyronie's disease (a condition that affects the genito-urinary tract and can cause sexual dysfunction in men). Bromelain has also been used successfully to heal wounds caused by burns and to increase the actions of antibiotics and chemotherapy drugs.

■ USES

- Reduces pain, bruising, and swelling from trauma (for example, sports injuries) or surgery and speeds the healing process
- Relieves the symptoms of gastrointestinal upset, aids in the healing of gastric ulcers, and is used as a digestive enzyme for pancreatic insufficiency
- Relieves the symptoms of angina, and because it inhibits clot formation and breaks down build-up of plaque in arteries, it is useful for thrombosis, thrombophlebitis, varicose veins, and atherosclerosis.
- Reduces joint inflammation in rheumatoid arthritis, osteoarthritis, sciatica, bursitis, tendinitis, and scleroderma
- Increases the actions of chemotherapy drugs and antibiotics
- Is useful in AIDS treatment as an antiviral agent
- Suppresses cough and decreases bronchial secretions, resulting in increased lung function in patients with upper respiratory tract infections. It is also effective in patients with sinusitis.
- Can prevent the thickening of the fibrous connective tissue in the penis associated with Peyronie's disease
- Used for healing burns
- Several studies suggest use as antimetastatic agent with chemotherapy.

■ DIETARY SOURCES

Bromelain is one of the simple digestive enzymes extracted from tropical fruit, in this case pineapple.

■ OTHER FORMS

Bromelain is available in tablet (500 mg) or capsule form for oral use.

■ HOW TO TAKE IT

For use as a digestive aid, 500 mg with meals is the recommended dosage. For other uses, the following dosages are recommended.

- Traumatic injuries—500 mg four times a day on an empty stomach
- Cardiovascular disease—500 to 750 mg three times a day on an empty stomach
- Joint inflammation—500 to 2,000 mg a day in two doses
- Antitumor activity—1,000 mg a day

For all other uses, consult your health care provider. You should take bromelain for only 8 to 10 days, but it may be tolerated for longer periods.

■ PRECAUTIONS

Bromelain may cause nausea, vomiting, diarrhea, and excessive menstrual bleeding, but no serious side effects have been reported in humans; however, allergic reactions, including skin reactions and asthma, may occur if you are allergic to pineapples. Experiments in animals have not shown bromelain to cause cancer or birth defects, but there have not been any studies concerning use of bromelain in pregnancy. Check with your health care provider if you have a blood-clotting disorder, liver or kidney disease, or hypertension.

■ POSSIBLE INTERACTIONS

Bromelain can increase your risk of bleeding if you take bromelain along with anticoagulants (blood-thinning agents). If you are taking antibiotics, such as tetracycline, bromelain can increase its effects. A rapid heart rate may result if you have high blood pressure.

■ CALCIUM

Calcium is a mineral important for strong bones and teeth. It also helps your heart, nerves, muscles, and other body systems work properly. Milk and dairy products, such as cheese and yogurt, give you most of the calcium you get from food, but you can also get it from nuts, green leafy vegetables, and calcium-enhanced orange juice. Vitamins A, C, D, and E help you use the calcium you get from food. Stress and lack of exercise can harm your calcium balance. Most people in the United States, especially women, do not get enough calcium in their diet.

■ USES

Getting enough calcium can help your body do the following.

- Develop strong bones and teeth
- Prevent osteoporosis and broken bones
- Reduce your blood pressure
- Lower your cholesterol levels
- Keep your heart regular
- Reduce cramps and moodiness from premenstrual syndrome
- Reduce irritability, insomnia, depression, and headaches during menopause
- Reduce risks of pregnancy, such as high blood pressure and preeclampsia
- Prevent gum disease
- Prevent cancer of the colon and rectum
- Prevent kidney stones

■ DIETARY SOURCES

The richest sources of calcium include cheeses (Parmesan, Romano, Gruyère, Swiss, Provolone, Monterey Jack, Edam, Cheddar, Muenster, Gouda, Tilsit, Colby, Caraway, Brick, Roquefort, Port du Salut, Cheshire, Havarti, Fontina, Mozzarella, Feta); wheat-soy flour; blackstrap molasses; and rennin.

Other good sources of calcium include almonds, bok choy, brazil nuts, broccoli, cabbage, caviar, dried figs, greens (dandelion, turnip, collard, mustard, kale), hazelnuts, ice cream, milk, oysters, sardines, soybean flour, and yogurt.

You can also get calcium from many herbs, spices, and seaweeds (for example, basil, chervil, cinnamon, dill weed, fennel, fenugreek, ginseng, kava kava, kelp, marjoram, oregano, parsley, poppy seed, sage, and savory).

■ OTHER FORMS

Calcium is available in many forms. Lead has been found in some types, so use caution when choosing a product. Lead is a toxic metal that can harm the brain and kidneys, and can reduce red blood cell production. Children are most at risk for lead poisoning. The following are some of the available forms of calcium.

- Calcium citrate. This is the most easily used form of calcium, and the most easily digested. Lead levels are safe. It is especially recommended for elderly persons, people taking ulcer medication, and people who want to lower their blood pressure.
- Calcium carbonate. This type is less expensive, and lead levels are safe if it is refined. Rolaids and Tums contain calcium carbonate. Other antacids contain aluminum and can harm your calcium balance.
- Calcium gluconate. This type is safe.
- Calcium lactate. This is another safe form.
- Calcium chloride. This is not recommended because it irritates the gastrointestinal tract.

You should be cautious with products that may contain harmful levels of lead. These include unrefined calcium carbonate from oyster shells or limestone, bone meal, and Dolomite.

■ HOW TO TAKE IT

You should take small doses throughout the day, and drink 6 to 8 cups of water throughout the day to avoid constipation.

- Adults ages 19 to 50 need 1,000 mg of calcium each day. After age 50, adults need 1,200 mg each day.
- Adolescents ages 9 to 18 need 1,300 mg each day.
- Children ages 6 to 8 need 800 mg each day; children ages 1 to 5 need 500 mg each day.

■ PRECAUTIONS

Do not take extremely large doses of calcium (5,000 mg per day, or 2,000 mg per day or more over a long period) without talking with your health care provider. High doses can cause kidney stones and other serious problems.

Avoid calcium products that contain harmful levels of lead (see above).

Talk with your provider about your calcium needs if you have any thyroid or kidney problems, or if you have hormone or vitamin deficiencies.

■ POSSIBLE INTERACTIONS

Some foods, drinks, and medications can cause you to lose calcium. These include sodium (salt), phosphorus (some soft drinks), aluminum-containing antacids, sugar, saturated fat, caffeine, alcohol, high protein intake from supplements or special diets (however, some protein is good for maintaining your calcium reserves), and fiber.

Some foods, drinks, and medicines make it hard for your body to get the calcium it needs. These include alcohol, aspirin, barbiturates, fiber, neomycin, strong sedatives, oxalic acid (found in chocolate, rhubarb, spinach, chard, sweet potatoes, dried beans), phytic acid (grains), and uronic acid (a type of fiber in fruits and vegetables).

Extra calcium can interfere with your body's use of other important minerals, such as iron, zinc, magnesium, iodine, manganese, and copper.

For additional information supporting this handout, please refer to our website: www.onemedicine.com/public/products/access

147

CARTILAGE

Cartilage is elastic, translucent connective tissue in people and animals. Most cartilage turns into bone as animals mature, but some remains in its original form in places such as the nose, ears, knees, and other joints. Two kinds of cartilage are used as nutritional supplements. Bovine cartilage (also called cow cartilage) comes from cattle, and shark cartilage comes from sharks. (Interestingly, sharks do not have any bones in their bodies, only cartilage.) Cartilage supplements started to be used to treat cancerous tumors when researchers observed that a protein in shark cartilage stopped the growth of new blood vessels. Since tumors get their nourishment from blood, they need to make new networks of blood vessels in order to grow. If shark cartilage could stop the blood vessels from being developed, researchers reasoned, then the cancer couldn't grow and might even shrink. However, studies to prove that the process works in humans have not yet been published. Bovine cartilage has been shown to speed up wound healing and reduce inflammation.

USES

Here is a partial list of the health problems cartilage helps to relieve.

- Cancer (including melanoma, lung cancers, and prostate, breast, and other cancers)
- Macular degeneration, a disease in which too many blood vessels grow in the eye or grow in the wrong places, eventually resulting in blindness
- Psoriasis, a skin disease that is also worsened by overgrowth of blood vessels
- Bone diseases, such as osteoporosis
- Rheumatoid arthritis
- Osteoarthritis
- Inflammation and pain, especially in joints
- Intestinal inflammation

DIETARY SOURCES

Not available; use commercially prepared cartilage for safety.

OTHER FORMS

Cartilage is sold in powdered form or in capsules that contain the powder.

New anticancer drugs are being developed to take advantage of the effective elements in cartilage supplements.

HOW TO TAKE IT

When using shark or bovine cartilage as a dietary supplement, 3 to 4,750 mg capsules per day.

When using shark or bovine cartilage to treat cancer, the normal supplement dose may increase by 3 fold, by mouth before meals. If the unpleasant taste causes nausea or stomach upset, you can take the same amount by enema.

PRECAUTIONS

- Whether you're using shark or bovine cartilage, buy from reputable manufacturers.
- Check labels carefully and choose only supplements that contain 100 percent pure shark cartilage.
- Check the color of the cartilage supplements before you take them. Any color other than white means the product is not pure and you should not consume it.
- Never give cartilage supplements to children.
- Pregnant women should not take cartilage.
- People who recently had surgery or recently survived a heart attack should not take cartilage supplements.

Cartilage can be used in addition to conventional treatments for cancer and arthritis, but it should not be a substitute for conventional treatments. Check with your health care provider, and if you're taking cartilage on your own, be sure to let your health care provider know what type and how much you're taking.

Cartilage supplements are expensive. Bovine cartilage costs about $160 for a month's supply, while shark cartilage is about $700 for a month's supply.

POSSIBLE INTERACTIONS

Cartilage is not known to interfere with other remedies or medicines.

People who take a large quantity of shark cartilage, which contains calcium, may need to take magnesium and potassium to help maintain the correct mineral balance in their bodies.

For more information about cartilage, consult your health care provider.

■ CHROMIUM

Chromium is an essential trace element for humans. In order for the body to use chromium, it must be converted to an active form. Glucose tolerance factor (GTF) is an active form of chromium that has been isolated from brewer's yeast. GTF chromium helps insulin pull glucose (blood sugar) from the bloodstream into the cells for energy. Insulin is very important for carbohydrate, protein, and fat metabolism. Not getting enough chromium in your diet can affect insulin's ability to process these nutrients.

It is estimated that as many as 90 percent of all Americans' diets are low in chromium. Eating a lot of highly processed foods may contribute to this problem because foods lose chromium during the refining process. Children with protein-calorie malnutrition, people who have diabetes, and older people may be especially at risk for chromium deficiency. Eating too many sugary foods, exercising strenuously, and having an infection or physical injury can cause your body to lose chromium. Low chromium levels can increase blood sugar and raise triglyceride (a type of fat) and cholesterol levels.

■ USES

Here is a list of some of the health problems associated with low chromium levels.

- Diabetes. People with diabetes cannot adequately process blood sugar. People who have type 1 diabetes need insulin shots to help them process blood sugar. Type 2 diabetics can often control their blood sugar with diet alone. Studies show that taking chromium supplements can improve the ability of people with type 2 diabetes to process blood sugar, especially if their body's store of chromium is low. Some people have higher than normal blood sugar (hyperglycemia), but are not considered diabetic. These people often have low chromium levels and can also benefit from taking chromium supplements. High blood sugar levels due to low chromium levels is a common problem among older people.
- Hypoglycemia. Hypoglycemia is the opposite of hyperglycemia and diabetes. People who have hypoglycemia have low blood sugar. Low chromium levels may be a contributing factor of hypoglycemia in some people. Taking 200 mcg of chromium a day may improve the symptoms of hypoglycemia.
- Cardiovascular disease. Low chromium levels are associated with increased blood cholesterol and a greater risk of developing heart disease. Taking chromium supplements has been shown to increase HDL ("good") cholesterol and lower triglyceride and total cholesterol levels in people with diabetes and people with high blood sugar.
- Glaucoma. Chromium affects insulin receptors in the eye. There is a strong association between low chromium levels and increased risk of glaucoma. Glaucoma is a common problem among people with diabetes.
- Obesity. Preliminary evidence suggests that taking chromium supplements may help reduce body fat and increase muscle tissue.
- Osteoporosis. Chromium picolinate has been shown to decrease urinary excretion of calcium and hydroxyproline in women, and may help preserve bone density in postmenopausal women.

■ DIETARY SOURCES

Brewer's yeast, lean meats (especially processed meats), cheeses, pork kidney, whole-grain breads and cereals, molasses, spices, and some bran cereals.

Brewer's yeast grown in chromium-rich soil is the best dietary source for chromium. Vegetables, fruits, and most refined and processed foods (except for some processed meats, which contain high amounts of chromium) contain low amounts of chromium. Hard tap water can supply 1 to 70 percent of your daily requirement. Cooking in stainless steel cookware increases the chromium content of food.

■ OTHER FORMS

Chromium is available commercially in several forms, including chromium polynicotinate, chromium picolinate, chromium-enriched yeast, and chromium chloride. Chromium is available in multivitamins and alone in tablet and capsule forms. Preparation doses are typically between 15 and 200 mcg chromium a day in multivitamins.

■ HOW TO TAKE IT

To prevent and treat disease, you should take between 100 to 200 mcg of chromium daily.

As with all medicines and supplements, check with a health care provider before giving chromium supplements to a child.

■ PRECAUTIONS

The form of chromium found in foods is generally nontoxic. However, extremely high amounts can cause toxicity and gastric irritation. High amounts or tissue accumulation of chromium can make insulin less effective. Check with your health care provider before taking chromium if you have diabetes, hyperglycemia, or hypoglycemia.

■ POSSIBLE INTERACTIONS

Chromium combines with niacin to form glucose tolerance factor (GTF). Calcium carbonate and antacids reduce the absorption of chromium.

■ COPPER

Copper is a metal that your body needs in small amounts. Even though you need very little, copper is an essential nutrient that helps make hemoglobin, the main component of red blood cells. It also produces energy and forms collagen, a key part of bones and connective tissue. Copper helps your nervous system operate properly, and helps protect nerve fibers.

We do not know all the ways copper helps people. Research has shown that copper may make your immune system stronger, may help relieve the symptoms of arthritis and other inflammatory conditions, and may even help lessen allergy symptoms.

Some people with arthritis wear copper bracelets to help reduce pain. Research has shown that these and other copper medications may provide relief of arthritis pain. If you have arthritis, talk with your health care provider about whether copper may be helpful to you.

Copper is available in many foods. Although you need very little copper, most people in the United States probably do not get as much copper as they should from their diet. However, very few people get so little copper that it causes health problems, so supplementation is probably unnecessary. You can improve your copper balance by including foods that contain copper, such as shellfish and nuts.

■ USES

You should talk with your provider before taking copper supplements. Copper may be helpful if you have the following conditions: arthritis, anemia, chemical hypersensitivity, high cholesterol, aneurysms, fatigue, allergies, and stomach ulcers

Pregnant women need more copper. As always, if you are pregnant, talk with your health care provider before taking any supplements.

■ DIETARY SOURCES

Copper is found in many varied food sources. The best sources include the following.

- Seafood (especially raw oysters; also squid, whelk, lobster, mussels, crab, and other shellfish)
- Organ meats (beef liver, kidneys, heart)
- Nuts (for example, cashews, filberts, macadamia nuts, pecans, almonds, pistachios)
- Legumes (especially lentils, navy beans, and peanuts)

- Chocolate (unsweetened or semisweet baker's chocolate, cocoa)
- Cereals (for example, bran flakes, shredded wheat, raisin bran)
- Fruits and vegetables (for example, dried fruits, mushrooms, tomatoes, potatoes, bananas, grapes, avocado)
- Blackstrap molasses
- Black pepper
- An additional source is from water that flows through copper pipes.

■ OTHER FORMS

Copper supplements are available, often combined with sulfate, picolinate, gluconate, and amino acids.

■ HOW TO TAKE IT

Daily dietary copper intake recommended by the National Research Council of the United States: 1.5 to 3.0 mg per day for adults. For children 2 to 11 years, 1.5 to 2.5 mg. Not recommended for children under 2.

The best way to get enough copper is to add foods to your diet that contain copper.

If you take copper supplements, you should also take zinc. You should take 8 to 15 mg of zinc for every 1 mg of copper you take.

■ PRECAUTIONS

You don't need a lot of copper. You should consult your health care provider before taking copper supplements. Too much copper can cause nausea, vomiting, stomach pain, headache, dizziness, weakness, and diarrhea. Dangerous levels of copper (copper poisoning) are extremely rare. However, severe cases can lead to heart problems, jaundice, coma, and even death.

You should avoid eating acidic foods that are stored in copper containers.

Keep copper supplements away from children.

■ POSSIBLE INTERACTIONS

Your copper balance could be hurt by alcohol, eggs, fructose, and molybdenum (a metallic element found in trace amounts in the human body).

Your body may have a hard time absorbing copper from food if you are ingesting too much calcium, iron, manganese, tin, zinc, vitamin B_6, vitamin C, or antacids.

■ CREATINE

Creatine has gained much popularity in recent years as an energy-enhancing supplement for athletes. Unlike anabolic steroids, the only documented side effect of taking creatine is weight gain. Creatine is a naturally occurring amino acid (protein building block) found in the skeletal muscles of your body. When you do high-intensity, short-duration exercise, such as lifting weights or sprinting, a special chemical reaction takes place to provide a burst of energy to your muscles. Creatine is fundamental to this reaction. Your body does not store very much creatine in your muscles for normal, everyday functions. If you desire to increase your muscle strength, improve your endurance, and delay fatigue for high-intensity, short-duration sports, then creatine supplements may help you achieve your goals. It is not for everyone, however. For example, it will not help you increase your performance for endurance (aerobic) sports such as running or biking. Also, some people don't respond well to creatine supplements because of various hereditary factors.

The market is flooded with numerous forms of creatine supplements. For maximum benefit, take a formula that supplies creatine monohydrate in combination with glucose (carbohydrate).

■ USES

Creatine can produce the following effects.
- Increases the availability of instant energy to your muscles
- Increases muscle strength
- Improves endurance for high-intensity, short-duration exercise
- Helps delay fatigue
- Promotes lean-muscle mass
- Reduces muscle wasting in post-surgical patients
- May benefit heart patients by increasing heart function and reducing heart spasms as well as allowing increased exercise capacity

■ DIETARY SOURCES

Your body manufactures about half the creatine you need for normal daily functions. The other half comes from your diet. The best dietary sources of creatine are red meat and fish. These foods provide about 1 g of creatine per half pound of raw meat. However, to gain energy-producing benefits, you can't get enough creatine from your diet alone, but need to take creatine monohydrate supplements.

■ OTHER FORMS

Creatine monohydrate is available in a variety of forms. The most common form is a powder you mix with juice or water. Manufacturers claim the new liquid preparations of creatine monohydrate are absorbed into the bloodstream faster and are more convenient to take than the powdered form. It is also more expensive than the powdered form. Creatine monohydrate is also available in tablets, capsules, energy bars, fruit-flavored chews, drink mixes, and other preparations. Taking creatine monohydrate in combination with glucose (a simple carbohydrate) has been shown to work better than taking creatine alone, so you will find many creatine-glucose combination products on the market. Consult your health care provider to determine which product is best for you.

■ HOW TO TAKE IT

In order to get maximum benefits from taking creatine supplements, it is necessary to "load" your muscles first to build up the creatine stores. A person who weighs 180 lbs. should take 5 g of creatine monohydrate four times a day (20 g total per day) for a week. Your muscles will then be "loaded" with creatine and you should begin to see some of the beneficial effects. Usually, a maintenance dose of 2 to 5 g per day is enough to replace whatever creatine you have used and keep your levels at the "loaded" point. If you weigh significantly more or less than 180 lbs, adjust the dosage up or down accordingly.

■ PRECAUTIONS

There have been no dangerous side effects shown from taking creatine monohydrate supplements to increase athletic performance. The only side effect documented in clinical studies is weight gain. This is due to an increase in water both inside and outside the muscle cells as well as an increase of lean-muscle tissue. It is not uncommon to gain 6 to 10 lbs. during the first two weeks of taking creatine supplements.

There are reports of other side effects from taking creatine supplements, such as muscle cramping, muscle strains and pulls, gastrointestinal problems, kidney malfunction, and liver damage. Some studies have already disproved these claims, and more research is being conducted. At this time, creatine supplementation is considered safe.

■ POSSIBLE INTERACTIONS

Avoid foods and beverages that contain caffeine, because it will cancel out the positive effects of taking supplemental creatine. Remember that caffeine is found not only in coffee, tea, and soft drinks, but also in chocolate and some over-the-counter cold remedies or pain relievers. Check the label to be sure.

■ DEHYDROEPIANDROSTERONE (DHEA)

Dehydroepiandrosterone (DHEA) is the most abundant androgen (a male steroid hormone) secreted by the adrenal glands, and to some extent, by the ovaries and testes. It is a precursor for other steroid hormones, such as testosterone and estrogen. Peak levels of DHEA occur at age 25. By age 80, DHEA levels decrease to 10 to 20 percent of the peak level. DHEA has been labeled an antiaging hormone because deficiencies in old age may make individuals more susceptible to cancer of the breast, prostate, and bladder; atherosclerosis; high blood pressure; autoimmune diseases (for example, diabetes, lupus erythematosus, rheumatoid arthritis); osteoporosis; high cholesterol; obesity; memory disturbances; chronic fatigue; and other manifestations of aging. Older individuals with higher DHEA levels are often in better heath than those with lower levels. Thus, the two most important factors concerning DHEA are that it declines in old age and that it is deficient in several diseases.

■ USES

- Heart disease. In one study, healthy men with low levels of DHEA were three times more likely to die of heart disease than those with high levels of DHEA.
- Aging. Significant positive changes (for example, less muscle wasting, less memory loss, improved mood, and energy) have been seen in some elderly men given DHEA, but more extensive research trials are necessary to determine extent of association.
- Osteoporosis. DHEA increases bone mass in postmenopausal women. However, supplementation is not recommended until more extensive human trials have been conducted.
- Autoimmune disease. Low levels of DHEA have been found in patients with autoimmune disorders (for example, lupus erythematosus, rheumatoid arthritis, multiple sclerosis, ulcerative colitis, AIDS). DHEA supplements in patients with autoimmune disorders improved their stamina and overall sense of well-being. In particular, patients with lupus treated with DHEA showed improved kidney function.
- Depression. DHEA has been used experimentally in depressed patients who demonstrated improvement in both depression and memory.
- AIDS. DHEA treatment in people with AIDS may have promise because low DHEA levels have been linked to decreased immune function. However, controlled clinical trials have not yet been conducted to investigate this hypothesis.
- Performance enhancement. Because DHEA is believed to build muscle mass, reduce fat, and reduce recovery time following injury, it is popular with athletes. However, human studies are needed to verify these claims. DHEA is also used to enhance sexual performance.

■ DIETARY SOURCES

Most of the DHEA on the market is made in laboratories from sterols (especially diosgenin) extracted from wild yams found in Mexico.

■ OTHER FORMS

Some extracts from wild yams are marketed as "natural DHEA." These extracts of diosgenin are believed by some to be converted into DHEA by the body. However, because it takes several chemical reactions to covert diosgenin into DHEA, it is unlikely that the body can make this conversion.

■ HOW TO TAKE IT

DHEA is available in capsules, chewing gum, and drops that are placed under the tongue. It is recommended that you take only "pharmaceutical grade" DHEA.

■ PRECAUTIONS

High doses of DHEA may inhibit the body's natural ability to synthesize DHEA and may be toxic to liver cells. Because DHEA increases the production of the male hormone testosterone, women should be aware of any signs of masculinization (for example, loss of hair on the head, hair growth on the face, weight gain around the waist, or acne), and men should be aware of signs of excess testosterone (for example, testicular wasting, sexual aggressiveness, aggressive tendencies, male pattern baldness, and high blood pressure).

Because DHEA is a precursor of estrogen and testosterone, patients with cancers stimulated by hormones (for example, breast, prostate, ovarian, testicular) should avoid DHEA.

DHEA is not recommended for people under 40 years of age, unless DHEA levels are known to be low (less than 130 mg/dL in women and less than 180 mg/dL in men).

The International Olympic Committee and National Football League recently banned the use of DHEA by athletes because its effects are very similar to those of anabolic steroids.

■ POSSIBLE INTERACTIONS

One study has indicated that vitamin E may protect against potential degenerative damage to the liver associated with DHEA treatment. Alcohol may increase the effects of DHEA.

■ ETHYLENEDIAMINETETRAACETIC ACID (EDTA)

EDTA chelation therapy is a nonsurgical treatment for heart disease. Doctors use a synthetic solution, called EDTA (ethylenediaminetetraacetic acid), to pull unsafe waste from your bloodstream. This cleaning process leaves you with an improved blood supply to your legs, heart, and other organs. EDTA chelation therapy can help you avoid heart and artery disease. If you already have such a disease, EDTA might be an alternative to bypass surgery.

Your health care provider may offer chelation therapy. EDTA is injected intravenously at your provider's office. Later, you get rid of the waste it removes from your bloodstream through urination. Hospitalization is not necessary, so this therapy is more comfortable and less expensive than a bypass operation. The American College of Advancement of Medicine (ACAM) offers training in this therapy.

The Food and Drug Administration (FDA) has not approved EDTA chelation therapy as an alternative to bypass surgery. However, more than 500,000 heart patients have been treated safely with EDTA chelation therapy. There are more government-led safety tests under way now, which may confirm the safety of EDTA and eventually lead to FDA approval.

EDTA chelation therapy is approved by the FDA as treatment for lead poisoning and other metal poisoning.

■ USES

Researchers originally came up with this method of cleaning the blood as a way to treat lead poisoning. The clean blood flow also seems to help people with heart disease. EDTA clears clogged arteries and improves blood flow to the heart. If you are at risk for heart disease or other vascular problems, using early chelation therapy reduces that risk. If your health care provider recommends a treatment like heart bypass surgery, EDTA may be another choice. If you do have a surgical procedure such as angioplasty or bypass, EDTA chelation therapy can help keep you healthy afterwards.

Chelation therapy is one of the only medically accepted treatments for lead, mercury, or arsenic poisoning. Research confirms that children with lead poisoning experience healthy growth spurts after undergoing EDTA chelation therapy.

EDTA may have a positive effect on Alzheimer's disease because it removes unsafe metals, such as aluminum, from the brain. Chelation therapy helps your immune system work better, perhaps helping you resist conditions such as cancer and lupus. If you are already ill, EDTA can help you recover. A strong immune system also helps you quickly recover from wounds. EDTA can prevent gangrene and helps many people avoid amputation. The improved blood flow also can help people with arthritis, Parkinson's disease, and multiple sclerosis. Studies have shown that chelation therapy improves vision problems like macular degeneration.

■ DIETARY SOURCES

EDTA is synthetic and not found naturally. It is usually combined with vitamins and minerals (such as vitamin C and magnesium), and delivered through an intravenous injection (directly into your bloodstream).

■ OTHER FORMS

N/A

■ HOW TO TAKE IT

You will receive your chelation therapy in a health care provider's office. It will be delivered slowly, over a period of three to four hours. Your health care provider will probably suggest two to three weekly EDTA treatments. Most people with heart disease need 20 to 30 such sessions.

You will follow a similar but shorter process if you are being treated for lead poisoning or an excess of other toxic heavy metals.

■ PRECAUTIONS

EDTA infusions must be given slowly. Treatments will be scheduled at least 24 hours apart in order to avoid potentially dangerous side effects. Overdose may lead to kidney failure, organ damage, seizures, or even death.

Your health care provider will monitor your blood pressure, blood glucose, cholesterol, organ function, and other vital statistics during your treatment with EDTA.

■ POSSIBLE INTERACTIONS

EDTA chelation therapy is most effective when you eat foods low in fat and unrefined foods. This means eating a wide variety of fresh foods that have not been canned, frozen, or commercially prepared. You should also add more fiber to your diet. Your health care provider might suggest an antioxidant supplement and a multivitamin, which will help you get the most out of EDTA chelation therapy.

■ FLAXSEED OIL

Flaxseed oil is rich in a type of fat called alpha-linolenic acid (ALA), an essential fatty acid used as a source of energy by the body. It also serves as the parent substance to compounds that regulate blood pressure, blood clotting, heart rate, blood vessel dilation, the immune response, and the breakdown of fats. Essential fatty acids are also used to make brain and nerve tissue.

ALA is a member of a family of fats called omega-3 fatty acids. Flaxseed oil and fish oils are the richest sources of omega-3 fatty acids. Canola oil and soybean oils also contain some omega-3 fatty acids. Corn, safflower, cottonseed, sesame, and sunflower oils are rich in fats called omega-6 fatty acids. These two families of fats have very important, but different, roles in the body. It is important to have a balance of omega-6 and omega-3 fatty acids in the diet. Excessive intake of either type of fat can cause health problems.

American diets are typically high in omega-6 fatty acids and low in omega-3 fatty acids. Taking in more omega-6 than omega-3 fatty acids through your diet may cause your body to produce substances that cause inflammation and negatively affect your body's response to disease. These imbalances may make you more susceptible to heart disease, inflammatory conditions such as arthritis and psoriasis, and infections, and can lower your immunity. You may gain significant health benefits by increasing the level of omega-3 fatty acids in your diet. This is especially true if you take in large amounts of omega-6 fatty acids.

■ USES

Here is a partial list of illnesses that may be prevented or treated with flaxseed oil.

- Skin disorders. Flaxseed oil may reduce the itching, swelling, and redness associated with certain skin disorders such as psoriasis.
- Hypertension. One tablespoon of flaxseed oil per day appears to be effective in lowering blood pressure.
- Heart disease. ALA may reduce the risk of heart disease by improving the function and integrity of arteries that carry blood throughout the body and to the brain. High doses of ALA may reduce blood cholesterol and triglyceride levels.
- Diabetes. Flaxseed oil may help reduce cholesterol and triglyceride levels in some people with diabetes. However, some people with type 2 diabetes cannot properly metabolize ALA, so flaxseed oil may be of no benefit to them.

- Autoimmune disorders. These disorders, such as rheumatoid arthritis and ulcerative colitis, cause immune cells to attack healthy tissue in the body. Flaxseed oil is converted to a substance in the body that can inhibit this autoimmune reaction.

■ DIETARY SOURCES

Flaxseed oil is found in flaxseed or flaxseed meal. Flaxseed oil is the richest source of omega-3 fatty acids, containing approximately 55 to 65 percent of the essential fatty acid ALA. It also contains the natural antioxidants beta-carotene (vitamin A) and carotenoids.

■ OTHER FORMS

Flaxseed oil is available in liquid and softgel capsule form, and, like any oil, should be refrigerated to prevent it from becoming rancid. Flaxseed oil requires special packaging because it is easily destroyed by heat, light, and oxygen. The highest quality flaxseed products are manufactured using fresh pressed seeds, are bottled in dark or opaque containers, and processed at low temperatures in the absence of light, extreme heat, or oxygen.

■ HOW TO TAKE IT

Because flaxseed oil is easily damaged by heat and light, it must be added to foods after they have been cooked. Use flaxseed oil as a salad dressing, in dips, sprayed over popcorn, or add it to hot or cold cereal.

For the prevention and treatment of disease adults should take 1 to 3 tsp. per day.

As with all dietary supplements, check with a health care provider before giving flaxseed oil to a child.

■ PRECAUTIONS

Flaxseed oil will add additional calories and fat to your diet unless you reduce your intake of other fats.

■ POSSIBLE INTERACTIONS

Flaxseed oil may increase your need for vitamin E. Because flaxseed oil may increase bleeding time, you should check with your health care provider if you are taking a blood-thinning medication or have a bleeding disorder.

■ GAMMA-LINOLENIC ACID

Gamma-linolenic acid (GLA) is an essential fatty acid that comes primarily from plant-based oils. Linoleic acid, which is found in cooking oils and processed foods, is converted into GLA in the body. GLA supplements are available in the form of evening primrose oil, black currant seed oil, and borage oil, which also provide linoleic acid. For example, evening primrose oil is 72 percent linoleic acid. The average North American diet provides more than 10 times the necessary amount of linoleic acid.

People who have diabetes are less able than healthy individuals to convert linoleic acid to GLA. Other conditions that appear to reduce the body's ability to convert linoleic acid to GLA include aging, alcoholism, atopic dermatitis, premenstrual syndrome, rheumatoid arthritis, cancer, and cardiovascular disease. Aging also appears to reduce conversion of linoleic acid to GLA. If you are an older person or have one of these conditions, you may want to talk to your provider about supplementing your diet with GLA.

If you have rheumatoid arthritis, you may benefit from GLA supplementation. It may enable you to take less non-steroidal anti-inflammatory drugs, which can cause stomach and intestinal problems. However, more research is needed to establish the proper dosage for long-term use.

Research has shown that GLA may help prevent cardiovascular disease by dilating blood vessels, lowering blood pressure, and preventing atherosclerosis.

Cancer is another condition where GLA may be useful. Studies in people with colon cancer, breast cancer, and melanoma show that GLA inhibits the growth of tumors and the spread of cancer.

For hemodialysis patients with uremic skin symptoms, studies show that skin conditions improved when the subjects used evening primrose oil supplements. Studies suggest that GLA is also helpful in increasing bone density and calcium absorption in people who have osteoporosis.

■ USES

- Rheumatoid arthritis. GLA may reduce inflammation.
- Diabetes. GLA supplementation assists nerve function and helps prevent nerve damage caused by diabetes.
- Cancer. GLA may help suppress tumor growth and spread of cancer, particularly in colon cancer, breast cancer, and melanoma.
- Heart disease. GLA may help prevent heart disease by inhibiting plaque formation, dilating blood vessels, and lowering blood pressure.

- Eyes. GLA is beneficial in Sjögren's syndrome and may be useful in other dry eye conditions.
- GLA supplements may help the symptoms of many conditions that occur with aging. It can also reduce the symptoms of alcoholism, atopic dermatitis, and osteoporosis.
- Menstrual problems (painful menstruation or no menstruation). Essential fatty acids such as those found in flaxseed, evening primrose, and borage oils reduce inflammation and support hormone production. Dosage is 1,000 to 1,500 mg one or two times per day.

■ DIETARY SOURCES

GLA is found in the plant-seed oils of evening primrose, black currant, borage, and fungal oils. GLA is also found in human milk and, in small amounts, in a wide variety of common foods, particularly organ meats.

■ OTHER FORMS

GLA supplements are available in several forms, including evening primrose oil, black current seed oil, borage oil, and borage oil capsules

Several manufacturing methods can destroy the nutrient value of GLA products. Some preferred methods use proprietary names for their process, generically known as "modified atmospheric packing methods." Generally, a high-quality oil will be certified as organic by a reputable third party, packaged in light-resistant containers, refrigerated, and marked with a freshness date.

■ HOW TO TAKE IT

There is no recommended dietary allowance (RDA) for GLA.

A recommended dosage for rheumatoid arthritis is 1.4 g per day. As the cost of oils can be high, and lower doses are usually effective, an acceptable clinical dosage of evening primrose, black currant, or borage oil would be 1,500 mg once or twice daily.

Studies have shown that up to 2.8 g of GLA per day is well tolerated. A healthy person eating a normal diet should consume fewer saturated fats and more polyunsaturated fats. Avoid products that contain hydrogenated fats. Discuss your total fat intake with your health care provider if you are thinking about taking GLA supplements.

■ PRECAUTIONS

GLA from dietary sources appears to be nontoxic. Talk to your health care provider about your regular diet, so he or she can help you decide if you should take GLA supplements, and what kind of supplements are best for you. Remember that GLA supplements are fats and contain a lot of calories.

■ POSSIBLE INTERACTIONS

None known

■ GLUTAMINE

Glutamine is an amino acid, one of the building blocks from which protein is made. Glutamine is found in plant and animal sources, as well as in supplement form. It helps the body maintain a healthy pH balance and is necessary for making and repairing cells.

As the most plentiful free amino acid in muscle tissue, glutamine plays an important role in all parts of the body. It speeds recovery and healing, helps curb cravings, and can improve mental acuity.

■ USES

Glutamine helps relieve the following health problems.

- Food cravings
- Alcoholism
- Problems with brain activity and mental functions
- Digestive tract problems, including ulcers, Crohn's disease, irritable bowel syndrome, and leaky gut syndrome
- Wounds, including those caused by surgery and leg ulcers (helps wounds heal faster)
- Autoimmune diseases
- Connective tissue diseases
- Arthritis
- Fibrosis
- The muscle wasting caused by conditions such as AIDS and cancer
- Damage caused by radiation therapy
- Developmental disabilities
- Schizophrenia
- Epilepsy
- Fatigue
- Impotence
- Stress

■ DIETARY SOURCES

Foods that contain a significant amount of glutamine include plant and animal protein foods, such as meats, milk, soy proteins, raw spinach, raw parsley, and cabbage. Cooking can destroy glutamine, especially in vegetables.

■ OTHER FORMS

Glutamine is available in some multivitamin complexes, protein supplements, and individual supplements. You can purchase it at most pharmacies and health food stores in the form of powders, capsules, tablets, or liquid.

Standard preparations are available in 500 mg tablets or capsules.

■ HOW TO TAKE IT

It is best to take glutamine for conditions such as peptic ulcers, arthritis, Crohn's disease, and impotence. You should consult your health care provider for many of the medical conditions that glutamine can help. Your health care provider can help you determine how much glutamine you should take and what other nutrients you should take with glutamine to help it work better.

Although your body normally has enough glutamine, it gets used up by extreme stress caused by surgery, disease, or a long illness, or even by vigorous exercise. When the body's own stores of glutamine run short, supplements or dietary sources of glutamine can help restore the balance and help you recover faster.

There is no recommended dietary requirement (RDA) yet for glutamine, so check with your health care provider to find out how much you need. He or she will probably recommend that you take between 500 to 1,500 mg a day, depending on what condition you have, what other medications you're taking, and other factors specific to you.

As with all medicines and supplements, check with your health care provider before giving glutamine supplements to a child.

■ PRECAUTIONS

People who have Reye's syndrome, kidney disease, cirrhosis of the liver, or other illnesses that cause ammonia to build up in the blood should not take glutamine.

■ POSSIBLE INTERACTIONS

- Glutamine works best when taken on an empty stomach before breakfast or between meals.
- Glutamine may work better if you take it with vitamins A, C, and E, and zinc, depending on your illness.
- You should not take glutamine with milk or other protein foods, for example, meat, fish, and beans.
- Deficiency may result from prolonged illness or extreme stress.

For more information about glutamine, consult your health care provider.

■ IRON

Iron performs many tasks in the human body. It delivers oxygen from the lungs to all parts of your body, helps your muscles work, and helps break down substances that can damage your body. Hemoglobin is the protein that carries iron and oxygen to all parts of your body. If your cells do not get enough iron, you can get anemia. There are several types of anemia, and the one associated with iron is called iron-deficient anemia. The most common symptoms of anemia are weakness and tiredness. Those at the highest risk of anemia are growing children (6 months to 4 years of age), adolescents (especially girls), and pregnant women.

■ USES

The most important use of iron supplements is to improve the symptoms of iron-deficient anemia. This kind of anemia can be caused by prolonged blood loss such as that from a bleeding ulcer or a malignant tumor; iron-poor diet or inefficient absorption of dietary iron; pregnancy; and the rapid growth that takes place during infancy, early childhood, and adolescence.

■ DIETARY SOURCES

The best dietary sources of iron are liver, lean red meat, poultry, fish, oysters, shellfish, and kidney. Iron from these sources is readily absorbed.

The following foods are also sources of iron: dried beans, fruits, and vegetables. Absorption of iron from these sources depends on other components of the diet. Vitamin C and meat products help iron absorption, while calcium (including all dairy products), bran, tea, and unprocessed whole grain products block absorption.

Iron is often added to these foods: egg yolks, dried fruits, dark molasses, whole-grain and enriched bread, wines, and cereals.

■ OTHER FORMS

Ferrous sulfate is the most common form of oral iron supplement. Other available include ferrous fumarate, ferrous succinate, ferrous gluconate, ferrous lactate, ferrous glutamate, and ferrous glycine. Slow-release preparations are also available. Supplemental iron should be taken only under the supervision of your health care provider. He or she will recommend the form that is best for you.

■ HOW TO TAKE IT

For treatment of iron-deficient anemia, adults should take 65 mg of an iron supplement three times a day with water. It is preferable to take the supplements between meals because they are absorbed better without food. As with all medications and supplements, check with a health care provider before giving iron supplements to a child.

■ PRECAUTIONS

Iron supplements must be kept in childproof bottles and out of the reach of children. If a child accidentally ingests iron supplements, it can be fatal.

■ POSSIBLE INTERACTIONS

Iron inhibits the absorption of the following drugs: disodium etidronate, levodopa, penicillamine, ciprofloxacin, norfloxacin, ofloxacin, and tetracycline. Antacids can reduce the absorption of iron supplements taken orally.

Take iron supplements at least two hours before or after taking any of the above drugs or antacids.

For more information about iron supplements, consult your health care provider.

■ LIPASE

Lipases are one of three categories of enzymes manufactured by the pancreas. The pancreas is a leaf-shaped gland about five inches long. Along with lipase, the pancreas secretes the hormones insulin and glucagon, which your body needs to metabolize sugar into the bloodstream. The other two enzymes include amylases, which break starch molecules into more simple sugars, and proteases, which break protein molecules into single amino acids. Lipases help your body digest fats by hydrolyzing (breaking up) triglycerides into base glycerol and fatty acid molecules creating free fatty acids and monoglycerides, which are more easily used by the body.

■ USES

Lipase can be used to treat digestive problems and conditions that cause you to have trouble absorbing nutrients from food. These conditions can result in nutrient deficiences. Lipase supplements can help your body absorb food more easily, keeping your body's nutrients at healthy levels.

Some consider pancreatic enzymes of value in treating autoimmune disorders (such as rheumatoid arthritis), inflammatory diseases, and food allergies. Pancreatic enzymes have been most studied in treating early diagnosed celiac disease (a condition that affects the intestinal tract and can cause nutrient deficiencies) by enhancing the benefit of a gluten-free diet.

■ DIETARY SOURCES

Lipase is manufactured by the pancreas. It does not come from your diet, but it can be supplemented with animal enzymes.

■ OTHER FORMS

Lipase produced by the pancreas is called pancreatic lipase. There is also gastric lipase (produced by the stomach) and hepatic lipase (produced by the liver).

■ HOW TO TAKE IT

Pancreatic enzymes are available in tablet and capsule form. Follow the package directions or your health care provider's instructions for the proper dose.

■ PRECAUTIONS

Most people produce plenty of pancreatic lipase. You are only considered to have a lipase deficiency when your pancreas produces 10 to 15 percent less than normal levels.

Lipase and other pancreatic enzyme supplements are not associated with side effects.

■ POSSIBLE INTERACTIONS

Lipase deficiency caused by pancreatitis (inflammation of the pancreas) can be a serious, even life-threatening condition. Self-treatment with lipase supplements is not recommended without medical supervision.

Tablets or capsules of lipase enzymes may be helpful, but you should also avoid alcohol (alcoholism is the leading cause of pancreatitis). Because the pancreas aids in the digestion of fats, a low-fat diet is often recommended.

■ LYSINE

Lysine is an essential amino acid that you must get from food because your body cannot make enough of it. Lysine helps your body process fatty acids, and it is particularly important for proper growth. Lysine also helps your body absorb calcium, and it plays an important role in the formation of collagen, a substance important to your bones and tissues.

A vegetarian diet may not provide sufficient lysine. Plants, although they are sources of protein, do not contain enough lysine. This is especially true of cereal grains as sources of protein. If you get too little lysine in your diet, your body may develop a poor nitrogen balance, and you may ultimately develop kidney stones. Signs of getting too little lysine include fatigue, nausea, dizziness, appetite loss, emotional agitation, bloodshot eyes, decreased immunity, slow growth, anemia, enzyme deterioration, reproductive disorders, pneumonia, and acidosis (a pH imbalance in the body).

■ USES

Lysine is used to treat herpes infections caused by both herpes simplex and herpes zoster viruses. Taking lysine supplements can speed your recovery time and reduce chances of reinfection.

Some studies have found lysine helpful in treating cardiovascular disease, osteoporosis, asthma, migraine, nasal polyps, and postepisiotomy pain. Consult your health care provider about taking lysine for these problems.

■ DIETARY SOURCES

Good sources of lysine include the following.
- Meat, particularly red meat
- Cheeses
- Poultry
- Sardines
- Nuts
- Eggs
- Soybeans

The most concentrated sources of lysine are torula yeast, dried and salted cod, soybean protein isolate, soybean protein concentrate, Parmesan cheese, pork loin (excluding fat), dried and frozen tofu, freeze-dried parsley, defatted and low-fat soybean flour, fenugreek seed, and dried spirulina seaweed.

■ OTHER FORMS

- L-lysine acetylsalicylate (LAS)
- Lysine clonixinate (LC)
- L-lysine monohydrochlorine (LMH)

■ HOW TO TAKE IT

The recommended dietary allowances for lysine include the following.
- Birth to 4 months: 103 mg per kilogram of body weight a day
- 5 months to 2 years: 69 mg per kilogram of body weight a day
- 3 to 12 years: 44 mg per kilogram of body weight a day
- Adults and teenagers: 12 mg per kilogram of body weight a day

Some experts say that adults need 30 mg per kilogram of body weight a day.

You should determine how much lysine your diet provides, and if you are not getting enough, discuss with your health care provider whether you should supplement your diet. He or she can help you decide how much lysine to take and what form would be best for you.

■ PRECAUTIONS

Lysine may increase cholesterol and triglyceride levels in your blood. If you have problems with cholesterol or triglyceride levels, or if you have cardiovascular disease, be sure to talk with your health care provider before taking supplements.

Lysine appears to be nontoxic.

■ POSSIBLE INTERACTIONS

Vitamin C aids lysine in collagen formation. No harmful interactions are known.

■ MAGNESIUM

The mineral magnesium is important for your heart, muscles, and kidneys. It is part of what makes up your teeth and bones. Most important, it activates enzymes, giving you energy and helping your body work properly. It can help reduce stress, depression, and insomnia. Vitamin B6 helps you get the magnesium you need and works with magnesium in many ways.

Magnesium is available in many foods. However, most people in the United States probably do not get as much magnesium as they should from their diet. Nutrition tables can give you only a rough idea of how much magnesium you are getting. Scientists have found that different ways of determining the amount of magnesium in foods produce different results. Also, many foods have not been thoroughly analyzed.

Certain medical conditions can upset your body's magnesium balance. For example, intestinal flu with vomiting or diarrhea can cause temporary deficiencies. Long-term deficiencies can be caused by stomach and bowel diseases, diabetes, pancreatitis, kidney malfunction, and diuretics. Talk with your health care provider about your magnesium needs if you have any of these conditions.

■ USES

Getting enough magnesium can help you in the following ways:
- Prevent hardening of the arteries (arteriosclerosis)
- Prevent strokes and heart attacks
- Reduce your blood pressure
- Lower your cholesterol and triglyceride levels
- Correct heart arrhythmias
- Stop acute asthma attacks
- Decrease your insulin needs if you have diabetes
- Prevent kidney stones
- Treat Crohn's disease
- Treat noise-induced hearing loss
- Improve your vision if you have glaucoma
- Reduce cramps, irritability, fatigue, depression, and water retention associated with menstruation
- Prevent serious complications of pregnancy, such as preeclampsia and eclampsia
- Restore your normal energy level
- Improve your sleep
- Reduce anxiety and depression
- Reduce the effects of stress

■ DIETARY SOURCES

The richest sources of magnesium are tofu, nuts (Brazil nuts, almonds, cashews, black walnuts, pine nuts), pumpkin and squash seeds, peanuts, green leafy vegetables, legumes, wheat bran, whole grains, soybean flour, blackstrap molasses.

Other good sources are whole wheat flour, oat flour, beet greens, spinach, shredded wheat, bran cereals, oatmeal, bananas, baked potatoes (with the skin), pistachio nuts.

You can also get magnesium from many herbs, spices, and seaweeds (for example, agar seaweed, coriander, dill weed, celery seed, sage, dried mustard, basil, cocoa powder, fennel seed, savory, cumin seed, tarragon, marjoram, and poppy seed).

■ OTHER FORMS

Magnesium is available in many forms. The best supplements are labeled "soluble," which means it's easier for your body to absorb the magnesium it needs. These come in gelatin capsules. Recommended types include magnesium citrate, magnesium gluconate, and magnesium lactate.

Other familiar sources of magnesium are milk of magnesia (magnesium hydroxide), often used as a laxative or antacid, Epsom salts (magnesium sulfate) used as a laxative or tonic, or added to a bath. Some magnesium can be absorbed through the skin.

■ HOW TO TAKE IT

You should take small doses of magnesium throughout the day, with a full glass of water with each dose to avoid diarrhea. These are the recommended daily amounts:
- Adult men ages 19 to 30: 400 mg; after age 30: 420 mg
- Adult women ages 19 to 30: 310 mg; after age 30: 320 mg
- Boys ages 14 to 18: 410 mg
- Girls ages 14 to 18: 360 mg
- Children ages 9 to 13: 240 mg; children ages 4 to 8: 130 mg; children ages 1 to 3: 80 mg

■ PRECAUTIONS

Do not take magnesium supplements if you have severe heart disease or kidney disease without talking with your health care provider.

Overuse of milk of magnesia (as a laxative or antacid) or Epsom salts (as a laxative or tonic) can cause you to ingest too much magnesium, especially if you have kidney problems. Too much magnesium can cause serious health problems and even death.

■ POSSIBLE INTERACTIONS

Some foods, drinks, and medications can cause you to lose magnesium. These include sodium (salt), sugar, caffeine, alcohol, fiber, riboflavin in high doses, insulin, diuretics, and digitalis.

Some foods, drinks, and medicines make it hard for your body to get the magnesium it needs. These include calcium, iron, manganese, phosphorus, zinc, and fat.

■ MANGANESE

Manganese is a metal that occurs widely in plant and animal tissues. It is called a trace element because it is found in very small quantities in the human body. Our bodies store approximatley 20 milligrams of manganese, mostly in the bones. Manganese aids in forming connective tissue, fats and cholesterol, bones, blood-clotting factors, and proteins. It is also necessary for normal brain function. Manganese is a component of manganese superoxide dismutase (MnSOD), an antioxidant that protects the body from toxic substances. It is easy to obtain adequate amounts of manganese from the diet.

■ USES

The following illnesses may be affected by manganese.

- Diabetes. People who have diabetes sometimes have significantly less manganese than healthy people. Manganese decreases blood sugar levels in some people with diabetes.
- Rheumatoid arthritis. People with rheumatoid arthritis (inflammation of the joints) can have low levels of MnSOD, which helps protect the joints from damage during inflammation. Manganese supplementation increases MnSOD activity.
- Epilepsy. An important study in the early 1960s demonstrated that manganese-deficient rats were more susceptible to seizures and had electroencephalograms (EEGs) consistent with seizure activity.
- Schizophrenia. People who have schizophrenia may also respond well to manganese supplementation.
- Osteoporosis. Bone loss occurs more rapidly after menopause and can lead to osteoporosis (brittle, thin, bones). Manganese, and other trace elements, increase bone density in postmenopausal women.
- Other conditions. Manganese is also used to treat hardening of the arteries (atherosclerosis), high cholesterol (hypercholesterolemia), tinnitus, and hearing loss.

■ DIETARY SOURCES

- Nuts (especially pecans and almonds)
- Wheat germ and whole grains
- Unrefined cereals
- Leafy vegetables
- Liver
- Kidney
- Legumes (peanuts, beans)
- Dried fruits

Refined grains, meats, and dairy products contain very small amounts of manganese. Unrefined foods, such as whole grain breads and cereals, are higher in manganese.

■ OTHER FORMS

Manganese is available in a wide variety of forms including manganese salts (sulfate and gluconate) and manganese chelates (aspartate, picolinate, fumarate, malate, succinate, citrate, and amino acid chelate). It is available in tablets or capsules, usually along with other vitamins and minerals.

■ HOW TO TAKE IT

There is no recommended dietary allowance (RDA) for manganese. Dietary recommendations are based on typical dietary intake and are intended to prevent deficiency symptoms. The average intake of manganese ranges from 2 mg to 9 mg per day. In some cases, people may require more manganese (10 mg per day) than is indicated below.

The estimated safe and adequate daily intakes for manganese are 2 to 5 mg for adults, 1 to 3 mg for children and adolescents, and 0.3 to 1 mg for infants.

■ PRECAUTIONS

Excessive intake of manganese can produce toxic effects. You should not regularly exceed the estimated safe and adequate daily intakes for manganese listed above.

■ POSSIBLE INTERACTIONS

Calcium, copper, iron, magnesium, and zinc compete for absorption in the small intestines. Excess intake of one can reduce the absorption of the others. Excess manganese may produce iron-deficiency anemia.

■ MELATONIN

Melatonin is an important hormone secreted by the pineal gland in the brain. Since its identification in 1958, studies have shown that melatonin actually regulates many of the other hormones in the body. These hormones control our circadian rhythm, the 24-hour patterns that our bodies respond to every day. The release of melatonin is stimulated by darkness and suppressed by light, so it helps control when we sleep and when we wake. Melatonin also controls the timing and release of female reproductive hormones, affecting menstrual cycles, menarche, and menopause. Overall levels of melatonin in the body also respond to the process of aging. Children have the highest levels of nocturnal melatonin; as adults age, their nocturnal melatonin levels get lower and lower, which means they go to sleep and wake up earlier, and may suffer from disrupted sleep patterns.

■ USES

- Jet lag. Melatonin is used to restore sleeping patterns and fatigue caused by cross time-zone travel.
- Insomnia. Melatonin can restore more regular sleep patterns in those who suffer from insomnia as a result of low melatonin levels (that is, older people and some children with sleep disorders that may be caused by autism, epilepsy, Down syndrome, or cerebral palsy).
- Cancer. Melatonin can help prevent and treat some cancers, particularly those that are related to hormones (for example, breast cancer, prostate cancer) and non–small cell lung cancer. It also greatly increases the effectiveness and lowers the side effects of some cancer drugs (for example, interferon and interleukin 2).
- Depression. Melatonin may be beneficial in treating depression related to low melatonin levels (for example, seasonal affective disorder)
- Preliminary studies show melatonin may be useful in treating multiple sclerosis, coronary heart disease, epilepsy, and post-menopausal osteoporosis; and in preventing sudden infant death syndrome.

■ DIETARY SOURCES
N/A

■ OTHER FORMS
Melatonin is available as tablets, capsules, and sublingual tablets.

■ HOW TO TAKE IT
There is no official dosage range for melatonin supplements. Different people will be more sensitive or less sensitive to melatonin. For those especially sensitive to it, lower dosages may work as effectively as the standard amount, while taking the standard amount or higher dosage could cause anxiety and irritability.

To treat insomnia, one dose of 3 mg an hour before bedtime is usually effective, although dosages as low as 0.1 to 0.3 mg may improve sleep for some people. If 3 mg a night is not effective after three days, try 6 mg one hour before bedtime. An individually effective dose should produce restful sleep with no daytime irritability or fatigue. For treatment of jet lag, take 5 mg of melatonin one hour before bedtime upon arrival at your destination, and take it for the first five days. Dosages for anticancer treatment may be much higher (10 to 50 mg per day). Do not take melatonin supplements long term without consulting your health care provider.

■ PRECAUTIONS
There are no known serious side effects to supervised melatonin use. Lack of sleep and insufficient exposure to darkness may suppress your body's natural production of melatonin. Some people may experience vivid dreams or nightmares when they take melatonin. Overuse or incorrect use of melatonin could disrupt circadian rhythms. Melatonin can cause drowsiness if taken during the day. If you experience morning drowsiness after taking melatonin at night, take less of it.

It may not be good for you to take melatonin if you have an autoimmune disorder, such as lupus or rheumatoid arthritis, or an immune system cancer, such as lymphoma or leukemia. If you are taking melatonin for depression, make sure you do so under your health care provider's care and advice. In some cases, melatonin can actually worsen the symptoms of depression instead of making them better.

If you take corticosteroids for anti-inflammatory or immune suppressive purposes (for example, you have had a transplant), use melatonin cautiously, and always under the supervision of your health care provider. Melatonin could interfere with fertility. Do not take it if you are pregnant or nursing.

■ POSSIBLE INTERACTIONS
- Vitamin B_{12} changes the level of production of melatonin. If you have low levels of melatonin, you will often have low vitamin B_{12} levels as well. Taking vitamin B_{12} (1.5 mg of methylcobalamin per day) can help sleeping disorders because it increases melatonin production.
- Protein, vitamin B_6, niacinamide, and acetyl carnitine all help your body produce melatonin.
- Nonsteroidal anti-inflammatory drugs (NSAIDs), such as aspirin and ibuprofen, reduce melatonin production levels in the body, so it is best not to take these right before bedtime. Beta blockers also keep melatonin levels from rising naturally at night.
- Some antidepressants increase the levels of brain melatonin. Benzodiazepines, like Xanax and Valium, interfere with melatonin production. Alcohol and caffeine can also interfere with melatonin production, as can diuretics and calcium channel blockers.

■ PHENYLALANINE

Phenylalanine is an essential amino acid that you need to get from food because your body cannot make enough of it. In healthy people, the body changes phenylalanine into tyrosine, which in turn makes important hormones, such as norepinephrine and epinephrine. Adults use about 90 percent of the phenylalanine consumed to make tyrosine, children about 40 percent. Phenylalanine may be used to treat pain, depression, multiple sclerosis, Parkinson's disease, rheumatoid arthritis, osteoarthritis, and even cancer.

Phenylketonuria (PKU) is a disorder in which the body fails to turn phenylalanine into tyrosine properly. This disease appears in infants about 3 to 6 months old, often causing severe mental retardation. It may also cause seizures and hyperactivity. Some people with PKU have a skin rash, such as eczema. PKU occurs in approximately 1 in 10,000 Caucasian infants and 1 in 132,000 African-American infants. In the United States, newborns are tested for PKU during the first 48 hours of life. PKU must be treated before the infant is 3 months old if it is to be treated successfully.

People with PKU must eat a phenylalanine-restricted, tyrosine-supplemented diet to have optimum brain development and growth. Experts disagree about whether people with PKU can discontinue this diet without problems and, if so, at what age. Mental performance and intelligence is better in those who have stayed on the diet, according to some studies. Consult your health care provider about the pros and cons of treatment.

Pregnant women with untreated PKU give birth to small infants with birth defects. These birth defects are often severe, and these infants may not live long. If you have PKU and you are, or may become, pregnant, you should be on a phenylalanine-restricted diet.

Too little phenylalanine may cause confusion, emotional agitation, depression, decreased alertness, decreased memory, behavioral changes, decreased sexual interest, bloodshot eyes, cataracts, decreased insulin, decreased skin melanin (pigment), and increased appetite. If you are getting too little phenylalanine, you should take supplemental phenylalanine and tyrosine. Otherwise, you may fail to gain weight or grow taller, lose your hair, have problems with your bones, get anemia, or even die.

■ USES

- Cancer: You may reduce tumor growth and metastasis, particularly in malignant melanoma (skin cancer), by getting less phenylalanine and tyrosine.
- Depression
- Inflammation
- Multiple sclerosis: You may improve bladder control, increase mobility, and reduce depression.
- Pain: You may be able to reduce chronic pain, particularly in osteoarthritis.
- Parkinson's disease: You may improve rigidity, walking disabilities, and speech difficulties.

- Vitiligo: You may improve the condition with a combination of oral L-phenylalanine, topical cream containing phenylalanine, and ultraviolet-A radiation.

■ DIETARY SOURCES

- Cheeses
- Nuts and seeds
- Milk chocolate
- Meat (excluding fat), particularly organ meats
- Poultry (excluding skin)
- Fish, including shellfish
- Milk
- Eggs
- Aspartame (Nutrasweet)

Some of the most concentrated sources of phenylalanine are torula yeast, soybean protein isolate and concentrate, peanut flour, dried spirulina seaweed, defatted and low-fat soybean flour, dried and salted cod, dried and frozen tofu, Parmesan cheese, almond meal, dry roasted soybean nuts, dried watermelon seeds, and fenugreek seeds.

■ OTHER FORMS

- D-phenylalanine
- L-phenylalanine
- D,L-phenylalanine (50/50 blend of D-phenylalanine and L-phenylalanine)
- Topical creams

■ HOW TO TAKE IT

The recommended dietary allowances for phenylalanine plus tyrosine include the following.

- Birth to 4 months: 125 mg per kilogram of body weight a day
- 5 months to 2 years: 69 mg per kilogram of body weight a day
- 3 to 12 years: 22 mg per kilogram of body weight a day
- Adults and teenagers: 14 mg per kilogram of body weight a day

Some experts say that adults need 39 mg per kilogram of body weight a day.

Talk with your health care provider about dosages for specific uses. Generally, nutritional doses are 0.75 to 2 g a day and therapeutic doses are 2 to 3 g a day. Supplements are usually taken 15 to 30 minutes before meals.

■ PRECAUTIONS

- Anxiety, headaches, and hypertension are possible side effects.
- People with PKU and women who are lactating or are pregnant should not take phenylalanine supplements.
- L-dopa competes with phenylalanine for absorption and should not be taken at the same time of day.
- Little is known about the use of aspartame (Nutrasweet) during pregnancy. Talk with your health care provider about using this artificial sweetener.
- Doses in excess of 5 g a day may be toxic.

■ POSSIBLE INTERACTIONS

Vitamins B_6 and C help the body absorb phenylalanine. Increased amounts of other amino acids will inhibit phenylalanine absorption.

■ PHOSPHORUS

An addition to food and water, your body needs certain vitamins and minerals to survive. Calcium and phosphorus are two of the most important minerals in the human body, working together to build strong bones and teeth. Phosphorus makes up about 1 percent of total body weight, so if you weigh 150 pounds you have a pound and a half of phosphorus in your body. Most of the phosphorus in your body (about 85 percent) is in your bones and teeth, where it combines with calcium to make bones hard and strong. The rest is in your cells and other tissues. In the kidneys, phosphorus is important in filtering out wastes. It also helps maintain the acid-base (pH) balance in your blood. Phosphorus controls the flow of energy in your body and helps reduce muscle pain after a hard workout. Your body needs phosphorus for the growth, maintenance, and repair of all your tissues and cells, and for the production of DNA and RNA. You also need phosphorus to make use of other vitamins and minerals, including vitamin D, calcium, iodine, magnesium, and zinc.

■ USES

We do not normally need to take phosphorus supplements because the foods we eat contain a lot of phosphorus. In some cases, however, such as in a person with kidney disease, a health care provider may prescribe phosphorus supplements. Sometimes athletes use phosphate supplements before competitions or heavy workouts to help reduce muscle pain and fatigue. Phosphorus and calcium can be used together to help heal bone fractures and to treat vitamin D deficiencies such as osteomalacia and rickets.

■ DIETARY SOURCES

Red meat and poultry contain significant amounts of phosphorus. Other sources include dried milk and milk products, hard cheeses, canned fish, nuts, eggs, and soft drinks.

■ OTHER FORMS

Elemental phosphorus, a white or yellow waxy substance that burns on contact with air is highly toxic and no longer used in medicine (although it is used in some homeopathic treatments and should be taken under the care of a qualified practitioner). Instead, health care providers may recommend using one or more of the following inorganic phosphates, which are not toxic.

- Dibasic potassium phosphate
- Monobasic potassium phosphate
- Dibasic sodium phosphate
- Monobasic sodium phosphate
- Tribasic sodium phosphate

■ HOW TO TAKE IT

If you are under 24 years old, or are pregnant or breastfeeding, you need 1,200 mg of phosphorus daily. For everyone else, 800 mg is the recommended dietary allowance (RDA) of phosphorus. Because most people get enough phosphorus from food, you don't normally need to worry about taking supplements. It is more important to pay attention to what you eat and to make sure that you get a good balance of calcium and phosphorus in your diet. Cutting down on meats and finding alternatives to soft drinks can help correct any imbalance between calcium and phosphorus in your body. At the same time, it is important to make sure you are getting enough calcium in your diet, which is somewhat more difficult.

■ PRECAUTIONS

Phosphates can be toxic at levels over 1 g per day. Too much phosphate can lead to diarrhea and calcification (hardening) of organs and soft tissue, and interfere with the body's ability to use iron, calcium, magnesium, and zinc. If you are an athlete taking supplements that contain phosphate, be sure to use them only occasionally.

Nutritionists recommend a balance of calcium and phosphorus from your diet, but the typical American diet is low in calcium and high in phosphorus, with two to four times as much phosphorus as calcium. It's easy to understand why. Meat and poultry contain 10 to 20 times as much phosphorus as calcium, and carbonated beverages such as colas have as much as 500 mg of phosphorus in one serving. When there is more phosphorus than calcium in your system, your body will draw on the calcium stored in your bones for normal functions. This can lead to reduced bone mass that makes bones brittle and fragile, or to gum and tooth problems. Low calcium to phosphorus ratios (low levels of calcium in relation to levels of phosphorus) may also increase your risk of high blood pressure and colorectal cancer. A balance of calcium and phosphorus in the foods you eat can help reduce stress, reduce the risk of osteoporosis, and relieve the symptoms of osteoarthritis and other problems that are related to the body's ability to use calcium.

■ POSSIBLE INTERACTIONS

The following can contribute to phosphorus deficiency.

- Aluminum-containing antacids
- Iron
- Magnesium
- Caffeine
- Inadequate vitamin D

For more information about phosphorus, consult your health care provider.

■ POTASSIUM

Potassium is a mineral that helps the kidneys function normally. It also plays a role in cardiac, skeletal, and smooth muscle contraction, making it an important nutrient for normal heart function. Recent studies have suggested that potassium helps lower blood pressure, and that it can help reduce the risk of death from an acute heart attack when administered by a health care provider along with insulin and glucose. If you take in too much potassium in your diet, you run the risk of getting hyperkalemia (having too much potassium in the blood). If you don't take in enough, you run the risk of getting hypokalemia (not having enough potassium in the blood).

For most people a healthy diet rich in vegetables and fruits is a safe way to get the amount of potassium you need. The elderly are at a high risk for hyperkalemia due to the decreased kidney function that occurs naturally as you age. Older people should be careful when taking any medication, because they can affect potassium levels in the body. Talk with your health care provider before taking potassium or any supplement.

■ USES

The most important use of potassium is to treat the symptoms of hypokalemia, which include weakness, lack of energy, stomach disturbances, an irregular heartbeat, and an abnormal EKG (electrocardiogram, a test that measures heart function).

Under a health care provider's supervision, potassium can also be used to lower blood pressure, prevent stroke, treat muscle weakness and diabetes mellitus, and help prevent death from an acute heart attack.

■ DIETARY SOURCES

The best dietary sources of potassium are fresh unprocessed foods, including meats, vegetables (especially potatoes), fruits (especially avocados), and citrus juices (such as orange juice). Most of our potassium needs can be met by eating a varied diet with adequate intake of milk, meats, cereals, vegetables, and fruits.

■ OTHER FORMS

There are several potassium supplements on the market, including potassium acetate, potassium bicarbonate and potassium citrate effervescent, potassium chloride, and potassium gluconate. Potassium can also be found in multivitamins.

■ HOW TO TAKE IT

You should not take a potassium supplement other than what's in a multivitamin unless your health care provider instructs you to do so. As with all medications and supplements, check with a health care provider before giving potassium supplements to a child. The average potassium intake estimated by the National Research Council is as follows. This amount is most likely provided by your daily diet.

- Infants: 780 mg a day
- Children: 1,600 mg a day
- Adults: 3,500 mg a day

There is no recommended increased intake of potassium during pregnancy and nursing.

■ PRECAUTIONS

If you have kidney problems, you should not take potassium supplements unless told to do so by your health care provider. If you are elderly, take potassium supplements under the supervision of your health care provider, because of decreased kidney function with age.

■ POSSIBLE INTERACTIONS

Certain drugs may affect potassium levels in your body. These include nonsteroidal anti-inflammatory drugs such as ibuprofen, beta-blocking drugs, heparin, and others. If you take any other medications or supplements, consult with your health care provider before taking potassium supplements.

■ PSYLLIUM

Psyllium is a soluble fiber used primarily as a gentle bulk laxative. It comes from a shrublike herb called plantain that grows worldwide. There are many species of plantain that can produce up to 15,000 tiny, mucilage-coated seeds per plant. The plantain herb that produces psyllium seed is not the same plant as edible plantains.

The seeds are odorless and have almost no taste. Psyllium makes stools softer, which helps relieve constipation, irritable bowel syndrome, hemorrhoids, and other intestinal problems. Its ability to speed waste matter through the digestive system helps reduce the risk of colon cancer and other intestinal diseases by shortening the amount of time toxins stay in the body. Unlike wheat bran and some other fiber supplements, psyllium does not cause excessive gas and bloating.

■ USES
Here is a partial list of the health problems psyllium helps relieve.
- Constipation
- Diarrhea
- Irritable bowel syndrome
- Hemorrhoids
- Crohn's disease
- High cholesterol (Psyllium helps prevent the colon from absorbing cholesterol.)
- Colon cancer and some other cancers, and diseases of the colon
- Obesity (Adding fiber to the diet aids weight reduction even if calories are not restricted; soluble fibers such as psyllium help dieters feel full so they eat less. Psyllium also helps control blood sugar and insulin, which is important to overweight people as well as to people who have diabetes.)
- Hypertension and heart disease (High-fiber foods help reduce heart disease risk.)

■ DIETARY SOURCES
- Psyllium seed or husk
- Combination fiber remedies that include psyllium, such as Metamucil

■ OTHER FORMS
Standard preparations of psyllium are available in dry seed or husk form, to be mixed with water as needed. Psyllium is an ingredient in some commercially prepared laxatives such as Metamucil. Psyllium is added to some cereals to increase fiber content.

■ HOW TO TAKE IT
Add $1/2$ to 2 tsp. of psyllium seed to 1 cup (8 oz.) of warm water. Mix well, then drink immediately before it becomes too thick to swallow comfort-ably. (Psyllium thickens rapidly when water is added to it.) If you're using a commercial product that contains psyllium, follow package directions.

If you're not accustomed to taking psyllium, start with a low dose, such as 1 tsp. in an 8-oz. glass of water once a day, then increase to 2 tsps. and two 8-oz. glasses of water per day, as needed.

Your health care provider may recommend higher doses of psyllium to treat certain conditions. For example, a recommended program for irritable bowel syndrome is to start with $1/2$ or 1 tsp. of psyllium in one glass of water each day, then gradually increase by adding a little more psyllium every third or fourth day until you're taking a total of four doses, each consisting of 1 tsp. of psyllium to an 8-oz. glass of water, a day.

It is very important to make sure you drink plenty of water when you take psyllium or any fiber supplement because fiber soaks up water from your digestive system. If you don't take in extra water to make up for that effect, fiber supplements can cause blockage or constipation. Be sure to drink at least six to eight glasses of water each day.

Take psyllium first thing in the morning or before bedtime. As a weight-loss aid, take at least 30 minutes before meals.

As with all medicines and supplements, check with a health care provider before giving psyllium to a child.

■ PRECAUTIONS
Don't take psyllium within an hour of the time you take other medications because it can interfere with how the drugs is absorbed and may make the medication less effective. Allow at least one hour between the time you take medicines or drugs and the time you take psyllium.

Always take psyllium with a full 8-oz. glass of water, and be sure to drink at least six to eight full glasses of water during the day.

Do not take guar, another fiber supplement that works the same way psyllium does, if you're taking psyllium. You can use one or the other, but don't use both at the same time.

■ POSSIBLE INTERACTIONS
Psyllium may block absorption or reduce the effectiveness of prescription and nonprescription medicines. It may also alter the way your body uses or absorbs minerals, so check with your health care provider if you suspect you have a mineral deficiency.

For more information about psyllium, consult your health care provider.

■ SELENIUM

Selenium is a trace mineral found in soil and food. It is an important antioxidant, which means it helps prevent harmful chemical reactions from occurring in the body's cells. Protected cells are better able to fight off diseases, including heart disease, cancer, and disorders associated with aging.

Most of us do not get enough selenium from food. When our selenium levels are low, we run a higher risk of getting a variety of illnesses because our immune systems may be sluggish and toxins build up in the blood.

If you need to add selenium to your diet, your health care provider will probably suggest that you take a selenium supplement in combination with vitamin E. Research shows that selenium taken together with vitamin E promotes overall health and prevents or treats many diseases.

■ USES

Selenium cures Keshan disease, a serious heart disorder common to women and children in China, where the farmland lacks minerals. However, clinical studies conclude that selenium also protects the body from more common illnesses, including the following.

- Cancer. Selenium reduces your risk of breast, colon, liver, skin, and lung cancers. Selenium keeps tumors from growing by helping to build healthy, cancer-fighting white blood cells.
- Heart disease. Studies show that selenium prevents heart attacks and strokes by lowering your bad (LDL) cholesterol. Selenium also keeps your arteries clear of dangerous fatty deposits, which makes it an important addition to your therapy after a heart attack.
- Weakened immune system. Selenium helps build up white blood cells, boosting your body's ability to fight illness and infection.

Selenium also helps with the following.

- Reproductive health, through increasing male fertility, as well as helping with proper fetal development
- Helps the liver, thyroid, and pancreas function normally
- Prevents premature aging, cataract formation and, possibly, sudden infant death syndrome (SIDS)
- Treats lupus, rheumatoid arthritis, and alcoholic cirrhosis of the liver
- Treats most skin disorders, including poor elasticity, acne, eczema, and psoriasis

■ DIETARY SOURCES

Much of your selenium comes from dietary sources. Brewer's yeast and wheat germ, liver, butter, fish and shellfish, garlic, grains, sunflower seeds, and Brazil nuts are all good sources of selenium. It's also found in alfalfa, burdock root, catnip, fennel seed, ginseng, raspberry leaf, and yarrow.

Selenium is destroyed when foods are refined or processed. You should try eating a wide variety of whole, unprocessed foods. This means eating foods in their original state, not canned, frozen, or commercially prepared.

■ OTHER FORMS

Your health care provider may recommend that you add selenium to your diet. You can do this by taking a vitamin-mineral supplement, a nutritional antioxidant formula, or a separate supplement. Selenium is also available in nutritional yeast.

■ HOW TO TAKE IT

Clinical trials suggest that you take 50 to 200 mcg of selenium daily to see real benefits. Men need at least 70 mcg daily; women at least 55 mcg. Pregnant and nursing mothers' needs increase to 65 to 75 mcg daily. Researchers say that most of us need to take more than 100 mcg of selenium supplements daily to see improvements in disease resistance and overall health.

As with all medicines and supplements, check with a health care provider before giving selenium supplements to a child.

Take selenium with vitamin E daily for best results. Ask your health care provider to recommend an appropriate dose. (1 mg selenium daily taken with 200 IUs of vitamin E is typical.)

Do not take vitamin C with selenium because it may make the selenium less effective and, possibly, more toxic.

■ PRECAUTIONS

Selenium is usually not toxic. However, high doses (more than 1,000 mcg a day) over time may produce fatigue, arthritis, hair or fingernail loss, garlicky breath or body odor, gastrointestinal disorders, or irritability. Researchers have also discovered high levels of selenium in children with behavioral problems.

■ POSSIBLE INTERACTIONS

Vitamin E increases selenium's effectiveness as an antioxidant. When you take the two together, you give your cells the best protection available.

Your body has a hard time absorbing and using selenium when taken with vitamin C. To avoid this, take your vitamin and mineral supplements at different times of the day. Remember that all supplements are best absorbed when taken with a meal.

You may need a higher than usual dose of selenium if you are undergoing chemotherapy.

■ SPIRULINA

Spirulina is a type of blue-green algae that has been consumed for thousands of years as a staple in the diet of Mexican (Aztecs, Mayans), African, and Asian peoples. It is a rich source of nutrients, especially protein, and thus is an important food for vegetarians. It is known for its antiviral and anticancer properties as well as its ability to stimulate the immune system.

■ USES

- AIDS and other viruses (for example, herpes simplex, human cytomegalovirus, influenza virus, mumps, measles). Spirulina prevents reproduction of viruses and stimulates the immune system.
- Cancer. Spirulina inhibits some cancers in laboratory animals and oral cancer in humans.
- Anemia. Spirulina promotes hematopoiesis (formation and development of red blood cells).
- Skin disorders. Spirulina helps to maintain healthy skin and treats several skin disorders, such as eczema and psoriasis.
- Vitamin A deficiency. Studies have determined that spirulina is an effective source of dietary vitamin A.

Spirulina can be used for general immune support, and as an easily absorbed protein supplement if you have a lack of appetite. It is also used in the treatment of Candida (yeast infections) and hypoglycemia (low blood sugar). Weight lifters often use it as a protein source.

■ DIETARY SOURCES

Spirulina is a microalgae that flourishes in warm climates and warm alkaline water. It is available dried and freeze-dried.

■ OTHER FORMS

Spirulina is available in pill or powder form. Most spirulina consumed in the United States is cultivated in a laboratory. There are many different spirulina species, only some of which are identified on labels of commercially available products. *Spirulina maxima* (cultivated in Mexico) and *Spirulina platensis* (cultivated in California) are the most popular.

■ HOW TO TAKE IT

Consult your health care provider for the correct dosage of spirulina. A standard dosage of spirulina is 4 to 6 tablets (500 mg each) per day.

■ PRECAUTIONS

None known. Talk with your health care provider before taking spirulina if you are pregnant or breast-feeding.

■ POSSIBLE INTERACTIONS

None reported

■ SULFUR

Sulfur is a mineral naturally occurring near hot springs and volcanic craters. The "rotten egg" smell of sulfur mineral baths is caused by sulfur dioxide gas escaping into the air. Sulfur has been used medicinally since ancient times, and it is contained in every cell in your body. It is a component of three different amino acids (the building blocks that make up protein). Approximately 0.25 percent of your total body weight is sulfur. It is most concentrated in keratin, which gives you strong hair, nails, and skin. It is known as "nature's beauty mineral" because your body needs it to manufacture collagen, which keeps your skin elastic and young-looking.

Sulfur is used primarily to ease the red, itchy rashes of conditions such as eczema and diaper rash. It also helps to protect your body against toxins in the environment. In addition, people with arthritis may find pain relief from taking a soothing bath in hot sulfur springs.

■ USES

- Used primarily to treat the red, itchy discomfort of eczema, diaper rash, dry scalp, hemorrhoids, and similar conditions
- Sulfur baths can help relieve arthritis pain.
- In recent years, the benefits of garlic have been widely studied. Research suggests that the beneficial effects of garlic in lowering cholesterol levels and blood pressure are likely due to the sulfur it contains.
- Necessary for the body to make collagen—the substance in your skin that keeps it elastic, young-looking, and wrinkle-free.
- Aids in certain digestive disorders, especially acid reflux, indigestion made worse by milk, chronic diarrhea, and vomiting in the morning.
- Can help gynecological problems such as premenstrual syndrome and menopausal discomforts.

■ DIETARY SOURCES

The elemental mineral form of sulfur is found in rocks near hot springs and volcanos. The form your body uses is found in protein-rich foods such as meat, organ meats, poultry, fish, eggs, cooked dried beans and peas, and milk and milk products. Other good sources include garlic, onions, brussels sprouts, asparagus, kale, and wheat germ.

■ OTHER FORMS

To ease skin rashes, there are ointments, creams, lotions, or dusting powders containing sulfur as the active ingredient. If you suffer from arthritis, soaking in a natural sulfur bath (the kind usually found at hot springs) can greatly ease the pain in your joints. Talk to your health care provider to see if you might benefit from this type of therapy. Organic sulfur (the kind our body uses) is available in the form of MSM (metylsulfonylmethane).

Sulfur is also available as a dietary supplement in tablets and capsules. However, you most likely do not need to take extra sulfur. If you are eating a well-balanced diet that includes the recommended daily allowance of protein, you should get all the sulfur you need to maintain your body's daily functions. Any extra sulfur will be excreted in your urine. Follow the advice of your health care provider in taking sulfur as a supplement.

■ HOW TO TAKE IT

If you have arthritis, an oral dose of 500 mg to 1,000 mg per day may decrease symptoms. Consult your health care provider before taking sulfur supplements.

■ PRECAUTIONS

Sulfur, by itself, is not toxic to our bodies. However, some people are highly allergic to relatives of sulfur such as sulfites and sulfa drugs. Sulfites are used as a food preservative and can trigger asthma and other allergic reactions in people who are sensitive. Sulfa drugs can cause hypoglycemia (low blood sugar), skin rashes, high fever, headache, fatigue, and gastric problems. Tell your health care provider if you think you may be allergic to sulfur-containing substances.

■ POSSIBLE INTERACTIONS

Too much selenium can compete with sulfur in your body because it substitutes for sulfur in some chemical reactions. Talk with your health care provider about maintaining a healthy balance of sulfur and selenium in your diet, and be sure to consult with him or her before taking either selenium or sulfur supplements.

■ TYROSINE

Tyrosine is a nonessential amino acid that is synthesized in the body from phyenylalanine. Because tyrosine is a precursor of the neuro-transmitters norepinephrine and dopamine, both of which regulate mood, a deficiency of tyrosine (leading to a deficiency of norepineph-rine) can result in depression.

Tyrosine aids in the the production of melanin (pigment responsible for hair and skin color) and in the functions of the adrenal, thryroid, and pituitary glands. Tyrosine deficiency has been linked to hypothy-roidism, low blood pressure, low body temperature, and restless leg syndrome.

Because tyrosine binds unstable molecules that can potentially cause damage to the cells and tissues, it is considered a mild antioxidant. Thus, it may be useful in heavy smokers and in people who have been exposed to harmful chemicals and radiation.

■ USES

- Depression. Tyrosine appears to be a safe and effective treatment for depression; however, symptoms of depression recur when tyrosine supplementation is discontinued. Most data on the efficacy of tyrosine in the treatment of depression are anecdotal and have not been proved in scientific studies.
- Stress. Tyrosine seems to relieve the physical symptoms of stress if administered before the stressful situation occurs, though studies on humans are limited.
- Premenstrual syndrome (PMS). Though most data are anecdotal, tyrosine may help reduce the irritability, depression, and fatigue associated with PMS.
- Low sex drive. Tyrosine appears to stimulate the libido.
- Parkinson's disease. Parkinson's disease is treated with L-dopa, which is made from tyrosine; thus, tyrosine supplementation is being studied in people with Parkinson's disease.
- Weight loss. Tyrosine is an appetite suppressant and helps reduce body fat.
- Chronic fatigue and narcolepsy (involuntary sleep). Tyrosine appears to have a mild stimulatory effect on the central nervous system.

- Drug detoxification. Tyrosine appears to be a successful adjunct for the treatment of cocaine abuse and withdrawal; it is often used in conjunction with tryptophan and imipramine (an antidepressant). Successful withdrawal from caffeine and nicotine has also been anecdotally reported.

■ DIETARY SOURCES

Although tyrosine is found in soy products, chicken, fish, almonds, avoca-dos, bananas, dairy products, lima beans, pumpkin seeds, and sesame seeds, it is difficult to get therapeutic amounts of tyrosine from food. It is also produced from phenylalanine in the body.

■ OTHER FORMS

Many tyrosine supplements are available.

■ HOW TO TAKE IT

Tyrosine should be taken 30 minutes before meals three times a day on an empty stomach (with juice or water). Tyrosine should not be taken with other amino acids or with proteins such as milk.

Tyrosine is more effective if it is taken with up to 25 mg of vitamin B_6.

■ PRECAUTIONS

Tyrosine should not be taken by patients who are taking monoamine oxidase (MAO) inhibitors for depression or by patients with high blood pressure because it can cause dangerous elevations of blood pressure. Tyrosine may also cause the growth of malignant melanoma (skin cancer) by promoting the division of cancer cells. Migraine headaches and gastrointestinal upset may occur after taking supplements.

■ POSSIBLE INTERACTIONS

- Tyrosine is often used with tryptophan and imipramine (an antidepres-sant) to treat cocaine abuse and withdrawal.
- Folic acid, niacin, vitamin C, and copper are needed if tyrosine is to metabolize into adrenaline, norepinephrine, and dopamine.
- Tyrosine should not be taken with other amino acids or with proteins such as milk.

◾ VANADIUM

Vanadium is an essential trace mineral. It is present in varying amounts in the soil and in many foods. It can also be inhaled from the air as a result of burning petroleum or petroleum products. At the end of the last century, vanadium was thought to be a cure for various diseases, but it turned out to be toxic at the high doses prescribed. Vanadium is necessary for bone and tooth development. Too little vanadium may result in high cholesterol and triglyceride levels, poor blood sugar control (for example, diabetes or hypoglycemia), and cardiovascular and kidney disease. However, the effects of vanadium deficiency in humans have not been studied.

◾ USES

- Vanadium improves blood sugar control in experimental animals with type 1 and type 2 diabetes mellitus; however, no human studies have been conducted to support these findings.
- High doses of vanadium improve the strength of bones and teeth in experimental animals.
- Studies have not been able to determine definitively any performance-enhancing effects of vanadium (for example, in body building).
- Vanadium may reduce cholesterol in experimental animals.
- Heart disease rates are low in areas of the world (for example, South America) where soils contain high levels of vanadium. No cause and effect relationship has been demonstrated, however.

◾ DIETARY SOURCES

The best sources of vanadium are sunflower, safflower, corn, and olive oils, as well as buckwheat, parsley, oats, rice, green beans, carrots, cabbage, pepper, and dill. It is important to note, however, that only about 5 percent of vanadium is absorbed by the body; most of it is eliminated in the feces. Vanadium supplementation is rarely, if ever, necessary. Eating any of the above foods, particularly vegetable oils, will provide a sufficient amount of vanadium. Some experts do not recommend taking vanadium supplements until more is known about how this mineral affects the human body.

◾ OTHER FORMS

Vanadium exists in several forms, including vanadyl and vanadate. Vanadyl sulfate is most commonly found in nutritional supplements. Because of its toxicity, some experts believe that vanadium should be considered a drug and not a nutritional supplement.

◾ HOW TO TAKE IT

Typical over-the-counter doses of vanadium are 30 to 60 mg per day in pill form.

◾ PRECAUTIONS

- Animal studies have not proven the efficacy or safety of vanadium in humans.
- Extremely high doses of inhaled vanadium (for example, in workers who clean petroleum storage tanks) irritate the lungs and turn the tongue green, but neither symptom causes any long-term or serious problems.
- High levels of vanadium may cause manic-depression.
- High levels of vanadium may contribute to some bone and kidney diseases.

◾ POSSIBLE INTERACTIONS

- The effects of vanadium are reduced by some psychiatric medications (for example, phenothiazines, monoamine oxidase inhibitors).
- Vitamin C, ethylenediaminetetraacetic acid (EDTA), and methylene blue decrease vanadium levels in the body. Therefore, they are effective in treating manic depression, where vanadium levels are high.
- Tobacco decreases vanadium uptake.
- Vanadium and chromium should not be taken together.

■ VITAMIN A (RETINOL)

Vitamin A is important in maintaining good vision, healthy skin, and healthy mucous membranes. Research has shown it is also necessary for proper immune system function. Vitamin A is also important for proper growth, bone formation, reproduction, and wound healing. Your liver can store up to a year's supply of vitamin A. The stored supply of this vitamin is used up more quickly if you become ill or have an infection.

■ USES

- Acne and psoriasis. Drugs including vitamin A successfully clear up acne and psoriasis. Even more recently, another drug made from vitamin A is helping to lessen scars and wrinkles on the skin, making them less noticeable, and helping to prevent wrinkles from forming.
- Immune system. Research has shown that vitamin A boosts the immune system to help fight off illness and infection, especially viral illness.
- Wound healing. Your body needs vitamin A, along with several other nutrients, when it is forming new tissue and skin.
- Measles. Reduces infant mortality from this disease
- Also used to treat night blindness and hyperkeratosis

■ DIETARY SOURCES

Vitamin A is found only in foods from animal sources, especially beef, calf, and chicken liver. Dairy products such as milk, butter, cheese, and ice cream are also good sources. However, beta-carotene, a nutrient found in fruits and vegetables, can be converted to vitamin A in the body as needed. Most dark-green leafy vegetables and most orange vegetables and fruits contain a lot of beta-carotene, and by eating these foods you will increase your body's supply of vitamin A. Vegetables such as sweet potatoes, carrots, and winter squash, and fruits such as cantaloupe and mango are all good sources of beta-carotene.

■ OTHER FORMS

You can buy natural vitamin A supplements either as retinol or retinyl palmitate. All forms of vitamin A are easily absorbed. Tablets or capsules are available in 10,000 IU, 25,000 IU, and 50,000 IU doses. Your health care provider will help you decide which vitamin A dosage is best for you. Most multivitamins contain the recommended dietary allowance (RDA) for vitamin A. If you are taking a multivitamin, you are probably getting more than enough vitamin A to meet your average needs. You should never take more than 25,000 IU per day (10,000 IU for children) without a health care provider's supervision.

In many cases, taking beta-carotene, the precursor form of vitamin A, is a safer alternative to taking vitamin A. Unlike vitamin A, beta-carotene is water-soluble and does not build up in the body, so it can be taken in larger amounts without the same risk. This makes it a better alternative for children, adults with liver or kidney disease, and pregnant women.

■ HOW TO TAKE IT

Vitamin A is a fat-soluble vitamin and is absorbed along with the fat in your diet. Supplements containing vitamin A should be taken during or shortly after a meal.

■ PRECAUTIONS

Pregnant women should never take vitamin A supplements, because they can cause birth defects. All prenatal vitamins contain some vitamin A, and taking any more would be dangerous to the fetus.

Too much vitamin A is toxic to the body and can even be fatal. You probably won't get toxic amounts of vitamin A from your daily diet, but taking vitamin A supplements without a health care provider's supervision is not recommended. Vitamin A is found in many different types of vitamin formulas. For example, supplements that say "wellness formula," "immune system formula," "cold formula," "eye health formula," "healthy skin formula," or "acne formula," all may contain vitamin A. If you take a variety of different formulas, you could put yourself at risk for vitamin A toxicity. Some of the symptoms of vitamin A toxicity are lasting headache, fatigue, muscle and joint pain, dry, cracking skin and lips, dry, irritated eyes, nausea or diarrhea, and hair loss.

Alcohol use makes vitamin A toxicity more likely. Consuming more than 25,000 IU of vitamin A per day (adults) and 10,000 IU per day (children) from either food or supplements or both can be toxic. Do not take vitamin A supplements if you are using Accutane, Retin-A or any vitamin A–derived drugs used to treat acne, psoriasis, and other skin problems.

■ POSSIBLE INTERACTIONS

- High doses of vitamin E cause the body to use more vitamin A.
- Zinc is needed in order for the body to use vitamin A.
- Zinc deficiency can cause the same symptoms as vitamin A deficiency, because the body is not able to use the vitamin A it has without zinc.
- Your body needs enough protein to use vitamin A. Adults should eat at least 7 oz. of protein each day, and children at least 4 oz. each day.
- Some medications, such as estrogens and oral contraceptives, may increase retinol levels in the blood. Talk with your health care provider before taking Vitamin A supplements if you regularly take any type of medication.

■ VITAMIN B₁ (THIAMINE)

Vitamin B₁ is also called thiamine. You need vitamin B₁ in your daily diet to help break down carbohydrates (starches). The energy produced by this process helps your body perform functions as basic as breathing and moving. Not getting enough vitamin B₁ in your daily diet leads to a disease called beri beri, which can affect your nervous system and heart. Alcoholics are at a high risk of developing beri beri because prolonged intake of large amounts of alcohol depletes your body's supply of vitamin B₁.

■ USES

The most important use of vitamin B₁ is to improve symptoms of beri beri. These symptoms include nervous system symptoms such as pain, swelling, and redness of the hands and feet, and a tickling or burning sensation in the hands and feet. Confusion and loss of memory are also potential symptoms.

Other symptoms of beri beri include difficulty in breathing, swelling of the legs, and rapid heart beat. Certain diuretics may cause you to lose Vitamin B₁ through urination, causing a deficiency.

Recent research suggests that vitamin B₁ may help manage congestive heart failure.

Vitamin B₁ may also play a negative role in cancer chemotherapy. Researchers have found that taking too much vitamin B₁ while undergoing chemotherapy may make tumors grow more quickly.

■ DIETARY SOURCES

Cereals and pork are excellent sources of vitamin B₁. Other good sources of vitamin B₁ are white enriched rice, sunflower seeds, peanuts, wheat germ, brewer's yeast, soy milk, beans, and pasta.

Milk, fruits, and vegetables are also good sources of vitamin B₁ if consumed in adequate amounts.

■ OTHER FORMS

Vitamin B₁ is labeled as thiamine hydrochloride and thiamine mononitrate. It is available as tablets or capsules in multivitamin form, including children's chewable and liquid forms, B-complex form, or by itself.

■ HOW TO TAKE IT

To avoid diseases of vitamin B₁ deficiency, adults should take between 1.1 mg and 1.5 mg of vitamin B₁ daily with water, preferably after eating. Pregnant women should take 1.5 mg daily, and women who are breast-feeding should take 1.6 mg of vitamin B₁ daily. As with all medications and supplements, check with a health care provider before giving vitamin B₁ supplements to a child. If you are pregnant, discuss taking vitamin B₁ with your health care provider before you begin taking it.

■ PRECAUTIONS

Vitamin B₁ is generally nontoxic. Stomach upset can occur at very high doses (much higher than the recommended daily doses).

■ POSSIBLE INTERACTIONS

Vitamin B₁ is depleted by excess alcohol intake.

For more information about vitamin B₁, consult your health care provider.

■ VITAMIN B₂ (RIBOFLAVIN)

Riboflavin, also known as vitamin B2, enables carbohydrates, proteins, and fats to release energy. Riboflavin is needed for normal reproduction, growth, and repair of skin, hair, nails, and joints. It is also important to the immune system, which protects your body against disease.

■ USES

Here is a partial list of the illnesses that riboflavin helps prevent, and those that it helps to treat.

- Migraine headache. Riboflavin may help prevent migraine headaches. Studies have suggested that supplementation with riboflavin is more effective than aspirin in preventing these severe headaches.
- Cataracts. Riboflavin deficiency may cause cataracts. Riboflavin is vital to the activity of an enzyme that protects your eyes. Riboflavin deficiency is fairly common in older people. Before taking more than the recommended dietary allowance (RDA) for riboflavin to prevent cataracts, speak to your health care provider.
- Riboflavin supplements may help in the treatment of sickle cell anemia. It may also enhance the effectiveness of iron supplements in the treatment of anemia.
- Rheumatoid arthritis. Too little riboflavin in your diet may put you at risk for rheumatoid arthritis. Supplementation with riboflavin may help improve your symptoms.

Riboflavin is also helpful in the following ways.
- May relieve symptoms of carpal tunnel syndrome
- Reduces the effects of stress
- Skin problems such as acne (especially acne rosacea), dermatitis, eczema, and ulcers may improve with riboflavin supplementation
- May improve muscle cramps
- May protect against certain types of cell damage that occur during a heart attack or stroke
- Enhances immune function

■ DIETARY SOURCES

The best sources of riboflavin include brewer's yeast, almonds, organ meats, whole grains, wheat germ, wild rice, mushrooms, soybeans, milk, and spinach.

Riboflavin is added to flours and cereals. Riboflavin is destroyed by light and alkalis such as baking soda. It is not destroyed by heat, although it will leach into cooking water. Foods should be stored away from light to help retain their riboflavin content.

■ OTHER FORMS

Riboflavin supplements are available in two forms: simple or activated. It is also found in multivitamin preparations and in B-complex vitamins, in 25-, 50-, and 100-mg tablets.

■ HOW TO TAKE IT

Recommended dietary allowances for riboflavin are listed below.
- Children 1 to 3 years: 0.5 mg/day
- Children 4 to 8 years: 0.6 mg/day
- Children 9 to 13 years: 0.9 mg/day
- Men 14 years and older: 1.3 mg/day
- Women 14 to 19 years: 1.0 mg/day
- Women during pregnancy: 1.4 mg/day
- Women during lactation: 1.6 mg/day

As with all medicines, check with a health care provider before giving riboflavin to a child.

■ PRECAUTIONS

Riboflavin toxicity is rare. Possible reactions to high doses include itching, numbness, burning or prickling sensations, and sensitivity to light. High doses of riboflavin can affect urinalysis test results.

■ POSSIBLE INTERACTIONS

- Sulfa drugs, antimalaria drugs, estrogen, cathartic agents, and alcohol can interfere with the effectiveness of riboflavin.
- In high doses, riboflavin may reduce the effectiveness of the anticancer drug methotrexate.
- Riboflavin's effects may be decreased by long-term use of barbiturates.
- Certain liver diseases can affect how well riboflavin works.
- Riboflavin is needed to activate vitamin B_6.

For more information on riboflavin, check with your health care provider.

■ VITAMIN B₃ (NIACIN)

Vitamin B₃, or niacin, is a member of the B-vitamin family. It is water-soluble, which means it is not stored in your body and needs to be frequently replenished. There are two forms of vitamin B₃, niacin (also known as nicotinic acid) and niacinamide (also known as nicotinamide). Both forms work the same way as an important nutrient in your body, but are used to treat different conditions.

Your body needs vitamin B₃ to turn carbohydrates into energy. Without B₃, your body systems would grind to a halt. B₃ is also involved in the breakdown of fat and cholesterol, which is why niacin (nicotinic acid) has been found to be a good cholesterol-lowering agent.

Your body uses vitamin B₃ to make various compounds, such as sex hormones and adrenal hormones. It can also help the body get rid of toxic and harmful chemicals, and it helps with blood sugar control.

Most people get enough of this vitamin just from the foods they eat. Your health care provider may prescribe a vitamin B₃ supplement for high cholesterol or other conditions. It is important that your health care provider closely monitors you while you are taking high doses of vitamin B₃ because it can cause serious side effects, such as liver damage, at these dosages.

■ USES

Niacin reduces LDL (bad) cholesterol and increases HDL (good) cholesterol. It can also enhance the effect of prescription cholesterol-lowering drugs. Use it for this purpose only under the close supervision of a health care provider.

Niacinamide can help treat osteoarthritis and rheumatoid arthritis, insulin-dependent diabetes, insomnia, and migraine headaches.

Either form may be used to treat or prevent vitamin B₃ deficiency (pellagra). People with cancer or tuberculosis, women who take oral contraceptives (birth control pills), and people suffering from protein deficiencies are more likely to have vitamin B₃ deficiency.

■ DIETARY SOURCES

Our bodies actually manufacture vitamin B₃ from protein, so if you are eating enough protein, you will also be getting enough vitamin B₃. The best sources of vitamin B₃ are found in protein-rich foods such as lean meats, chicken, fish, eggs, cooked dried beans and peas, liver, nonfat or lowfat milk and cheese, soybeans, and nuts.

Other good sources include brewer's yeast, wheat germ, enriched breads and cereals, whole grains (except corn), mushrooms, and green vegetables. Vitamin B₃ can be lost in cooking water, so you should steam, bake, or stir-fry vegetables when possible.

■ OTHER FORMS

If your health care provider advises you to take extra vitamin B₃, you can purchase niacin or niacinamide supplements in a variety of forms, including tablets in strengths of 25 mg, 50 mg, 100 mg, 250 mg, and 500 mg. Although timed-release tablets and capsules are available, and have advantages, there are studies showing that timed-release niacin may cause liver damage. Niacin is also available as inositol hexaniacinate, a preparation developed in Europe. Inositol hexaniacinate is a sustained-release delivery method that is not thought to lead to liver disorders.

■ HOW TO TAKE IT

It is important to take niacin supplements with food to avoid stomach upset and to decrease the risk of developing stomach ulcers.

■ PRECAUTIONS

High doses (75 mg or more) of niacin can cause side effects. The most common side effect is called "niacin flush." You may feel a burning, tingling sensation in your face and chest, and your skin will get red or "flushed." It is harmless unless you have asthma; so people with asthma should not take niacin supplements at high dosages. At very high doses like those used to lower cholesterol, liver damage and stomach ulcers can occur. If you have had liver disease or stomach ulcers, you should not take niacin supplements. If you have diabetes, gallbladder disease, or gout, you can take supplements under the close supervision of your health care provider.

■ POSSIBLE INTERACTIONS

Keep in mind the following facts about niacin.
- Works with other B-vitamins to keep the body's "engine" running.
- May be used together with other cholesterol-lowering drugs.
- Be careful if taking with high blood pressure medication. (Follow your health care provider's instructions closely.)
- Alcohol can interfere with your body's absorption of vitamin B₃ as well as many other vitamins and minerals.

For additional information supporting this handout, please refer to our website: www.onemedicine.com/public/products/access
Copyright ©2000 Integrative Medicine Communications • 1029 Chestnut St., Newton, MA 02464 • T 877-426-6633 • F 877-426-6630

■ VITAMIN B₅ (PANTOTHENIC ACID)

All the cells in your body need vitamin B₅, or pantothenic acid. It is a water-soluble B vitamin that is converted by the body into a compound called coenzyme A, which your body needs to change food into energy. Vitamin B₅ is also known as the "antistress" vitamin because it supports the healthy functioning of your adrenal glands, the organs that help your body cope with all types of stress. Vitamin B₅ is needed for proper nerve and muscle action, and it is vital to maintaining a healthy immune system. It also seems to help decrease the painful symptoms of rheumatoid arthritis.

■ USES

- Some health care providers recommend taking vitamin B₅ for fatigue, allergies, asthma, psoriasis, or other chronic illness, or if you have a very active or stressful lifestyle. Vitamin B₅ has not been proved useful for these conditions.
- Taking vitamin B₅ seems to help reduce the pain, swelling, and stiffness of rheumatoid arthritis and to improve wound healing, especially after surgery.
- Pantethine seems to help lower blood lipids (fats, cholesterol, and triglycerides) and speed up the detoxification process.

■ DIETARY SOURCES

Pantothenic acid gets its name from the Greek work *pantos,* meaning "everywhere," because it is available in a wide variety of foods. A lot of vitamin B₅ is lost in processing, so fresh meats, vegetables, and whole unprocessed grains have more vitamin B₅ than refined, canned, and frozen food. The best sources are brewer's yeast, whole-grain breads and cereals, mushrooms, liver, dried beans and peas, avocados, fish, chicken, nuts (pecans, hazelnuts), peanuts, cauliflower, milk and cheese, potatoes, oranges, bananas, and eggs.

■ OTHER FORMS

Vitamin B₅ is included in most B-complex vitamins. It is also available in single supplement form as calcium pantothenate, which is 92 percent pantothenic acid and 8 percent calcium. It is available in 100-, 250-, and 500-mg capsules.

■ HOW TO TAKE IT

For general adrenal support or stress relief, 250 to 500 mg daily is probably adequate. For treating rheumatoid arthritis, 1,000 mg twice daily (2,000 mg a day) is the recommended amount. To lower blood lipid levels (cholesterol or triglycerides), the recommended dose of pantethine is 300 mg three times daily (900 mg a day). Take with water, preferably after eating, or according to your health care provider's recommendation.

■ PRECAUTIONS

There are no known interactions or side effects associated with taking vitamin B₅ supplements. It is recommended that you take vitamin B₅ along with other B vitamins to reduce the possibility of a B-vitamin imbalance in your system.

■ POSSIBLE INTERACTIONS

There are no known adverse interactions with any other vitamins, herbs, or drugs.

■ VITAMIN B₆ (PYRIDOXINE)

Vitamin B₆ is a water-soluble vitamin. Our bodies use three forms of vitamin B₆: pyridoxine (PN), pyridoxal (PL), and pyridoxamine (PM). Most of the time you will hear vitamin B₆ referred to as pyridoxine. Vitamin B₆ performs several functions in our body, including breaking down carbohydrates for energy production, and forming hemoglobin and other substances that our bodies need to perform properly.

■ USES

The uses of vitamin B₆ include the following:

- To improve the symptoms of vitamin B₆ deficiency. These symptoms include inflammation (redness, swelling, pain) of the mouth, chapped lips, irritability, depression, and confusion.
- To treat anemia and nervous systems disorders caused by tuberculosis drugs
- To treat patients who have taken an overdose of the tuberculosis drug isoniazid
- To reduce the symptoms of premenstrual syndrome (PMS)
- To reduce nausea and vomiting during pregnancy
- To prevent heart disease. Recent studies have shown that vitamin B₆, vitamin B₁₂, and folate can lower blood levels of homocysteine, a substance that is an independent risk factor for heart disease.

■ DIETARY SOURCES

Chicken, fish, kidney, liver, eggs, and pork are excellent sources of vitamin B₆. The following are also good sources of vitamin B₆: yeast, wheat germ, whole grain cereals, beans, potatoes, bananas, and oatmeal. Vitamin B₆ can be lost from food that's frozen or processed (example: luncheon meats).

■ OTHER FORMS

Vitamin B₆ is available in the form of pyridoxine hydrochloride. It is available as tablets in multivitamin form (including children's chewable), B-complex form, or by itself in dosages ranging from 1 mg to 150 mg. Vitamin B₆ is also found in children's multivitamin liquid drops.

■ HOW TO TAKE IT

To avoid vitamin B₆ deficiency, men should get 2.0 mg and women 1.5 mg of vitamin B₆ daily. Pregnant women need 2.2 mg of vitamin B₆ daily, and women who are breast-feeding need 2.1 mg daily. People who eat a balanced diet containing the sources of vitamin B₆ listed above should be able to meet the daily requirement without taking a supplement. Consult your health care provider if you have questions about your daily requirement of vitamin B₆. When taking a vitamin supplement, always take it with water, preferably after a meal. As with all medications and supplements, check with a health care provider before giving vitamin B₆ supplements to a child.

■ PRECAUTIONS

Vitamin B₆ can cause neurological disorders when taken in high doses (200 mg per day or greater) over a long period of time. Discontinuing high doses usually leads to a complete recovery.

■ POSSIBLE INTERACTIONS

Vitamin B₆ inhibits the effectiveness of the Parkinson's disease drug levodopa. For more information about vitamin B₆, consult your health care provider.

VITAMIN B₉ (FOLIC ACID)

Folic acid, also called folate or vitamin B₉, is critical to many body processes, including the health of your nervous system, blood, and cells. It protects against heart disease, birth defects, osteoporosis, and certain cancers.

USES

Folic acid protects the body against, and helps treat, many disorders, including the following.

- Birth defects. Low levels of folic acid have been linked with birth defects. Half of neural tube defects (such as spina bifida) are believed to be preventable if women of childbearing age supplement their diets with folic acid. Studies suggest that the amount of folic acid needed to prevent neural tube defects is more easily reached with supplements than from dietary sources alone.
- Heart attacks and stroke. Folic acid is essential to a process that clears a substance called homocysteine from the blood. High homocysteine levels have been linked with increased risk of heart disease and stroke.
- Cancers. Low levels of folic acid may play a role in cancer development, particularly cancers of the cervix, lung, and colon.
- Osteoporosis. Lack of folic acid, and the resulting increase in homocysteine levels, weakens bones, making them more likely to fracture.
- Depression and other mental problems. Folic acid is important for brain function. It helps regulate mood, sleep, and appetite. Increasing levels of folic acid has reversed negative mental or psychological symptoms in some people, particularly older people. Folic acid has a mild antidepressant effect, and taking folic acid supplements has been shown to improve the effect of the drug Prozac.

Folic acid is also beneficial in the following ways: prevents anemia, which can decrease the function and number of red blood cells, helps treat headaches, may relieve rheumatoid arthritis, can help with infertility treatment, may help acne, and may be useful for people with AIDS.

DIETARY SOURCES

Foods that contain a significant amount of folic acid include liver, lentils, rice germ, brewer's yeast, soy flour, black-eyed peas, navy beans, kidney beans, peanuts, spinach, turnip greens, lima beans, whole wheat, and asparagus.

Food processing (for example, boiling, heating) can destroy folic acid. Storing food at room temperature for long periods of time can also destroy its folic acid content. As of January 1998, commercial grain products are fortified with folic acid.

OTHER FORMS

B₉ supplements are available as both folic acid and folinic acid. While folate is more stable, folinic acid is the most efficient form for raising body stores of the nutrient.

HOW TO TAKE IT

Folic acid comes as tablets, or as an injection that you get from your health care provider. Tablets are available in doses from 40 mcg to 1,000 mcg. The recommended dietary allowance (RDA) for folic acid depends on your age and sex (see below). Unless you are pregnant, you will likely get enough folic acid from your diet. Check with your health care provider before you start taking supplements and before giving folic acid supplements to a child.

The RDA for folic acid is as follows.

- Infants under 6 months: 25 mcg
- 6 to 12 months: 35 mcg
- Children 1 to 3 years: 50 mcg
- Children 4 to 6 years: 75 mcg
- Children 7 to 10 years: 100 mcg
- Male and female 11 to 14: 150 mcg
- Males 15 years and older: 400 mcg
- Females 15 years and older: 400 mcg
- Pregnant females: 400 mcg
- Lactating females: 280 mcg

PRECAUTIONS

Folic acid toxicity is rare. High doses (above 15 mg) can cause stomach problems, sleep problems, skin reactions, and seizures. Folic acid supplementation can mask vitamin B₁₂ deficiency, which can cause permanent damage to your nervous system. Folic acid supplementation should always include vitamin B₁₂.

POSSIBLE INTERACTIONS

- May reduce zinc absorption
- Absorption and function decreases with estrogens, alcohol, various chemotherapy drugs (notably methotrexate), sulfasalazine, barbiturates, and anticonvulsant drugs
- If you take aspirin, ibuprofen, or acetaminophen for long periods, you will need more folic acid

Folic acid works best when taken with vitamin B₁₂, niacin, choline, and vitamin C.

For more information about folic acid, consult your health care provider.

■ VITAMIN B$_{12}$ (COBALAMIN)

Vitamin B$_{12}$ is also called cobalamin. We need vitamin B$_{12}$ in our daily diet to help the cells in our bodies grow and maintain normal function. It is an especially important vitamin for healthy bone marrow (where blood cells are formed) and the nervous system. Not getting enough vitamin B$_{12}$ leads to a disease called pernicious anemia, which results in red blood cells not getting enough oxygen and causing disorders of the nervous system. The elderly are at higher risk for developing pernicious anemia because aging causes a decrease in the amount of vitamin B$_{12}$ that the body is able to absorb from food.

■ USES

The most important use of vitamin B$_{12}$ is to improve the symptoms of pernicious anemia. These symptoms include weakness, pallor, and neurologic symptoms such as burning or prickling of the hands and feet, loss of balance, confusion, loss of memory, and moodiness.

Recent studies suggest a role for vitamin B$_{12}$ in the prevention of heart disease. Patients taking a combination of folic acid, vitamin B$_{12}$, and vitamin B$_6$ lowered their blood levels of homocysteine, a substance that seems to be associated with a higher risk of heart disease.

■ DIETARY SOURCES

Vitamin B$_{12}$ is present in foods containing animal protein. The richest sources of it are liver and kidney. Other good sources of vitamin B$_{12}$ include milk, eggs, fish, and cheese.

■ OTHER FORMS

Vitamin B$_{12}$ can be found in vitamin form as cyanocobalamin. It is available as tablets, softgels, or lozenges in multivitamin form (including children's chewable and liquid drops), B-complex form, or by itself.

■ HOW TO TAKE IT

To avoid disorders of vitamin B$_{12}$ deficiency, adults should get 2.0 mcg of vitamin B$_{12}$ daily. People whose daily diet includes meat, milk, and other dairy products should be able to meet the 2.0 mcg recommended daily requirement without taking a vitamin supplement. Vegetarians who do not eat animal protein products should take a vitamin supplement with water, preferably after eating. Pregnant women should get 2.2 mcg of vitamin B$_{12}$ daily and women who are breast-feeding should get 2.6 mcg of vitamin B$_{12}$ daily. As with all medications and supplements, check with your health care provider before giving vitamin B$_{12}$ supplements to a child. Elderly people may need more than 2.0 mcg of vitamin B$_{12}$ daily because of decreasing ability to absorb vitamin B$_{12}$ from our diet as we age. Elderly people should check with their health care provider to find out what dosage best fits their needs.

■ PRECAUTIONS

Vitamin B$_{12}$ is non-toxic, but there is no known benefit to healthy individuals of taking more than the 2.0 mcg recommended daily allowance.

■ POSSIBLE INTERACTIONS

Vitamin B$_{12}$ can have its absorption decreased by the drug metformin, which is used to treat hyperglycemia (high blood sugar). It also can be destroyed by megadoses (500 mg or greater) of vitamin C.

■ VITAMIN C (ASCORBIC ACID)

Your body does not store vitamin C so you must consume enough each day to maintain good health. Vitamin C is needed for the growth and repair of tissues in all parts of your body. It is necessary to form collagen, an important protein used to make skin, scar tissue, tendons, ligaments, and blood vessels. Because of this, your body uses a lot of vitamin C to repair wounds. Vitamin C is also needed to form and repair cartilage, bones, and teeth. Large amounts of vitamin C are used by your body during any kind of healing process, whether it's from a cold, infection, disease, injury, or surgery. In these cases you may need extra vitamin C. Vitamin C helps reduce the damage to the body caused by toxic chemicals and pollutants like drugs and cigarette smoke. Smokers especially need extra vitamin C. Research has shown that vitamin C can help prevent cancer and is necessary for a healthy immune system. It also helps maintain good vision as you get older.

■ USES

Vitamin C can have many positive effects on your body, including the following.

- Boosts immune system functions
- Protects against cancer
- Necessary for wound healing
- Helps prevent cataracts
- Increases HDL (good) cholesterol
- Decreases risk of heart disease
- Reduces blood pressure
- Useful in treating allergies
- Maintains healthy blood vessels
- Counteracts asthma spasms
- Helps overcome male infertility
- Helps protect diabetics against long-term complications
- Protects against sunburn and its effects.
- Can assist treatment of bleeding gums, easy bruising, and arthritis
- Assists treatment of arthritis and other inflammatory conditions

If you eat many cured, processed, or preserved meats like bacon, sausage, ham, hot dogs, or sliced luncheon meat, you should know that Vitamin C helps prevent these foods from forming cancer-causing "nitrosamines" in the stomach. It's a good idea to eat foods rich in vitamin C, or take vitamin C supplements, at the same time you eat processed meats.

■ DIETARY SOURCES

Vitamin C is present in many fruits and vegetables. Foods that are excellent sources of vitamin C include orange juice, green peppers, watermelon, papaya, grapefruit, cantaloupe, strawberries, mango, broccoli, tomato juice, brussels sprouts, cauliflower, and cabbage. Vitamin C is also found in raw and cooked leafy greens (turnip greens, spinach), canned and fresh tomatoes, potatoes, winter squash, raspberries, and pineapple. Vitamin C is sensitive to light, air, and heat. Eating vegetables raw, or minimally cooked, increases their vitamin C content.

■ OTHER FORMS

You can purchase either natural or synthetic vitamin C, also called ascorbic acid, in a wide variety of supplement forms. Tablets, capsules, and chewable tablets are probably the most popular, but vitamin C also comes in powdered crystalline, effervescent tablet and liquid form. You can purchase dosages ranging from 25 mg to 1,000 mg per tablet. "Buffered" vitamin C is available if you find that regular ascorbic acid bothers your stomach. "Ester-C" is a form of vitamin C which the manufacturer claims is better absorbed by the body. Laboratory testing concluded that this claim is not true, and has shown that regular vitamin C is absorbed just as well.

■ HOW TO TAKE IT

Vitamin C is not stored in the body, so it must be replaced as it gets used. The best way to take supplements is with meals two or three times per day, depending on the dosage. The Recommended Daily Allowance (RDA) of vitamin C is 60 mg for adults, 70 mg for pregnant women, 95 mg for breast-feeding women, 100 mg for smokers, 40 mg for young children, and 50 mg for older children. Some studies suggest that adults should take between 250 mg and 500 mg twice a day for maximum benefit. Be sure to check with your health care provider before taking more than 1,000 mg of vitamin C on a daily basis.

■ PRECAUTIONS

Vitamin C is generally non-toxic. In high doses (more than 2,000 mg daily) it can cause diarrhea, gas, or stomach upset. Check with your health care provider before taking vitamin C supplements if you have any kidney problems. Infants born to mothers taking 6 g or more of vitamin C may develop rebound scurvy due to sudden drop in daily intake.

■ POSSIBLE INTERACTIONS

Vitamin C can have the following affects in the body.

- Increases iron absorption from food and iron supplements or multivitamin/mineral supplements
- Decreases copper absorption
- Interferes with blood test for vitamin B_{12}, inform your provider if you are having blood tests and you take extra vitamin C
- No known adverse interactions with any drugs or herbs

Vitamin C is used by the liver to detoxify drugs and other chemicals. If you are currently taking regular medication, check with your health care provider before starting any vitamin supplements.

■ VITAMIN D

Vitamin D is essential to build and maintain healthy bones throughout life. Calcium, the main element of bone, can be absorbed into the body only when vitamin D is present. Vitamin D and calcium are involved in many body functions, including keeping your immune and nervous systems healthy.

■ USES

Getting enough vitamin D can help prevent a number of serious health conditions, including those listed below.

- Osteoporosis: a preventable condition of soft, fragile, easily fractured bones. Vitamin D protects against the preventable bone diseases of rickets, osteomalacia, osteoporosis, and osteopenia. Seniors in northern climates and people who do not receive direct sunlight daily need to take a vitamin D supplement to keep their bones strong. Calcium supplements will not help prevent or treat osteoporosis if your vitamin D level is low.
- Cancer: Vitamin D is involved in cell growth and has been shown to decrease the growth of leukemia, colon cancer, skin cancer, and breast cancer cells. Researchers have found that people with adequate levels of vitamin D have a lowered risk of prostate and colorectal cancers.
- Diabetes: Vitamin D may help regulate blood sugar to prevent diabetes or to help control it.
- Multiple sclerosis: Vitamin D may help protect against this condition.
- Heart disease: Vitamin D may help prevent hardening of the arteries (arteriosclerosis) and lower blood pressure.

Vitamin D is also helpful in the following ways.
- Helps control blood sugar
- May help an overactive parathyroid
- Reduces cartilage damage in people with osteoarthritis and may decrease the severity of rheumatoid arthritis
- Has been successful in treating psoriasis

You may benefit from taking a vitamin D supplement if the following applies to you.
- You are on anticonvulsant drug therapy or glucocorticoid therapy.
- You eat a strict vegan diet.

■ DIETARY SOURCES

Foods that contain vitamin D include the following.
- Cod liver oil
- Salmon
- Tuna
- Fortified milk
- Oysters
- Mushrooms
- Fortified cereals
- Egg yolk

Sunlight is a natural source of vitamin D. If you are fair-skinned, 20 to 30 minutes a day in bright sunlight will meet your vitamin D needs. If you are dark-skinned, you need three hours to get the same benefit. Clouds, smog, clothing, sunscreen, and window glass all decrease the amount of vitamin D you get from sunlight.

■ OTHER FORMS

Vitamin D is included in many multivitamins. It can be found in over-the-counter preparations in strengths from 50 IU to 1,000 IU as softgel capsules, tablets, and liquid. Higher-dose prescription preparations are available. If you have trouble digesting fat, vitamin D injections are also available by prescription.

■ HOW TO TAKE IT

To prevent disease, adults who do not get regular exposure to bright sunlight should take between 200 IU and 400 IU daily. Discuss your supplement regimen regularly with your health care provider. As with all medications, check with your health care provider before giving vitamin D to a child.

■ PRECAUTIONS

Taking too much vitamin D (more than 1,000 IU daily) can make you very ill. Symptoms include excessive thirst, metal taste, bone pain, tiredness, sore eyes, itching skin, vomiting, diarrhea, a need to urinate, and muscle problems. Getting too much sunlight will not give you too much vitamin D.

Check with your doctor before taking vitamin D if you have high blood calcium or phosphorus levels or if you have a cardiac or kidney disease.

■ POSSIBLE INTERACTIONS

The following decreases the amount of vitamin D you get.
- Cholestyramine
- Mineral oil
- Alcohol
- Some anticonvulsant therapies

You may also have mineral imbalances from using vitamin D if you take magnesium-containing antacids, digitalis glycosides, verapamil, and thiazide diuretics. For more information about vitamin D, talk with your health care provider.

■ VITAMIN E

Research has shown that vitamin E helps the body ward off many diseases, and it protects cells from certain kinds of damage, which helps them live longer. The effect of this protection over time is that vitamin E helps slow down the cell damage that happens naturally as we age.

■ USES

Vitamin E protects the body against some disorders and helps treat others. This is a partial list of these disorders.

- Cancer. Vitamin E plays an important role in cancer treatment, including cancers of the skin, mouth and throat, stomach, colon, breast, and prostate gland. It may also reduce the risk of cancers of the lung, esophagus, and cervix. Vitamin E seems to interfere with the oxygen-controlled signals that make cancer cells grow. It also protects normal cells from the damaging effects of chemotherapy, but leaves cancer cells vulnerable.
- Heart attacks and strokes. Research suggests that vitamin E helps prevent arteries from clogging by blocking the conversion of cholesterol into its most dangerous form. Vitamin E is also a powerful anti-clotting agent, which helps blood flow more easily through arteries when fatty plaques (fat deposits that stick to blood vessel walls) are present.
- Immune system disorders. These disorders lower the body's defenses against illness, but vitamin E can bring your level of immunity up again.
- Aging-related diseases. Vitamin E can prevent the progress of these diseases, such as Alzheimer's disease, which can cause physical and mental decline.
- Cataracts and macular degeneration. Vitamin E can counteract these conditions, which affect your eyesight and can lead to blindness.
- Diabetes. Vitamin E can help reduce the risk of heart disease in people with diabetes.

Vitamin E also helps in other ways.
- Slows the aging of all cells and tissues
- Protects against environmental pollutants
- Keeps red blood cells healthy and helps prevent anemia
- Treats disorders related to trouble digesting fats
- Serves in the treatment of most skin diseases
- Helps wounds heal faster
- Promotes the treatment of reproductive disorders
- Reduces premenstrual discomforts
- Decreases symptoms of lupus

■ DIETARY SOURCES

Foods that contain a significant amount of vitamin E include: nuts (including almonds, hazelnuts, and walnuts) as well as sunflower seeds, corn-oil margarine, mayonnaise, cold-pressed vegetable oils, including corn, safflower, soybean, cottonseed, canola, and wheat germ (the richest one), spinach and kale, sweet potatoes, and yams.

■ OTHER FORMS

You can choose between natural and synthetic forms of vitamin E. Health care providers usually recommend natural vitamin E (d-alpha-tocopherol). The synthetic form is called dl-alpha-tocopherol.

Vitamin E comes as softgels, tablets and capsules. You will find them in doses that include 50 IU, 100 IU, 200 IU, 400 IU, 500 IU, 600 IU, and 1,000 IU.

For people who have trouble digesting fats, vitamin E succinate ("dry-E") is best.

■ HOW TO TAKE IT

For the prevention and treatment of disease, adults should take between 200 IU and 400 IU of vitamin E daily with water, preferably after eating.

As with all medicines and supplements, check with a health care provider before giving vitamin E supplements to a child.

■ PRECAUTIONS

Vitamin E is generally nontoxic. In high doses (more than 1,200 IU daily) it can cause nausea, gas, diarrhea, and heart palpitations.

Check with your health care provider before taking vitamin E under the following conditions.
- If you have high blood pressure
- If you are taking blood-thinners such as coumadin or warfarin

■ POSSIBLE INTERACTIONS

Possible interactions involving vitamin E include:
- Inhibits the absorption of vitamin K which promotes clotting of blood
- Can increase the risk of abnormal bleeding in people taking anti-coagulants
- Can be destroyed by iron supplements, can have its absorption decreased by the drugs cholestyramine and colestipol
- Enhances the use of the body's vitamin A supplies; excess intake of vitamin E can deplete vitamin A stores in the body
- Is enhanced by selenium, a trace element in foods
- Is depleted by heavy alcohol use

◾ VITAMIN H (BIOTIN)

Vitamin H, more commonly known as biotin, enables the body to use the energy in food. Biotin is also important to cell health and reproduction. People with diabetes may improve their blood sugar control with biotin. Hair and nails also need biotin to be healthy.

◾ USES

Here is a partial list of the health problems biotin helps treat.

- Diabetes. Biotin supplements may help improve blood sugar control in people with diabetes by improving insulin usage and increasing blood sugar usage.
- Hair and nails. Biotin supplements may improve thin or splitting toenails or fingernails and improve hair health. Biotin has also been used to combat premature graying of hair, though it is likely to be useful only for those with a low biotin level.
- Genetic problems. Some babies cannot use biotin well and need biotin supplements.
- Skin problems. Some skin disorders, such as "cradle cap," improve with biotin supplements.
- Muscular dystrophy. Biotin has been used as part of the treatment for certain types of this muscle-related illness.
- Nutritional health. Biotin has been used for people in weight-loss programs to help them metabolize fat more efficiently.
- Infections. Biotin has been used to treat intestinal candidiasis (a yeast infection).

◾ DIETARY SOURCES

These foods contain a significant amount of biotin.

- Liver
- Nuts
- Kidney
- Egg yolks
- Brewer's yeast
- Chocolate
- Whole grain products
- Beans
- Fish

Food-processing techniques can destroy biotin. Less-processed versions of the foods listed above will contain more biotin.

◾ OTHER FORMS

Biotin is available in multivitamin and B-vitamin complexes, and as individual supplements.

Standard preparations are available in 10 mcg, 50 mcg, and 100 mcg tablets and contain either simple biotin or a complex with brewer's yeast.

◾ HOW TO TAKE IT

Your body makes biotin in the intestines, so a recommended dietary requirement (RDA) has not been set. An adequate amount of biotin is about 30 to 100 mcg daily. Most Americans get 28 to 42 mcg daily. Doses of up to 2,500 mcg have been used safely to treat hair and nail problems.

As with all medicines and supplements, check with your health care provider before giving biotin supplements to a child.

◾ PRECAUTIONS

Biotin is nontoxic. No side effects have been noted, even with high doses.

◾ POSSIBLE INTERACTIONS

- Works best when taken with B-vitamins
- May lessen the symptoms of pantothenic acid and zinc deficiencies
- Is not absorbed in the presence of raw egg whites
- Requirements may rise if a person takes sulfa drugs or estrogen or drinks alcohol
- Deficiency may result from prolonged use of anticonvulsant drugs or long-term use of antibiotics

For more information about biotin, talk with your health care provider.

▪ VITAMIN K

Vitamin K is best known for its role in helping blood clot properly, and in preventing excessive bleeding. It also plays an important role in bone health.

▪ USES

Vitamin K protects the body against the following.

- Bleeding. Vitamin K is used to reduce risk of bleeding in liver disease, jaundice, malabsorption, or in association with long-term use of aspirin or antibiotics. Vitamin K has been used in the treatment of heavy menstrual bleeding, and with vitamin C to treat morning sickness. Babies are sometimes given a vitamin K injection soon after birth, because in certain cases, such as in premature infants, they are at increased risk for bleeding.
- Osteoporosis. Vitamin K is needed for bones to use calcium. Vitamin K supplements may improve bone mass in postmenopausal women. Vitamin K deficiency is linked to osteoporosis because low levels have been found in those with the condition. Supplements of vitamin K have been used to treat osteoporosis.

Vitamin K also helps in the following ways.
- Vitamin K may prevent kidney stones.
- A vitamin K analog, K compound 5, may stop liver cancer growth.
- Some forms (water-soluble chlorophyll) help control body, fecal, and urinary odor.
- Water-soluble forms are used to treat skin wounds.

▪ DIETARY SOURCES

Foods that contain a significant amount of vitamin K include chlorophyll, green tea, turnip greens, broccoli, spinach, cabbage, asparagus, and dark green lettuce.

Freezing foods may destroy vitamin K, but heating does not affect it.

▪ OTHER FORMS

- Vitamin K supplements are available in both natural and synthetic forms.
- Supplements of fat-soluble chlorophyll are an excellent source of vitamin K.
- Water-soluble chlorophyll is the most common form of vitamin K

found over the counter. The water-soluble form is not absorbed into the body, and is useful for treatment of skin, and to reduce body odor.
- Vitamin K is available in multivitamin complexes, and as 5-mg tablets.

▪ HOW TO TAKE IT

The recommended dietary allowance (RDA) for vitamin K is 80 mcg for men, and 65 mcg for women. To help prevent and treat disease, increase the amount of dark green leafy vegetables you eat, and supplement your diet with up to 500 mcg of vitamin K each day.

As with all medications and supplements, check with a health care provider before giving vitamin K supplements to a child.

▪ PRECAUTIONS

- Vitamin K can interfere with the action of anticoagulants such as warfarin or coumadin.
- X-rays and radiation can raise vitamin K requirements.
- Vitamin K is excreted in breast milk, and crosses the placenta. Pregnant women and women who are breast-feeding should consult their health care provider before starting vitamin K supplements.
- Your body may need more vitamin K if you are taking aspirin, cholestyramine, phentoin, or mineral oil laxatives.
- Some snake venoms destroy vitamin K, which helps blood clot properly. Vitamin K may be injected to stop the bleeding from snakebite.
- Extended use of antibiotics may result in vitamin K deficiency. These drugs kill not only harmful bacteria, but also beneficial, vitamin K-activating bacteria.

▪ POSSIBLE INTERACTIONS

- Natural vitamin K taken orally is generally nontoxic.
- Large doses of the synthetic form of vitamin K, which you may get to prevent bleeding in certain conditions, may cause anemia and liver damage.
- Injections of vitamin K can cause flushing, sweats, chest pain, and constricted breathing.
- Blood problems, jaundice, and liver problems have been seen in newborns after they are given vitamin K.
- Intramuscular injections of vitamin K may cause pain, swelling, and eczema.

■ ZINC

Zinc is an essential trace mineral, which, next to iron, is the second most abundant trace mineral in the body. Zinc is stored primarily in muscle but is also found in red and white blood cells, the retina of the eye, bones, skin, kidneys, liver, and pancreas. In men, the prostate gland contains more zinc than any other organ.

Recent research has attempted to determine the true value of zinc lozenges in preventing or reducing cold symptoms, with some studies showing good results. You can buy zinc lozenges in any pharmacy now to treat the common cold.

■ USES

Zinc supplements can help the body in the following ways.
- Helps prevent cancer
- Prevents and treats colds
- Boosts the activity of immune system
- Speeds healing of wounds
- Treats and may prevent acne
- May prevent macular degeneration (eyesight deterioration that happens as people age)
- Treats some cases of anorexia nervosa (anorexia is a symptom of zinc deficiency, and the teenage population is at higher risk for zinc deficiency due to poor dietary habits)
- Improves male fertility, especially among smokers
- Treats rheumatoid arthritis (may have anti-inflammatory effects)
- Treats Wilson's disease (a disorder of excess copper storage)
- Decreases changes in the sense of taste during cancer treatments
- Heightens sense of taste and smell

Some conditions may affect how your body absorbs zinc, or may increase your need for zinc. If you have one of the following conditions, you may benefit from zinc supplements.
- Acrodermatitis eteropathica (the inherited disease that causes zinc malabsorption)
- Alcoholism
- Diabetes
- Kidney disease
- Celiac disease
- Inflammatory bowel disease, ulcerative colitis
- Chronic diarrhea
- Pancreatic conditions
- Prostate problems (BPH, prostatitis, cancer)

Women who are pregnant or are breast-feeding, and those who take oral contraceptives may also have an increased need for zinc.

■ DIETARY SOURCES

We absorb 20 to 40 percent of the zinc that is in our food. Zinc from animal foods like red meat, fish, and poultry is the most readily absorbed form. Zinc in vegetables is less available to our bodies, and vegetable fiber itself lessens how much zinc we can absorb and use. Dairy products and eggs contain fair amounts of zinc, but it is less easily absorbed from these sources.

The following foods are the best sources of usable zinc: oysters (richest source), red meats, shrimp, crab, and other shellfish.

Other good, though less easily absorbed sources, include legumes (especially lima beans, black-eyed peas, pinto beans, soybeans, peanuts), whole grains, miso, tofu, brewer's yeast, cooked greens, mushrooms, green beans, and pumpkin seeds.

■ OTHER FORMS

Zinc sulfate is the most frequently used supplement. This is the least expensive form, but it is the least easily absorbed and may cause stomach upset. Health care providers usually prescribe 220 mg zinc sulfate, which contains approximately 55 mg of elemental zinc. More easily absorbed forms are available: zinc picolinate, zinc citrate, zinc acetate, zinc glycerate, and zinc monomethionine.

These different forms contain different amounts of zinc in the "compound." Always look for the "amount of elemental zinc" listed in milligrams on the label. Usually this will be between 30 and 50 mg of elemental zinc. Remember that you take in about 10 to 15 mg of zinc from food every day. Your health care provider should take this into account when prescribing how much supplemental zinc you should take. Zinc lozenges are also available in most drug stores and grocery stores, and are used for treating colds. Zinc lozenges are also available for the treatment of colds.

■ HOW TO TAKE IT

Talk to your health care provider or nutritionist before you take zinc supplements. You get the most benefit from zinc supplements if you take them with water or juice (not milk) in between meals, and don't take them at the same time that you take iron or calcium supplements. If this bothers your stomach, you can take the zinc with a meal.

■ PRECAUTIONS

Most trace minerals are toxic if you take too much, and this is true of zinc. Symptoms of toxicity are stomach upset and vomiting, usually occurring if 2,000 mg or more has been swallowed. Studies have stated that up to 150 mg is fairly safe, but that much is usually not needed and may interfere with your body's use of other minerals. Research has shown that less than 50 mg a day is a safe amount to take over time, but researchers are not sure what happens if you take more than that over a long period. Talk with your health care provider before taking zinc or any other supplement.

One known negative side effect of too much zinc is that it lowers HDL (good) cholesterol and raises LDL (bad) cholesterol. Some research has shown that megadoses of zinc lower immune function, but other studies have not confirmed this. If zinc sulfate causes stomach irritation, try another form, such as zinc citrate. Check with your health care provider first. Other reported side effects of zinc toxicity are dizziness, headache, drowsiness, increased sweating, uncoordination of muscles, alcohol intolerance, hallucinations, and anemia.

■ POSSIBLE INTERACTIONS

Because zinc interacts with some other nutrients, you may want to take a multivitamin or mineral preparation that contains zinc, copper, iron, and folate. This will help keep these nutrients in balance with one another. Too much zinc can interfere with copper absorption and cause a copper deficiency. This affects the iron status in your body and can lead to anemia. Too much copper and too much iron interfere with zinc absorption. Zinc interferes with folate absorption. Talk with you health care provider before taking zinc or any other supplement.

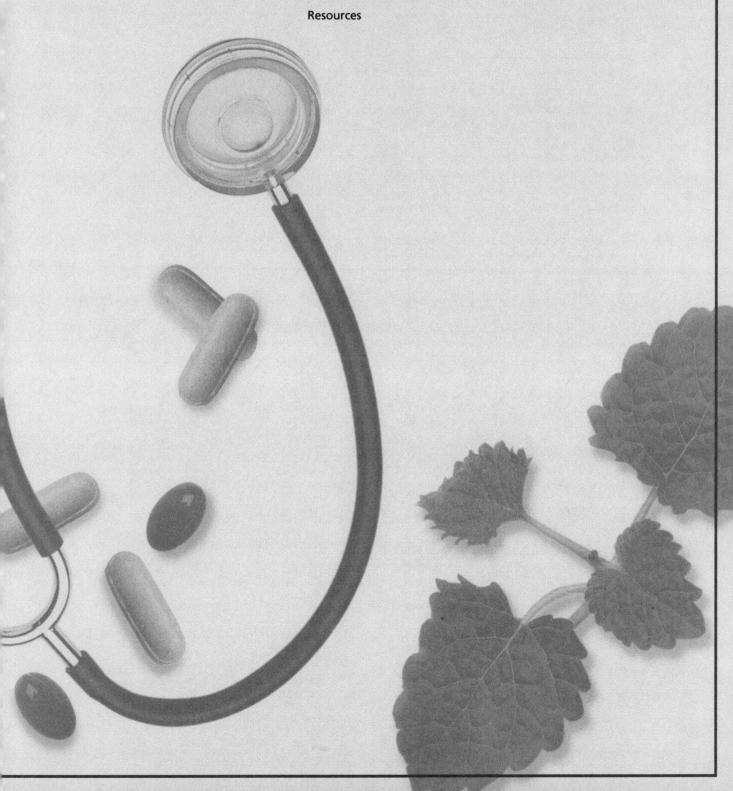

QUICK Access

APPENDICES

Quick Reference Guide

Resources

This comprehensive Quick Reference Guide allows for a quick search of category lists drawn from the *Quick Access* monographs. At a glance, you can review the herbs or supplements used in treating a particular condition, the contraindications of using a particular herb or supplement, and much more. Once you have found what you are looking for in the Quick Reference Guide, refer to the appropriate monograph for detail.

As an example, you may care to quickly review all of the herbs and supplements that may be used to treat benign prostatic hyperplasia. Using one of the many search lists included, you will find a list that includes vitamins, amino acids, herbs, and micro-nutrients. Reference back to the monograph on BPH to review more detail, or reference back to the monograph on the individual herb or supplement mentioned. The majority of those most often used or prescribed herbs and supplements are currently in the *Quick Access* monograph system, with future editions supplying even more.

There are thirteen separate lists that can be searched in this Quick Reference Guide, allowing easy and targeted access to the information you are looking for.

- Conditions by Medical Category
- Conditions by Signs and Symptoms
- Conditions by Herb and Supplement Treatment Options
- Herbs by Uses and Indications
- Herbs by Warnings, Precautions, Contraindications
- Herbs by Side Effects
- Herbs by Interactions with Other Drugs, Herbs, Supplements
- Herbs by Taxonomic Cross-Reference
- Supplements by Uses and Indications
- Supplements by Warnings, Precautions, Contraindications
- Supplements by Side Effects
- Supplements by Interactions with Other Drugs, Herbs, Supplements
- Combined Herb and Supplement Treatment Options by Condition

■ CONDITIONS BY MEDICAL CATEGORY

This list takes the condition monograph topics and organizes them into respective medical systems or categories.

BRAIN AND NERVOUS SYSTEM CONDITIONS
dementia
headache, migraine
headache, sinus
headache, tension
Parkinson's disease
seizure disorders

DIGESTION AND ABSORPTION CONDITIONS
cirrhosis of the liver
constipation
diarrhea
dysphagia
gallbladder disease
gastritis
gastroesophageal reflux disease
hepatitis, viral
intestinal parasites
irritable bowel syndrome
peptic ulcer
ulcerative colitis

ENDOCRINE CONDITIONS
diabetes mellitus
hyperthyroidism
hypothyroidism
thyroiditis

EYE/EAR/NOSE/THROAT CONDITIONS
allergic rhinitis
conjunctivitis
laryngitis
otitis media
pharyngitis
sinusitis

GENITOURINARY CONDITIONS
benign prostatic hyperplasia
prostatitis
urethritis
urinary incontinence
urolithiasis

GYNECOLOGIC CONDITIONS
amenorrhea
dysmenorrhea
endometriosis
menopause
preeclampsia
urinary tract infection in women
vaginitis

HEART and CIRCULATORY CONDITIONS
angina
atherosclerosis
congestive heart failure
hypertension
endocarditis
myocardial infarction
pericarditis

INFECTIOUS DISEASES
candidiasis
herpes zoster (varicella-zoster) virus
herpes simplex virus
HIV and AIDS
Reiter's syndrome
Roseola

INTEGUMENTARY CONDITIONS
alopecia
burns
cutaneous drug reactions
dermatitis
eczema
insect bites
psoriasis
warts

MUSCULOSKELETAL CONDITIONS
bursitis
gout
low back pain
osteoarthritis
osteomyelitis
osteoporosis
rheumatoid arthritis
sprains and strains
tendinitis

PSYCHIATRIC CONDITIONS
anorexia nervosa
anxiety
depression-unipolar mood disorders

PULMONARY CONDITIONS
asthma
bronchitis
chronic obstructive pulmonary disease
common cold
cough
influenza
pertussis
primary pulmonary hypertension
pulmonary edema

OTHER CONDITIONS
anemia
attention-deficit/hyperactivity disorder
chronic fatigue syndrome
edema
fever of unknown origin
fibromyalgia syndrome
food allergy
hemorrhoids
hypercholesterolemia
hyperkalemia
hypoglycemia
infantile colic
insomnia
motion sickness
obesity
Raynaud's phenomenon
sexual dysfunction
sleep apnea

■ CONDITIONS BY SIGNS AND SYMPTOMS

This list extracts the individual signs and symptoms included in each condition monograph and combines them to create a collection of all medical conditions that may be considered when a particular sign or symptom presents.

ABDOMINAL CRAMPING
allergic rhinitis
diarrhea
food allergy
insect bites
ulcerative colitis

ABDOMINAL CRAMPING, LOW
dysmenorrhea
irritable bowel syndrome
urinary tract infection in women

ABDOMINAL DISCOMFORT
hepatitis, viral

ABDOMINAL PAIN
anemia
cirrhosis of the liver
gastritis
HIV and AIDS
hypercholesterolemia
seizures

ABDOMINAL PAIN, LOW
benign prostatic hyperplasia

ABDOMINAL PAIN, RADIATING ANTERIORLY
urolithiasis

ABDOMINAL PAIN, UPPER RIGHT
preeclampsia

ABDOMINAL SWELLING
constrictive pericarditis

ABDOMINAL TENDERNESS
endometriosis

ABSCESS
candidiasis

ABSCESS, TISSUE AROUND PAINFUL BONE
osteomyelitis

ABSENTMINDEDNESS
seizures

ACHE RADIATING TO LOWER BACK, GROIN, LEGS
dysmenorrhea

ACHILLES TENDINITIS
Reiter's syndrome

ACNE
amenorrhea

ACNEIFORMS
cutaneous drug reactions

AGITATION
hyperthyroidism, thyroid storm

AGNOSIA
dementia

ALERTNESS, CHANGE IN
sleep apnea

ALLERGIES
chronic fatigue syndrome

ALLODYNIA
fibromyalgia syndrome

AMENORRHEA
menopause

ANAL FISSURES
hemorrhoids

ANAL INFECTIONS
herpes simplex virus, genital

ANAPHYLAXIS
insect bites

ANEMIA
ulcerative colitis

ANEMIA, NORMOCHROMIC
rheumatoid arthritis

ANEMIA, NORMOCYTIC
rheumatoid arthritis

ANGINA
anemia
pulmonary edema

ANGIOEDEMA
food allergy
insect bites

ANGIOMAS, SPIDER
cirrhosis of the liver

ANOREXIA
amenorrhea
cirrhosis of the liver
congestive heart failure
gallbladder disease
gastritis
hepatitis, viral
pericarditis
pertussis
Reiter's syndrome
ulcerative colitis

ANTERIOR FONTANELLE, BULGING
roseola

ANXIETY
congestive heart failure
dementia
hypoglycemia
myocardial infarction
pericarditis
pulmonary edema
sexual dysfunction

ANXIETY, ANTICIPATORY
insomnia

AORTITIS
Reiter's syndrome

APHASIA
dementia
endocarditis

APHONIA
laryngitis

APNEA
pertussis
seizures

APNEA SYNDROME, INFANTS
gastroesophageal reflux disease

APPETITE, INCREASED
hyperthyroidism

APPETITE LOSS
allergic rhinitis
severe herpes simplex virus
neonatal herpes simplex virus
oral-facial herpes zoster
 (varicella-zoster)
influenza

APRAXIA
dementia

ARCHED BACK AND CLENCHED FISTS
infantile colic

ARRHYTHMIA
myocardial infarction
Reiter's syndrome

ARTERIES, HARDENED FEEL OF
atherosclerosis

ARTHRALGIAS
chronic fatigue syndrome
hepatitis, viral
ulcerative colitis

ARTHRITIC DISORDERS
Reiter's syndrome

ARTHRITIS (THREE JOINTS OR MORE)
rheumatoid arthritis

ARTHUS REACTION
insect bites

ASCITES, PORTAL HYPERTENSION
cirrhosis of the liver

ASPIRATION
dysphagia, oropharyngeal

ASPIRATION, RECURRENT
gastroesophageal reflux disease

ASTHMA
insect bites

ASYMMETRICAL SIGNS
Reiter's syndrome

AURA
migraine headache
seizures

AUTOMATISMS
seizures

AVERSION TO CIGARETTES
hepatitis, viral

BACK PAIN
anemia
endocarditis
low back pain
osteoporosis
prostatitis

BACK PAIN, PERSISTENT
osteomyelitis

BALANCE, POOR
Parkinson's disease

BALDNESS, FEMALE DIFFUSE
alopecia

BALDNESS, MALE PATTERN
alopecia

BALD PATCHES
alopecia

BELCHING
gastroesophageal reflux disease
infantile colic

BILIARY COLIC
gallbladder disease

BIZARRE BEHAVIOR
hypoglycemia

BLADDER FUNCTION PAIN
endometriosis

BLADDER OUTLET OBSTRUCTION
benign prostatic hyperplasia
prostatitis

BLEPHAROSPASM
Parkinson's disease

BLINDNESS
herpes simplex virus, eye

BLINKING, INFREQUENT
hyperthyroidism

BLISTERS
burns
dermatitis
psoriasis

BLOATING
constipation
edema
intestinal parasites
irritable bowel syndrome

BLOOD PRESSURE, HIGH
preeclampsia
seizures

BLOOD PRESSURE, RAPID DROP
food allergy

BLOOD PRESSURE ABNORMALITIES
amenorrhea

BLURRED VISION
diabetes
herpes simplex virus
HIV and AIDS
hypoglycemia

**BODY-MASS INDEX (BMI)
OVER 25 OR 30**
obesity

**BONE PAIN AND SENSATION
OF HEAT**
osteomyelitis

BONY CREPITUS
osteoarthritis

BONY HYPERTROPHY
osteoarthritis

**BOWEL EMPTYING,
INCOMPLETE**
constipation
irritable bowel syndrome

BOWEL FUNCTION PAIN
endometriosis

BOWEL HABIT CHANGES
irritable bowel syndrome

**BOWEL MOVEMENT, RELIEF
OF PAIN AFTER**
irritable bowel syndrome

**BOWEL MOVEMENT, UPON
WAKING OR AFTER EATING**
irritable bowel syndrome

**BOWEL MOVEMENTS,
DIFFICULTY**
constipation

**BOWEL MOVEMENTS, MUCUS
DISCHARGE**
ulcerative colitis

BRADYKINESIA
Parkinson's disease

BREAST ENLARGEMENT
amenorrhea

BREATH, SHORTNESS OF
asthma
bronchitis
food allergy
endocarditis

BREATHING DIFFICULTY
edema
HIV and AIDS
hyperkalemia
laryngitis
Parkinson's disease
pharyngitis

BREATHING SPLINTED
pericarditis

**BRONCHIAL INFECTION,
RECURRENT**
chronic obstructive
  pulmonary disease

**BRONCHITIS-LIKE
SYMPTOMS**
pertussis

BRONCHOSPASM
gastroesophageal reflux disease

BRUIT, OVER THYROID GLAND
hyperthyroidism

BRUIT OVER NARROWED VESSEL
atherosclerosis

CARDIOVASCULAR FAILURE
insect bites

CARPAL TUNNEL SYNDROME
hypothyroidism

CERVICAL ADENOPATHY
herpes simplex virus, oral-facial

CERVICAL LESIONS
herpes simplex virus, genital

CERVICITIS
urethritis in women

CHEST, BURNING SENSATION
bronchitis

CHEST, HYPERINFLATED
asthma

**CHEST, PRESSURE
SENSATION**
dysphagia, esophageal

CHEST PAIN
angina
atherosclerosis
gastroesophageal reflux disease
HIV and AIDS
myocardial infarction
pericarditis

CHEST PAIN, PLEURITIC
primary pulmonary hypertension

CHEST TIGHTNESS
asthma
pulmonary edema

CHILLS
chronic fatigue syndrome
cough
diarrhea
gout
endocarditis
influenza
pharyngitis
prostatitis
urinary tract infection in women
urolithiasis

CHOKING
dysphagia
oropharyngeal
pertussis

CIRCINATE BALANITIS
Reiter's syndrome

CIRCULATORY COLLAPSE
herpes simplex virus, neonatal

CIRRHOSIS
amenorrhea

CIRRHOSIS OF LIVER
alcoholism

COLD, DAMP WEATHER PAIN
sinus headache

**COLD AND CYANOSED FEET
AND HANDS**
migraine headache

COLD HANDS AND FEET
menopause

COLD INTOLERANCE
hypothyroidism

COMA
diabetes
hypoglycemia
seizures

CONCENTRATION, IMPAIRED
anxiety
chronic fatigue syndrome
depression-unipolar mood
  disorders

CONFUSION
hyperthyroidism
hypothyroidism

CONGESTIVE HEART FAILURE
cough

CONJUNCTIVITIS
herpes simplex virus, eye
Reiter's syndrome

CONSCIOUSNESS, ALTERING
pericardial effusion

CONSCIOUSNESS, LOSS OF
seizures

CONSCIOUSNESS, LOSS OF, INFANTS
pertussis

CONSTANT MOTION TO LESSEN PAIN
urolithiasis

CONSTANT STARE
hyperthyroidism

CONSTIPATION
dysmenorrhea
hemorrhoids
hypothyroidism
irritable bowel syndrome
Parkinson's disease
seizures

CORNEAL LESIONS
herpes simplex virus, eye

CORNEAL ULCERATION
Reiter's syndrome

CORONARY HEART DISEASE
menopause

COSTOCHONDRITIS
Reiter's syndrome

COUGH
asthma
chronic obstructive pulmonary
  disease
common cold
HIV and AIDS
endocarditis
primary pulmonary hypertension
sinusitis
sleep apnea

COUGH, BLOOD
edema

COUGH, CHRONIC
gastroesophageal reflux disease

COUGH, INCREASING
pertussis

**COUGH, MUCUS OR PUS
PRODUCED BY**
bronchitis

COUGH, NONPRODUCTIVE
influenza

COUGH, ORTHOPNEIC
congestive heart failure

COUGH, RESIDUAL
pertussis

COUGH, WHILE SWALLOWING
dysphagia, oropharyngeal

COUGH PAROXYSMS
pertussis

CREPITUS
tendinitis

CRYING, INFANT
otitis media

CRYING, INCONSOLABLE
infantile colic

CUSHING'S SYNDROME
amenorrhea

CUTANEOUS DISEASE
candidiasis

CYANOSIS
asthma
bronchitis
chronic obstructive pulmonary disease
herpes simplex virus, neonatal
pericardial effusion
pulmonary edema
Raynaud's phenomenon
seizures

CYSTITIS
Reiter's syndrome

DEATH THOUGHTS
depression-unipolar mood
  disorders

**DECLINING SCHOOL
PERFORMANCE**
seizures

DEFECATION, FREQUENT NEED
diarrhea
ulcerative colitis

DEFECATION, STRAINING
hemorrhoids

DEHYDRATION
diabetes

DELERIUM
hyperthyroidism, thyroid storm
endocarditis

DEMENTIA
HIV and AIDS
hypothyroidism
Parkinson's disease

DENGUE FEVER
insect bites

DEPRESSION
anorexia
HIV and AIDS
hypoglycemia
hypothyroidism
menopause
seizures
sexual dysfunction
sleep apnea
tension headache

DERMAL DISEASE
herpes simplex virus

DERMAL TISSUE NECROSIS
cutaneous drug reactions

DERMATITIS, ATOPIC
food allergy

DERMIS, EPIDERMIS, AND DEEPER LAYERS
burns, third degree

DIAPHORESIS
pulmonary edema

DIAPHRAGM, FLATTENED
asthma

DIARRHEA
allergic rhinitis
dysmenorrhea
food allergy
HIV and AIDS
influenza
insect bites
irritable bowel syndrome
otitis media
roseola
seizures
ulcerative colitis

DIARRHEA, BLOODY
ulcerative colitis

DIARRHEA, MALODOROUS
intestinal parasites

DIARRHEA, VIOLENT
ulcerative colitis

DIGITAL PERIOSITIS
Reiter's syndrome

DISINHIBITED BEHAVIOR
dementia

DISTORTED PERCEPTION OF PHYSICAL SELF
anorexia

DIZZINESS
anxiety
fibromyalgia syndrome
menopause
motion sickness
myocardial infarction

DROWSINESS, DAYTIME
insomnia
sleep apnea

DYSENTERY
intestinal parasites

DYSMENORRHEA
endometriosis

DYSPAREUNIA
endometriosis

DYSPEPSIA
gastritis

DYSPHAGIA
gastroesophageal reflux disease
laryngitis
thyroiditis, Riedel's
thyroiditis, subacute

DYSPNEA
anemia
anxiety
asthma
chronic obstructive pulmonary disease
congestive heart failure
constrictive pericarditis
myocardial infarction
pericardial effusion
pulmonary edema
thyroiditis, Riedel's

DYSPNEA, EXERTIONAL
primary pulmonary hypertension

DYSURIA
herpes simplex virus, genital
prostatitis

EARDRUM, BULGING
otitis media

EAR INFECTIONS
allergic rhinitis

EARLY-MORNING WAKING
insomnia

EAR PAIN
otitis media

EATING, EXTENDED TIME REQUIRED
dysphagia, esophageal

EATING, RELUCTANCE
anorexia

ECZEMATOUS REACTION
cutaneous drug reactions

EDEMA
candidiasis
herpes simplex virus, eye
herpes simplex virus, finger or hand
insect bites
sprains and strains
tendinitis

EDEMA, HANDS AND FACE
preeclampsia

EDEMA, LOWER EXTREMITY
pulmonary edema

EDEMA, LOWER EXTREMITY
pulmonary edema

EDEMA, PERIPHERAL
chronic obstructive pulmonary disease
cirrhosis of the liver
congestive heart failure

EJACULATION, PAINFUL
prostatitis

EJACULATION, PREMATURE OR RETARDED
sexual dysfunction

ELECTROCARDIOGRAM, ABNORMAL
angina

EMACIATION
anorexia

EMBOLUS
atherosclerosis

EMESIS, RECURRENT, INFANTS
gastroesophageal reflux disease

EMOTIONAL EXPRESSION, RESTRAINED
anorexia

EMOTIONAL STRESS
tension headache

ENERGY LOSS
depression-unipolar mood disorders

EPIDERMIS, RED AND PAINFUL
burns, first degree

EPIDERMIS, RED AND PAINFUL WITH BLISTERS
burns, second degree

EPIGASTRIC PAIN
peptic ulcer

EPIGASTRIC PAIN, UPPER RIGHT QUADRANT
gallbladder disease

ERECTION, INABILITY TO MAINTAIN
sexual dysfunction

ERYTHEMA
bursitis
eczema
herpes simplex virus, finger or hand
insect bites

ERYTHEMA, VULVAR
candidiasis

ERYTHEMA MULTIFORME/NODOSUM
cutaneous drug reactions

ERYTHEMATOUS BUCCAL MUCOSA
candidiasis

ERYTHROCYTE SEDIMENTATION RATE, ELEVATED
rheumatoid arthritis

ESOPHAGEAL LESIONS
candidiasis

ESOPHAGUS, SENSATION OF FOOD STUCK
dysphagia, esophageal

EUNUCHOIDISM/GIGANTISM (TALL STATURE)
amenorrhea

EXCORIATIONS
dermatitis

EXECUTIVE FUNCTIONING DISTURBANCE
dementia

EXERCISE INTOLERANCE
congestive heart failure

EXERTION, PAIN BROUGHT ON BY
angina

EXTREMITIES, SWOLLEN
edema

EXTREMITY, LOWER, EDEMA
pulmonary edema

EXTREMITY NUMBNESS
diabetes
Raynaud's phenomenon

EXTREMITY PAIN
endocarditis

EXTREMITY TINGLING
diabetes

EYEBROWS, LOSS OF
hypothyroidism

EYE DISCHARGE
conjunctivitis

EYE ITCHING, TEARING, BURNING
conjunctivitis

EYE PAIN
herpes simplex virus, eye

EYE REDNESS
conjunctivitis

EYES, GRITTY SENSATION
conjunctivitis

EYES, OVERNIGHT CRUSTING
conjunctivitis

EYES, SWELLING
thyroiditis, Hashimoto's

EYES, SWOLLEN, REDDENED, BULGING
hyperthyroidism

FACIAL LESIONS
herpes simplex virus, oral-facial

FACIAL PAIN, LOCALIZED
sinus headache

FACIAL PUFFINESS
edema
hypothyroidism

FACIAL SWELLING
food allergy

FAILURE TO THRIVE, INFANTS
gastroesophageal reflux disease

FATIGUE
allergic rhinitis, severe
anemia
anxiety
bronchitis
congestive heart failure
constrictive pericarditis
depression-unipolar mood
 disorders
diabetes
fibromyalgia syndrome
hepatitis, viral
hyperkalemia
hypoglycemia
endocarditis
influenza
intestinal parasites
motion sickness
osteomyelitis
sleep apnea

FATIGUE, EXCESSIVE
primary pulmonary hypertension

FATIGUE, SEVERE
chronic fatigue syndrome

FATTY FOOD INTOLERANCE
gallbladder disease

FEELINGS OF INEFFECTIVENESS
anorexia
depression

FEELINGS OF UNREALITY
anxiety

FEVER
bronchitis
bursitis
candidiasis
cough

diarrhea
fever of unknown origin
gout
hepatitis, viral
herpes simplex virus, finger
 or hand
herpes simplex virus, genital
herpes simplex virus, neonatal
herpes simplex virus, oral-facial
HIV and AIDS
hyperthyroidism, thyroid storm
endocarditis
laryngitis
osteomyelitis
otitis media
pericarditis
pharyngitis
prostatitis
Reiter's syndrome
roseola
sinus headache
sinusitis
ulcerative colitis
urinary tract infection in women
urolithiasis

FEVER, LOW-GRADE
chronic fatigue syndrome
herpes zoster (varicella–zoster)
pertussis
rheumatoid arthritis
thyroiditis, subacute

FEVER, SUDDEN ONSET
influenza

FEVER (CHILDREN)
common cold

FINGERNAILS/TOENAILS, PITTED AND DISCOLORED
psoriasis

FINGERTIP PAIN (OSLER NODE)
endocarditis

FINGERTIPS, ULCERS
Raynaud's phenomenon

FISSURING, SKIN
dermatitis

FLANK PAIN, SEVERE
urolithiasis

FLATULENCE
food allergy

FLUSHING
pericarditis

FRACTURE, WITHOUT TRAUMA
osteoporosis

GAIT DISTURBANCES
Parkinson's disease

GANGRENE
atherosclerosis

GASSINESS
infantile colic
intestinal parasites
irritable bowel syndrome

GASTRITIS, ANTRAL
peptic ulcer

GASTROESOPHAGEAL REFLUX DISEASE
cough
dysphagia, esophageal

GASTROESOPHAGEAL VARICES, BLEEDING
cirrhosis of the liver

GASTROINTESTINAL BLEEDING
gastritis

GASTROINTESTINAL DISTRESS
cirrhosis of the liver
dysmenorrhea

GASTROINTESTINAL LESIONS
candidiasis

GENITALIA, EXTERNAL, RED AND SWOLLEN
vaginitis

GENITAL LESIONS, EXTERNAL
herpes simplex virus, genital

GINGIVA
herpes simplex virus, oral-facial

GINGIVOSTOMATITIS
herpes simplex virus, oral-facial

GLOBUS SENSATION, NECK
gastroesophageal reflux disease

GLOSSITIS
anemia

GLYCOSURIA
diabetes

GOITER
amenorrhea
iodine deficiency

GROWTH RETARDATION, CHILDREN
hypothyroidism

GUILT, INAPPROPRIATE
depression-unipolar mood
 disorders

GYNECOMASTIA
cirrhosis of the liver

HAIR, DRY, SCALY, THICK, AND COARSE
hypothyroidism

HAIRS, BROKEN OR EASILY REMOVED
alopecia

HALLUCINATIONS
dementia

HAND JOINTS, PAIN
rheumatoid arthritis

HEADACHE
allergic rhinitis
amenorrhea
anemia
chronic fatigue syndrome
dysmenorrhea
fever of unknown origin
fibromyalgia syndrome
food allergy
hepatitis, viral
herpes simplex virus, genital
herpes zoster (varicella–zoster)
HIV and AIDS
hypertension
hypoglycemia
hypothyroidism
endocarditis
influenza
menopause
motion sickness
pharyngitis
seizures
sinusitis

HEADACHE, BIFRONTAL OR OCCIPITAL
tension headache

HEADACHE, FRONTAL
sinus headache

HEADACHE, MORNING
sleep apnea

HEAD FULLNESS, HEAD SHAKING
otitis media

HEAD PAIN, STEADY AND DULL
tension headache

HEARING DIFFICULTY
otitis media

HEARING DISTURBANCES
migraine headache

HEARTBEAT, RAPID
thyroiditis, silent

HEARTBURN
cough
gastroesophageal reflux disease

HEART RATE, RAPID INCREASE
food allergy

HEAVINESS, TIGHTNESS, BURNING IN CHEST
myocardial infarction

HEBERDEN'S NODULES OF DISTAL INTERPHALANGEAL JOINTS
osteoarthritis

HEIGHT, LOSS OF
osteoporosis

HELICOBACTER PYLORI
peptic ulcer

HEMGOLOBINURIA
anemia

HEMIPARESIS
endocarditis

HEMOPTYSIS
congestive heart failure
primary pulmonary hypertension

HEPATIC ENCEPHALOPATHY
cirrhosis of the liver

HEPATOMEGALY
cirrhosis of the liver
herpes simplex virus, neonatal

HERPES
HIV and AIDS

HERPETIC WHITLOW
herpes simplex virus, finger or hand

HIRSUITISM, FACIAL
menopause

HIVES
allergic rhinitis
food allergy

HOARSENESS
common cold
gastroesophageal reflux disease
hypothyroidism
laryngitis
thyroiditis, Riedel's

HOARSENESS, SUDDEN
food allergy

HOT FLUSHES
amenorrhea
menopause

HYPERACTIVITY
attention-deficit/
  hyperactivity disorder
depression-unipolar mood
  disorders
thyroiditis, silent

HYPERGLYCEMIA
diabetes

HYPERLIPIDEMIA
diabetes

HYPERSALIVATION
motion sickness

HYPERSOMNIA
depression-unipolar mood
  disorders

HYPERTENSION
hyperthyroidism
myocardial infarction
obesity
sleep apnea

HYPERTENSION, PORTAL
cirrhosis of the liver

HYPERVIGILANCE
anxiety

HYPOTENSION
candidiasis
myocardial infarction

HYPOTENSION, RELATIVE
pericardial effusion

HYPOTENSION, SECONDARY TO ANAPHYLACTIC SHOCK
insect bites

HYPOTHERMIA
herpes simplex virus, neonatal

IMPAIRED FUNCTIONING
insomnia

IMPOTENCE
sexual dysfunction
sleep apnea

IMPULSIVITY
attention-deficit/hyperactivity
  disorder

INACTIVITY
depression-unipolar mood
  disorders

INATTENTION
attention-deficit/hyperactivity
  disorder

INCONTINENCE
dementia
menopause
Parkinson's disease
seizures

INCOORDINATION
hypoglycemia

INDURATION
eczema

INFECTION, INCREASED SUSCEPTIBILITY TO
diabetes

INFECTIONS, CHRONIC
HIV and AIDS

INFERTILITY
endometriosis

INFLAMMATION
arthritis
burns
candidiasis
gout
insect bites
laryngitis
osteomyelitis
tendinitis
sprains and strains

INFLUENZA
hepatitis, viral

INITIATIVE, RESTRAINED
anorexia

INSOMNIA
anorexia
anxiety
congestive heart failure
depression-unipolar mood
  disorders
tension headache

INSPIRATIONS, SUDDEN FORCEFUL
pertussis

INTERCOURSE, PAIN DURING
sexual dysfunction

INTESTINAL PAIN
endometriosis

IRITIS
Reiter's syndrome

IRRITABILITY
allergic rhinitis, severe
anorexia
anxiety
common cold
depression-unipolar mood
  disorders
herpes simplex virus, oral-facial
hypoglycemia
hypoglycemia
menopause
migraine headache
osteomyelitis
otitis media
seizures
sleep apnea

IRRITABLE BOWEL SYNDROME
fibromyalgia syndrome

ITCHING
eczema
herpes simplex virus, genital
psoriasis
warts

ITCHING, MUCOUS MEMBRANES
allergic rhinitis

ITCHING, PENILE OPENING
urethritis

JAUNDICE
cirrhosis of the liver
hepatitis, viral

JAUNDICE, EPISODIC
anemia

JAUNDICE, PROGRESSIVE
herpes simplex virus, neonatal

JOINT, SHINY RED OR PURPLE COLORATION
gout

JOINT INSTABILITY
sprains and strains

JOINT PAIN
fibromyalgia syndrome
gout
endocarditis
osteoarthritis
psoriasis

JOINT SWELLING, HEAT, AND STIFFNESS
gout

JUGULAR VEIN DISTENSION
constrictive pericarditis

KAPOSI SARCOMA
HIV and AIDS

KERATITIS
Reiter's syndrome

KERATODERMAL BLENNORRHAGICA
Reiter's syndrome

KETOACIDOSIS
diabetes

KOILONYCHIA
anemia

LANGUAGE DETERIORATION
dementia

LARYNGITIS
gastroesophageal reflux disease

LARYNGOEDEMA
insect bites

LEG CRAMPS
atherosclerosis
diabetes

LEG FATIGUE
low back pain

LETHARGY
depression-unipolar mood
  disorders
herpes simplex virus, neonatal
hypothyroidism
seizures

LIBIDO, DIMINISHED
anorexia
depression-unipolar mood
  disorders

LICHENOID
cutaneous drug reactions

LID LAG
hyperthyroidism
hypothyroidism

LIGHTHEADEDNESS
anemia
anxiety

LIP LESIONS
herpes simplex virus, oral-facial

LIPS, SWELLING OR ITCHING
food allergy

LIVER, ENLARGEMENT
hypercholesterolemia

LOUD P2
primary pulmonary hypertension

LUPUS ERYTHEMATOSUS WITH MALAR ERYTHEMA
cutaneous drug reactions

LYME DISEASE
insect bites

LYMPHADENOPATHY
chronic fatigue syndrome
rheumatoid arthritis

LYMPHADENOPATHY, AXILLARY
herpes simplex virus, finger or hand

LYMPHADENOPATHY, INGUINAL
herpes simplex virus, genital

LYMPHADENOPATHY, PERSISTENT
HIV and AIDS

LYMPH NODE ENLARGEMENT
pharyngitis

MACULOPAPULAR ERUPTIONS
cutaneous drug reactions

MACULOPAPULES
herpes zoster (varicella–zoster)

MALAISE
candidiasis
cirrhosis of the liver
diarrhea
fever of unknown origin
hepatitis, viral
herpes simplex virus, genital
herpes simplex virus, oral-facial
herpes zoster (varicella-zoster)
   virus
endocarditis
laryngitis
motion sickness
osteomyelitis
pericarditis
prostatitis
Reiter's syndrome
rheumatoid arthritis
sinusitis
thyroiditis, subacute
ulcerative colitis

MALARIA
insect bites

MALIGNANCIES
HIV and AIDS

MEMORY IMPAIRMENT
dementia

MEMORY LAPSES
dementia
fibromyalgia

MEMORY LOSS
dementia
Parkinson's disease
sleep apnea

MENSTRUAL DISORDERS
hypothyroidism

MENSTRUAL IRREGULARITIES
cirrhosis of the liver

MENSTRUAL PAIN
dysmenorrhea

MENSTRUATION, ALTERED
hyperthyroidism

MENSTRUATION, HEAVY
dysmenorrhea

MENSTRUATION, PELVIC PAIN CYCLING WITH
endometriosis

MENTAL CONFUSION
dementia
hypoglycemia

MENTAL DEFICIENCY, CHILDREN
hypothyroidism

MENTAL STATUS, SUDDEN CHANGE
edema

MICROABSCESS
candidiasis

MIDEPIGASTRIC PAIN/ TENDERNESS
intestinal parasites

MOOD DISTURBANCES
dementia

MOODINESS
sleep apnea

MOTOR ACTIVITIES, IMPAIRMENT
dementia

MOTOR DISTURBANCES
dementia

MOUTH, DRY
sleep apnea

MOUTH, SWELLING AND ITCHING
food allergy

MOUTH FISSURES
candidiasis

MOUTH INFLAMMATION
Reiter's syndrome

MUCOSAL DISEASE
herpes simplex virus

MUSCLE ACHES
influenza

MUSCLE ATROPHY
atherosclerosis

MUSCLE PAIN
endocarditis

MUSCLES, NECK AND SHOULDERS, TIGHT AND SORE
tension headache

MUSCLE SPASM, TOTAL BODY
seizures

MUSCLE TENSION
anxiety

MUSCLE TONE, POSTURAL, LOSS OF
seizures

MUSCLE WEAKNESS
chronic fatigue syndrome
endocarditis

MUSCULAR PAIN
edema

MYALGIAS
chronic fatigue syndrome
fever of unknown origin
hepatitis, viral
herpes simplex virus, oral-facial
pericarditis

MYIASIS
insect bites

MYOCARDIAL INFARCTION
endocarditis

MYOCLONIC LIMB JERKS
seizures

NASAL CONGESTION
allergic rhinitis
common cold
sinusitis

NASAL DISCHARGE, PURULENT
sinus headache

NASAL MUCOSA, INFLAMMATION
sinusitis

NASAL OBSTRUCTION
allergic rhinitis
influenza

NASAL PASSAGES, RED AND TURGESCENT
sinus headache

NAUSEA
amenorrhea
congestive heart failure
dysmenorrhea
food allergy
gallbladder disease
gastritis
hepatitis, viral
hypertension, severe
influenza
intestinal parasites
migraine headache
motion sickness
myocardial infarction
peptic ulcer
urolithiasis

NECK VEINS, DISTENDED
congestive heart failure

NECROSIS, CUTANEOUS
insect bites

NERVOUSNESS
anxiety
hyperthyroidism
thyroiditis, silent

NEURALGIA
postherpetic
herpes zoster (varicella–zoster)
   virus

NEURALGIA, FACIAL
herpes simplex virus, oral-facial

NEURITIS, ACUTE
herpes zoster (varicella–zoster)

NEUROLOGICAL SIGNS, ABNORMAL
edema

NEUROLOGICAL SYMPTOMS
anemia

NOCTURIA
congestive heart failure
menopause
prostatitis

NOSE, RUNNY AND ITCHING
food allergy

NUMBNESS
endocarditis
Raynaud's phenomenon

OBSESSIVE-COMPULSIVE BEHAVIOR
anorexia

OCULAR ABNORMALITIES
Parkinson's disease

ODYNOPHAGIA
gastroesophageal reflux disease
pericarditis

ORGASM, DIFFICULTY
sexual dysfunction

OSTEOPOROSIS
menopause

PAIN
herpes simplex virus, genital
infantile colic
internal hemorrhoids
Raynaud's phenomenon
Reiter's syndrome
sprains and strains
tendinitis
ulcerative colitis

PAIN, ACUTE ONSET
bursitis
myocardial infarction

PAIN, EXQUISITE
gout

PAIN, LOCALIZED
bursitis

PAIN, THYROID AREA
thyroiditis, suppurative

PAIN FOLLOWING MEALS
gallbladder disease

PAIN REFERRED TO LABIUM
urolithiasis

PAIN REFERRED TO TESTES
urolithiasis

PALATE LESIONS
herpes simplex virus, oral-facial

PALLOR
endocarditis
motion sickness
Raynaud's phenomenon
seizures

PALMAR ERYTHEMA
cirrhosis of the liver

PALPITATIONS
anemia
anxiety
hyperkalemia
hyperthyroidism
hypoglycemia
menopause
primary pulmonary hypertension

PANCREATITIS SYMPTOMS
hypercholesterolemia

PAPULES
eczema

PAPULES, FLESH-TONE
warts

**PAPULES, ROUGH, THICKENED,
SCARCELY ELEVATED**
Plantar warts

PAPULES, TINY AND FLAT
genital warts

PARALYSIS
hyperkalemia
endocarditis
stroke

PARESTHESIA
fibromyalgia
hyperkalemia

PAROTID ENLARGEMENT
cirrhosis of the liver

**PELVIC INFLAMMATORY
DISEASE**
urethritis in women

PELVIC PAIN
endometriosis
pelvic inflammatory disease

PERIANAL INFECTIONS
herpes simplex virus, genital

PERIANAL LUMP
external hemorrhoids

PERICARDITIS
Reiter's syndrome
rheumatoid arthritis

PERINEAL IRRITATION
urinary incontinence

PERIODONTAL DISEASE
osteoporosis

PERIPHERAL EDEMA
constrictive pericarditis
primary pulmonary hypertension

PERLECHE
candidiasis

**PERSONAL CONTROL,
EXCESSIVE NEED FOR**
anorexia

PERSONALITY OR BEHAVIOR CHANGE
sleep apnea

PETECHIAE
endocarditis

**PHARYNGEAL MUCUS
MEMBRANE INFLAMMATION**
pharyngitis

PHARYNGITIS
herpes simplex virus, oral-facial
sinusitis

PHOTOSENSITIVITY
cutaneous drug reactions

PHYSICAL ACTIVITY, PAIN WITH
fibromyalgia
tension headache

**PHYSICAL STRESSORS, INCREASED
SUSCEPTIBILITY**
dementia

PICA
anemia

PLANTAR FASCITIS
Reiter's syndrome

PLEURAL EFFUSION
rheumatoid arthritis

PNEUMONIA
herpes simplex virus

POLYDIPSIA
diabetes

POLYPHAGIA
diabetes

POLYURIA
amenorrhea
diabetes

POSTEXERTIONAL PAIN
fibromyalgia

POSTICTAL CONFUSION
seizures

POSTNASAL DRIP
cough
sinusitis

POSTURAL ABNORMALITIES
osteoporosis
Parkinson's disease

PREMENSTRUAL SYNDROME
dysmenorrhea
tension headache

PREOCCUPATION WITH BODY IMAGE
anorexia

PREOCCUPATION WITH FOOD
anorexia

PROSTATITIS
Reiter's syndrome

PROTEIN, IN URINE
preeclampsia

PROTEINURIA
congestive heart failure

PRURITIC PAPULES
insect bites

PRURITIS
candidiasis
dermatitis
diabetes
external hemorrhoids
herpes zoster (varicella–zoster)
insect bites

**PRURITIS, VAGINAL AND
VULVAR**
vaginitis

PSYCHOLOGICAL DISTURBANCES
anxiety
dementia
depression-unipolar mood
   disorders
fibromyalgia

PULMONARY CONGESTION
constrictive pericarditis

PULMONARY EDEMA
congestive heart failure

PULMONARY FIBROSIS
gastroesophageal reflux disease

PULMONARY INFARCTION
endocarditis

PULMONIC INSUFFICIENCY
primary pulmonary hypertension

PULSE, LOWERED OR ABSENT
atherosclerosis

PULSE, RAPID
hyperthyroidism, thyroid storm
seizures

PULSE, SLOW
hypothyroidism
thyroiditis, Hashimoto's

PUPILS, DILATED
seizures

PUSTULAR LESIONS
herpes simplex virus, finger or
   hand

RALES
pulmonary edema

RANGE OF MOTION, LIMITED
osteoarthritis

RASHES
allergic rhinitis
herpes zoster (varicella–zoster)
HIV and AIDS
roseola

**RASHES, DERMATOSOMAL
DISTRIBUTION**
herpes zoster (varicella–zoster)
   virus

RASHES, PERIRECTAL OR VULVAR
intestinal parasites

RAYNAUD'S PHENOMENON
fibromyalgia

**RECOGNITION OF OBJECTS,
IMPAIRED**
dementia

REFLEXES, SLOW
thyroiditis, Hashimoto's

REGURGITATION
cough
gastroesophageal reflux disease

**REGURGITATION, LIQUID THROUGH
NOSE**
dysphagia, oropharyngeal

RENAL FAILURE
amenorrhea

RESPIRATORY ARREST
pulmonary edema

RESPIRATORY DISTRESS
food allergy
herpes simplex virus, neonatal

RESPIRATORY FAILURE
insect bites

RESPIRATORY SYMPTOMS
roseola

**RESPIRATORY TRACT
INFECTION, UPPER**
cough
pertussis
sinus headache

RESTLESS LEG SYNDROME
fibromyalgia

RESTLESSNESS
common cold
depression-unipolar mood
   disorders
migraine headache

RETINOPATHY
hypertension, severe

**RETROSTERNAL BURNING
SENSATION**
gastroesophageal reflux disease

**RETROSTERNAL FULLNESS AFTER
SWALLOWING**
dysphagia, esophageal

RHEUMATOID NODULES
rheumatoid arthritis

RHINITIS
pertussis

RHINORRHEA
common cold
influenza

RHINORRHEA, YELLOW OR GREEN
sinus headache

RHONCHI
pulmonary edema

RIGHT VENTRICULAR LIFT
primary pulmonary hypertension

RIGHT VENTRICULAR S4
primary pulmonary hypertension

RIGIDITY
Parkinson's disease

RIGID THINKING
anorexia

ROCKY MOUNTAIN FEVER
insect bites

RUBOR
Raynaud's phenomenon

SALIVATION, INCREASED
seizures

SALPINGITIS
urethritis in women

SATELLITE LESIONS, SPREAD TO THIGHS AND ANUS
vaginitis

SCABS
herpes zoster (varicella–zoster)

SCALES
dermatitis
eczema

SCALP ARTERIES, PROMINENT
migraine headache

SCLERITIS
Reiter's syndrome

SEIZURES
dementia
hypertension, severe
hypoglycemia
endocarditis
roseola

SELF-REPROACH
depression-unipolar mood
  disorders

SEMEN, BLOODY
prostatitis

SENSATION, LOSS OF
anemia

SENSATION OF FULLNESS
internal hemorrhoids

SENSE OF IMPENDING DOOM/ EXCESSIVE WORRY
anxiety

SENSITIVITY TO LIGHT
conjunctivitis
hyperthyroidism
migraine headache
Reiter's syndrome

SEXUAL DESIRE, LACK OF
sexual dysfunction

SEXUAL DYSFUNCTION
prostatitis

SIGHING RESPIRATION
anxiety

SINUS PAIN AND TENDERNESS
sinusitis

SINUS SYMPTOMS
allergic rhinitis

SITTING DISCOMFORT
hemorrhoids
low back pain

SKIN
erythematous lesions
candidiasis

SKIN, COLOR CHANGES
Raynaud's phenomenon

SKIN, COOL AND DRY
thyroiditis, Hashimoto's

SKIN, INCREASED TEMPERATURE
bursitis, septic

SKIN, LARGE LOCAL REACTION
insect bites

SKIN, MOIST WITH INCREASED PERSPIRATION
hyperthyroidism

SKIN, PALE OR BROWNISH YELLOW AND LEATHERY
burns, third degree

SKIN, RAISED AND THICKENED
hyperthyroidism
hypothyroidism

SKIN, RED
dermatitis

SKIN, STINGING OR BURNING
dermatitis

SKIN, THICKENED AND LICHENIFIED
dermatitis

SKIN, WARMTH AND REDNESS
gout
tendinitis

SKIN CHARRING
burns, third degree

SKIN DARKENING
amenorrhea

SKIN ERUPTIONS, FIXED
cutaneous drug reactions

SKIN LESIONS
eczema
HIV and AIDS

SKIN LESIONS, AFTER INJURIES
psoriasis

SKIN LESIONS, CRUSTING AND INFECTION
insect bites

SKIN LESIONS, RAISED
psoriasis

SKIN LESIONS, VESICULAR
herpes simplex virus, neonatal

SKIN LESIONS (JANEWAY)
endocarditis

SLEEP, DEEP
seizures

SLEEP, IMPAIRED MAINTENANCE
insomnia

SLEEP, IMPAIRED ONSET
insomnia

SLEEP DISORDERS
fibromyalgia

SLEEP DISTURBANCES
anxiety
chronic fatigue syndrome
dementia
hyperthyroidism
menopause
otitis media
Parkinson's disease
sleep apnea

SLEEPINESS, DAYTIME
sleep apnea

SMELL, LOSS OF
sinusitis

SNEEZING
allergic rhinitis
common cold
influenza

SNORING, LOUD AND IRREGULAR
sleep apnea

SOCIAL SPONTANEITY, LIMITED
anorexia

SOCIAL WITHDRAWAL
anorexia

SORES, OPEN
edema

SPATIAL DISORIENTATION
dementia

SPEECH, SLOWED
hypothyroidism

SPEECH, SLURRED
hypoglycemia

SPEECH PROBLEMS
Parkinson's disease

SPINAL DEFORMITY/ HUNCHED BACK
osteoporosis

SPITTING UP AFTER FEEDING
infantile colic

SPLEEN, ENLARGEMENT
hypercholesterolemia

SPLENOMEGALY
cirrhosis of the liver
herpes simplex virus, neonatal

SPLENOMEGALY WITH LEUKOPENIA
rheumatoid arthritis

SPONDYLOARTHROPATHY
Reiter's syndrome

SPUTUM, BLOODY
endocarditis

SPUTUM, EXCESSIVE
chronic obstructive pulmonary
  disease

SPUTUM, PINK AND FROTHY
pulmonary edema

STANDING, DIFFICULTY
low back pain

STENOSIS, ARTERIAL
atherosclerosis

STIFFNESS
diabetes
gout
low back pain
osteoarthritis
Reiter's syndrome
rheumatoid arthritis
sprains and strains

STIFFNESS, MORNING
fibromyalgia
Reiter's syndrome

STOMACH, SWOLLEN OR DISTENDED
infantile colic

STOOL, BLOOD AND MUCUS IN
ulcerative colitis

STOOL, COLORLESS
hepatitis, viral

STOOL, DIFFICULT PASSAGE
constipation

STOOL, HARD
constipation

STOOL, LOOSE
diarrhea

STOOL, MUCUS IN
hemorrhoids
irritable bowel syndrome

STOOL, PASSAGE OF WORM
intestinal parasites

STOOL, TARRY OR RED
peptic ulcer

STRAINING DURING DEFECATING
hemorrhoids

SUBLUXATION
osteoarthritis

SUICIDAL BEHAVIOR
dementia
depression

SUICIDAL THOUGHTS
depression-unipolar mood
    disorders

SWALLOWING DIFFICULTY
dysphagia, oropharyngeal
Parkinson's disease

SWALLOWING PAIN
pharyngitis

SWEATING
anxiety

SWEATING, COLD
motion sickness

SWEATING, EXCESSIVE
hypoglycemia

SWEATING, INCREASED
seizures
thyroiditis, silent

SWEATING, NIGHT
cough
HIV and AIDS
endocarditis
menopause
ulcerative colitis

SWELLING
Reiter's syndrome
sprains and strains

SWELLING, BASE OF NECK
hyperthyroidism

SWELLING, LOCALIZED
bursitis

SWELLING, MUSCULAR
edema

SWELLING, PATCHES OF
food allergy

SWELLING, SOFT TISSUE
osteoarthritis

**SWELLING AND
TENDERNESS, BONE**
osteomyelitis

**SYNCOPE, EXERTIONAL
OR NEAR**
primary pulmonary hypertension

SYNCOPE, NEAR
anxiety
migraine headache

TACHYARRHYTHMIA
hyperthyroidism

TACHYCARDIA
anxiety
hyperthyroidism
pericardial effusion

TEETH, ACHING
allergic rhinitis

TEETH GRINDING
tension headache

TENDERNESS, LOCALIZED
bursitis
gout
osteoarthritis
rheumatoid arthritis
tendinitis

TENESMUS, DISTRESSING
ulcerative colitis

**TERMINAL FAT PADS,
ATROPHY OF**
Raynaud's phenomenon

TESTICULAR ATROPHY
cirrhosis of the liver

THIGH PAIN
dysmenorrhea

THIRST
amenorrhea

**THROAT, ITCHING OR
TIGHTNESS**
food allergy

THROAT, SORE
bronchitis
chronic fatigue syndrome
common cold
gastroesophageal reflux disease
influenza
pharyngitis
sleep apnea

**THROAT, TICKLING, SCRATCHINESS,
RAWNESS**
laryngitis

**THROAT CLEARING,
CONSTANT**
laryngitis

THROBBING, SEVERE
migraine headache
Raynaud's phenomenon

THROMBOSIS
atherosclerosis

THRUSH
candidiasis
HIV and AIDS

**THYROID GLAND,
ASYMMETRICALLY ENLARGED**
thyroiditis, Riedel's

**THYROID GLAND, ENLARGED AND
PAINFUL**
thyroiditis, subacute

**THYROID GLAND, MODERATELY
ENLARGED**
thyroiditis, silent

**THYROID GLAND,
SYMMETRICALLY ENLARGED**
thyroiditis, Hashimoto's

TOE TIP PAIN (OSLER NODE)
endocarditis

TONGUE, SWELLING OR ITCHING
food allergy

TONGUE LESIONS
herpes simplex virus, oral-facial

TONIC CONTRACTIONS
seizures

TONSIL ENLARGEMENT
pharyngitis

TOOTHACHE
sinusitis

TOPHI
gout

TREMBLING
anxiety

TREMOR
dementia
hyperthyroidism
Parkinson's disease

TREMULOUSNESS
hypoglycemia

TRICUSPID MURMUR
primary pulmonary hypertension

**TRIGLYCERIDES, HIGH
LEVELS**
hypercholesterolemia

TUBERCULOSIS, PULMONARY
cough

**TURNER'S SYNDROME (SHORT
STATURE)**
amenorrhea

TYMPANIC MEMBRANES, INFLAMED
roseola

ULCER, DUODENAL
peptic ulcer

**ULCER, GANGRENOUS,
FINGERTIPS**
Raynaud's phenomenon

ULCER, GASTRIC
peptic ulcer

ULCERATION
insect bites

URETHRAL DISCHARGE
herpes simplex virus, genital

**URETHRAL DISCHARGE, PURULENT
OR WHITISH-MUCUS**
urethritis, in men

URETHRAL LESIONS
herpes simplex virus, genital

URETHRITIS
Reiter's syndrome

URINARY TRACT ATROPHY
menopause

URINARY TRACT INFECTION
candidiasis

**URINARY TRACT INFECTION,
RECURRENT**
prostatitis

**URINATION, BURNING
SENSATION**
benign prostatic hyperplasia
urethritis in men
urinary tract infection in women

**URINATION, COMPLETE
INABILITY**
benign prostatic hyperplasia

URINATION, DRIBBLING AFTER
benign prostatic hyperplasia

URINATION, FREQUENT
allergic rhinitis
benign prostatic hyperplasia
dysmenorrhea
prostatitis

**URINATION, FREQUENT AND
UNUSUAL URGE**
urinary incontinence
urinary tract infection in women

URINATION, INVOLUNTARY
urinary incontinence

URINATION, PAINFUL
urethritis in women

URINE, BLOOD AND PUS IN
urinary tract infection in women

URINE, BLOOD IN
benign prostatic hyperplasia
endocarditis

URINE, DARK
hepatitis, viral

URINE, DIFFICULTY STARTING STREAM
benign prostatic hyperplasia

URINE, REDUCTION IN AMOUNT
preeclampsia

URINE, STRONG-SMELLING
urinary tract infection in women

URTICARIA
cutaneous drug reactions
food allergy

URTICARIA, GENERALIZED
insect bites

URTICARIAL PAPULES
insect bites

VAGINAL ATROPHY
menopause

VAGINAL DISCHARGE
urethritis in women
vaginitis

VAGINAL DRYNESS
menopause
sexual dysfunction

VAGINAL MUCOUS MEMBRANES, RED AND SWOLLEN
vaginitis

VASCULITIS
cutaneous drug reactions
rheumatoid arthritis

VASOMOTOR SYMPTOMS
menopause

VERTIGO
hypoglycemia
migraine headache

VESICLES
dermatitis
herpes zoster (varicella–zoster)

VESICLES, OOZING AND CRUSTING
eczema

VESICULAR LESIONS
herpes simplex virus, finger or hand

VISCERAL DISEASE
herpes simplex virus

VISION DISTURBANCES
migraine headache
preeclampsia

VISUAL FIELD ABNORMALITIES
amenorrhea

VOICE, UNNATURAL CHANGES
laryngitis

VOICE, WEAK
dysphagia, oropharyngeal

VOICE, WEAK
dysphagia, esophageal

VOMITING
congestive heart failure
dysmenorrhea
food allergy
gallbladder disease
gastritis
hepatitis, viral
herpes simplex virus, neonatal
HIV and AIDS
hypertension, severe
influenza
intestinal parasites
migraine headache
motion sickness
myocardial infarction
otitis media
peptic ulcer
pertussis
urolithiasis

VOMITING, BLOOD
peptic ulcer

VULVAR ERYTHEMA
candidiasis

VULVOVAGINITIS
candidiasis

WALKING PROBLEMS
Parkinson's disease

WATER BRASH
gastroesophageal reflux disease

WEAKNESS
chronic fatigue syndrome
cirrhosis of the liver
diabetes
fibromyalgia
hyperkalemia
low back pain
myocardial infarction

WEIGHT GAIN
bronchitis
chronic obstructive pulmonary disease
depression-unipolar mood disorders
hypothyroidism

WEIGHT GAIN, SUDDEN AND EXCESSIVE
preeclampsia

WEIGHT LOSS
anorexia
chronic obstructive pulmonary disease, late stages
cirrhosis of the liver
depression-unipolar mood disorders
diarrhea
dysphagia, oropharyngeal
HIV and AIDS
hyperthyroidism
intestinal parasites
peptic ulcer
Reiter's syndrome
rheumatoid arthritis
thyroiditis, silent
ulcerative colitis

WEIGHT LOSS, RAPID
diabetes

WHEEZING
asthma
bronchitis
chronic obstructive pulmonary disease
cough
gastroesophageal reflux disease

WITHDRAWAL
depression-unipolar mood disorders

WORTHLESSNESS, FEELINGS OF
depression-unipolar mood disorders

WRIST JOINTS
rheumatoid arthritis

XANTHOMAS, TENDONS AND SKIN
hypercholesterolemia

ZOSTER OPHTHALMICUS
herpes zoster (varicella–zoster) virus

■ **CONDITIONS BY HERB AND SUPPLEMENT TREATMENT OPTIONS**
This extracts the items included in the Herb and Nutrition sections of each condition monograph and combines them to create a collective list of herbs and supplements, each with a respective list of conditions where their use may be considered. Some herbs and supplements listed may not yet have a monograph created in the Quick Access *system.*

N-ACETYL CYSTEINE
allergic rhinitis
asthma
bronchitis
chronic obstructive pulmonary disease
hepatitis, viral
HIV and AIDS
peptic ulcer

ACIDOPHILUS
hepatitis, viral
herpes simplex virus
HIV and AIDS
infantile colic
intestinal parasites
irritable bowel syndrome
osteomyelitis
peptic ulcer
vaginitis

S-ADENOSYLMETHIONINE
osteoarthritis

ALANINE
benign prostatic hyperplasia

ALFALFA
anemia
hypercholesterolemia
hypothyroidism
thyroiditis

ALGAE, BLUE GREEN
alopecia

ALOE
burns
cutaneous drug reactions

ALPHA-LIPOIC ACID
Parkinson's disease

AMINO ACIDS
benign prostatic hyperplasia
Parkinson's disease

ANGELICA
menopause

ANISE SEED
infantile colic
irritable bowel syndrome
pertussis

ANTIMICROBIALS
osteomyelitis

ANTIOXIDANTS
atherosclerosis
cirrhosis of the liver
congestive heart failure
dementia
low back pain
myocardial infarction
Parkinson's disease
Reiter's syndrome
rheumatoid arthritis

ARNICA OIL
sprains and strains

ARTICHOKE LEAVES
edema

ASHWAGANDA
rheumatoid arthritis

ASHWAGANDA ROOT
chronic fatigue syndrome
fibromyalgia

ASPARTATE
osteoporosis

ASTRAGALUS
alopecia
common cold
herpes simplex virus
osteomyelitis
pertussis

ASTRAGALUS ROOT
chronic fatigue syndrome
fibromyalgia
hepatitis, viral

BALM OF GILEAD
cough

BARBERRY
candidiasis
cirrhosis of the liver
diarrhea
intestinal parasites
osteomyelitis
peptic ulcer

BAUME DE CANADA
cough

BEARBERRY
infective endocarditis
prostatitis

BELLADONNA
asthma

BERGAMOT
anxiety

BETA-CAROTENE
bronchitis
burns
chronic fatigue syndrome
common cold
cough
dermatitis
eczema
endometriosis
fever of unknown origin
food allergy
hepatitis, viral

herpes simplex virus
herpes zoster (varicella–zoster) virus
HIV and AIDS
infective endocarditis
influenza
intestinal parasites
myocardial infarction
pertussis
pharyngitis
Reiter's syndrome
roseola
sinus headache
sinusitis
sprains and strains
tension headache
ulcerative colitis
urethritis
urinary tract infection in women
vaginitis
warts

BETAINE
atherosclerosis
congestive heart failure
hypertension

BILBERRY
allergic rhinitis
diabetes mellitus
edema
osteoarthritis
Reiter's syndrome

BIOFLAVONOIDS
allergic rhinitis
dermatitis
eczema
hemorrhoids
migraine headache
sprains and strains
tendinitis

BIOTIN
alopecia
candidiasis
dementia
depression-unipolar mood
  disorders
ulcerative colitis

BISMUTH SUBCITRATE
gastritis
peptic ulcer

BLACKBERRY LEAF
diarrhea

BLACK COHOSH
alopecia
amenorrhea
depression-unipolar mood
  disorders
dysmenorrhea
endometriosis
fibromyalgia
infective endocarditis
menopause
osteoarthritis
osteoporosis
sprains and strains

BLACK HAW
low back pain

BLACK HOREHOUND
motion sickness

BLACK STRAP MOLASSES
anemia

BLACK WALNUT
intestinal parasites

BLADDERWRACK
amenorrhea
hypothyroidism
obesity
osteoporosis
thyroiditis

BLUEBERRIES
urethritis
urinary incontinence
urinary tract infection in women

BLUE FLAG
endometriosis
hypercholesterolemia
osteoporosis
rheumatoid arthritis

BLUE MONKSHOOD
pericarditis

BLUE VERVAIN
hypercholesterolemia

BONESET
bronchitis

BORAGE OIL
amenorrhea
dermatitis
dysmenorrhea
eczema
food allergy

BORON
amenorrhea
osteoarthritis
osteoporosis

BOSWELLIA
osteoarthritis
rheumatoid arthritis

BRAN, RAW
irritable bowel syndrome

BREWER'S YEAST
diabetes mellitus
diarrhea

BROMELAIN
angina
atherosclerosis
burns
bursitis
chronic obstructive pulmonary
  disease
cutaneous drug reactions
dermatitis
eczema
endocarditis
food allergy
gout
hyperthyroidism
insect bites
low back pain

myocardial infarction
Reiter's syndrome
rheumatoid arthritis
sinus headache
sinusitis
sprains and strains
tendinitis
thyroiditis
ulcerative colitis

BROOM
edema
pulmonary edema

BUCHU
edema
urethritis
urinary tract infection in women

BUGLEWEED
hyperthyroidism
thyroiditis

BUPLEURUM
Parkinson's disease

BURDOCK
anemia
constipation
psoriasis

BURDOCK ROOT
eczema
herpes zoster (varicella–zoster) virus
hypercholesterolemia
osteomyelitis

BUTCHER'S BROOM
edema

CALCIUM
amenorrhea
anxiety
attention-deficit/hyperactivity
  disorder
candidiasis
depression-unipolar mood disorders
edema
endometriosis
herpes zoster (varicella–zoster) virus
hyperthyroidism
hypothyroidism
osteoporosis
Raynaud's phenomenon
tension headache
ulcerative colitis

CALCIUM CITRATE
osteoporosis

CALCIUM/MAGNESIUM
dementia
insomnia
low back pain
menopause
tendinitis
tension headache
thyroiditis
urinary incontinence

CALIFORNIA POPPY
burns

CAPRYLIC ACID
candidiasis

CARNITINE
atherosclerosis
cirrhosis of the liver
congestive heart failure

L-CARNITINE
angina
chronic fatigue syndrome
chronic obstructive
   pulmonary disease
HIV and AIDS
myocardial infarction
primary pulmonary hypertension
pulmonary edema

CAROB POWDER
diarrhea

CASCARA SAGRADA
constipation

CASTOR OIL
cough

CATECHIN
cirrhosis of the liver
dermatitis
eczema
hemorrhoids

CATNIP
attention-deficit/hyperactivity disorder
fever of unknown origin
food allergy
infantile colic
peptic ulcer
pertussis
roseola

CAYENNE
diabetes mellitus
tension headache

CELANDINE
food allergy
warts

CERNILTON
prostatitis

CHAMOMILE
attention-deficit/hyperactivity disorder
candidiasis
conjunctivitis
cutaneous drug reactions
dermatitis
diarrhea
eczema
food allergy
herpes simplex virus
herpes zoster (varicella–zoster) virus
insomnia
motion sickness
peptic ulcer
pertussis
roseola

CHAMOMILE OIL
insomnia

CHAMOMILE TEA
dysmenorrhea

CHASTE TREE
alopecia

amenorrhea
dysmenorrhea
endometriosis
menopause
osteoporosis
sexual dysfunction

CHICKWEED
cutaneous drug reactions
dermatitis
eczema

CHICORY
food allergy

CHOLAGOGUE
HIV and AIDS

CHOLINE
cirrhosis of the liver
gallbladder disease
hepatitis, viral
migraine headache
obesity
Parkinson's disease
primary pulmonary hypertension
pulmonary edema

CHROMIUM
atherosclerosis
depression-unipolar mood disorders
hypercholesterolemia
osteoporosis
sleep apnea

CHROMIUM PICOLINATE
diabetes mellitus
fibromyalgia
hypoglycemia
obesity

CITRONELLA OIL
insect bites

CLARY SAGE
fibromyalgia

CLEAVERS
allergic rhinitis
burns
dermatitis
eczema
edema
endocarditis
insect bites
osteomyelitis
otitis media
urethritis

COD LIVER OIL
eczema
otitis media

COENZYME Q10
angina
atherosclerosis
chronic obstructive
   pulmonary disease
congestive heart failure
dementia
diabetes mellitus
edema
endocarditis
fibromyalgia
HIV and AIDS

hypercholesterolemia
hypertension
hyperthyroidism
obesity
pericarditis
primary pulmonary hypertension
pulmonary edema
Raynaud's phenomenon

COLEUS
psoriasis

COLTSFOOT
asthma
chronic obstructive
   pulmonary disease
cough

COMFREY
cutaneous drug reactions
dermatitis
eczema
hemorrhoids
herpes zoster (varicella–zoster) virus
tendinitis

COMFREY ROOT
burns

CONDURANGO
anorexia nervosa

CONEFLOWER
allergic rhinitis
bronchitis
burns
common cold
cutaneous drug reactions
endocarditis
fever of unknown origin
hepatitis, viral
herpes simplex virus
herpes zoster (varicella–zoster) virus
influenza
insect bites
laryngitis
osteomyelitis
otitis media
pertussis
pharyngitis
prostatitis
sinus headache
sinusitis
ulcerative colitis
urethritis
urinary tract infection in women
warts

COPPER
Reiter's syndrome

CORN SILK
endocarditis
prostatitis
urethritis
urinary tract infection in women
urolithiasis

COUCHGRASS
edema
urethritis
urinary tract infection in women

CRAMP BARK
endometriosis

hypertension
pertussis
preeclampsia
sprains and strains
ulcerative colitis
urolithiasis

CRAMP BARK TINCTURES
dysmenorrhea

CRANBERRIES
urethritis
urinary incontinence
urinary tract infection in women

CURCUMA
allergic rhinitis

CURCUMIN
tendinitis

CYANOCOBALAMINE
anemia

DAMIANA
sexual dysfunction

DANDELION
anemia
congestive heart failure
food allergy
HIV and AIDS
obesity

DANDELION LEAF
edema
endocarditis
hypertension
pulmonary edema

DANDELION ROOT
amenorrhea
constipation
edema
endometriosis
gallbladder disease
hypercholesterolemia
osteoporosis
sexual dysfunction

DESSICATED LIVER EXTRACT
cirrhosis of the liver
hepatitis, viral

DEVIL'S CLAW
gout
low back pain
osteoarthritis
rheumatoid arthritis

DIGESTIVE ENZYMES
constipation
intestinal parasites
irritable bowel syndrome
psoriasis

DIMETHYLAMINOETHANOL (DMAE)
Parkinson's disease

DIMETHYL GLYCINE
seizures

ECHINACEA
alopecia
warts

ECLIPTA ALBA
hepatitis, viral

EICOSAPENTAENOIC ACID (EPA)
gout

ELDER
edema
fever of unknown origin
influenza
insect bites
roseola

ELDERBERRY
allergic rhinitis
common cold
cough
otitis media

ELECAMPANE
asthma
bronchitis
cough
pertussis

ETHYLENEDIAMINETETRAACETIC ACID (EDTA)
dementia

EUCALYPTUS OIL
chronic obstructive
  pulmonary disease
cough
insect bites
sinus headache
sinusitis

EVENING PRIMROSE
amenorrhea
candidiasis
cirrhosis of the liver
dysmenorrhea
eczema
tension headache

EVENING PRIMROSE OIL
dermatitis
diabetes mellitus
food allergy
hypertension

EYEBRIGHT
allergic rhinitis
conjunctivitis
otitis media
Reiter's syndrome
sinus headache
sinusitis

FATTY ACIDS, ESSENTIAL
alopecia
amenorrhea
angina
atherosclerosis
attention-deficit/hyperactivity
  disorder
benign prostatic hyperplasia
candidiasis
chronic fatigue syndrome
congestive heart failure
dementia
depression-unipolar mood disorders
endometriosis
hyperthyroidism
hypothyroidism

migraine headache
obesity
osteoporosis
otitis media
Parkinson's disease
peptic ulcer
prostatitis
psoriasis
Reiter's syndrome
sleep apnea
tendinitis
tension headache
thyroiditis
ulcerative colitis

FENNEL
chronic obstructive pulmonary
  disease
cough
food allergy
roseola

FENNEL SEED
conjunctivitis
constipation
infantile colic
irritable bowel syndrome

FENUGREEK
anorexia nervosa
diabetes mellitus

FERROUS FUMERATE
anemia

FEVERFEW
migraine headache
sprains and strains

FIBER
obesity
ulcerative colitis

FIREWEED
candidiasis

FISH OIL
diabetes mellitus
otitis media

FLAVANOIDS
rheumatoid arthritis

FLAX MEAL
conjunctivitis
constipation
gallbladder disease
hemorrhoids
irritable bowel syndrome
ulcerative colitis

FLAX OIL
hypertension
pericarditis

FLAXSEED
amenorrhea
candidiasis
cirrhosis of the liver
eczema
tension headache

FLAXSEED OIL
cough
cutaneous drug reactions

dermatitis
dysmenorrhea
food allergy

FOLATE
candidiasis
cirrhosis of the liver
depression-unipolar mood
  disorders
diabetes mellitus
psoriasis

FOLIC ACID
anemia
atherosclerosis
congestive heart failure
gout
hepatitis, viral
hypertension
migraine headache
seizures
ulcerative colitis
urolithiasis
warts

FRANKINCENSE
asthma
cough

GAMMA-AMINOBUTYRIC ACID (GABA)
Parkinson's disease

GAMMA-LINOLENIC ACID (GLA)
alopecia

GAMMA-ORYZANOL
menopause

GANA DERMA
rheumatoid arthritis

GARLIC
bronchitis
candidiasis
cough
diabetes mellitus
endocarditis
HIV and AIDS
hypercholesterolemia
intestinal parasites
osteomyelitis
pertussis
primary pulmonary hypertension
pulmonary edema
sinus headache
vaginitis

GARLIC/GINGER TEA
influenza
pharyngitis
roseola
sinusitis

GARLIC OIL
intestinal parasites
otitis media

GELSEMIUM
asthma
burns
endometriosis

GENTIAN
atherosclerosis

HIV and AIDS
obesity

GERANIUM
ulcerative colitis

GINGER
angina
bronchitis
chronic obstructive pulmonary
  disease
constipation
cough
dementia
hypercholesterolemia
laryngitis
migraine headache
rheumatoid arthritis
sinus headache

GINGER ROOT
allergic rhinitis
asthma
burns
dysmenorrhea
endometriosis
hypoglycemia
irritable bowel syndrome
motion sickness
osteoarthritis
pertussis
Raynaud's phenomenon
sexual dysfunction

GINGER ROOT TEA
gastritis

GINKGO BILOBA
alopecia
angina
asthma
atherosclerosis
dementia
depression-unipolar mood
  disorders
edema
low back pain
menopause
migraine headache
osteomyelitis
Parkinson's disease
primary pulmonary hypertension
Raynaud's phenomenon
sexual dysfunction
tension headache
thyroiditis

GINSENG
rheumatoid arthritis

GINSENG, SIBERIAN
alopecia
anorexia nervosa
chronic fatigue syndrome
dementia
depression-unipolar mood
  disorders
fibromyalgia
HIV and AIDS
hypoglycemia

GLOBE ARTICHOKE
gallbladder disease
hepatitis, viral
Parkinson's disease

GLUCOSAMINE SULFATE
bursitis
osteoarthritis
Reiter's syndrome

GLUTAMIC ACID
benign prostatic hyperplasia
Parkinson's disease

GLUTAMINE
diarrhea
peptic ulcer

L-GLUTAMINE
burns
HIV and AIDS
obesity

GLUTATHIONE
cirrhosis of the liver
hepatitis, viral
Parkinson's disease

GLYCERATE
anemia

GLYCINATE
anemia

GLYCINE
benign prostatic hyperplasia

GLYCYRRHIZIC ACID
herpes simplex virus

GOLDENROD
edema

GOLDENSEAL
anorexia nervosa
burns
candidiasis
common cold
conjunctivitis
cutaneous drug reactions
diarrhea
hepatitis, viral
herpes zoster (varicella–zoster) virus
HIV and AIDS
influenza
intestinal parasites
laryngitis
osteomyelitis
peptic ulcer
pharyngitis
prostatitis
sinus headache
sinusitis
ulcerative colitis
urethritis
urinary tract infection in women
warts

GOLDENSEAL POWDER
insect bites

GOLDENSEAL ROOT
endocarditis
osteomyelitis

GOTU KOLA
burns
chronic fatigue syndrome
dermatitis
fibromyalgia

hypoglycemia
hypothyroidism
Parkinson's disease
rheumatoid arthritis
sexual dysfunction
thyroiditis

GRAPE SEED EXTRACT
diabetes mellitus
Parkinson's disease

GRAVEL ROOT
urolithiasis

GREATER CELANDINE
gallbladder disease
hypercholesterolemia

GREEN TEA
alopecia
asthma
hemorrhoids
hepatitis, viral

GRIFOLD FRONDOSA
rheumatoid arthritis

GRINDELIA
asthma

GUGGUL
hypothyroidism

GUMWEED
cough

HAWTHORN
angina
atherosclerosis
bronchitis
bursitis
chronic obstructive pulmonary
   disease
congestive heart failure
dementia
edema
endocarditis
hyperkalemia
hypertension
hypothyroidism
obesity
osteoarthritis
Parkinson's disease
pericarditis
primary pulmonary hypertension
pulmonary edema
sexual dysfunction
sprains and strains

HAWTHORN BERRIES
hypercholesterolemia
hyperthyroidism
preeclampsia
Raynaud's phenomenon

HESPERIDIN
cutaneous drug reactions
dermatitis
eczema
menopause

**HESPERIDIN METHYL
CHALCONE**
menopause

HOREHOUND
cough

HORSE CHESTNUT
edema

HORSETAIL
alopecia
amenorrhea
edema
hypothyroidism
osteoporosis
Reiter's syndrome
rheumatoid arthritis
thyroiditis
urethritis
urinary incontinence
urinary tract infection in women

HORSETAIL HERB
congestive heart failure

HUANG QI
HIV and AIDS

HYDROCHLORIC ACID
eczema

**HYDROCHLORIC ACID
SUPPLEMENTS**
asthma

HYDROXYCOBALAMIN
asthma

5-HYDROXYTRYPTOPHAN
fibromyalgia
insomnia
migraine headache
obesity

HYSSOP
pertussis

INDIAN TOBACCO
angina
asthma
bronchitis
congestive heart failure
cough
hypertension
pertussis
preeclampsia
primary pulmonary hypertension
pulmonary edema

INDIAN TOBACCO OIL
otitis media

INOSITOL
primary pulmonary hypertension

IODINE
amenorrhea
thyroiditis

IRISH MOSS
hypothyroidism

IRON
depression-unipolar mood disorders
endometriosis

IRON, ELEMENTAL
ulcerative colitis

JAMAICAN DOGWOOD
burns
bursitis
dysmenorrhea
endometriosis
herpes zoster (varicella–zoster)
   virus
insomnia
low back pain
migraine headache
sinus headache
sinusitis
sprains and strains
tension headache
urolithiasis

JASMINE
anxiety

JASMINE OIL
chronic fatigue syndrome
fibromyalgia

JUNIPER
Reiter's syndrome

KAVA KAVA
anxiety
attention-deficit/hyperactivity
   disorder
fibromyalgia
insomnia
sexual dysfunction
tension headache
urethritis
urolithiasis

KELP
amenorrhea
hypothyroidism
obesity
osteoporosis

KHELLA
asthma

LACTOBACILLUS
irritable bowel syndrome

**LACTOBACILLUS
ACIDOPHILUS**
candidiasis

LACTOBACILLUS SPECIES
diarrhea

LADY'S MANTLE
amenorrhea
osteoporosis

LAVENDER
anxiety
asthma
attention-deficit/hyperactivity disorder
chronic fatigue syndrome
fibromyalgia
obesity

LAVENDER ESSENCE OIL
candidiasis

LAVENDER OIL
chronic obstructive pulmonary
   disease
insect bites

insomnia
intestinal parasites
sinus headache
sinusitis

LECITHIN
cirrhosis of the liver
gallbladder disease
hepatitis, viral
obesity
Parkinson's disease

LEMON BALM
anorexia nervosa
anxiety
attention-deficit/hyperactivity
    disorder
dementia
depression-unipolar mood
    disorders
fever of unknown origin
fibromyalgia
herpes simplex virus
herpes zoster (varicella–zoster) virus
hyperthyroidism
infantile colic
insomnia
Parkinson's disease
peptic ulcer
sexual dysfunction
ulcerative colitis

LEOPARD'S BANE
low back pain

LICORICE
amenorrhea
anorexia nervosa
candidiasis
chronic obstructive pulmonary
    disease
common cold
depression-unipolar mood
    disorders
dysphagia
gastroesophageal reflux disease
HIV and AIDS
hyperthyroidism
influenza
laryngitis
menopause
osteomyelitis
osteoporosis
pharyngitis
Reiter's syndrome
sinus headache
sinusitis
tendinitis

**LICORICE,
DEGLYCYRRHIZINATED**
gastritis
peptic ulcer

LICORICE ROOT
asthma
bronchitis
chronic fatigue syndrome
constipation
cough
diarrhea
hepatitis, viral
herpes simplex virus
herpes zoster (varicella–zoster)
    virus

hypoglycemia
insect bites
pertussis
ulcerative colitis
warts

LILY OF THE VALLEY
congestive heart failure
edema
endocarditis
hyperkalemia
hypertension
pulmonary edema

LINDEN FLOWER
angina
atherosclerosis
attention-deficit/hyperactivity
    disorder
bronchitis
congestive heart failure
cough
dysphagia
edema
endocarditis
gastroesophageal reflux disease
hypertension
infantile colic
pericarditis
primary pulmonary hypertension
pulmonary edema

LIPASE
gallbladder disease

LIPOIC ACID
atherosclerosis

LIPOTROPIC AGENTS
gallbladder disease

LITHIUM
hyperthyroidism

LOBELIA
low back pain

LOMATIUM
bronchitis
herpes simplex virus
osteomyelitis
warts

LOMATIUM ROOT
chronic fatigue syndrome

LUNGWORT
bronchitis

L-LYSINE
herpes simplex virus

MAGNESIUM
alopecia
amenorrhea
anxiety
asthma
atherosclerosis
attention-deficit/hyperactivity
    disorder
candidiasis
chronic obstructive pulmonary
    disease
congestive heart failure
cutaneous drug reactions

depression-unipolar mood
    disorders
diabetes mellitus
dysmenorrhea
edema
fibromyalgia
herpes zoster (varicella-zoster) virus
HIV and AIDS
hypercholesterolemia
hyperkalemia
hypertension
hyperthyroidism
hypoglycemia
endocarditis
irritable bowel syndrome
migraine headache
osteoporosis
preeclampsia
pulmonary edema
seizures
sexual dysfunction
tension headache
ulcerative colitis

MAGNESIUM ASPARTATE
chronic fatigue syndrome
pulmonary edema

MAGNESIUM CITRATE
urolithiasis

MA HUANG
asthma
obesity

MALE FERN
intestinal parasites

MAGNESIUM ASPARTATE
primary pulmonary hypertension

MANGANESE
diabetes mellitus
osteoporosis
Parkinson's disease
seizures
tension headache

MARIGOLD
burns
candidiasis
conjunctivitis
cutaneous drug reactions
dermatitis
eczema
hemorrhoids
herpes zoster (varicella–zoster) virus
insect bites
laryngitis
otitis media

MARSHMALLOW ROOT
burns
cutaneous drug reactions
diarrhea
gastritis
irritable bowel syndrome
ulcerative colitis
urethritis
urinary incontinence
urinary tract infection in women

MARSHMALLOW ROOT POWDER
peptic ulcer

MARSHMALLOW ROOT TEA
eczema
food allergy

MAX EPA
hypertension

MEADOWSWEET
bursitis
food allergy
irritable bowel syndrome
migraine headache
osteoarthritis
peptic ulcer
Reiter's syndrome
tension headache
ulcerative colitis

MELATONIN
fibromyalgia
insomnia

METHIONINE
cirrhosis of the liver
hepatitis, viral
obesity

MILK THISTLE
amenorrhea
cirrhosis of the liver
edema
endometriosis
food allergy
gallbladder disease
hepatitis, viral
HIV and AIDS
hypercholesterolemia
hyperthyroidism
irritable bowel syndrome
obesity
osteoporosis
Parkinson's disease
preeclampsia
psoriasis
seizures
sexual dysfunction

MINT
asthma

MISTLETOE
angina
atherosclerosis
congestive heart failure
hypertension

MONKSHOOD
angina
endometriosis

MONKSHOOD OIL
otitis media

MOTHERWORT
angina
congestive heart failure
edema
endocarditis
endometriosis
hypertension
hyperthyroidism
pulmonary edema
thyroiditis

MULLEIN
chronic obstructive pulmonary
   disease
cough
pertussis

MULLEIN FLOWER OIL
otitis media

MUSTARD OIL
cough

MYRRH
endocarditis
laryngitis

NERVINE HERBS
Parkinson's disease

NETTLES
allergic rhinitis
eczema
osteoporosis

NIACIN *(see Vitamin B₃)*
gout
hypercholesterolemia

NIACINAMIDE
(see Vitamin B₃)
dysmenorrhea
hypoglycemia
insomnia
osteoarthritis

NIGHT-BLOOMING CEREUS
angina
edema
endocarditis
hypertension
pulmonary edema

OATMEAL BATHS
cutaneous drug reactions

OATS
Parkinson's disease

OATSTRAW
amenorrhea
anorexia nervosa
anxiety
depression-unipolar mood
   disorders
edema
hypothyroidism
insect bites
osteoporosis
thyroiditis

OMEGA-3 FATTY ACIDS
anemia
atherosclerosis
attention-deficit/hyperactivity disorder
bursitis
candidiasis
chronic obstructive pulmonary
   disease
cirrhosis of the liver
hypercholesterolemia
migraine headache
osteoarthritis
preeclampsia
psoriasis
Raynaud's phenomenon

rheumatoid arthritis
tension headache

OMEGA-6 FATTY ACIDS
attention-deficit/hyperactivity
   disorder
candidiasis
chronic obstructive pulmonary
   disease
cirrhosis of the liver
eczema
psoriasis
tension headache

ONION
cough
diabetes mellitus

OREGANO OIL
cough

OREGON GRAPE
dermatitis
intestinal parasites
peptic ulcer

OREGON GRAPE ROOT
candidiasis

OSHA
warts

PALMITATE
asthma
dermatitis
eczema
food allergy

PANCREATIN
food allergy

PANTHENINE
hypercholesterolemia

PANTOTHENIC ACID
(see Vitamin B₅)
chronic fatigue syndrome
hypoglycemia
ulcerative colitis

PAPAIN
intestinal parasites

PARSLEY
edema
obesity

PASSIONFLOWER
anxiety
attention-deficit/hyperactivity
   disorder
chronic fatigue syndrome
depression-unipolar mood disorders
fibromyalgia
food allergy
hypertension
hyperthyroidism
insomnia
irritable bowel syndrome
peptic ulcer
preeclampsia
seizures
sexual dysfunction
thyroiditis
ulcerative colitis

PAU D'ARCO BARK
candidiasis

PAU D'ARCO TEA
vaginitis

PENNYROYAL OIL
insect bites

PEPPERMINT
cutaneous drug reactions
dermatitis
eczema
food allergy
infantile colic
insect bites
laryngitis
motion sickness
obesity
peptic ulcer
roseola

PEPPERMINT LEAF
dermatitis

PEPPERMINT OIL
chronic fatigue syndrome
gallbladder disease
irritable bowel syndrome
tension headache
ulcerative colitis

PETASITES
low back pain

PHOSPHATIDYL CHOLINE
fibromyalgia
Parkinson's disease

PHOSPHATIDYL SERINE
fibromyalgia

PHYLLANTHUS AMARUS
hepatitis, viral

PILL BEARING SPURGE
bronchitis

PINE OILS
cough

PIPSISSEWA
urethritis
urinary tract infection in women
urolithiasis

PLANTAIN
asthma
burns
conjunctivitis
cough
peptic ulcer
urethritis
urinary incontinence
urinary tract infection in women

PLANTAIN LEAVES
insect bites

PLEURISY ROOT
bronchitis

POKE ROOT
endometriosis
sprains and strains

POTASSIUM
peptic ulcer
pulmonary edema
tension headache

POTASSIUM ASPARTATE
edema
primary pulmonary hypertension
pulmonary edema

POTATO, FRESH GRATED
conjunctivitis
hemorrhoids

PRICKLY ASH BARK
alopecia
burns
dermatitis
Raynaud's phenomenon
sexual dysfunction

PRO-FLORA SUPPLEMENTS
food allergy
ulcerative colitis

PROPOLIS
laryngitis
pharyngitis

PSYLLIUM
irritable bowel syndrome
ulcerative colitis

PUMPKIN SEEDS
benign prostatic hyperplasia
prostatitis

PURPLE CONEFLOWER
cough

PYCNOGENOL
diabetes mellitus
Parkinson's disease

PYRIDOXAL-5-PHOSPHATE
asthma

PYRIDOXINE
hypoglycemia
urolithiasis

QUASSIA
intestinal parasites

QUERCETIN
allergic rhinitis
cutaneous drug reactions
dermatitis
diarrhea
eczema
food allergy
hyperthyroidism
insect bites
peptic ulcer
psoriasis
rheumatoid arthritis
sinusitis
sprains and strains
thyroiditis
ulcerative colitis

RAW HEART CONCENTRATE
pulmonary edema

RAW THYMUS GLANDULAR
fibromyalgia

RED ALDER BARK
dermatitis

RED CLOVER
cutaneous drug reactions
dermatitis
eczema
edema
insect bites
osteomyelitis
psoriasis

RED RASPBERRY
dysmenorrhea
endometriosis

RED ROOT
edema
endometriosis

RIBOFLAVIN *(see Vitamin B₂)*
ulcerative colitis

ROSE HIPS
allergic rhinitis
asthma
dermatitis
dermatitis
eczema
food allergy
hemorrhoids

ROSEMARY
alopecia
atherosclerosis
congestive heart failure
dementia
edema
endocarditis
fibromyalgia
primary pulmonary hypertension
pulmonary edema
Raynaud's phenomenon
sexual dysfunction

ROSEMARY LEAF
chronic fatigue syndrome
low back pain

ROSEMARY OIL
chronic fatigue syndrome
chronic obstructive pulmonary
   disease
insomnia

RUE
edema

RUTIN
dermatitis
eczema

SACROMYCES BOLARDII
diarrhea

SAGE
amenorrhea
asthma
laryngitis

SARSAPARILLA
dermatitis

psoriasis
rheumatoid arthritis

SAW PALMETTO
alopecia
anorexia nervosa
benign prostatic hyperplasia
prostatitis

SCHIZANDRA BERRY
chronic fatigue syndrome
fibromyalgia
hepatitis, viral

SELENIUM
amenorrhea
atherosclerosis
benign prostatic hyperplasia
candidiasis
chronic obstructive pulmonary
   disease
cirrhosis of the liver
congestive heart failure
dermatitis
endocarditis
endometriosis
food allergy
hepatitis, viral
herpes simplex virus
HIV and AIDS
hypercholesterolemia
hypothyroidism
Parkinson's disease
primary pulmonary hypertension
prostatitis
psoriasis
pulmonary edema
Reiter's syndrome
rheumatoid arthritis
tension headache
thyroiditis
ulcerative colitis
warts

SKULLCAP
anxiety
asthma
chronic fatigue syndrome
dysphagia
fibromyalgia
gastroesophageal reflux disease
migraine headache
Parkinson's disease
seizures
sexual dysfunction

SKUNK CABBAGE
asthma

SLIPPERY ELM
osteomyelitis

SLIPPERY ELM POWDER
burns
cutaneous drug reactions
diarrhea
dysphagia
gastritis
gastroesophageal reflux disease
herpes zoster (varicella–zoster) virus
irritable bowel syndrome
laryngitis
peptic ulcer
pharyngitis
ulcerative colitis

SOY
menopause

SPEARMINT
fever of unknown origin
infantile colic

SPIRULINA
anemia

SQUAW VINE
amenorrhea
endometriosis
osteoporosis

ST. JOHN'S WORT
anorexia nervosa
anxiety
burns
dementia
depression-unipolar mood
   disorders
dysphagia
gastroesophageal reflux disease
herpes simplex virus
herpes zoster (varicella–zoster) virus
HIV and AIDS
influenza
insomnia
low back pain
obesity
osteomyelitis
Parkinson's disease
sexual dysfunction
sinus headache
sinusitis

ST. JOHN'S WORT OIL
otitis media

STINGING NETTLE ROOT
benign prostatic hyperplasia

SULPHUR
peptic ulcer

SUNDEW
bronchitis

SWEET CLOVER
edema
SWEET VIOLET
cough

TANSY
intestinal parasites

TAURINE
congestive heart failure
primary pulmonary hypertension
pulmonary edema
seizures

L-TAURINE
angina
hypercholesterolemia

TEASEL ROOT
osteoarthritis
TEA TREE OIL
candidiasis
intestinal parasites

THIAMINE *(see Vitamin B₁)*
edema

obesity
ulcerative colitis

THUJA LEAF
warts

THYME
cough
intestinal parasites
pertussis

THYME LEAF
asthma
bronchitis
pulmonary edema
urethritis
urinary tract infection in women

THYME OIL
chronic obstructive pulmonary
   disease
cough
intestinal parasites
sinus headache
sinusitis

THYMUS EXTRACT
hepatitis, viral
herpes simplex virus

TURMERIC
burns
bursitis
cutaneous drug reactions
edema
gallbladder disease
hepatitis, viral
hyperthyroidism
insect bites
low back pain
osteoarthritis
rheumatoid arthritis
sprains and strains
thyroiditis

TYROSINE
amenorrhea

L-TYROSINE
hypothyroidism
thyroiditis

USNEA LICHEN
pertussis

UVA URSI
Reiter's syndrome
urethritis
urinary tract infection in women

VALERIAN
anorexia nervosa
asthma
burns
bursitis
depression-unipolar mood
   disorders
dysphagia
endometriosis
fibromyalgia
gastroesophageal reflux disease
herpes zoster (varicella–zoster) virus
hypertension
insomnia
irritable bowel syndrome

low back pain
obesity
osteomyelitis
peptic ulcer
pertussis
rheumatoid arthritis
seizures
sprains and strains
tension headache
ulcerative colitis

VANADIUM
diabetes mellitus

VANADYL SULFATE
hypoglycemia

VERVAIN
amenorrhea
endometriosis
osteoporosis
sexual dysfunction

VITAMIN A
allergic rhinitis
amenorrhea
common cold
conjunctivitis
diarrhea
gout
herpes simplex virus
herpes zoster (varicella–zoster) virus
hypothyroidism
endocarditis
influenza
osteoarthritis
osteomyelitis
peptic ulcer
pericarditis
tendinitis
thyroiditis
ulcerative colitis
vaginitis
warts

VITAMIN B$_1$
edema
depression-unipolar mood
  disorders
obesity
ulcerative colitis

VITAMIN B$_2$
depression-unipolar mood
  disorders
hypothyroidism
migraine headache
ulcerative colitis

VITAMIN B$_3$
dysmenorrhea
gout
hypercholesterolemia
hypothyroidism
hypoglycemia
insomnia
osteoarthritis

VITAMIN B$_5$
allergic rhinitis

VITAMIN B$_6$
allergic rhinitis
alopecia
amenorrhea
asthma
atherosclerosis
benign prostatic hyperplasia
congestive heart failure
depression-unipolar mood disorders
edema
hypothyroidism
migraine headache
seizures
sexual dysfunction

VITAMIN B$_{12}$
anemia
asthma
atherosclerosis
congestive heart failure
depression-unipolar mood disorders
herpes zoster (varicella–zoster) virus
HIV and AIDS
hypertension
psoriasis
seizures
ulcerative colitis

VITAMIN B-COMPLEX
anxiety
attention-deficit/hyperactivity
  disorder
candidiasis
chronic fatigue syndrome
cirrhosis of the liver
dementia
diabetes mellitus
dysmenorrhea
fibromyalgia
food allergy
hepatitis, viral
herpes zoster (varicella–zoster) virus
HIV and AIDS
hypercholesterolemia
hypertension
hypoglycemia
hypothyroidism
insect bites
insomnia
laryngitis
low back pain
obesity
osteoporosis
Parkinson's disease
Raynaud's phenomenon
sexual dysfunction
tension headache
thyroiditis
ulcerative colitis
warts

**VITAMIN B-COMPLEX WITH
EXTRA B$_{12}$**
cutaneous drug reactions

VITAMIN C
allergic rhinitis
amenorrhea
anemia
angina
asthma

atherosclerosis
attention-deficit/hyperactivity
  disorder
bronchitis
burns
candidiasis
chronic fatigue syndrome
chronic obstructive pulmonary
  disease
cirrhosis of the liver
common cold
congestive heart failure
conjunctivitis
cough
cutaneous drug reactions
dementia
depression-unipolar mood
  disorders
dermatitis
diabetes mellitus
diarrhea
eczema
edema
endocarditis
endometriosis
fever of unknown origin
fibromyalgia
food allergy
gallbladder disease
gastritis
gout
hemorrhoids
hepatitis, viral
herpes simplex virus
herpes zoster (varicella–zoster) virus
HIV and AIDS
hypercholesterolemia
hyperthyroidism
hypoglycemia
hypothyroidism
influenza
insect bites
intestinal parasites
laryngitis
low back pain
menopause
migraine headache
myocardial infarction
obesity
osteoarthritis
osteomyelitis
otitis media
Parkinson's disease
peptic ulcer
pericarditis
pertussis
pharyngitis
primary pulmonary hypertension
prostatitis
pulmonary edema
Raynaud's phenomenon
Reiter's syndrome
rheumatoid arthritis
roseola
sexual dysfunction
sinus headache
sinusitis
sprains and strains
tendinitis
tension headache
thyroiditis
ulcerative colitis
urethritis
urinary incontinence

urinary tract infection in women
vaginitis
warts

VITAMIN C WITH BIOFLAVONOIDS
bursitis

VITAMIN D
amenorrhea
ulcerative colitis

VITAMIN E
allergic rhinitis
alopecia
amenorrhea
atherosclerosis
burns
candidiasis
chronic obstructive pulmonary disease
cirrhosis of the liver
congestive heart failure
cutaneous drug reactions
dementia
dermatitis
diabetes mellitus
dysmenorrhea
edema
endocarditis
endometriosis
gallbladder disease
hemorrhoids
hepatitis, viral
herpes zoster (varicella–zoster)virus
HIV and AIDS
hypertension
hyperthyroidism
hypoglycemia
low back pain
menopause
migraine headache
myocardial infarction
osteoarthritis
osteomyelitis
Parkinson's disease
peptic ulcer
primary pulmonary hypertension
psoriasis
pulmonary edema
Raynaud's phenomenon
Reiter's syndrome
sexual dysfunction
sprains and strains
tendinitis
tension headache
thyroiditis
vaginitis
warts

VITAMIN K
amenorrhea
cirrhosis of the liver
hepatitis, viral
osteoporosis
ulcerative colitis

WHITE BYRONY
endometriosis

WHITE HOREHOUND
bronchitis

WHITE WILLOW
bursitis

WHITE WILLOW BARK
fever of unknown origin
low back pain
tension headache

WILD CHERRY BARK
asthma
bronchitis
cough

WILD INDIGO
endocarditis
sinus headache
sinusitis

WILD LETTUCE
herpes zoster (varicella–zoster)virus

WILD YAM
amenorrhea
anorexia nervosa
dysmenorrhea
dysphagia
endometriosis
gastroesophageal reflux disease
irritable bowel syndrome
low back pain
osteoporosis
rheumatoid arthritis
ulcerative colitis
urolithiasis

WILLOW
tendinitis

WITCH HAZEL
hemorrhoids
insect bites

WORMSEED
intestinal parasites

WORMWOOD
intestinal parasites

YARROW
alopecia
burns
cutaneous drug reactions
dermatitis
eczema
edema
endometriosis
fever of unknown origin
herpes simplex virus
endocarditis
influenza
osteomyelitis
roseola

YELLOW DOCK
anemia
constipation
eczema
osteomyelitis
psoriasis

YELLOW JASMINE
angina
herpes zoster (varicella–zoster) virus

YOHIMBE BARK
sexual dysfunction

YUCCA
osteoarthritis

ZINC
allergic rhinitis
alopecia
amenorrhea
anorexia nervosa
benign prostatic hyperplasia
bronchitis
burns
common cold
conjunctivitis
cough
cutaneous drug reactions
dementia
dermatitis
diabetes mellitus
eczema
endocarditis
endometriosis
fever of unknown origin
fibromyalgia
food allergy
gastritis
hepatitis, viral
herpes simplex virus
herpes zoster (varicella-zoster) virus
HIV and AIDS
hypertension
hypoglycemia
hypothyroidism
influenza
intestinal parasites
osteomyelitis
osteoporosis
peptic ulcer
pertussis
pharyngitis
prostatitis
psoriasis
Raynaud's phenomenon
Reiter's syndrome
rheumatoid arthritis
roseola
seizures
sinus headache
sinusitis
sprains and strains
tension headache
thyroiditis
ulcerative colitis
urethritis
urinary incontinence
urinary tract infection in women
vaginitis
warts

ZINC LOZENGES
laryngitis

■ HERBS BY USES AND INDICATIONS
This list extracts the items included in the Uses/Indications section of each herb monograph and combines them to create a collection of herbs that may be considered for a particular application or condition.

ABRASIONS
goldenseal

ABSCESS
chamomile, German
echinacea
goldenseal

ACHES AND PAINS
eucalyptus

ACNE
Brewer's yeast
cat's claw
evening primrose

ACNE, INFANT
chamomile, German

ACROCYANOSIS
grape seed extract

ADAPTOGEN
ginseng, American
ginseng, Asian
licorice

ADRENOCORTICAL INSUFFICIENCY, PRIMARY
licorice

AGING-RELATED DISORDERS
evening primrose

AIDS
bromelain
cat's claw
St. John's wort

ALCOHOLISM
evening primrose

ALLERGIES
cat's claw
devil's claw
feverfew
flaxseed oil
ginkgo biloba
licorice
stinging nettle

ALTERATIVE
barberry
echinacea
ginseng, American
ginseng, Asian
stinging nettle

ALZHEIMER'S DISEASE
ginkgo biloba

ANALGESIC
celery seed
devil's claw

ANALGESIC, TOPICAL
cayenne
peppermint

ANEMIA
feverfew
stinging nettle

ANESTHETIC
kava kava

ANGINA PECTORIS
bilberry
bromelain
hawthorn

ANODYNE
ginseng, Asian
valerian root

ANOGENITAL INFLAMMATION
chamomile, German

ANOREXIA
chamomile, Roman
devil's claw
ginseng, Siberian
St. John's wort

ANTIARRHYTHMIAS
hawthorn

ANTIARTERIOSCLEROTIC
green tea

ANTIBACTERIAL
cayenne
chamomile, German
green tea
lemon balm
peppermint

ANTIBIOTICS, POTENTIATION OF
bromelain

ANTICHOLESTEREMIC
garlic
green tea

ANTIDEPRESSANT
ginkgo biloba
ginseng, Asian
St. John's wort

ANTIDIARRHEAL
bilberry

ANTIDOTE TO STINGS
stinging nettle

ANTIEMETIC
ginger root
peppermint

ANTIFUNGAL
green tea

ANTIHELMINTIC
garlic

ANTIHEPATOTOXIN
licorice

ANTIHISTAMINE
garlic
stinging nettle

ANTIHYPERTENSIVE
cayenne
garlic

ANTI-INFECTIVE
echinacea

ANTI-INFLAMMATORY
barberry
bilberry
cat's claw
celery seed
chamomile, German
comfrey
echinacea
evening primrose
feverfew
flaxseed
licorice
saw palmetto

ANTILIPIDAEMIC
garlic

ANTIMETASTATIC AGENT
bromelain

ANTIMICROBIAL
chamomile, German
echinacea
garlic
licorice
St. John's wort

ANTIMITOTIC
comfrey

ANTIMUTAGENIC
green tea

ANTIOXIDANT
bilberry
cayenne
green tea

ANTIPARASITIC
peppermint

ANTIPATHOGENIC
goldenseal

ANTIPHOLIGISTIC
chamomile, German

ANTIPYRETIC
devil's claw
licorice

ANTIRHEUMATIC
devil's claw

ANTISEPTIC
barberry
eucalyptus
ginger root

ANTISEPTIC, URINARY
saw palmetto

ANTISPASMODIC
black cohosh

chamomile, German
chamomile, Roman
ginger root
kava kava
licorice
peppermint
valerian root

ANTITHROMBOTIC
ginkgo biloba

ANTITUMOR
licorice

ANTITUSSIVE
flaxseed

ANTIVIRAL
cat's claw
eucalyptus
green tea
licorice

ANXIETY
kava kava
St. John's wort
valerian root

APATHY
St. John's wort

APHRODISIAC
celery seed
ginseng, Asian

APPETITE LOSS
(see anorexia)

APPETITE STIMULANT
barberry
ginseng, Asian

AROMATIC
chamomile, German
peppermint

ARTERIAL WALL PLAQUE DEPOSITS
bilberry
bromelain

ARTERIES, STRENGTHENING OF
cayenne

ARTERIOSCLEROSIS
devil's claw

ARTHRITIS *(see also osteoarthritis, rheumatoid arthritis)*
barberry
burdock
cat's claw
celery seed
devil's claw
evening primrose
feverfew
flaxseed oil
ginger root
licorice

ASTHMA
aloe
cat's claw
evening primrose
flaxseed oil

green tea
licorice

ASTRINGENT
barberry
bilberry
comfrey
eucalyptus
goldenseal
green tea
hawthorn

ATHEROSCLEROSIS
bromelain
cayenne
ginkgo biloba
ginseng, Siberian

ATHEROSCLEROSIS, PREVENTION
green tea

ATTENTION DEFICIT/ HYPERACTIVITY DISORDER
ginseng, Siberian

AUTOIMMUNE REACTION
flaxseed oil
licorice

BACTERIAL ILLNESS
licorice

BACTERICIDE
valerian root

BACTERIOSTATIC
chamomile, German

BEDSORES
chamomile, Roman

BENIGN PROSTATIC HYPERPLASIA
saw palmetto
stinging nettle

BILE PRODUCTION
milk thistle

BITTER TONIC
barberry
feverfew
ginseng, American
goldenseal

BLADDER DISORDERS
devil's claw

BLADDER INFLAMMATION
flaxseed

BLOATING AND FULLNESS
chamomile, Roman
lemon balm

BLOOD CHOLESTEROL, LOWERING OF
Brewer's yeast
flaxseed
green tea

BLOOD PRESSURE DISORDERS
ginseng, Siberian

BLOOD PRESSURE REDUCTION
black cohosh
cayenne
evening primrose

BLUNT INJURIES
comfrey

BOILS
echinacea
goldenseal

BONE PAIN
cat's claw

BRONCHIAL INFLAMMATION/ INFECTION
barberry
comfrey
eucalyptus

BRONCHIAL IRRITATION
flaxseed

BRONCHITIS
licorice

BRONCHODILATOR
green tea

BRUISING
comfrey
evening primrose

BURNS
aloe
chamomile, Roman
flaxseed
milk thistle
St. John's wort
stinging nettle

BURSITIS
bromelain

CALCULI *(see also kidney stones)*
celery seed

CANCER
cat's claw
evening primrose
ginseng, American
ginseng, Asian
green tea

CANCER, PREVENTION
celery seed
flaxseed
green tea

CANDIDIASIS, CHRONIC
barberry

CAPILLARY FRAGILITY
bilberry
cayenne
grape seed extract

CAPILLARY WALL FORMATION AND STRENGTH
bilberry

CARBUNCLES
echinacea

CARDIAC INSUFFICIENCY WITH EDEMA
stinging nettle

CARDIAC WEAKNESS
hawthorn

CARDIOTONIC
ginseng, Asian
hawthorn

CARDIOVASCULAR DISEASE
bromelain

CARDIOVASCULAR DISEASE, PREVENTION
flaxseed

CARMINATIVE
cayenne
chamomile, German
ginger root
ginseng, Asian
lemon balm
peppermint
valerian root

CARPAL TUNNEL SYNDROME
cayenne

CATARACTS
bilberry

CATARRH, RESPIRATORY
lemon balm
peppermint
saw palmetto

CEREBRAL VASCULAR INSUFFICIENCY
ginkgo biloba

CHEMOTHERAPEUTIC AGENTS, POTENTIATION OF
bromelain

CHEST CONGESTION
eucalyptus

CHICKEN POX
chamomile, German

CHOLAGOGUE
barberry
ginger root
goldenseal
milk thistle

CHOLANGITIS
milk thistle

CHOLERETIC
milk thistle
peppermint

CHRONIC FATIGUE SYNDROME
evening primrose
ginseng, Siberian

CIRCULATORY DISORDERS
barberry
bilberry
ginkgo biloba

CIRCULATORY STIMULANT
cayenne
ginger root
ginkgo biloba
stinging nettle

CIRRHOSIS
cat's claw
milk thistle

CLAUDICATION, INTERMITTENT
evening primrose
ginkgo biloba

COCHLEAR DEAFNESS
ginkgo biloba

COLD, COMMON
echinacea
eucalyptus
ginger root
ginseng, American
ginseng, Asian
goldenseal
green tea

COLD, COMMON, PREVENTION
garlic

COLD SORES, HERPES SIMPLEX SYMPTOM
lemon balm

COLIC
chamomile, German
chamomile, Roman (folk
   remedy)

COLIC, INFANTILE
chamomile, Roman

COLIC, INTESTINAL
ginger root

COLLAGEN STABILIZATION
bilberry

COLON, IRRITABLE
peppermint

COLON DISORDERS, LAXATIVE ABUSE
flaxseed

CONCENTRATION, IMPAIRED
ginseng, Asian
ginseng, Siberian

CONGESTIVE HEART FAILURE
evening primrose
hawthorn

CONJUNCTIVITIS
goldenseal

CONSTIPATION
aloe
peppermint

CONSTIPATION, CHRONIC
flaxseed

CONSTIPATION, SPASTIC
chamomile, Roman

CONVALESCENCE, HELP DURING
cat's claw
ginseng, Asian
ginseng, Siberian

CONVULSIONS
valerian root

CORONARY ARTERIOSCLEROSIS
ginseng, Siberian

CORONARY ARTERY DISEASE
hawthorn

COUGH
flaxseed
green tea
licorice

COUGH, DRY
peppermint

COUGH, SPASMODIC
chamomile, German

CRAMPS, NIGHT LEG
valerian root

CRAMPS, STOMACH OR INTESTINAL
valerian root

CYSTITIS
saw palmetto

CYSTITIS, CHRONIC
kava kava

CYSTS
cat's claw

DEBILITY
cat's claw
ginseng, Siberian
saw palmetto

DECONGESTANT
eucalyptus
peppermint

DEMENTIA
ginkgo biloba

DEMULCENT
comfrey
evening primrose
flaxseed
licorice
milk thistle

DEODORANT
chamomile, German
eucalyptus

DEPRESSION
Brewer's yeast
cat's claw
ginkgo biloba
St. John's wort

DEPRESSION (MENOPAUSE)
black cohosh

DEVELOPMENTAL DISORDERS
evening primrose

DIABETES
aloe
bilberry
Brewer's yeast
cat's claw
evening primrose
flaxseed oil
ginseng, American
ginseng, Asian
goldenseal

DIABETES, NON-INSULIN DEPENDENT
Brewer's yeast
stinging nettle

DIABETIC NEUROPATHY
cayenne
evening primrose

DIABETIC RETINOPATHY
bilberry
ginkgo biloba

DIAPHORETIC
barberry
cayenne
chamomile, German
chamomile, Roman
ginger root
lemon balm

DIARRHEA
bilberry
goldenseal
green tea
peppermint

DIARRHEA, CHRONIC
barberry

DIGESTIVE DISORDERS
cat's claw
celery seed
chamomile, German

DIGESTIVE ENZYME
bromelain

DIURETIC
barberry
celery seed
chamomile, German
devil's claw
ginseng, Siberian
hawthorn
kava kava
saw palmetto
stinging nettle

DIVERTICULITIS
flaxseed

DOUCHE
garlic
goldenseal

DRUG RESISTANCE, TUMOR CELL
flaxseed oil

DRUG SIDE EFFECTS
cat's claw

DYSENTERY
barberry
cat's claw
green tea

DYSMENORRHEA
bilberry
flaxseed oil
ginger root
peppermint

DYSMENORRHEA, CONGESTIVE
feverfew

DYSPEPSIA
cayenne
devil's claw

DYSPEPSIA, FLATULENT
cayenne

EAR INFLAMMATION
chamomile, Roman
goldenseal

ECZEMA
chamomile, German
evening primrose
milk thistle

ECZEMA, INFANTILE
evening primrose

EDEMA
ginseng, American
ginseng, Asian

EMMENAGOGUE
black cohosh
celery seed
feverfew
peppermint

EMOLLIENT
comfrey
flaxseed

EMPHYSEMA
cayenne

ENTERITIS
goldenseal

ENTERITIS, MUCILAGE FOR
flaxseed

EPILEPSY, UNCONTROLLED
kava kava

ERYTHEMA
milk thistle

ESOPHAGEAL INFLAMMATION, CHRONIC
licorice

EXPECTORANT
barberry

cayenne
flaxseed
garlic
ginger root
ginseng, Asian
licorice
saw palmetto

EXPECTORANT, RELAXING
comfrey

EYE AILMENTS
barberry

EYE DISORDERS
bilberry

EYE IRRITATION
goldenseal

FATIGUE
Brewer's yeast
ginseng, American
ginseng, Asian
ginseng, Siberian

FATTY ACIDS, ESSENTIAL, DEFICIENCY
evening primrose

FEBRIFUGE
eucalyptus
lemon balm

FEELINGS OF WORTHLESSNESS
St. John's wort

FEVER
barberry
burdock
cayenne
valerian root

FIBROCYSTIC BREAST DISEASE
evening primrose

FIBROMYALGIA
St. John's wort

FIBROSITIS
devil's claw

FISTULAE
cat's claw
chamomile, German

FLATULENCE
chamomile, German
ginger root
lemon balm
peppermint

FOOD SENSITIVITIES
goldenseal

FRACTURES
comfrey

FRONTAL SINUS CATARRH
chamomile, Roman

FUNGAL ILLNESS
echinacea

FUNGUS
cat's claw

FURUNCULOSIS
echinacea

GALACTAGOGUE
celery seed
milk thistle
stinging nettle

GALLBLADDER DISORDERS
chamomile, Roman
devil's claw
milk thistle

GALLSTONES
milk thistle
peppermint

GASTRIC INFLAMMATION, CHRONIC
licorice

GASTRIC MUCUS STIMULATION
bilberry

GASTRITIS
cat's claw
chamomile, Roman
goldenseal

GASTRITIS, CHRONIC
licorice

GASTRITIS, MUCILAGE FOR
flaxseed

GASTROINTESTINAL DISORDERS
devil's claw
lemon balm

GASTROINTESTINAL STIMULANT
cayenne

GASTROINTESTINAL TRACT INFLAMMATION/INFECTION
barberry
chamomile, German

GASTROINTESTINAL UPSET
bromelain

GINGIVITIS
chamomile, German

GLANDULAR SWELLING
goldenseal

GLAUCOMA
bilberry

GONORRHEA
cat's claw
kava kava

GOUT
celery seed
devil's claw
stinging nettle

HAIR, STRENGTHEN
Brewer's yeast

HAY FEVER
chamomile, Roman

HEADACHE
aloe
devil's claw
ginger root
ginkgo biloba
lemon balm
peppermint

HEADACHE, CLUSTER
cayenne

HEADACHE, MENOPAUSE
black cohosh

HEADACHE, MIGRAINE
cayenne
evening primrose
feverfew
kava kava
valerian root

HEARTBURN
chamomile, German
chamomile, Roman
devil's claw

HEART DISEASE
cat's claw

HEART FAILURE
hawthorn

HELICOBACTER PYLORI
barberry

HEMORRHAGE
barberry

HEMORRHOIDS
aloe
bilberry
cat's claw
chamomile, German
chamomile, Roman
evening primrose
stinging nettle

HEPATITIS
barberry
milk thistle

HEPATORESTORATIVE
milk thistle

HERPES
cat's claw

HERPES SIMPLEX
St. John's wort

HERPES SIMPLEX, COLD SORES
lemon balm

HIRSUTISM
saw palmetto

HIV
aloe
cat's claw

HIVES
aloe

chamomile, German
peppermint

HORMONE RESTORATIVE
ginseng, Asian

HOT FLUSHES (MENOPAUSE)
black cohosh

HYPERCHOLESTEROLEMIA
evening primrose
ginseng, American
ginseng, Asian

HYPERSOMNIA
St. John's wort

HYPERTENSION
cat's claw
celery seed
flaxseed oil

HYPERTENSION, ESSENTIAL
hawthorn

HYPNOTIC, MILD
valerian root

HYPOGLYCEMIC
stinging nettle

HYPOTENSIVE
hawthorn

IMMUNE FUNCTION, NORMALIZATION OF
licorice

IMMUNE SYSTEM DISORDERS
cat's claw

IMMUNE SYSTEM ENHANCEMENT
aloe

IMMUNOSTIMULATION
echinacea

IMPETIGO
chamomile, German

IMPOTENCE
ginkgo biloba

INDIGESTION
barberry
cayenne
ginger root

INFANTILE ERUPTIONS
evening primrose

INFECTION
garlic

INFERTILITY
ginseng, American
ginseng, Asian

INFLAMMATION
flaxseed oil

INFLAMMATION, ARTHRITIS AND RHEUMATISM
black cohosh

INFLUENZA
echinacea
eucalyptus
ginger root
goldenseal
lemon balm
St. John's wort

INFLUENZA, PREVENTION
garlic

INSECT BITES
feverfew
lemon balm
stinging nettle

INSOMNIA
chamomile, German
ginseng, Siberian
kava kava
lemon balm
St. John's wort
valerian root

INTESTINAL INFLAMMATION
goldenseal

INTESTINAL PARASITES
feverfew

INTESTINAL ULCERATION OR EROSION
comfrey

IRRITABILITY
black cohosh
Brewer's yeast

IRRITABLE BOWEL SYNDROME
flaxseed
peppermint

JAUNDICE
barberry

JET LAG
kava kava

JOINT ACHES
ginger root

JOINT INFLAMMATION
bromelain

JOINTS, ARTHRITIC
stinging nettle

KIDNEY DISORDERS
devil's claw
ginseng, Siberian

KIDNEY INFLAMMATION/ INFECTION
barberry

KIDNEY STONES (see also calculi)
aloe
stinging nettle

LACERATIONS
goldenseal

LACTATION
saw palmetto

LAXATIVE
barberry
goldenseal
licorice

LAXATIVE, BULKING
flaxseed

LAXATIVE ABUSE, COLON PROBLEMS
flaxseed

LEUKOPENIA, RADIOTHERAPY- AND CHEMOTHERAPY-INDUCED
ginseng, Siberian

LIGAMENT STRAINS (see also sprains and strains)
comfrey

LIVER DAMAGE
milk thistle

LIVER DISORDERS
barberry
celery seed
chamomile, Roman
devil's claw
milk thistle

LOCOMOTIVE SYSTEM DISORDERS
devil's claw

LOW BACK PAIN
barberry
ginseng, Siberian

LUMBAGO
devil's claw

LUPUS SCLERODERMA
licorice

LYMPHEDEMA
grape seed extract

MACULAR DEGENERATION
bilberry
ginkgo biloba
grape seed extract

MASTALGIA
evening primrose

MASTECTOMY PAIN
cayenne

MEMBRANE STABILIZATION
bilberry

MEMORY LOSS, SHORT-TERM
ginkgo biloba

MENOPAUSE
black cohosh
ginseng, Asian
kava kava

MENSTRUAL DISORDERS
cat's claw
chamomile, Roman

devil's claw
feverfew
kava kava
lemon balm

MENSTRUAL PAIN
black cohosh
garlic
ginger root
lemon balm

MENSTRUATION, DELAYED
ginger root
lemon balm

MENTAL STAMINA
cat's claw
ginseng, American
ginseng, Asian

METABOLIC DISORDERS
evening primrose

MICTURITION
stinging nettle

MIGRAINE (see headache, migraine)

MILK PRODUCTION (see also lactation)
milk thistle

MONONUCLEOSIS
St. John's wort

MORNING SICKNESS
peppermint

MOTION SICKNESS
ginger root

MOUTH INFLAMMATION
chamomile, German
goldenseal

MOUTH PAIN
cayenne
chamomile, German

MOUTH SORES
barberry

MOUTHWASH
garlic
goldenseal

MUCUS, EXCESS
goldenseal

MULTIPLE SCLEROSIS
evening primrose
St. John's wort

MUSCLE RELAXANT
bilberry
kava kava

MUSCLE SPASMS
celery seed
valerian root

MUSCLE STRAINS (see also sprains and strains)
comfrey
ginger root

211

MUSCLE WASTING
saw palmetto

MUSCULOSKELETAL CONDITIONS, DEGENERATIVE
devil's claw

MUSCULOTROPIC
chamomile, German

MYALGIC CONDITIONS
devil's claw
peppermint

MYOCARDIAL INFARCTION, POST
hawthorn

NAILS, STRENGTHEN
Brewer's yeast

NASAL CONGESTION
peppermint

NASAL MUCOSITIS
chamomile, Roman

NASOPHARYNGEAL INFLAMMATION
echinacea

NAUSEA
chamomile, Roman
ginger root
peppermint

NEPHRITIS
flaxseed oil

NERVINE
black cohosh
celery seed
ginseng, Asian
kava kava
valerian root

NERVOUSNESS
valerian root

NERVOUSNESS, MENOPAUSE
black cohosh

NERVOUS UNREST
lemon balm

NEURALGIA
cat's claw
devil's claw
stinging nettle
valerian root

NEURALGIA, POSTHERPETIC
cayenne

NEURALGIA, TRIGEMINAL
cayenne

NEURALGIC CONDITIONS
peppermint

NEUROMUSCULAR INFLAMMATION
St. John's wort

NEWALL PAINFUL ARTHROSES
devil's claw

NICOTINE POISONING
devil's claw

NUTRITION, POOR
evening primrose

NUTRITIVE
stinging nettle

OBESITY
evening primrose

ORAL MUCOSA INFLAMMATION
peppermint

OSTEOARTHRITIS
bromelain
cayenne

PAIN RELIEF
kava kava

PALPITATIONS, MENOPAUSE
black cohosh

PECTORAL TONIC
comfrey

PELVIC CONGESTION
ginger root

PERICHOLANGITIS
milk thistle

PERIPHERAL ARTERIAL INSUFFICIENCY
ginkgo biloba

PEYRONIE'S DISEASE
bromelain

PHARYNGEAL MUCOSITIS
chamomile, Roman

PHYSICAL STAMINA
cat's claw
ginseng, American
ginseng, Asian

PLATELET AGGREGATION, REDUCTION OF
bilberry
bromelain
evening primrose
garlic
green tea

POLYCYSTIC OVARY DISEASE
saw palmetto

PREMENSTRUAL SYNDROME
black cohosh
evening primrose
ginkgo biloba

PSORIASIS
cayenne
chamomile, German
evening primrose
flaxseed oil
milk thistle

PSYCHOLOGICAL DISORDERS
evening primrose

PULMONARY CATTARH
burdock

PYORRHEA
echinacea

RADIATION DAMAGE
evening primrose
green tea

RADIATION SIDE EFFECTS
cat's claw

RASHES
aloe
chamomile, Roman

RASHES, DIAPER
chamomile, German

RASHES, HEAT
chamomile, German

RAYNAUD'S PHENOMENON
evening primrose
ginkgo biloba

RED BLOOD CELL DEPLETION
ginseng, Asian

REHABILITATION
hawthorn

REHABILITATION AFTER ACUTE ILLNESS
ginseng, American

RELAXANT
feverfew
saw palmetto

REPRODUCTIVE SYSTEM, TONIC
saw palmetto

RESPIRATORY INFECTION, CHRONIC
echinacea

RESPIRATORY INFLAMMATION
chamomile, German

RESPIRATORY TRACT CATARRH
eucalyptus

RESPIRATORY TRACT INFECTIONS
bromelain

RESPIRATORY TRACT IRRITATION
chamomile, German

RESTLESSNESS
kava kava

RESTORATIVE
ginseng, American
ginseng, Asian

RHEUMATIC CONDITIONS
burdock
feverfew
stinging nettle

RHEUMATIC PAIN
eucalyptus

RHEUMATISM
barberry
cat's claw
celery seed
devil's claw
licorice
stinging nettle

RHEUMATOID ARTHRITIS
bilberry
bromelain
cayenne
evening primrose
flaxseed oil
ginseng, Siberian

RINGWORM
eucalyptus

ROMEHELD'S SYNDROME
chamomile, Roman

RUBEFACIENT, TOPICAL
cayenne
ginger root
stinging nettle

SALPINGITIS
saw palmetto

SCIATICA
bromelain
stinging nettle

SCLERODERMA
bromelain

SCURVY
burdock

SEBORRHEIC DERMATITIS
Brewer's yeast

SEDATIVE
black cohosh
celery seed
devil's claw
ginseng, Asian
lemon balm
valerian root

SEDATIVE, MILD
chamomile, German

SEPTICEMIA
echinacea

SHINGLES
cat's claw
cayenne

SIALOGOGUE
ginseng, Asian

SJOGREN'S SYNDROME
evening primrose

SKIN, AGING
milk thistle

SKIN, DRY
aloe
evening primrose

SKIN ABRASIONS
chamomile, German

SKIN DISORDERS
flaxseed oil

SKIN ERUPTIONS
goldenseal

SKIN IRRITATION
chamomile, German
flaxseed

SKIN PROBLEMS
burdock

SKIN ULCERATION
echinacea

SLEEP DISORDERS, NERVOUS
lemon balm

SLEEPLESSNESS, CHILDHOOD
chamomile, German

SOPORIFIC
chamomile, Roman

SPASMOLYTIC
lemon balm

SPASMS
barberry

SPLEEN DISORDERS
barberry

SPRAINS AND STRAINS
comfrey
stinging nettle

STIFFNESS
kava kava

STIMULANT
eucalyptus
ginseng, Asian
ginseng, Siberian
peppermint

STOMACHACHE
feverfew

STOMACH BACTERIAL INFECTION
barberry

STOMACHIC
cayenne
chamomile, Roman
evening primrose
ginseng, Asian

STRESS
Brewer's yeast
ginseng, Siberian
kava kava
valerian root

STROKE
ginkgo biloba

STROKE, ISCHEMIC
bilberry

SWELLING REDUCTION
St. John's wort

TELANGIECTASES
grape seed extract

TENDINITIS
bromelain
devil's claw
stinging nettle

THROAT INFLAMMATION
eucalyptus
ginger root
goldenseal

THROMBOPHLEBITIS
bromelain

THROMBOSIS
bromelain
hawthorn

TINNEA
eucalyptus

TINNITUS
feverfew
ginkgo biloba

TINNITUS, MENOPAUSE
black cohosh

TONIC
ginseng, Siberian

TONSILLITIS
echinacea

TRAUMA, INJURIES AND SURGERY
bromelain

TRIGLYCERIDES, ELEVATED
flaxseed
green tea

TUMORS
cat's claw
lemon balm

ULCER
bilberry
bromelain
cat's claw
cayenne
chamomile, German
chamomile, Roman
ginseng, American
ginseng, Asian

ULCER, PEPTIC
aloe
chamomile, German
goldenseal
licorice

ULCERATIVE (BLOOD PURIFIER)
black cohosh

ULCERATIVE COLITIS
flaxseed oil

URETHRITIS
saw palmetto

URINARY TRACT, TONIC
saw palmetto

URINARY TRACT DISORDERS
kava kava

URINARY TRACT INFLAMMATION/INFECTION
barberry
cat's claw
celery seed
flaxseed
stinging nettle

URINARY TRACT INFLAMMATION/INFECTION, IRRIGATION
stinging nettle

VAGINAL DRYNESS
black cohosh

VAGINAL INFLAMMATION
chamomile, German

VARICOSE VEINS
bilberry
bromelain
grape seed extract
hawthorn

VASCULAR DISORDERS
bilberry

VASCULAR FRAGILITY
ginkgo biloba

VASCULAR TONIC
bilberry

VASODILATOR
bilberry
feverfew
garlic
hawthorn

VASODILATOR, PERIPHERAL
ginger root

VEINS, STRENGTHENING OF
cayenne

VENEREAL ERUPTIONS
burdock

VENOUS INSUFFICIENCY, CHRONIC
grape seed extract

VERTIGO
feverfew
ginkgo biloba

VERTIGO, MENOPAUSE
black cohosh

VIRAL ILLNESS
echinacea
ginseng, American

ginseng, Asian
St. John's wort

VIRILITY ENHANCEMENT
ginseng, Siberian

VISUAL FUNCTION, IMPAIRED
grape seed extract

VOMITING
ginger root

VULNERARY *(see wound healing)*

WEIGHT LOSS
Brewer's yeast

WOUND DEBRIDEMENT
bromelain

WOUND HEALING
aloe
cat's claw
chamomile, German
chamomile, Roman
comfrey
echinacea
evening primrose
flaxseed
goldenseal
lemon balm
milk thistle
St. John's wort

■ HERBS BY WARNINGS, PRECAUTIONS, CONTRAINDICATIONS

This list extracts the items included in the Warnings, Precautions, Contraindications section of each herb monograph and combines them to create a collection of herbs that must be considered with caution under particular circumstances, or in general due to issues of safety or toxicity.

ABDOMINAL PAIN
aloe

AIDS
burdock

ALLERGIC REACTION
bromelain

ALLERGIC REACTION, RAGWEED
chamomile, German
chamomile, Roman

APPENDICITIS
aloe

ASTHMA
bromelain

BACTERIAL FLORA OF DIGESTIVE TRACT
goldenseal

BILE DUCT INFLAMMATION
eucalyptus

BILIARY TRACT OBSTRUCTION
peppermint oil

BLOOD CLOTTING, SLOW
garlic

BLOOD PRESSURE DISORDERS
ginseng, American
ginseng, Asian

CARDIOVASCULAR DISORDERS
ginseng, American
ginseng, Asian
green tea

CHILDREN UNDER 2 YEARS
cayenne

CHILDREN UNDER 3 YEARS
burdock

CHOLECYSTITIS
peppermint oil

CHOLESTATIC LIVER DISEASE
licorice

CIRRHOSIS
licorice

COAGULATION DISORDERS
bromelain

COLITIS
aloe

CONTACT DERMATITIS
burdock

DERMATITIS
echinacea

DIABETES
ginseng, American
ginseng, Asian

DIET, CALORIE- AND FAT-RESTRICTED
flaxseed oil

DIVERTICULITIS
aloe

DIVERTICULOSIS
aloe

EDEMA
stinging nettle irrigation therapy

ELECTROLYTE IMBALANCE
aloe

EPILEPSY, TEMPORAL LOBE, TRIGGERING OF
evening primrose

ESOPHAGEAL STRICTURE
flaxseed

GALLSTONES
ginger root

GASTROINTESTINAL INFLAMMATION
eucalyptus

GASTROINTESTINAL IRRITATION
aloe
barberry
cayenne

GASTROINTESTINAL SENSITIVITY
green tea

GASTROINTESTINAL STRICTURE
flaxseed

HEART DISORDERS
licorice

HEMORRHAGIC COMPLICATIONS IN SURGERY
garlic

HEMORRHOIDS
aloe

HIV PATIENTS
burdock

HYPERTENSION
bromelain
ginseng, Siberian
goldenseal
licorice

HYPERTONIA
licorice

HYPOKALEMIA
licorice

INFANTS AND YOUNG CHILDREN
eucalyptus
peppermint oil

INTESTINAL INFLAMMATION
flaxseed

INTESTINAL OBSTRUCTION
aloe

IRRITABLE BOWEL SYNDROME
aloe

KIDNEY DISORDERS
bromelain
green tea
licorice

KIDNEY INFLAMMATION
celery seed

LACTATION
aloe
burdock
chamomile, German, excessive use
comfrey
eucalyptus
feverfew
garlic
kava kava
peppermint oil
saw palmetto
St. John's wort
stinging nettle irrigation therapy

LIVER DISEASE, SEVERE
eucalyptus
peppermint oil

LIVER DISORDERS
bromelain
milk thistle

MENSTRUATION
feverfew
garlic
stinging nettle irrigation therapy

ORGAN TRANSPLANT PATIENTS
burdock

OSTEOPOROSIS
Brewer's yeast

PANIC ATTACKS
green tea

PHENOTHIAZINE USE
evening primrose

PREGNANCY
aloe
barberry
black cohosh
burdock
celery seed
chamomile, German, excessive use

comfrey
eucalyptus
feverfew
garlic
ginger root, dried
ginseng, American
ginseng, Asian
ginseng, Siberian
goldenseal
hawthorn
kava kava
lemon balm
licorice
peppermint oil
saw palmetto
St. John's wort
stinging nettle irrigation therapy

SCHIZOPHRENIA
evening primrose

SELF-MEDICATION
hawthorn
saw palmetto

SKIN, BROKEN
comfrey

SKIN GRAFT PATIENTS
burdock

SKIN REACTIONS
bromelain
burdock
cayenne

SPASM
green tea

SYSTEMIC DISEASES
echinacea

TANNING BOOTH
celery seed

THYROID, OVERACTIVE
green tea

TOXICITY
licorice

TUBERCULOSIS PATIENTS
burdock

ULCER
aloe

ULTRAVIOLET THERAPY
celery seed

VITAMIN B
goldenseal, absorption with

YEAST PRODUCTS
Brewer's yeast

■ HERBS BY SIDE EFFECTS

This list extracts the items included in the Side Effects section of each herb monograph and combines them to create a collection of herbs that produce a particular side effect.

ABDOMINAL CRAMPS
aloe

ABDOMINAL PAIN
black cohosh
evening primrose
feverfew
St. John's wort

ABDOMINAL SPASM
green tea

ABORTION
chamomile, Roman

ALLERGIC CONTACT DERMATITIS
garlic

ALLERGIC REACTION
aloe
echinacea
kava kava
stinging nettle

ANXIETY
ginseng, Siberian

APPETITE LOSS
green tea

ATROPINE POISONING
comfrey consumption

BLOATING
St. John's wort

BLOOD PRESSURE, HIGH
ginseng, Siberian
St. John's wort

BRADYCARDIA
black cohosh
peppermint oil

BREATHING DIFFICULTY
barberry
evening primrose toxicity

BURNING SENSATION/ REDNESS
cayenne

CARDIAC ARREST
licorice

CONSTIPATION
St. John's wort

CONTACT URTICARIA
stinging nettle

CONVULSIONS
goldenseal

DIARRHEA
aloe
barberry

cat's claw
eucalyptus leaf
feverfew
goldenseal
green tea

DIZZINESS
black cohosh
ginkgo biloba
kava kava
St. John's wort

EDEMA
stinging nettle

EMESIS
chamomile, German
chamomile, Roman

EXCITABILITY
valerian root

EXTREMITY NUMBNESS
licorice

EYE IRRITATION
barberry

FLATULENCE
feverfew

GASTROINTESTINAL DISTRESS
eucalyptus leaf
garlic
ginkgo biloba
kava kava
saw palmetto
stinging nettle
valerian root

GASTROINTESTINAL IRRITATION
feverfew

HEADACHE
black cohosh
evening primrose
ginkgo biloba
ginseng, Siberian
green tea
kava kava
licorice

HEADACHE, MIGRAINE
hawthorn

HEARTBURN
ginger root
peppermint oil

HIVES
St. John's wort

HYDROQUINONE POISONING
bilberry

HYPERMENORRHEA
bromelain

HYPERSENSITIVITY REACTIONS
peppermint

HYPERTENSION
licorice

ILEUS
flaxseed

INDIGESTION
feverfew

INSOMNIA
ginseng, Siberian
green tea
valerian root

INTRACRANIAL HEMORRHAGE
ginkgo biloba

IRRITABILITY
ginseng, Siberian
green tea

ITCHING
St. John's wort

JOINT PAIN
black cohosh

KIDNEY DAMAGE
eucalyptus leaf

KIDNEY FAILURE, ACUTE
peppermint oil

KIDNEY IRRITATION
barberry

LAXATIVE EFFECT
milk thistle

LETHARGY
barberry
licorice

LIP SWELLING
feverfew

LIVER DAMAGE
eucalyptus leaf

MELANCHOLY
ginseng, Siberian

METRORRHAGIA
bromelain

MOUTH, DRY
St. John's wort

MOUTH IRRITATION
goldenseal

MOUTH ULCERATION
feverfew

MUSCLE TREMORS
peppermint oil

MUSCULAR WEAKNESS
licorice

MYOGLOBINURIA
licorice

NAUSEA
barberry
black cohosh
bromelain
eucalyptus leaf
evening primrose
feverfew
hawthorn
St. John's wort

NEPHRITIS, HEMORRHAGIC
barberry

NEPHRITIS, INTERSTITIAL
peppermint oil

NERVOUSNESS
feverfew
valerian root

NERVOUS SYSTEM OVERSTIMULATION
goldenseal

NOSE BLEED
barberry

OLIGURIA
stinging nettle

PALPITATIONS
ginseng, Siberian
green tea
hawthorn

PERICARDIAL PAIN
ginseng, Siberian

PHOTOSENSITIVITY
St. John's wort

POTASSIUM SECRETION, ELEVATED
licorice

PSEUDOALDOSTERONISM
licorice

RASHES, SKIN
kava kava
peppermint oil
St. John's wort

REFLEX EXCITABILITY, HEIGHTENED
green tea

RESPIRATORY PARALYSIS
barberry

RESTLESSNESS
green tea

SEDATION
evening primrose toxicity

SKIN, BURNING SENSATION
stinging nettle

SKIN IRRITATION
aloe
barberry

SKIN LESIONS, BURN-LIKE
garlic

215

SLEEP PROBLEMS
St. John's wort

SODIUM RETENTION
licorice

STOOLS, SOFT
evening primrose
hawthorn

TASTE, LOSS OF
feverfew

THROAT IRRITATION
goldenseal

TIREDNESS
St. John's wort

TONGUE SWELLING
feverfew

TREMOR
black cohosh
evening primrose toxicity
green tea

ULCERATION, INTERNAL AND EXTERNAL
goldenseal

VERTIGO
green tea

VISUAL DIMNESS
black cohosh

VOMITING
barberry
black cohosh
bromelain
eucalyptus leaf
feverfew
goldenseal
green tea
St. John's wort

WATER RETENTION
licorice

WEIGHT GAIN
licorice

WHITE BLOOD CELL COUNT, ELEVATED
goldenseal

▪ HERBS BY INTERACTIONS WITH OTHER DRUGS, HERBS, SUPPLEMENTS

This list extracts the items included in the Interactions section of each herb monograph and combines them to create a collection of herbs that interact in some way, positively or negatively, with a particular drug, other herb, or supplement.

ALCOHOL
kava kava

ALKALINES
green tea

ANALGESICS
valerian root

ANIMAL PROTEIN DRUGS
cat's claw

ANIMAL SERA
cat's claw

ANTIARRHYTHMICS
aloe

ANTICOAGULANTS
bromelain
garlic
ginger root

ANTICOAGULATION THERAPY
chamomile, German
chamomile, Roman

ANTIDIABETIC DRUGS
ginger root
ginseng, American
ginseng, Asian
St. John's wort

ANTIEPILEPTIC DRUGS
valerian root

ANTIHYPERTENSIVE DRUGS
cayenne
ginseng, American
ginseng, Asian

ANTIPSYCHOTIC DRUGS
ginseng, American
ginseng, Asian
ginseng, Siberian

ANTITHROMBOTIC DRUGS
feverfew

ANXIOLYTIC DRUGS
valerian root

ASPIRIN
feverfew
garlic

BARBITURATES
kava kava

BLOOD PLASMA, FRESH
cat's claw

BLOOD THINNERS
flaxseed oil

CAFFEINE
ginseng, American
ginseng, Asian
ginseng, Siberian

CARDIAC GLYCOSIDES
aloe

CARDIAC MEDICATIONS
ginger root

CENTRAL NERVOUS SYSTEM DEPRESSIVE DRUGS
St. John's wort

CORTICOSTEROIDS
aloe

CRYOPRECIPITATES
cat's claw

DIGITALIS
hawthorn
licorice

DRUG ABSORPTION
flaxseed

EPILEPTOGENICS
evening primrose

ESTROGEN, SYNTHETIC
black cohosh

FLUOXETINE
St. John's wort

FURAZOLIDONE
St. John's wort

GOTU KOLA
goldenseal

GRAVES' DISEASE THERAPY
lemon balm

HOPS
valerian root

HORMONE REPLACEMENT THERAPY
saw palmetto

HORMONES
ginseng, Siberian
saw palmetto

5-HYDROXYTRYPTOPHAN
St. John's wort

HYPERGLYCEMICS
St. John's wort

HYPERIMMUNOGLOBULIN THERAPY, INTRAVENOUS
cat's claw

HYPNOTICS
valerian root

HYPOGLYCEMICS
burdock

eucalyptus extract and oil
St. John's wort

IMMUNIZATIONS
cat's claw

IMMUNOSUPPRESSANT THERAPY
echinacea

INSULIN, BOVINE/PORCINE
cat's claw

ISOCARBOXAZID
St. John's wort

KAVA KAVA
alcohol
barbiturates
valerian root

L-DOPA
St. John's wort

LEMON BALM
valerian root

LICORICE
aloe
thiazide diuretics

MOCLOBEMIDE
St. John's wort

MONOAMINE OXIDASE INHIBITORS (MAOs)
cayenne
St. John's wort

ORAL CONTRACEPTIVES
black cohosh
saw palmetto

PAROXETINE
St. John's wort

PASSIONFLOWER
valerian root

PEPTIDE HORMONES
cat's claw

PHENELZINE (NARDIL)
ginseng, American
ginseng, Asian

POPPY
valerian root

SELECTIVE SEROTONIN REUPTAKE INHIBITORS (SSRI)
St. John's wort

SERTRALINE
St. John's wort

SKULLCAP
valerian root

STEROIDS
ginseng, American
ginseng, Asian
ginseng, Siberian

STIMULANTS
ginseng, American
ginseng, Asian
ginseng, Siberian

TETRACYCLINES
bromelain

THIAZIDE DIURETICS
aloe
licorice

THYMIC EXTRACTS, INTRAVENOUS
cat's claw

THYROID TREATMENTS
lemon balm

VALERIAN ROOT
kava kava
lemon balm
passionflower
poppy
skullcap

VITAMIN B
barberry

WARFARIN
feverfew

■ HERBS BY TAXONOMIC CROSS-REFERENCE
This list was produced to facilitate quick location of an herb monograph if only the botanical, pharmacopeial, or plant family name is known.

ALOE
Aloe vera/Aloe barbadensis/Aloe ferox (Botanical)
Liliaceae (Plant family)
Aloe barbadensis/capensis (Pharmacopeial)

BARBERRY/BARBERRY BARK/ BARBERRY ROOT/ BARBERRY ROOT BARK
Berberis vulgaris (Botanical)
Berberidaceae (Plant family)
Berberis vulgaris/Berberidis cortex/Berberidis radix/Berberidis radicis cortex (Pharmacopeial)

BILBERRY
Vaccinium myrtillus (Botanical)
Ericaceae (Plant family)
Myrtilli fructus/Myrtilli folium (Pharmacopeial)

BLACK COHOSH
Cimicifuga racemosa (Botanical)
Ranunculaceae (Plant family)
Cimicifugae racemosae rhizoma (Pharmacopeial)

BURDOCK
Arctium lappa/Arctium minus/Arctium tomentosum (Botanical)
Asteraceae (Plant family)
Bardanae radix (Pharmacopeial)

CAT'S CLAW
Uncaria tomentosa (Botanical)
Rubiaceae (Plant family)

CAYENNE (PAPRIKA)
Capsicum frutescens/Capsicum spp. (Botanical)
Solanaceae (Plant family)
Capsicum (Pharmacopeial)

CELERY SEED
Apium graveolens (Botanical)
Apiaceae (Plant family)
Apii fructus (Pharmacopeial)

CHAMOMILE, GERMAN
Matricaria recutita (Botanical)
Asteraceae (Plant family)
Matricariae flos (Pharmacopeial)

CHAMOMILE, ROMAN
Chamaemelum nobile (Botanical)
Asteraceae (Plant family)
Chamomillae romanae flos (Pharmacopeial)

COMFREY
Symphytum officinale (Botanical)
Boraginazeae (Plant family)
Symphyti folium/Symphyti radix (Pharmacopeial)

DEVIL'S CLAW *(Devil's Claw root)*
Harpagophytum procubens (Botanical)
Pedaliaceae (Plant family)
Harpagophyti radix (Pharmacopeial)

ECHINACEA *(Echinacea herb-root)*
Echinacea angustifolia herb-root/Echinacea pallida herb-root/Echinacea purpura herb-root (Botanical)
Asteraceae (Plant family)
Echinacea angustofoliae herba-radix/Echinacea pallidae herba-radix/Echinacea purpureae herba-radix (Pharmacopeial)

EUCALYPTUS *(Eucalyptus leaf, Eucalyptus oil)*
Eucalyptus globulus/Eucalyptus fructice-torum/Eucalyptus polybractea/smithii (Botanical)
Myrtaceae (Plant family)
Eucalypti folium/Eucalypti aetheroleum (Pharmacopeial)

EVENING PRIMROSE
Oenothera biennis (Botanical)
Onagraceae (Plant family)

FEVERFEW
Tanacetum parthenium/ Chrysanthemum parthenium (Botanical)
Compositae (Plant family)
Tanaceti parthenii herba (Pharmacopeial)

FLAXSEED
Linum usitatissimum (Botanical)
Linaceae (Plant family)
Lini semen (Pharmacopeial)

GARLIC
Allium sativum (Botanical)
Alliaceae (Plant family)
Allii sativi bulbus (Pharmacopeial)

GINGER
Zingiber officinale (Botanical)
Zingiberaceae (Plant family)
Zingiberis rhizoma (Pharmacopeial)

GINKGO BILOBA
Ginkgo biloba (Botanical)
Ginkgoaceae (Plant family)
Ginkgo folium (Pharmacopeial)

GINSENG, AMERICAN
Panax quinquefolium (Botanical)
Araliaceae (Plant family)
Ginseng radix (Pharmacopeial)

GINSENG, ASIAN
Panax ginseng (Botanical)
Araliaceae (Plant family)
Ginseng radix (Pharmacopeial)

GINSENG, SIBERIAN
Eleutherococcus senticosus/ Acanthopanax senticosus (Botanical)
Araliaceae (Plant family)
Eleutherococci radix (Pharmacopeial)

GOLDENSEAL
Hydrastis canadensis (Botanical)
Ranunculaceae (Plant family)
Hydrastis rhizoma (Pharmacopeial)

GRAPE SEED EXTRACT
Vitis vinifera (Botanical)
Vitaceae (Plant family)

GREEN TEA
Camellia sinensis (Botanical)
(Plant family)
(Pharmacopeial)

HAWTHORN *(Hawthorn Berry/Hawthorn Flower/Hawthorn Leaf/Hawthorn Leaf with Flower)*
Crataegus monogyna/Crataegus laevigata (Botanical)
Rosaceae (Plant family)
Crataegi fructus/crataegi flos/crataegi folium/cratagi folium cum flore (Pharmacopeial)

KAVA KAVA
Piper methysticum (Botanical)
Piperaceae (Plant family)
Piperis methystici rizoma (Pharmacopeial)

LEMON BALM
Melissa officinalis (Botanical)
Lamiaceae (Plant family)
Melissae folium (Pharmacopeial)

LICORICE
Glycyrrhiza glabra (Botanical)
Fabaceae (Plant family)
Liquiritiae radix (Pharmacopeial)

MILK THISTLE *(Milk Thistle fruit/Milk Thistle herb)*
Silybum marianum (Botanical)
Asteraceae (Plant family)
Cardui mariae fructus/Cardui mariae herba (Pharmacopeial)

PEPPERMINT *(Peppermint leaf, Peppermint oil)*
Mentha x piperita (Botanical)
Lamiaceae (Plant family)
Menthae piperitae folium/Menthae piperi-tae aetheroleum (Pharmacopeial)

SAW PALMETTO *(Saw Palmetto berry)*
Serenoa repens/Sabal serrulata (Botanical)
Aracaceae (Plant family)
Sabal fructus (Pharmacopeial)

ST. JOHN'S WORT
Hypericum perforatum (Botanical)
Hypericaceae (Plant family)
Hyperici herba (Pharmacopeial)

STINGING NETTLE *(Stinging nettle herb, Stinging nettle leaf, Stinging nettle root)*
Urtica dioica/Urtica urens (Botanical)
Urticaceae (Plant family)
Urticae herba/Urticae folium/Urticae radix (Pharmacopeial)

VALERIAN *(Valerian root)*
Valeriana officinalis
Valerianaceae (Plant family)
Valerianae radix (Pharmacopeial)

■ SUPPLEMENTS BY USES AND
INDICATIONS
*This list extracts the items included in
the Uses/Indications section of each
supplement monograph and combines
them to create a collection of supplements that may be considered for a particular application or condition.*

ACNE
selenium
sulfur
vitamin A (retinol)
vitamin B$_2$ (riboflavin)
vitamin B$_9$ (folic acid)
vitamin E
zinc

**ACRODERMATITIS
ENTEROPATHICA**
zinc

**ADOLESCENCE, IRON
REQUIREMENT**
iron

AGING
dehydroepiandrosterone (DHEA)
gamma-linolenic acid (GLA)
vitamin E

AIDS
dehydroepiandrosterone (DHEA)
glutamine
spirulina
vitamin B$_9$ (folic acid)

AIRWAY SPASMS
vitamin C

ALCOHOL DETOXIFICATION
vitamin B$_5$ (pantothenic acid)

ALCOHOLISM
gamma-linolenic acid (GLA)
niacinamide
vitamin B$_1$
zinc

ALLERGIES
alpha-linolenic acid (ALA)
copper
vitamin B$_5$ (pantothenic acid)
vitamin C

ALZHEIMER'S DISEASE
ethylenediaminetetraacetic acid (EDTA)
vitamin E

AMANITA POISONING
alpha-lipoic acid

AMENORRHEA
gamma-linolenic acid (GLA)

ANALGESIC ACTIVITY
creatine

ANEMIA
spirulina

ANEMIA, HEMOLYTIC
vitamin E

ANEMIA, MACROCYTIC
vitamin B$_9$ (folic acid)

ANEMIA, PERNICIOUS
vitamin B$_{12}$

ANEMIA, SIDEROBLASTIC
vitamin B$_6$

ANGINA
magnesium

ANOREXIA NERVOSA
zinc

ANTICLOTTING AGENT
vitamin E

**ANTICONVULSANT DRUG
THERAPY**
vitamin D

ANTIFUNGAL ACTIONS
pau d'arco

ANTI-INFLAMMATORY ACTIONS
creatine
vitamin C

ANTIMICROBIAL ACTIONS
pau d'arco

ANTINEOPLASTIC ACTIONS
pau d'arco

ANTIOXIDANTS, PROTECTION
vitamin C

ANTIVIRAL ACTIONS
pau d'arco

ANXIETY
magnesium
niacinamide

APNEA, RECURRENT IN INFANTS
magnesium

APPETITE SUPPRESSANT
tyrosine

ARSENIC POISONING
ethylenediaminetetraacetic acid (EDTA)

**ARTERIOSCLEROSIS,
PREVENTION**
vitamin D

**ARTERIOSCLEROTIC BRAIN
DISEASE**
vitamin E

ARTHRITIS
cartilage
copper
vitamin C

ASTHMA
lysine
magnesium
pau d'arco
vitamin B$_5$ (pantothenic acid)
vitamin C

ATHEROSCLEROSIS
manganese
vitamin E

**ATHEROSCLEROSIS,
PREVENTION**
magnesium

ATHLETIC PERFORMANCE
vitamin B$_5$ (pantothenic acid)

ATOPIC DERMATITIS
gamma-linolenic acid (GLA)

AUTOIMMUNE DISORDERS
alpha-linolenic acid (ALA)
dehydroepiandrosterone (DHEA)
lipase
vitamin D

**BENIGN PROSTATIC
HYPERPLASIA**
zinc

BERI BERI, DRY
vitamin B$_1$

BERI BERI, INFANTILE
vitamin B$_1$

BERI BERI, WET
vitamin B$_1$

BIPOLAR DISORDER
5-hydroxytryptophan (5-HTP)

**BLEEDING, EXCESSIVE,
PREVENTION**
vitamin K

BLEEDING GUMS
vitamin C

BLOATING
spirulina

BLOOD BUILDER
pau d'arco

BLOOD GLUCOSE CONTROL
vitamin H (biotin)

BLOOD LIPID REDUCTION
creatine

BLOOD LOSS, CHRONIC
iron

BLOOD PRESSURE, HIGH
magnesium
vitamin C
vitamin D

BODY BUILDING
vanadium

BODY ODOR
sulfur
vitamin K

BONE FRACTURES
vitamin D

BONE LOSS
calcium

BONE MINERALIZATION
vanadium
vitamin K

BRAIN DISORDERS
alpha-lipoic acid

BREAST CANCER
pau d'arco

**BREAST CANCER,
PREVENTION**
vitamin D

BRONCHITIS
pau d'arco

BRUISING
vitamin C

BURNS, SEVERE
vitamin A (retinol)

CADMIUM POISONING
selenium

CADMIUM TOXICITY
manganese

CANCER
alpha-linolenic acid (ALA)
cartilage
dehydroepiandrosterone (DHEA)
gamma-linolenic acid (GLA)
glutamine
manganese
phenylalanine
selenium
spirulina
vitamin E

CANCER, HORMONALLY RELATED
melatonin

CANCER, PREVENTION
vitamin C

CANCER INHIBITOR
psyllium

CANDIDA
spirulina

***CANDIDA ALBICANS*
INFECTION**
pau d'arco

CANDIDIASIS
sulfur
vitamin B$_9$ (folic acid)

CANDIDIASIS, INTESTINAL
vitamin H (biotin)

CAPILLARY FRAGILITY
vitamin C

**CARCINOGENESIS,
PREVENTION**
vitamin E

CARDIAC ARRHYTHMIAS
magnesium
potassium

CARDIOMYOPATHY, ALCOHOLIC
selenium

CARDIOVASCULAR DISORDERS
alpha-linolenic acid (ALA)
calcium
chromium
copper
magnesium
vitamin B_1
vitamin B_3 (niacin)

CARDIOVASCULAR DISORDERS, PREVENTION
vitamin C

CARPAL TUNNEL SYNDROME
vitamin B_2 (riboflavin)

CATARACTS
vitamin B_9 (folic acid)
vitamin B_2 (riboflavin)

CATARACTS, PREVENTION
selenium
vitamin C
vitamin E

CELIAC DISEASE
lipase
vitamin D
vitamin E
zinc

CERVICAL CANCER, PREVENTION
vitamin B_9 (folic acid)

CERVICAL DYSPLASIA
vitamin B_9 (folic acid)
vitamin C

CHEILOSIS
vitamin B_6

CHEMICAL HYPERSENSITIVITY
copper

CHEMOTHERAPY, MOUTH PAIN IN
glutamine

CHOLESTEROL, LOWERING OF
magnesium
psyllium
vanadium
vitamin B_5 (pantothenic acid)

CHRONIC OBSTRUCTIVE PULMONARY DISEASE
magnesium

CIRRHOSIS OF THE LIVER
selenium

COLITIS
glutamine
spirulina

COLON, CLEANSING AND HEALING OF
psyllium

COLON CANCER, PREVENTION
vitamin B_9 (folic acid)
vitamin D

COMA
vitamin B_1

CONFUSION
vitamin B_6

CONGENITAL DEFECTS
vitamin B_1

CONSTIPATION
phosphorus
psyllium
vitamin B_9 (folic acid)

CORONARY HEART DISEASE
melatonin

COUGH
phosphorus

CRITICAL ILLNESS
glutamine

CROHN'S DISEASE
glutamine

CYSTIC FIBROSIS
vitamin D
vitamin E

CYSTITIS
pau d'arco

DEGENERATIVE BRAIN DISEASE
vitamin E

DEPRESSION
dehydroepiandrosterone (DHEA)
5-hydroxytryptophan (5-HTP)
magnesium
melatonin
niacinamide
phenylalanine
sulfur
tyrosine
vitamin B_6
vitamin B_9 (folic acid)

DERMATITIS
vitamin B_2 (riboflavin)

DIABETES
alpha-lipoic acid
chromium
gamma-linolenic acid (GLA)
magnesium
manganese
niacinamide
potassium
vanadium
vitamin C
vitamin D
zinc

DIABETES, TYPE II
vitamin E

DIABETIC KETOACIDOSIS
phosphorus

DIABETIC NEUROPATHY
alpha-lipoic acid
vitamin H (biotin)

DIALYSIS PATIENTS
zinc

DIARRHEA
psyllium
vitamin B_1

DIARRHEA, CHRONIC
zinc

DIGESTION, IMPAIRED
lipase

DIGESTIVE DISORDERS
sulfur

DIVERTICULAR DISEASE
psyllium

DRUG DETOXIFICATION
tyrosine

DRUG TOXICITY
alpha-lipoic acid

DUCHENNE MUSCULAR DYSTROPHY
vitamin H (biotin)

DYSMENORRHEA
gamma-linolenic acid (GLA)

ECZEMA
alpha-linolenic acid (ALA)
selenium
spirulina
sulfur
vitamin B_2 (riboflavin)
vitamin E

ELDERLY
vitamin B_9 (folic acid)

ELDERLY PATIENTS
vitamin D

ENDURANCE, IMPROVEMENT IN
creatine

ENERGY
vitamin B_5 (pantothenic acid)

ENTERITIS, REGIONAL
cartilage

ENVIRONMENTAL POLLUTANTS, PROTECTION
vitamin E

EPILEPSY
manganese
melatonin

EYE HEALTH
sulfur

EYES, DRY
gamma-linolenic acid (GLA)

EYESIGHT
selenium

FATIGUE
copper
magnesium
melatonin

FATIGUE, CHRONIC
tyrosine

FATIGUE, PMS
magnesium

FAT MALABSORPTION DISORDERS
vitamin D
vitamin E

FAT METABOLISM
vitamin H (biotin)

FECAL ODOR
vitamin K

FIBER SUPPLEMENT
psyllium

FIBROCYSTIC BREAST DISEASE
vitamin E

FIBROMYALGIA
5-hydroxytryptophan (5-HTP)

FOOD ALLERGIES
lipase

FOOD ALLERGIES, HEADACHES
magnesium

FOOD CRAVINGS
glutamine

FORGETFULNESS
sulfur

FREE RADICAL DAMAGE
alpha-lipoic acid
ethylenediaminetetraacetic acid (EDTA)
vitamin B_2 (riboflavin)

GANGRENE
ethylenediaminetetraacetic acid (EDTA)

GAS
spirulina

GASTRIC MUCOSAL METABOLISM
glutamine

GASTRITIS
pau d'arco

GASTROENTERITIS, ACUTE
phosphorus

GASTROINTESTINAL DISORDERS
vitamin B_1

GASTROINTESTINAL DISTURBANCES, CHRONIC
iron

GASTROINTESTINAL HYPOTONIA
vitamin B_1

GENETIC ABNORMALITIES, INFANTS
vitamin H (biotin)

GENITOURINARY INFECTIONS
pau d'arco

GINGIVITIS
calcium

GLAUCOMA
chromium
magnesium

GLOSSITIS
vitamin B_6

GLUCOCORTICOID THERAPY
vitamin D

GLUCOSE INTOLERANCE
potassium

GLUCOSE METABOLISM IMPROVEMENT
creatine

GONORRHEA
pau d'arco

HAIR, GRAY
vitamin H (biotin)

HAIR, REJUVENATION
vitamin B_5 (pantothenic acid)

HEADACHE
vitamin B_9 (folic acid)

HEADACHE, CHILDREN
5-hydroxytryptophan (5-HTP)

HEADACHE, MIGRAINE
5-hydroxytryptophan (5-HTP)
lysine
magnesium

HEADACHE, MIGRAINE, PREVENTION
vitamin B_2 (riboflavin)

HEARING
magnesium

HEARING LOSS
manganese

HEART DISEASE
dehydroepiandrosterone (DHEA)
ethylenediaminetetraacetic acid (EDTA)
gamma-linolenic acid (GLA)
selenium
vanadium

HEART DISEASE, PREVENTION
vitamin B_9 (folic acid)

HEART IRREGULARITY
calcium

HEART SURGERY
vitamin E

HEAVY METAL DETOXIFICATION
alpha-lipoic acid

HEAVY METAL TOXICITY
selenium

HEMORRHAGE, NEWBORNS
vitamin K

HEMORRHAGE, PREVENTION
vitamin K

HEMORRHOIDS
iron
psyllium
sulfur

HEPATITIS, CHRONIC
alpha-lipoic acid

HERNIA
pau d'arco

HERPES
lysine
pau d'arco

HERPES SIMPLEX VIRUS
spirulina

HIGH-DENSITY LIPOPROTEIN LEVELS
vitamin B_3 (niacin)
vitamin C

HODGKINS DISEASE
pau d'arco

HOMOCYSTEINE, HIGH PLASMA LEVELS
vitamin B_6
vitamin B_{12}

HUMAN CYTOMEGALOVIRUS
spirulina

HYPERCHOLESTEROLEMIA
manganese

HYPERKERATOSIS
vitamin A (retinol)

HYPERTENSION
calcium
potassium

HYPOGLYCEMIA
chromium
niacinamide
spirulina

HYPOKALEMIA
potassium

IMMUNE SUPPORT
spirulina
zinc

IMMUNE SYSTEM ENHANCEMENT
vitamin A (retinol)
vitamin B_2 (riboflavin)
vitamin C

IMMUNOCOMPETENCE
manganese

IMMUNODEPRESSION
selenium

INFANCY, IRON REQUIREMENT
iron

INFERTILITY
vitamin B_9 (folic acid)

INFLAMMATION
phenylalanine

INFLAMMATORY BOWEL DISEASE
zinc

INFLAMMATORY BOWEL DISEASE, PREVENTION
vitamin D

INFLAMMATORY CONDITIONS
alpha-linolenic acid (ALA)
lipase
selenium

INFLUENZA VIRUS
spirulina

INSOMNIA
5-hydroxytryptophan (5-HTP)
melatonin
niacinamide

INSULIN SECRETION
vitamin D

IRON-DEFICIENT ANEMIA
iron

IRRITABILITY
sulfur
vitamin B_6

IRRITABLE BOWEL SYNDROME
psyllium

ISONIAZID OVERDOSE
vitamin B_6

JET LAG
melatonin

KIDNEY CALCIUM OXALATE STONES, PREVENTION
vitamin K

KIDNEY DISEASE
zinc

LACK OF APPETITE
spirulina

LACTATE ACIDOSIS, CONGENITAL
vitamin B_1

LACTATION
zinc

LAXATIVE, BULK
psyllium

LAXATIVE, MILD
phosphorus

LEAD POISONING
ethylenediaminetetraacetic acid (EDTA)
selenium

LEAKY GUT SYNDROME
glutamine

LEUKEMIA CELLS, INHIBITION
vitamin D

LEUKOPENIA
copper

LIBIDO, STIMULATION OF
tyrosine

LIVER CANCER
pau d'arco
vitamin K

LIVER DISORDERS
pau d'arco
selenium

LONG QT SYNDROME, CONGENITAL
magnesium

LOW-DENSITY LIPOPROTEIN LEVELS
vitamin B_3 (niacin)
vitamin E

LUNG CANCER, NON-SMALL CELL
melatonin

LUNG CANCER, PREVENTION
vitamin B_9 (folic acid)

LUNG FUNCTION
magnesium

LUPUS
alpha-linolenic acid (ALA)
dehydroepiandrosterone (DHEA)
pau d'arco
selenium
vitamin E

MACULAR DEGENERATION
cartilage
ethylenediaminetetraacetic acid (EDTA)
vitamin E

MACULAR DEGENERATION, PREVENTION
zinc

MALABSORPTION
lipase
spirulina

MALE FERTILITY
selenium
vitamin C
zinc

MALIGNANCY
iron

MANIC DEPRESSION
5-hydroxytryptophan (5-HTP)

MAPLE SYRUP DISEASE
vitamin B_1

MEASLES
spirulina

MEASLES, INFANT MORTALITY FROM
vitamin A (retinol)

MEMORY IMPROVEMENT
dehydroepiandrosterone (DHEA)

MENOPAUSE, SYMPTOMS OF
calcium
sulfur

MENSTRUAL BLEEDING
vitamin K

MENSTRUAL CRAMPS
calcium
magnesium

MENTAL HEALTH
magnesium

MENTAL ILLNESS
niacinamide

MERCURY POISONING
ethylenediaminetetraacetic acid (EDTA)
selenium

METAL TOXICITY
ethylenediaminetetraacetic acid (EDTA)

METHYLMALOIC ACIDURIA
vitamin B_{12}

MORNING SICKNESS
vitamin K

MOUTH PAIN
glutamine

MULTIPLE SCLEROSIS
alpha-linolenic acid (ALA)
dehydroepiandrosterone (DHEA)
melatonin
vitamin D

MUMPS
spirulina

MUSCLE CRAMPS
vitamin B_2 (riboflavin)

MUSCLE LOADING
creatine

MUSCLE WASTING
creatine

MUSCLE WEAKNESS
potassium

MUSCULAR CONDITIONS
selenium

MYOCARDIAL INFARCTION
magnesium

MYOCARDIAL INFARCTION, ACUTE
potassium

**MYOCARDIAL METABOLISM,
INCREASE IN**
creatine

MYOTONIC DYSTROPHY
selenium

NAILS, FRAIL, SPLITTING, OR THIN
vitamin H (biotin)

NARCOLEPSY
tyrosine

NASAL POLYPS
lysine

NAUSEA, IN PREGNANCY
vitamin B_6

**NECROTIZING
ENCEPHALOPATHY, SUBACUTE**
vitamin B_1

NERVOUSNESS
magnesium

**NEURAL TUBE BIRTH DEFECTS,
PREVENTION**
vitamin B_9 (folic acid)

NEURITIS OF PREGNANCY
vitamin B_1

NIGHT BLINDNESS
vitamin A (retinol)

OBESITY
chromium
dehydroepiandrosterone (DHEA)
5-hydroxytryptophan (5-HTP)

ORAL CONTRACEPTIVES
zinc

ORAL LEUKOPLAKIA
spirulina

ORAL THRUSH CANDIDIASIS
pau d'arco

OSTEOARTHRITIS
cartilage
niacinamide
sulfur

**OSTEOARTHRITIS,
CARTILAGE DAMAGE**
vitamin D

OSTEOARTHRITIS, PAIN
phenylalanine

OSTEOMALACIA
phosphorus, with calcium
vitamin D

OSTEOPENIA
vitamin D

OSTEOPOROSIS
calcium
chromium

dehydroepiandrosterone (DHEA)
gamma-linolenic acid (GLA)
manganese
melatonin
phosphorus, with calcium
vitamin D
vitamin K

**OSTEOPOROSIS,
PREVENTION**
vitamin B_9 (folic acid)

PAIN, CHRONIC
phenylalanine

PAIN, POSTEPISIOTOMY
lysine

PANCREATIC DISEASE
vitamin D
vitamin E

PARASITES
iron

PARATHYROID, OVERACTIVE
vitamin D

PARENTERAL NUTRITION
vitamin B_1

PARKINSON'S DISEASE
phenylalanine
tyrosine

PERFORMANCE ENHANCEMENT
dehydroepiandrosterone (DHEA)
vanadium

PERIODONTAL DISEASE
calcium

PERIPHERAL NEURITIS
vitamin B_6

PERNICIOUS ANEMIA
vitamin B_{12}

PHENYLKETONURIA (PKU)
tyrosine

PREECLAMPSIA, PREVENTION
calcium
magnesium

PREGNANCY
iron
magnesium
zinc

**PREGNANCY, HYPERTENSION
INDUCED BY**
calcium

PREMENSTRUAL SYNDROME (PMS)
calcium
gamma-linolenic acid (GLA)
magnesium
sulfur
tyrosine
vitamin B_6
vitamin E

PROSTATE CANCER
pau d'arco
zinc

PROSTATE FUNCTION
selenium

PROSTATITIS
pau d'arco
zinc

PROTEIN SOURCE
spirulina

PSORIASIS
alpha-linolenic acid (ALA)
cartilage
selenium
spirulina
vitamin A (retinol)
vitamin B_5 (pantothenic acid)
vitamin E

PSYCHIATRIC SYMPTOMS, ELDERLY
vitamin B_9 (folic acid)

**RADIATION DAMAGE,
GASTROINTESTINAL**
glutamine

RADIATION THERAPY EFFECTS
sulfur

RASHES, DIAPER
sulfur

**RECOVERY AFTER SURGERY
OR TRAUMA**
glutamine

**RECOVERY FROM
PROLONGED ILLNESS**
glutamine

RED BLOOD CELL INTEGRITY
vitamin E

REPRODUCTIVE DISORDERS
vitamin E

RHEUMATISM
pau d'arco
sulfur

RHEUMATOID ARTHRITIS
cartilage
dehydroepiandrosterone (DHEA)
gamma-linolenic acid (GLA)
manganese
phenylalanine
selenium
sulfur
vitamin B_9 (folic acid)
vitamin B_5 (pantothenic acid)
vitamin B_2 (riboflavin)
vitamin D
zinc

RICKETS
phosphorus, with calcium

RICKETS, PREVENTION
vitamin D

RINGWORM
pau d'arco

SCALP, DRY
sulfur

SCHIZOPHRENIA
niacinamide

SEBORRHEIC DERMATITIS
vitamin H (biotin)

SEIZURES, PYRIDOXINE-DEPENDENT
vitamin B_6

SEXUAL FUNCTION, MALE
zinc

SHORT BOWEL SYNDROME
vitamin D

SICKLE CELL ANEMIA
vitamin B_9 (folic acid)
vitamin B_2 (riboflavin)

SJOGREN'S SYNDROME
gamma-linolenic acid (GLA)

SKIN, REJUVENATION
vitamin B_5 (pantothenic acid)

SKIN, WOUND TREATMENT
vitamin K

SKIN CANCER, PREVENTION
vitamin D

SKIN DISORDERS
selenium
spirulina
vitamin A (retinol)
vitamin E
vitamin H (biotin)

SKIN PROBLEMS
vitamin B_2 (riboflavin)

SLEEP DISTURBANCES
sulfur

SLEEP PATTERNS, RESTORATION OF
melatonin

SMELL, IMPROVEMENT
zinc

SPERM MOTILITY
selenium

STAMINA INCREASE
vitamin B_5 (pantothenic acid)

STOMATITIS
pau d'arco
vitamin B_6

STOOL SOFTENER
psyllium

STRENGTH, IMPROVEMENT IN
creatine

STRESS
tyrosine
vitamin B_2 (riboflavin)

STRESS, EXTREME
glutamine

STROKE
alpha-lipoic acid

STROKE, PREVENTION
magnesium
potassium
vitamin B_9 (folic acid)
vitamin D

SUDDEN INFANT DEATH SYNDROME (SIDS)
melatonin
selenium

SUNBURN
vitamin C

TASTE, IMPROVEMENT
zinc

TASTE ALTERATION, CANCER TREATMENT
zinc

TEETH, LOOSE
calcium

TEETH, MINERALIZATION OF
vanadium

TINNITUS
manganese

TONIC
pau d'arco

TORSADE DE POINTES
magnesium

TRANSPLANT REJECTION
vitamin D

TRAUMA
glutamine

TRIGLYCERIDE LEVELS
magnesium
vitamin B_3 (niacin)

TUBERCULOSIS, PREVENTION
vitamin D

ULCER
copper
pau d'arco

ULCER, PEPTIC
glutamine

ULCER, PEPTIC, BLEEDING
iron

ULCER, SKIN
vitamin B_2 (riboflavin)

ULCERATIVE COLITIS
dehydroepiandrosterone (DHEA)
vitamin B_1
zinc

URINE ODOR
vitamin K

VAGINAL CANDIDIASIS
pau d'arco

VASCULITIS
selenium

VEGAN DIET
vitamin D

VIRAL INFECTIONS
vitamin A (retinol)

VITAMIN A DEFICIENCY
spirulina

VITILIGO
copper
phenylalanine

VOMITING, IN PREGNANCY
vitamin B_6

WATER RETENTION, PMS
magnesium

WEIGHT LOSS
tyrosine

WEIGHT REDUCTION
psyllium

WERNICKE'S ENCEPHALOPATHY
vitamin B_1

WILSON'S DISEASE
zinc

WOUND HEALING
ethylenediaminetetraacetic acid (EDTA)
vitamin B_5 (pantothenic acid)
vitamin C
vitamin E
zinc

WOUNDS, SEVERE
vitamin A (retinol)

WOUND TREATMENT
vitamin K

■ **SUPPLEMENTS BY WARNINGS, PRECAUTIONS, CONTRAINDICATIONS**
This list extracts the items included in the Warnings, Precautions, Contraindications section of each supplement monograph and combines them to create a collection of supplements that must be considered with caution under particular circumstances, or in general due to issues of safety or toxicity.

ALCOHOL
vitamin A toxicity

ALCOHOLICS
sulfur

ALLERGIC DERMATITIS
chromium

ALTERED MENTAL STATE
5-hydroxytryptophan (5-HTP)

ANTICOAGULANT DRUGS
vitamin K

ANTIDEPRESSANT DRUGS
5-hydroxytryptophan (5-HTP)

ASTHMA
vitamin B_3 (niacin)

ATRIOVENTRICULAR BLOCK, HIGH-GRADE
magnesium

AUTOIMMUNE DISORDERS
melatonin

AUTONOMIC DYSFUNCTION
5-hydroxytryptophan (5-HTP)

BEHAVIORAL PROBLEMS
selenium

BIRTH DEFECTS
vitamin A (retinol)

BLEEDING TIME, PROLONGED
vitamin E

BLOOD-CLOTTING CONDITIONS
pau d'arco

BLOOD COMPOUNDS, MONITORING
ethylenediaminetetraacetic acid (EDTA)

BLOOD PRESSURE, HIGH
tyrosine
vitamin E

BLOOD PRESSURE, MONITORING OF
ethylenediaminetetraacetic acid (EDTA)

BONE MASS, REDUCED
phosphorus

BREAST CANCER
dehydroepiandrosterone (DHEA)

BRONCHOGENIC CARCINOMA
chromium

CALCIFICATION, SOFT TISSUE
calcium

CALCIUM, DRAIN OF
phosphorus

CALCIUM, HIGH BLOOD LEVELS
vitamin D

CANCER, HORMONE-SENSITIVE
dehydroepiandrosterone (DHEA)

CHEMOTHERAPY
vitamin B_1

CHILDREN
psyllium
shark cartilage

CHOLESTEROL, INCREASED LEVEL
lysine

CORTICOSTEROIDS
melatonin

CORTICOSTEROIDS, LONG-TERM USE
sulfur

COUMADIN
vitamin K

CYANOCOBALAMIN
vitamin B_{12} deficiency

DEPRESSION
melatonin

DIABETES
alpha-lipoic acid
vitamin B_3 (niacin)

DROWSINESS
melatonin

ELDERLY PATIENTS
potassium
sulfur

ENDURANCE
creatine

EPILEPSY
vitamin B_9 (folic acid)

FAT INTAKE
alpha-linolenic acid (ALA)

FERTILITY
melatonin

GALLBLADDER DISORDERS
vitamin B_3 (niacin)

GASTRIC IRRITATION
chromium

GLUCOSE, BLOOD, MONITORING OF
vitamin B_3 (niacin)

GOUT
vitamin B_3 (niacin)

HEART ATTACK PATIENTS
shark cartilage

HEART DISEASE
vitamin D

HEART DISEASE, SEVERE
magnesium

HEMODIALYSIS
copper

HYPERTENSION
vitamin E

HYPOCALCEMIA
calcium chloride

IMMUNE SYSTEM CANCERS
melatonin

KIDNEY DISEASE
magnesium
vitamin D

KIDNEY DISEASE, CHRONIC
vitamin A

KIDNEY DISORDERS
vitamin C

KIDNEY FUNCTION, IMPAIRED
sulfur

KIDNEY FUNCTION, MONITORING
ethylenediaminetetraacetic acid (EDTA)

KIDNEY STONES
calcium

LACTATION
melatonin
phenylalanine
vitamin K

L-DOPA
phenylalanine

LEAD TOXICITY
calcium

LEARNING DISABILITIES
selenium

LEUKEMIA
melatonin

LEVODOPA
vitamin B_6

LIVER DAMAGE
vitamin B_3 (niacin)

LIVER DISEASE, CHRONIC
vitamin A

LIVER FUNCTION, IMPAIRED
sulfur

LUNG IRRITATION
vanadium

LYMPHOMA
melatonin

MALIGNANT MELANOMA
tyrosine

MINERAL DEFICIENCY
magnesium

MOISTURE
glutamine powder

MONOAMINE OXIDASE (MAO) INHIBITORS
tyrosine

MULTIVITAMINS
zinc

NAUSEA
vitamin B_6

NEUROMUSCULAR ABNORMALITIES
5-hydroxytryptophan (5-HTP)

NEUROTOXICITY
vitamin C

ORGAN FUNCTION, MONITORING
ethylenediaminetetraacetic acid (EDTA)

OSTEOPOROSIS
phosphorus

OVARIAN CANCER
dehydroepiandrosterone (DHEA)

PARENTERAL IRON THERAPY
iron

PARKINSON'S DISEASE
vitamin B_6

PATIENTS UNDER 40 YEARS OF AGE
dehydroepiandrosterone (DHEA)

PHENYLKETONURIA
phenylalanine

PHOSPHORUS, HIGH BLOOD LEVELS
vitamin D

PREGNANCY
melatonin
phenylalanine
shark cartilage
sulfur
vitamin A
vitamin B_6
vitamin K

PREMENSTRUAL SYNDROME
vitamin B_6

PROSTATE CANCER
dehydroepiandrosterone (DHEA)

RADIATION
vitamin K

RENAL IMPAIRMENT, SEVERE
potassium

RENAL INSUFFICIENCY
potassium

SCURVY, INFANTS
vitamin C

SKIN ULCER
chromium

SULFITE ALLERGY
sulfur

SURGERY
sulfur

SURGICAL PATIENTS
shark cartilage

TESTICULAR CANCER
dehydroepiandrosterone (DHEA)

TONGUE, GREEN COLOR
vanadium

TOXICITY
chromium
magnesium
manganese
selenium
vitamin A
vitamin B_3 (niacin)

TOXICOSIS
copper

TRANSPLANT PATIENTS
melatonin

TRIGLYCERIDE, INCREASED LEVEL
lysine

ULCER, PEPTIC
vitamin B_3 (niacin)

URINE DISCOLORATION
vitamin B_2 (riboflavin)

VASCULAR FUNCTION, MONITORING
ethylenediaminetetraacetic acid (EDTA)

VITAMIN B_{12} DEFICIENCY
vitamin B_9 (folic acid)

VOMITING
vitamin B_6

WARFARIN
vitamin E
vitamin K

X-RAYS
vitamin K

∎ SUPPLEMENTS BY SIDE EFFECTS

This list extracts items included in the Side Effects section of each supplement monograph and combines them to create a collection of supplements that produce a particular side effect.

ABDOMINAL PAIN
vitamin A (retinol)

ACNE
dehydroepiandrosterone (DHEA)

AGGRESSIVE TENDENCIES
dehydroepiandrosterone (DHEA)

ALCOHOL INTOLERANCE
zinc

ALLERGIC REACTIONS
sulfur
vitamin B_1

ALOPECIA
vitamin A (retinol)

ANAPHYLAXIS
iron
psyllium

ANEMIA
zinc

ANEMIA, HEMOLYTIC
vitamin K

ANOREXIA
vitamin A (retinol)

ANXIETY
phenylalanine

ARTHRALGIAS
iron

ARTHRITIS
selenium

ASTHMA
sulfur

ATAXIA
vitamin B_6

BETA CELL DAMAGE
vanadium

BLOOD PRESSURE, LOW
vitamin B_3 (niacin)

BLOOD PRESSURE ELEVATION
dehydroepiandrosterone (DHEA)
manganese
tyrosine
vanadium

BODY ODOR
selenium

BONE FRACTURES
vitamin A (retinol)

BONE PAIN
vitamin D

BRADYCARDIA
potassium

BREATHING, CONSTRICTED
vitamin K

BREATHING DIFFICULTY
potassium

BURNING
vitamin B_2 (riboflavin)

CALCIUM, ABSORPTION
phosphorus

CANCER CELL DIVISION
tyrosine

CARDIAC ARRHYTHMIA
potassium

CARDIOVASCULAR FAILURE
vitamin D

CHEST PAIN
vitamin K

CIRCADIAN RHYTHMS, DISRUPTION
melatonin

CONDUCTION DISTURBANCES
potassium

CONJUNCTIVITIS
vitamin A (retinol)

CONSTIPATION
iron

DEPRESSION
selenium

DIARRHEA
copper poisoning
iron
phosphorus
potassium
vitamin A (retinol)
vitamin B_3 (niacin)
vitamin C
vitamin D
vitamin E

DIARRHEA, BLOODY
iron

DIZZINESS
copper poisoning
zinc

DROWSINESS
zinc

ECZEMA FROM INTRAMUSCULAR INJECTIONS
vitamin K

EPIGASTRIC PAIN
copper poisoning

EYES, DRY
vitamin A (retinol)

EYES, SORE
vitamin D

FAINTING
vitamin B_3 (niacin)

FATIGUE
selenium
sulfur
vitamin A (retinol)
vitamin D

FEELINGS OF FULLNESS
5-hydroxytryptophan (5-HTP)

FEVER
iron
sulfur

FINGERNAIL LOSS
selenium

FLATULENCE
5-hydroxytryptophan (5-HTP)
potassium
vitamin E

FLUSHING
vitamin B_3 (niacin)
vitamin K

GARLICKY BREATH
selenium

GAS
vitamin C

GASTRIC DISTRESS
sulfur
vitamin B_1
vitamin C in excess

GASTRIC HYPOMOTILITY
potassium

GASTRIC IRRITATION
zinc

GASTRIC UPSET, MILD
tyrosine

GASTROINTESTINAL DISORDERS
5-hydroxytryptophan (5-HTP)
iron
selenium
vitamin B_9 (folic acid)

GASTROINTESTINAL IRRITATION
zinc

GASTROINTESTINAL UPSET
vanadium

HAIR GROWTH ON THE FACE
dehydroepiandrosterone (DHEA)

HAIR LOSS
dehydroepiandrosterone (DHEA)
selenium

HALLUCINATIONS
zinc

HEADACHE
copper poisoning
iron
phenylalanine
sulfur
vitamin A (retinol)
zinc

HEADACHE, MIGRAINE
tyrosine

HEARTBURN
5-hydroxytryptophan (5-HTP)
iron
vitamin B_3 (niacin)

HEMOCHROMATOSIS
iron

HEMOLYSIS
vitamin K

HEMORRHAGIC NECROSIS OF THE GASTROINTESTINAL TRACT
iron

HEPATOTOXICITY
dehydroepiandrosterone (DHEA)

HYPERBILIRUBINEMIA
vitamin K

HYPERCALCEMIA
calcium
vitamin D

HYPERKALEMIA
potassium

HYPERPARATHYROIDISM
phosphorus

HYPERTENSION
copper poisoning
phenylalanine

HYPOGLYCEMIA
sulfur

IMMUNE FUNCTION, DEPRESSION OF
zinc

INSULIN, INHIBITION
chromium

INTESTINAL DISTURBANCES
vitamin C

INTRACRANIAL PRESSURE
vitamin A (retinol)

IRON ABSORPTION
phosphorus

IRON TOXICITY
iron

IRRITABILITY
selenium

ITCHING
vitamin B_2 (riboflavin)
vitamin D

JAUNDICE
copper poisoning
vitamin K

JOINT PAIN
vitamin A (retinol)

KIDNEY FAILURE
ethylenediaminetetraacetic acid (EDTA)

LETHARGY
potassium

LEUKOCYTOSIS
vitamin A (retinol)

LIPS, DRY CRACKING
vitamin A (retinol)

LIVER DAMAGE
vitamin K

LIVER MALFUNCTION
vitamin B_3 (niacin)

LIVER TOXICITY
vitamin B_3 (niacin)

LYMPHADENOPATHY
iron

MAGNESIUM ABSORPTION
phosphorus

MALAISE
iron

MALE PATTERN BALDNESS
dehydroepiandrosterone (DHEA)

MANGANESE TOXICITY
manganese

MANIC DEPRESSION
vanadium

MASCULINIZATION
dehydroepiandrosterone (DHEA)

**MEDICATION, INTERFERENCE
WITH ABSORPTION**
psyllium

METALLIC TASTE
copper poisoning
vitamin D

MUSCLE FUNCTION, IMPAIRED
vitamin D

MUSCLE PAIN
vitamin A (retinol)

MUSCLE WEAKNESS
potassium

MUSCULAR INCOORDINATION
zinc

NAUSEA
cartilage

copper poisoning
5-hydroxytryptophan (5-HTP)
iron
pau d'arco
potassium
vitamin A (retinol)
vitamin B_3 (niacin)
vitamin E

NIGHTMARES
melatonin

NUMBNESS
vitamin B_2 (riboflavin)

NUTRITIONAL TOXICITY
magnesium

ORGAN CALCIFICATION
phosphorus

ORGAN DAMAGE
ethylenediaminetetraacetic acid (EDTA)
iron

OSTEOPOROSIS
calcium
vitamin D

**PAIN FROM INTRAMUSCULAR
INJECTIONS**
vitamin K

PALPITATIONS
vitamin E

PARALYSIS
potassium

PHLEBITIS
iron

PRICKLING SENSATIONS
vitamin B_2 (riboflavin)

**PROTEIN SYNTHESIS,
INHIBITION OF**
vanadium

**PSYCHIATRIC
ABNORMALITIES**
manganese

PULMONARY IRRITATION
vanadium

RASHES
sulfur

RENAL FAILURE
vitamin D

RHEUMATOID ARTHRITIS
iron

RUMBLING SENSATIONS
5-hydroxytryptophan (5-HTP)

SEIZURE
ethylenediaminetetraacetic acid (EDTA)

SENSITIVITY TO LIGHT
vitamin B_2 (riboflavin)

SENSORY NEUROPATHY
vitamin B_6

SEXUAL AGGRESSIVENESS
dehydroepiandrosterone (DHEA)

SKIN, ALLERGIC REACTIONS
vitamin B_9 (folic acid)

SKIN, DRY CRACKING
vitamin A (retinol)

SLEEP PROBLEMS
vitamin B_9 (folic acid)

SOFT TISSUE ABSORPTION
phosphorus

STOMACH PAIN
potassium

SWEATING
vitamin K
zinc

**SWELLING FROM
INTRAMUSCULAR INJECTIONS**
vitamin K

TACHYCARDIA
copper poisoning

TASTE, UNPLEASANT
cartilage

TESTICULAR ATROPHY
dehydroepiandrosterone (DHEA)

THIRST, EXCESSIVE
vitamin D

TINGLING SENSATION
vitamin B_3 (niacin)

TISSUE NECROSIS
potassium

TOXICITY
vitamin D
zinc

TREMOR
vanadium

ULCERS
vitamin B_3 (niacin)

UPPER GASTRIC DISCOMFORT
iron

UREMIA
copper poisoning

URINARY URGENCY
vitamin D

URTICARIA
iron

VIVID DREAMS
melatonin

VOMITING
copper poisoning
iron

potassium
vitamin B_3 (niacin)
vitamin D
zinc

WEAKNESS
copper poisoning
potassium

WEIGHT GAIN
creatine

WEIGHT GAIN AROUND THE WAIST
dehydroepiandrosterone (DHEA)

ZINC
phosphorus

■ SUPPLEMENTS BY INTERACTIONS WITH OTHER DRUGS, HERBS, SUPPLEMENTS

This list extracts the items included in the Interactions section of each supplement monograph and combines them to create a collection of supplements that interact, positively or negatively, with a particular drug, herb, or other supplement.

ACE INHIBITORS
potassium

ACETAMINOPHEN
vitamin B_9 (folic acid)

ACETAZOLAMIDE
potassium

ACETYL CARNITINE
melatonin

ADRIAMYCIN
vitamin B_3 (niacin)

ALCOHOL
calcium
copper
dehydroepiandrosterone (DHEA)
magnesium
melatonin
vitamin B_1
vitamin B_9 (folic acid)
vitamin B_3 (niacin)
vitamin B_2 (riboflavin)
vitamin D
vitamin E
vitamin H (biotin)

ALUMINUM-CONTAINING ANTACIDS
calcium

AMILORIDE
potassium

AMINO ACIDS
phenylalanine
sulfur
tyrosine

ANTACIDS
chromium

ANTACIDS, VERY HIGH AMOUNTS
copper

ANTIBIOTICS
vitamin B_2 (riboflavin)
vitamin H (biotin)
vitamin K

ANTICOAGULANT DRUGS
vitamin E

ANTICONVULSANT DRUGS
vitamin B_9 (folic acid)
vitamin H (biotin)

ANTIDEPRESSANT DRUGS
vitamin B_2 (riboflavin)

ANTIHYPERTENSIVE DRUGS
vitamin B_3 (niacin)

ANTI-MALARIAL DRUGS
vitamin B_2 (riboflavin)

ARSENIC POISONING
sulfur

ASCORBIC ACID
vanadium

ASPIRIN
calcium
vitamin B_9 (folic acid)
vitamin K

AVIDIN
vitamin H (biotin)

BARBITURATES
calcium
vitamin B_9 (folic acid)
vitamin B_2 (riboflavin)

BETA-BLOCKERS
melatonin
potassium

BETA-CAROTENE
vitamin C

BILIRUBIN
vitamin C

BRAN, WHEAT
psyllium

BUMETANIDE
potassium

CAFFEINE
calcium
creatine
magnesium
melatonin
phosphorus

CALCIUM
copper
magnesium
manganese
zinc

CALCIUM CARBONATE
chromium

CALCIUM CHANNEL BLOCKERS
melatonin

CATHARTIC AGENTS
vitamin B_2 (riboflavin)

CHEMOTHERAPY DRUGS
vitamin B_9 (folic acid)

CHOLESTYRAMINE
vitamin D
vitamin E
vitamin K

CHOLINE
vitamin B_9 (folic acid)

CHROMIUM
vanadium

CIPROFLOXACIN
iron

COENZYME Q10
vitamin H (biotin)

COLESTIPOL
vitamin E

COPPER
calcium
manganese

COPPER ABSORPTION
vitamin C

COPPER DEFICIENCY
zinc

CYCLOSERINE
vitamin B_6

CYSTEINE
copper

DIGITALIS
magnesium
vitamin D

DIGOXIN
potassium

DISODIUM ETIDRONATE
iron

DIURETICS
magnesium
melatonin
ethylenediaminetetraacetic acid (EDTA)
glutamine
iron
lysine
phenylalanine
selenium
vitamin B_{12}
vitamin B_9 (folic acid)

EGG
copper

EGG WHITE
vitamin H (biotin)

ESTROGENS
vitamin A (retinol)
vitamin B_9 (folic acid)
vitamin B_2 (riboflavin)
vitamin H (biotin)

ETHACYNIC ACID
potassium

ETHYLENEDIAMINETETRAACETIC ACID (EDTA)
vanadium

FAT
magnesium
vitamin A (retinol)

FATTY ACIDS
alpha-linolenic acid (ALA)

FIBER
magnesium
psyllium

FIBER, HIGH
ethylenediaminetetraacetic acid (EDTA)

FIBER DIETARY
zinc

FOLATE ABSORPTION
zinc

FOLIC ACID
magnesium
vitamin H (biotin)

FRUCTOSE
copper

FUROSEMIDE
potassium
vitamin B_1

GLUCOSE
creatine

GLUCOSE TOLERANCE FACTOR (GTF)
chromium

GLUTATHIONE
alpha-lipoic acid

HEPARIN
potassium

H_2 INHIBITORS
iron

HYDRALAZINE
vitamin B_6

IBUPROFEN
vitamin B_9 (folic acid)

INSULIN
magnesium

IODINE
calcium

IRON
calcium
copper
magnesium
manganese
phosphorus
vitamin E
zinc

IRON ABSORPTION
vitamin C

ISONIAZID
vitamin B_6

LEUCINE
vitamin B_3 (niacin)

LEVODOPA
iron

LIPID-REDUCING DRUGS
vitamin B_3 (niacin)

LITHIUM
vanadium

MAGNESIUM
calcium
ethylenediaminetetraacetic acid (EDTA)
5-hydroxytryptophan (5-HTP)
manganese
phosphorus

MAGNESIUM-CONTAINING ANTACIDS
vitamin D

MAGNESIUM SHARK CARTILAGE
cartilage

MAGNESIUM TRISILICATE
iron

MANGANESE
calcium
copper
magnesium

METFORMIN
vitamin B$_{12}$

METHOTREXATE
vitamin B$_2$ (riboflavin)

METHYLENE BLUE
vanadium

MINERAL OIL
vitamin D

MINERAL OIL LAXATIVES
vitamin K

MOLYBDENUM
copper

MONOAMINE OXIDASE INHIBITORS
melatonin
vanadium

NEOMYCIN
calcium

NIACIN
chromium
5-hydroxytryptophan (5-HTP)
vitamin B$_9$ (folic acid)

NIACINAMIDE
melatonin

NORFLOXACIN
iron

NSAIDs
potassium

OFLOXACIN
iron

ORAL CONTRACEPTIVES
vitamin A (retinol)

OXALIC ACID
calcium

PANTOTHENIC ACID
vitamin D
vitamin H (biotin)

PENICILLAMINE
iron
vitamin B$_6$

PHENOBARBITOL
vitamin B$_3$ (niacin)

PHENOTHIAZINES
vanadium
vitamin B$_2$ (riboflavin)

PHENYTOIN
vitamin D
vitamin K

PHOSPHORUS
calcium
magnesium

PHYTATES
copper

PHYTIC ACID
calcium

POTASSIUM SHARK CARTILAGE
cartilage

PRIMIDONE
vitamin B$_3$ (niacin)

PROTEIN
melatonin
vitamin A (retinol)

PROTEIN, HIGH INTAKE
calcium

PROTEINS, MILK
tyrosine

PROTON PUMP INHIBITORS
iron

PYRAZINAMIDE
vitamin B$_6$

RIBOFLAVIN IN HIGH DOSAGES
magnesium

SATURATED FATS
calcium
ethylenediaminetetraacetic acid (EDTA)

SEDATIVES, STRONG
calcium

SELENIUM
sulfur
vitamin C
vitamin E

SNAKE VENOMS
vitamin K

SODIUM
calcium
magnesium

SODIUM-POTASSIUM PUMP
vanadium

SPIRONOLACTONE
potassium

ST. JOHN'S WORT
5-hydroxytryptophan (5-HTP)

SUGAR
calcium
magnesium

SULFA DRUGS
vitamin B$_2$ (riboflavin)
vitamin H (biotin)

SULFASALAZINE
vitamin B$_9$ (folic acid)

TETRACYCLINE
iron

THIAZIDE DIURETICS
potassium
vitamin D

TIN
copper

TOBACCO
vanadium

TRANQUILIZERS
vitamin B$_2$ (riboflavin)

TRIAMTERENE
potassium

TRICYCLICS
melatonin

TRIMETHOPRIM
potassium

TRYPTOPHAN
vitamin B$_3$ (niacin)
vitamin B$_2$ (riboflavin)

URONIC ACID
calcium

VALIUM
melatonin

VERAPAMIL
vitamin D

VITAMIN A
vitamin A (retinol)
vitamin E
vitamin K

VITAMIN B$_2$
vitamin B$_3$ (niacin)

VITAMIN B$_6$
copper
glutamine
5-hydroxytryptophan (5-HTP)
melatonin
phenylalanine
tyrosine

VITAMIN B$_{12}$

melatonin
vitamin B$_9$ (folic acid)
vitamin C
vitamin H (biotin)

VITAMIN B$_3$ (NIACIN)
vitamin B$_2$ (riboflavin)

VITAMIN B$_6$ (PYRIDOXINE)
vitamin B$_2$ (riboflavin)

VITAMIN B$_1$ (THIAMINE)
vitamin B$_2$ (riboflavin)

VITAMIN C
alpha-lipoic acid

VITAMIN C HIGH LEVELS
copper

VITAMIN D
phosphorus

VITAMIN E
alpha-lipoic acid
dehydroepiandrosterone (DHEA)
selenium
vitamin A (retinol)
vitamin C
vitamin K

VITAMIN K DEFICIENCY
vitamin E

XANAX
melatonin

ZINC
calcium
copper
magnesium
manganese
selenium
vitamin A (retinol)
vitamin B$_9$ (folic acid)
vitamin H (biotin)

■ COMBINED HERB AND SUPPLEMENT TREATMENT BY CONDITION

This extracts the items included in the Herb and Nutrition sections in each condition monograph and combines them to create a collective list of all conditions in the Quick Access system, with the respective herbs and supplements that may be considered in treating them. Some of the herbs and supplements listed may not yet have a monograph created in the Quick Access system.

ALLERGIC RHINITIS
N-acetyl cysteine
bilberry
bioflavonoids
cleavers
coneflower
curcuma
elderberry
eyebright
ginger root
nettles
quercetin
rose hips
vitamin A
vitamin B_5
vitamin B_6
vitamin C
vitamin E
zinc

ALOPECIA
algae, blue green
astragalus
biotin
black cohosh
chaste tree
echinacea
fatty acids, essential
gamma-linolenic acid (GLA)
ginkgo biloba
ginseng, Siberian
green tea
horsetail
magnesium
prickly ash bark
rosemary
saw palmetto
vitamin B_6
vitamin E
yarrow
zinc

AMENORRHEA
black cohosh
bladderwrack
borage oil
boron
calcium
chaste tree
dandelion root
evening primrose
fatty acids, essential
flaxseed
horsetail
iodine
kelp
lady's mantle
licorice
magnesium
milk thistle

oatstraw
sage
selenium
squaw vine
tyrosine
vervain
vitamin A
vitamin B_6
vitamin C
vitamin D
vitamin E
vitamin K
wild yam
zinc

ANEMIA
alfalfa
black strap molasses
burdock
cyanocobalamine (vitamin B_{12})
dandelion
ferrous fumerate
folic acid
glycerate
glycinate
omega-3 fatty acids
spirulina
vitamin B_{12}
vitamin C
yellow dock

ANGINA
bromelain
L-carnitine
coenzyme Q10
fatty acids, essential
ginger
ginkgo biloba
hawthorn
indian tobacco
linden flower
mistletoe
monkshood
motherwort
night-blooming cereus
L-taurine
vitamin C
yellow jasmine

ANOREXIA NERVOSA
condurango
fenugreek
ginseng, Siberian
goldenseal
lemon balm
licorice
multivitamins
oatstraw
protein supplements
saw palmetto
St. John's wort
valerian
wild yam
zinc

ANXIETY
bergamot
calcium
jasmine
kava kava
lavender
lemon balm
magnesium
oatstraw
passionflower

skullcap
St. John's wort
vitamin B-complex

ASTHMA
N-acetyl cysteine
belladonna
coltsfoot
elecampane
frankincense
gelsemium
ginger root
ginkgo biloba
green tea
grindelia
hydrochloric acid supplements
hydroxcobalamin
indian tobacco
khella
lavender
licorice root
magnesium
ma huang
mint
palmitate
plantain
pyridoxal-5-phosphate
rose hips
sage
skullcap
skunk cabbage
thyme leaf
valerian
vitamin B_6
vitamin B_{12}
vitamin C
wild cherry bark

ATHEROSCLEROSIS
antioxidants
betaine
bromelain
carnitine
chromium
coenzyme Q10
fatty acids, essential
folic acid
gentian
ginkgo biloba
hawthorn
linden flower
lipoic acid
magnesium
mistletoe
omega-3 fatty acids
rosemary
selenium
vitamin B_6
vitamin B_{12}
vitamin C
vitamin E

ATTENTION-DEFICIT/ HYPERACTIVITY DISORDER
calcium
catnip
chamomile
fatty acids, essential
kava kava
lavender
lemon balm
linden flower
magnesium
omega-3 fatty acids
omega-6 fatty acids

passionflower
vitamin B-complex
vitamin C

BENIGN PROSTATIC HYPERPLASIA
alanine
amino acids
fatty acids, essential
glutamic acid
glycine
pumpkin seeds
saw palmetto
selenium
stinging nettle root
vitamin B_6
zinc

BRONCHITIS
N-acetyl cysteine
beta-carotene
boneset
coneflower
elecampane
garlic
ginger
hawthorn
indian tobacco
licorice root
linden flower
lomatium
lungwort
pill bearing spurge
pleurisy root
sundew
thyme leaf
vitamin C
white horehound
wild cherry bark
zinc

BURNS
aloe
beta-carotene
bromelain
california poppy
cleavers
comfrey root
coneflower
gelsemium
ginger root
L-glutamine
goldenseal
gotu kola
jamaican dogwood
marigold
marshmallow root
plantain
prickly ash bark
slippery elm powder
St. John's wort
turmeric
valerian
vitamin C
vitamin E
yarrow
zinc

BURSITIS
bromelain
glucosamine sulfate
hawthorn
jamaican dogwood
meadowsweet
omega-3 fatty acids
proteolytic enzymes

turmeric
valerian
vitamin C with bioflavonoids
white willow

CANDIDIASIS
antifungal spices
barberry
biotin
calcium
caprylic acid
chamomile
evening primrose
fatty acids, essential
fireweed
flaxseed
folate
garlic
goldenseal
lactobacillus acidophilus
lavender essence oil
licorice
magnesium
marigold
omega-3 fatty acids
omega-6 fatty acids
oregon grape root
pau d'arco bark
selenium
tea tree oil
vitamin B-complex
vitamin C
vitamin E

CHRONIC FATIGUE SYNDROME
ashwaganda root
astragalus root
beta-carotene
L-carnitine
fatty acids, essential
ginseng, Siberian
gotu kola
jasmine oil
lavender
licorice root
lomatium root
magnesium aspartate
pantothenic acid
passionflower
peppermint oil
rosemary leaf
rosemary oil
schizandra berry
skullcap
vitamin B-complex
vitamin C

**CHRONIC OBSTRUCTIVE
PULMONARY DISEASE**
N-acetyl cysteine
bromelain
L-carnitine
coenzyme Q10
coltsfoot
eucalyptus oil
fennel
ginger
hawthorn
lavender oil
licorice
magnesium
mullein
omega-3 fatty acids
omega-6 fatty acids
rosemary oil

selenium
thyme oil
vitamin C
vitamin E

CIRRHOSIS OF THE LIVER
antioxidants
barberry
carnitine
catechin
choline
dessicated liver extract
evening primrose
flaxseed
folate
glutathione
lecithin
methionine
milk thistle
omega-3 fatty acids
omega-6 fatty acids
selenium
vitamin B-complex
vitamin C
vitamin E
vitamin K

COMMON COLD
astragalus
beta-carotene
coneflower
echinacea
elderberry
goldenseal
licorice
vitamin A
vitamin C
zinc

CONGESTIVE HEART FAILURE
antioxidants
betaine
carnitine
coenzyme Q10
dandelion
fatty acids, essential
folic acid
hawthorn
horsetail herb
indian tobacco
lily of the valley
linden flower
magnesium
mistletoe
motherwort
rosemary
selenium
taurine
vitamin B_6
vitamin B_{12}
vitamin C
vitamin E

CONJUNCTIVITIS
chamomile
eyebright
fennel seed
flax meal
goldenseal
marigold
plantain
potato, fresh grated
vitamin A
vitamin C
zinc

CONSTIPATION
burdock
cascara sagrada
dandelion root
digestive enzymes
fennel seed
flax meal
ginger
licorice root
yellow dock

COUGH
balm of Gilead
baume de Canada
beta-carotene
castor oil
coltsfoot
elderberry
elecampane
eucalyptus oil
fennel
flaxseed oil
frankincense
garlic
ginger
gumweed
horehound
indian tobacco
licorice root
linden flower
mullein
mustard oil
onion
oregano oil
pine oils
plantain
purple coneflower
sweet violet
thyme
thyme oil
vitamin C
wild cherry bark
zinc

CUTANEOUS DRUG REACTIONS
aloe
bromelain
chamomile
chickweed
comfrey
coneflower
flaxseed oil
goldenseal
hesperidin
magnesium
marigold
marshmallow root
oatmeal baths
peppermint
quercetin
red clover
slippery elm powder
turmeric
vitamin B-complex with extra B_{12}
vitamin C
vitamin E
yarrow
zinc

DEMENTIA
antioxidants
biotin
calcium/magnesium
coenzyme Q10
ethylenediaminetetraacetic acid (EDTA)

fatty acids, essential
ginger
ginkgo biloba biloba
ginseng, Siberian
hawthorn
lemon balm
rosemary
St. John's wort
vitamin B-complex
vitamin C
vitamin E
zinc

**DEPRESSION-UNIPOLAR MOOD
DISORDERS**
biotin
black cohosh
calcium
chromium
fatty acids, essential
folate
ginkgo biloba
ginseng, Siberian
iron
lemon balm
licorice
magnesium
multivitamins
oatstraw
passionflower
St. John's wort
valerian
vitamin B_1
vitamin B_2 (riboflavin)
vitamin B_6
vitamin B_{12}
vitamin C

DERMATITIS
beta-carotene
bioflavonoids
borage oil
bromelain
catechin
chamomile
chickweed
cleavers
comfrey
evening primrose oil
flaxseed oil
gotu kola
hesperidin
marigold
oregon grape
palmitate
peppermint
peppermint leaf
prickly ash bark
quercetin
red alder bark
red clover
rose hips
rutin
sarsaparilla
selenium
vitamin C
vitamin E
yarrow
zinc

DIABETES MELLITUS
bilberry
brewer's yeast
cayenne
chromium picolinate
coenzyme Q10
evening primrose oil
fenugreek
fish oil
folate
garlic
grape seed extract
magnesium
manganese
onion
pycnogenol
vanadium
vitamin B-complex
vitamin C
vitamin E
zinc

DIARRHEA
barberry
blackberry leaf
brewer's yeast
carob powder
chamomile
glutamine
goldenseal
lactobacillus species
licorice root
marshmallow root
quercetin
sacromyces bolardii
slippery elm powder
vitamin A
vitamin C

DYSMENORRHEA
black cohosh
borage oil
chamomile tea
chaste tree
cramp bark tinctures
evening primrose
flaxseed oil
ginger root
jamaican dogwood
magnesium
niacinamide
red raspberry
vitamin B-complex
vitamin E
wild yam

DYSPHAGIA
licorice
linden flower
skullcap
slippery elm powder
St. John's wort
valerian
wild yam

ECZEMA
beta-carotene
bioflavonoids
borage oil
bromelain
burdock root
catechin
chamomile
chickweed
cleavers

cod liver oil
comfrey
evening primrose
flaxseed
hesperidin
hydrochloric acid
marigold
marshmallow root tea
nettles
omega-6 fatty acids
palmitate
peppermint
quercetin
red clover
rose hips
rutin
vitamin C
yarrow
yellow dock
zinc

EDEMA
artichoke leaves
bilberry
broom
buchu
butcher's broom
calcium
cleavers
coenzyme Q10
couchgrass
dandelion leaf
dandelion root
elder
ginkgo biloba
goldenrod
hawthorn
horse chestnut
horsetail
lily of the valley
linden flower
magnesium
milk thistle
motherwort
night-blooming cereus
oatstraw
parsley
potassium aspartate
red clover
red root
rosemary
rue
sweet clover
thiamine (vitamin B_1)
turmeric
vitamin B_6
vitamin C
vitamin E
yarrow

ENDOCARDITIS
bearberry
beta-carotene
black cohosh
bromelain
cleavers
coenzyme Q10
coneflower
corn silk
dandelion leaf
garlic
goldenseal root
hawthorn
lily of the valley
linden flower

magnesium
motherwort
myrrh
night-blooming cereus
rosemary
selenium
vitamin A
vitamin C
vitamin E
wild indigo
yarrow
zinc

ENDOMETRIOSIS
beta-carotene
black cohosh
blue flag
calcium
chaste tree
cramp bark
dandelion root
fatty acids, essential
gelsemium
ginger root
iron
jamaican dogwood
milk thistle
monkshood
motherwort
poke root
red raspberry
red root
selenium
squaw vine
valerian
vervain
vitamin C
vitamin E
white byrony
wild yam
yarrow
zinc

FEVER OF UNKNOWN ORIGIN
beta-carotene
catnip
coneflower
elder
lemon balm
spearmint
vitamin C
white willow bark
yarrow
zinc

FIBROMYALGIA
ashwaganda root
astragalus root
black cohosh
chromium picolinate
clary sage
coenzyme Q10
ginseng, Siberian
gotu kola
5-hydroxytryptophan
jasmine oil
kava kava
lavender
lemon balm
magnesium
melatonin
passionflower
phosphatidyl choline
phosphatidyl serine
raw thymus glandular

rosemary
schizandra berry
skullcap
valerian
vitamin B-complex
vitamin C
zinc

FOOD ALLERGY
beta-carotene
borage oil
bromelain
catnip
celandine
chamomile
chicory
dandelion
evening primrose oil
fennel
flaxseed oil
marshmallow root tea
meadowsweet
milk thistle
palmitate
pancreatin
passionflower
peppermint
pro-flora supplements
quercetin
rose hips
selenium
vitamin B-complex
vitamin C
zinc

GALLBLADDER DISEASE
choline
dandelion root
flax meal
globe artichoke
greater celandine
lecithin
lipase
lipotropic agents
milk thistle
peppermint oil
turmeric
vitamin C
vitamin E

GASTRITIS
bismuth subcitrate
ginger root tea
licorice, deglycyrrhizinated
marshmallow root
slippery elm powder
vitamin C
zinc

GASTROESOPHAGEAL REFLUX DISEASE
licorice
linden flower
skullcap
slippery elm powder
St. John's wort
valerian
wild yam

GOUT
bromelain
devil's claw
eicosapentaenoic acid (EPA)
folic acid (vitamin B_9)
niacin (vitamin B_3)

vitamin A
vitamin C

HEMORRHOIDS
bioflavonoids
catechin
comfrey
flax meal
green tea
marigold
potato, fresh grated
rose hips
vitamin C
vitamin E
witch hazel

HEPATITIS, VIRAL
N-Acetyl cysteine
acidophilus
astragalus root
beta-carotene
chinese thoroughwax
choline
coneflower
dessicated liver extract
eclipta alba
folic acid (vitamin B_9)
globe artichoke
glutathione
goldenseal
green tea
lecithin
licorice root
methionine
milk thistle
phyllanthus amarus
schizandra berry
selenium
thymus extract
turmeric
vitamin B-complex
vitamin C
vitamin E
vitamin K
zinc

HERPES SIMPLEX VIRUS
acidophilus
astragalus
beta-carotene
chamomile
coneflower
glycyrrhizic acid
lemon balm
licorice root
lomatium
L-lysine
selenium
St. John's wort
thymus extract
vitamin A
vitamin C
yarrow
zinc

**HERPES ZOSTER (varicella–
zoster) virus**
beta-carotene
burdock root
calcium
chamomile
comfrey
coneflower
goldenseal
jamaican dogwood

lemon balm
licorice root
magnesium
marigold
slippery elm powder
St. John's wort
valerian
vitamin A
vitamin B_{12}
vitamin B-complex
vitamin C
vitamin E
wild lettuce
yellow jasmine
zinc

HIV AND AIDS
N-acetyl cysteine
acidophilus
beta-carotene
L-carnitine
cholagogue
coenzyme Q10
dandelion
garlic
gentian
ginseng, Siberian
L-glutamine
goldenseal
huang qi
licorice
magnesium
milk thistle
multivitamins
selenium
St. John's wort
vitamin B_{12}
vitamin B-complex
vitamin C
vitamin E
zinc

HYPERCHOLESTEROLEMIA
alfalfa
blue flag
blue vervain
burdock root
chromium
coenzyme Q10
dandelion root
garlic
ginger
greater celandine
hawthorn berries
magnesium
milk thistle
niacin (vitamin B_3)
omega-3 fatty acids
panthenine
selenium
L-taurine
vitamin B-complex
vitamin C

HYPERKALEMIA
hawthorn
lily of the valley
magnesium

HYPERTENSION
betaine
coenzyme Q10
cramp bark
dandelion leaf
evening primrose oil

flax oil
folic acid (vitamin B_9)
hawthorn
indian tobacco
lily of the valley
linden flower
magnesium
mistletoe
motherwort
night-blooming cereus
passionflower
valerian
vitamin B_{12}
vitamin B-complex
vitamin E
zinc

HYPERTHYROIDISM
bromelain
bugleweed
calcium
coenzyme Q10
fatty acids, essential
hawthorn berries
lemon balm
licorice
lithium
magnesium
milk thistle
motherwort
passionflower
quercetin
Rebmania glutinosa
Stephania tetranda
turmeric
vitamin C
vitamin E

HYPOGLYCEMIA
chromium picolinate
ginger root
ginseng, Siberian
gotu kola
licorice root
magnesium
niacinamide (vitamin B_3)
pantothenic acid (vitamin B_5)
pyridoxine (vitamin B_6)
vanadyl sulfate
vitamin B-complex
vitamin C
vitamin E
zinc

HYPOTHYROIDISM
alfalfa
bladderwrack
calcium
coleus foreskohlii
fatty acids, essential
gotu kola
guggul
hawthorn
horsetail
irish moss
kelp
oatstraw
selenium
L-tyrosine
vitamin A
vitamin B_2 (riboflavin)
vitamin B_3
vitamin B_6
vitamin B-complex

vitamin C
zinc

INFANTILE COLIC
acidophilus
anise seed
catnip
fennel seed
lemon balm
linden flower
peppermint
spearmint

INFLUENZA
beta-carotene
coneflower
elder
garlic/ginger tea
goldenseal
licorice
St. John's wort
vitamin A
vitamin C
yarrow
zinc

INSECT BITES
bromelain
citronella oil
cleavers
coneflower
elder
eucalyptus oil
goldenseal powder
lavender oil
licorice root
marigold
oatstraw
pennyroyal oil
peppermint
plantain leaves
quercetin
red clover
turmeric
vitamin B-complex
vitamin C
witch hazel

INSOMNIA
calcium/magnesium
chamomile
chamomile oil
5-Hydroxytryptophan (5-HTP)
jamaican dogwood
kava kava
lavender oil
lemon balm
melatonin
niacinamide
passionflower
rosemary oil
St. John's wort
valerian
vitamin B-complex

INTESTINAL PARASITES
acidophilus
barberry
beta-carotene
black walnut
digestive enzymes
garlic
garlic oil
goldenseal
lavender oil

male fern
oregon grape
papain
quassia
tansy
tea tree oil
thyme
thyme oil
vitamin C
wormseed
wormwood
zinc

**IRRITABLE BOWEL
SYNDROME**
acidophilus
anise seed
bran, raw
digestive enzymes
fennel seed
flax meal
ginger root
lactobacillus
magnesium
marshmallow root
meadowsweet
milk thistle
passionflower
peppermint oil
psyllium
slippery elm powder
valerian
wild yam

LARYNGITIS
coneflower
ginger
goldenseal
licorice
marigold
myrrh
peppermint
propolis
sage
slippery elm powder
vitamin B-complex
vitamin C
zinc lozenges

LOW BACK PAIN
antioxidants
black haw
bromelain
calcium/magnesium
devil's claw
ginkgo biloba
jamaican dogwood
leopard's bane
lobelia
petasites
rosemary leaves
St. John's wort
turmeric
valerian
vitamin B-complex
vitamin C
vitamin E
white willow bark
wild yam

MENOPAUSE
angelica
black cohosh
calcium/magnesium
chaste tree

gamma-oryzanol
ginkgo biloba
hesperidin
hesperidin methyl chalcone
licorice
soy
vitamin C
vitamin E

MIGRAINE HEADACHE
bioflavonoids
choline
fatty acids, essential
feverfew
folic acid (vitamin B_9)
ginger
ginkgo biloba
5-Hydroxytryptophan
jamaican dogwood
magnesium
meadowsweet
omega-3 fatty acids
skullcap
vitamin B_2 (riboflavin)
vitamin B_6
vitamin C
vitamin E

MOTION SICKNESS
black horehound
chamomile
ginger root
peppermint

MYOCARDIAL INFARCTION
antioxidants
beta-carotene
bromelain
L-carnitine
vitamin C
vitamin E

OBESITY
bladderwrack
choline
chromium picolinate
coenzyme Q10
dandelion
fatty acids, essential
fiber
gentian
L-glutamine
hawthorne
5-Hydroxytryptophan (5-HTP)
kelp
lavender
lecithin
ma huang
methionine
milk thistle
multivitamins
parsley
peppermint
St. John's wort
thiamine (vitamin B_1)
valerian
vitamin B-complex
vitamin C

OSTEOARTHRITIS
S-Adenosylmethionine
bilberry
black cohosh
boron
boswellia

devil's claw
ginger root
glucosamine sulfate
hawthorn
meadowsweet
niacinamide
omega-3 fatty acids
teasel root
turmeric
vitamin A
vitamin C
vitamin E
yucca

OSTEOMYELITIS
acidophilus
analgesics
antimicrobials
astragalus
barberry
burdock root
cleavers
coneflower
garlic
ginkgo biloba
goldenseal
goldenseal root
licorice
lomatium
red clover
slippery elm
St. John's wort
valerian
vitamin A
vitamin C
vitamin E
yarrow
yellow dock
zinc

OSTEOPOROSIS
aspartate
black cohosh
bladderwrack
blue flag
boron
calcium citrate
chaste tree
chromium
dandelion root
fatty acids, essential
horsetail
kelp
lady's mantle
licorice
magnesium
manganase
milk thistle
nettles
oatstraw
squaw vine
vervain
vitamin B-complex
vitamin K
wild yam
zinc

OTITIS MEDIA
cleavers
cod liver oil
coneflower
elderberry
eyebright
fatty acids, essential
fish oil

garlic oil
indian tobacco oil
marigold
monkshood oil
mullein flower oil
St. John's wort oil
vitamin C

PARKINSON'S DISEASE
alpha-lipoic acid
amino acids
antioxidants
choline
dimethylaminoethanol (DMAE)
fatty acids, essential
gamma-aminobutyric acid (GABA)
ginkgo biloba
globe artichoke
glutamic acid
glutathione
gotu kola
grape seed extract
hawthorn
lecithin
lemon balm
manganese
milk thistle
nervine herbs
oats
phosphatidyl choline
pycnogenol
selenium
skullcap
St. John's wort
vitamin B-complex
vitamin C
vitamin E

PEPTIC ULCER
N-acetyl cysteine
acidophilus
barberry
bismuth subcitrate
catnip
chamomile
fatty acids, essential
glutamine
goldenseal
lemon balm
licorice, deglycyrrhizinated
marshmallow root powder
meadowsweet
oregon grape
passionflower
peppermint
plantain
potassium
quercetin
slippery elm powder
sulphur
valerian
vitamin A
vitamin C
vitamin E
zinc

PERICARDITIS
blue monkshood
coenzyme Q10
flax oil
hawthorn
linden flower
vitamin A
vitamin C

PERTUSSIS
anise seed
astragalus
beta-carotene
catnip
chamomile
coneflower
cramp bark
elecampane
garlic
ginger root
hyssop
indian tobacco
licorice root
mullein
thyme
usnea lichen
valerian
vitamin C
zinc

PHARYNGITIS
beta-carotene
coneflower
garlic/ginger tea
goldenseal
licorice
propolis
slippery elm powder
vitamin C
zinc

PREECLAMPSIA
cramp bark
hawthorn berries
indian tobacco
magnesium
milk thistle
omega-3 fatty acids
passionflower

PRIMARY PULMONARY HYPERTENSION
L-carnitine
choline
coenzyme Q10
garlic
ginkgo biloba
hawthorn
indian tobacco
inositol
linden flower
magnesium aspartate
potassium aspartate
rosemary
selenium
taurine
vitamin C
vitamin E

PROSTATITIS
bearberry
cernilton
coneflower
corn silk
fatty acids, essential
goldenseal
pumpkin seeds
saw palmetto
selenium
vitamin C
zinc

PSORIASIS
burdock
coleus
digestive enzymes
fatty acids, essential
folate
milk thistle
omega-3 fatty acids
omega-6 fatty acids
quercetin
red clover
sarsaparilla
selenium
vitamin B_{12}
vitamin E
yellow dock
zinc

PULMONARY EDEMA
broom
L-carnitine
choline
coenzyme Q10
dandelion leaf
garlic
hawthorn
indian tobacco
lily of the valley
linden flower
magnesium
magnesium aspartate
motherwort
night-blooming cereus
potassium
potassium aspartate
raw heart concentrate
rosemary
selenium
taurine
thyme leaf
vitamin C
vitamin E

RAYNAUD'S PHENOMENON
calcium
coenzyme Q10
ginger root
ginkgo biloba
hawthorn berries
omega-3 fatty acids
prickly ash bark
rosemary
vitamin B-complex
vitamin C
vitamin E
zinc

REITER'S SYNDROME
antioxidants
beta-carotene
bilberry
bromelain
copper
eyebright
fatty acids, essential
glucosamine sulfate
horsetail
juniper
licorice
meadowsweet
selenium
uva ursi
vitamin C
vitamin E
zinc

RHEUMATOID ARTHRITIS
antioxidants
ashwaganda
blue flag
boswellia
bromelain
devil's claw
flavanoids
gana derma
ginger
ginseng
gotu kola
grifold frondosa
horsetail
nightshades
omega-3 fatty acids
quercetin
sarsaparilla
selenium
turmeric
valerian
vitamin C
wild yam
zinc

ROSEOLA
beta-carotene
catnip
chamomile
elder
fennel
garlic/ginger tea
peppermint
vitamin C
yarrow
zinc

SEIZURES
dimethyl glycine
folic acid (vitamin B_9)
magnesium
manganese
milk thistle
passionflower
skullcap
taurine
valerian
vitamin B_6
vitamin B_{12}
zinc

SEXUAL DYSFUNCTION
chaste tree
damiana
dandelion root
ginger root
ginkgo biloba
gotu kola
hawthorn
kava kava
lemon balm
magnesium
milk thistle
passionflower
prickly ash bark
rosemary
skullcap
St. John's wort
vervain
vitamin B_6
vitamin B-complex
vitamin C
vitamin E
yohimbe bark

SINUS HEADACHE
beta-carotene
bromelain
coneflower
eucalyptus oil
eyebright
garlic
ginger
goldenseal
jamaican dogwood
lavender oil
licorice
St. John's wort
thyme oil
vitamin C
wild indigo
zinc

SINUSITIS
beta-carotene
bromelain
coneflower
eucalyptus oil
eyebright
garlic/ginger tea
goldenseal
jamaican dogwood
lavender oil
licorice
quercetin
St. John's wort
thyme oil
vitamin C
wild indigo
zinc

SLEEP APNEA
chromium
fatty acids, essential

SPRAINS AND STRAINS
arnica oil
beta-carotene
bioflavonoids
black cohosh
bromelain
cramp bark
feverfew
hawthorn
jamaican dogwood
poke root
quercetin
turmeric
valerian
vitamin C
vitamin E
zinc

TENDINITIS
bioflavonoids
bromelain
calcium/magnesium
comfrey
curcumin
fatty acids, essential
licorice
vitamin A
vitamin C
vitamin E
willow

TENSION HEADACHE
beta-carotene
calcium
calcium/magnesium

cayenne
evening primrose
fatty acids, essential
flaxseed
ginkgo biloba
jamaican dogwood
kava kava
magnesium
manganese
meadowsweet
omega-3 fatty acids
omega-6 fatty acids
peppermint oil
potassium
selenium
valerian
vitamin B-complex
vitamin C
vitamin E
white willow bark
zinc

THYROIDITIS
alfalfa
bladderwrack
bromelain
bugleweed
calcium/magnesium
fatty acids, essential
ginkgo biloba
gotu kola
horsetail
iodine
motherwort
oatstraw
passionflower
quercetin
selenium
turmeric
L-tyrosine
vitamin A
vitamin B-complex
vitamin C
vitamin E
zinc

ULCERATIVE COLITIS
beta-carotene
biotin
bromelain
calcium
coneflower
cramp bark
fatty acids, essential
fiber
flax meal
folic acid (vitamin B$_9$)
geranium
goldenseal
iron, elemental
lemon balm
licorice root
magnesium
marshmallow root
meadowsweet
pantothenic acid (vitamin B$_5$)
passionflower
peppermint oil
pro-flora supplements
psyllium
quercetin
vitamin B$_2$ (riboflavin)
selenium
slippery elm powder
thiamine (vitamin B$_1$)

valerian
vitamin A
vitamin B$_{12}$
vitamin B-complex
vitamin C
vitamin D
vitamin K
wild yam
zinc

URETHRITIS
beta-carotene
blueberries
buchu
cleavers
coneflower
corn silk
couchgrass
cranberries
goldenseal
horsetail
kava kava
marshmallow root
plantain
thyme leaf
uva ursi
vitamin C
zinc

URINARY INCONTINENCE
blueberries
calcium/magnesium
cranberries
horsetail
marshmallow root
plantain
vitamin C
zinc

**URINARY TRACT INFECTION
IN WOMEN**
beta-carotene
blueberries
buchu
coneflower
corn silk
couchgrass
cranberries
goldenseal
horsetail
marshmallow root
plantain
thyme leaf
uva ursi
vitamin C
zinc

UROLITHIASIS
corn silk
cramp bark
folic acid (vitamin B$_9$)
gravel root
jamaican dogwood
kava kava
magnesium citrate
pyridoxine
wild yam

VAGINITIS
acidophilus
beta-carotene
garlic
pau d'arco tea
vitamin A
vitamin C

vitamin E
zinc

WARTS
beta-carotene
celandine
coneflower
echinacea
folic acid (vitamin B$_9$)
goldenseal
licorice root
lomatium
osha
selenium
thuja leaf
vitamin A
vitamin B-complex
vitamin C
vitamin E
zinc

■ RESOURCES - CONDITIONS

ALLERGIC RHINITIS

The Burton Goldberg Group. *Alternative Medicine: The Definitive Guide.* Tiburon, Calif: Future Medicine Publishing, Inc; 1997.

Ferri FF. *Ferri's Clinical Advisor: Instant Diagnosis and Treatment.* St Louis, Mo: Mosby-Year Book; 1999.

Fisher C. Nettles: an aid to the treatment of allergic rhinitus. *Eur J Herbal Med.* p. 34–35.

Morrison R. *Desktop Guide to Keynotes and Confirmatory Symptoms.* Albany, Calif: Hahnemann Clinic Publishing; 1993.

Noble J, ed. *Textbook of Primary Care Medicine.* 2nd ed. St Louis, Mo: Mosby-Year Book; 1996.

Tierney LM Jr, McPhee SJ, Papadakis MA, eds. *Current Medical Diagnosis and Treatment 1994.* Norwalk, Conn: Appleton & Lange; 1994.

ALOPECIA

Guendert DV. *Management of Alopecia.* February 1, 1995. Department of Otolaryngology, UTMB. Accessed at Neuropathy Research at the Medical College of Georgia, http://npntserver.mcg.edu/html/alopecia/documents/BALDNESS_95.html on January 13, 1999.

Hay IC, Jamieson M, Ormerod AD. Randomized trial of aromatherapy: successful treatment for alopecia areata. Arch Dermatol. 1998;134:1349–1352.

Lebwohl M. New treatments for alopecia areata. Lancet. 1997;349:222–223.

Whiting DA. The Diagnosis of Alopecia. Dallas, Tex: University of Texas. Baylor Hair Research and Treatment Center. Accessed at Neuropathy Research at the Medical College of Georgia, http://npntserver.mcg.edu/html/alopecia/documents/DiagnosisAA.html on January 13, 1999.

AMENORRHEA

Mowrey DB. *The Scientific Validation of Herbal Medicine.* New Canaan, Conn: Keats Publishing; 1988.

National Institutes of Health: Accessed at www.nih.gov on January 16, 1999.

Tierney LM, McPhee SJ, Papadakis MA, eds. *Current Medical Diagnosis & Treatment 1999.* 38th ed. Stamford, Conn: Appleton & Lange; 1999.

Tyler VE. *Herbs of Choice.* New York, NY: Pharmaceutical Products Press; 1994.

Ullman D. *Discovering Homeopathy.* Berkeley, Calif: North Atlantic Books; 1991.

ANEMIA

Branch Jr WT. *Office Practice of Medicine.* Philadelphia, Pa: WB Saunders Company; 1994.

Fauci AS, Braunwald E, Isselbacher KJ et al, eds. *Harrison's Principles of Internal Medicine.* 14th ed. New York, NY: McGraw-Hill; 1998.

Kelley WN, ed. *Textbook of Internal Medicine.* 3rd ed. Philadelphia, Pa: Lippincott-Raven; 1997.

Tyler TE. *The Honest Herbal: A Sensible Guide to the Use of Herbs and Related Remedies.* 3rd ed. New York, NY: Pharmaceutical Products Press; 1993.

ANGINA

Ballegard S, et al. Acupuncture in angina pectoris: does acupuncture have a specific effect? *J Intern Med.* 1991; 229:357–362.

Caligiuri G, et al. Immune system activation follows inflammation in unstable angina: pathogenetic implications. *J Am Coll Cardiol.* 1998;32:1295–1304.

Cohen M, et al. A comparison of low-molecular weight heparin with unfractionated heparin for unstable coronary artery disease. *N Engl J Med.* 1997;337:447–452.

Kruzel T. *The Homeopathic Emergency Guide.* Berkeley, Calif: North Atlantic Books; 1992:58–60.

Werbach M. *Nutritional Influences on Illness.* New Canaan, Conn: Keats Publishing; 1988:40–77.

Zhou XP, Liu JX. Metrological analysis for efficacy of acupuncture on angina pectoris [in Chinese]. *Chung-Kuo Chung His I Chieh Ho Tsa Chih.* 1993;13:212–214.

ANOREXIA NERVOSA

Balch JF, Balch PA. *Prescription for Nutritional Healing.* 2nd ed. Garden City Park, NY: Avery Publishing Group; 1997.

Diagnostic and Statistical Manual of Mental Disorders. 4th ed. Washington, DC: American Psychiatric Association; 1994.

Garner DM, Garfinkel PE, eds. *Handbook of Treatment for Eating Disorders.* 2nd ed. New York, NY: The Guilford Press; 1997.

The Harvard Mental Health Letter. October & November, 1997.

Kalasky KL, ed. *The Alternative Health & Medicine Encyclopedia.* 2nd ed. Detroit, MI: Gale Research; 1998.

Kaplan AS, Garfinkel PE, eds. *Medical Issues and the Eating Disorders—The Interface.* New York, NY: Brunner/Mazel Publishers; 1993.

Shils ME, Olson JA, Shike M, ed. *Modern Nutrition in Health and Disease.* 8th ed. Philadelphia, Pa: Lea & Febiger; 1994:2.

Werbach MR. *Nutritional Influences on Illness.* New Canaan, Conn: Keats Publishing Inc; 1987.

ANXIETY

American Council on Collaborative Medicine. *Dr. Victor Bagnall's Nutritional Therapy.* Accessed at: http://www.nutrimed.com/anxiety.htm on December 2, 1998.

American Psychiatric Association. *Diagnostic and Statistical Manual of Mental Disorders.* 4th ed. Washington, DC: American Psychiatric Association; 1994.

Andreoli TE, Bennett JC, Carpenter CCJ. *Cecil Essentials of Medicine.* 3rd ed. Philadelphia, Pa: WB Saunders; 1993.

Barker LR, Burton JR, Zieve PD, eds. *Principles of Ambulatory Medicine.* 4th ed. Baltimore, Md: Williams & Wilkins; 1995:139–154.

Blumenthal M, ed. *The Complete German Commission E Monographs.* Boston, Mass: Integrative Medicine Communications; 1998:422, 463–464.

Dr. Bower's Complementary and Alternative Medicine Home Page. Available at: http://avery.med.virginia.edu/~pjb3s.

Goldberg RJ. Anxiety reduction by self-regulation: theory, practice, and evaluation. *Ann Intern Med.* 1982;96:483.

Health and Healing News. Accessed at: http://hhnews.com/kava_update.htm on Dec. 2, 1998.

Herbal Alternatives. Accessed at: http://herbalalternatives.com/kava.htm on December 2, 1998.

Jussofie A, Schmiz A, Hiernke C. Kavapyrone enriched extract from *Piper methysticum* as modulator of the GABA binding site in different regions of the rat brain. *Psychopharmacology.* 1994;116:469–474.

Kinzler E, Kromer J, Lehmann E. Effect of a special kava extract in patients with anxiety-, tension-, and excitation states of non-psychotic genesis. Double blind study with placebos over four weeks [in German]. *Arzneimforsch.* 1991;41:584–588.

Lehmann E, et al. Efficacy of special kava extract *(Piper methysticum)* in patients with states of anxiety, tension and excitedness of non-mental origin-A double blind placebo controlled study of four weeks treatment. *Phytomedicine.* 1996;3:113–119.

Lindenberg Von D, Pitule-Schodel H. D, L-Kavain in comparison with oxazepam in anxiety states. Double-blind clinical trial. *Forschr Med.* 1990;108:50–54.

Morrison R. *Desktop Guide to Keynotes and Confirmatory Symptoms.* Albany, Calif: Hahnemann Clinic Publishing; 1993:4, 40, 293.

Stein JH, ed. *Internal Medicine.* 4th ed. St. Louis, Mo: Mosby-Year Book; 1994.

Volz HP, Kieser M. Kava kava extract WS 1490 versus placebo in anxiety disorders-a randomized placebo controlled 25 week outpatient trial. *Pharmacopsychiatry.* 1997;30:1–5.

ASTHMA

Bartram T. *Encyclopedia of Herbal Medicine.* Dorset, England: Grace Publishers; 1995:40–41.

Hope BE, Massey DB, Fournier-Massey G. Hawaiian materia medica for asthma. *Hawaii Med J.* 1993;52:160–166.

Kruzel T. *The Homeopathic Emergency Guide.* Berkeley, Calif: North Atlantic Books; 1992:21–27.

Middleton E, ed. *Allergy: Principles and Practice.* 5th ed. St. Louis, Mo: Mosby-Year Book, Inc; 1998.

Monteleone CA, Sherman AR. Nutrition and asthma. *Arch Intern Med.* 1997;157:23–24.

Murray MT, Pizzorno JE. *Encyclopedia of Natural Medicine.* Rocklin, Calif: Prima Publishing; 1998:150–155.

Rakel RE, ed. *Conn's Current Therapy.* 50th ed. Philadelphia, Pa: WB Saunders; 1998.

ATHEROSCLEROSIS

Bartram T. *Encyclopedia of Herbal Medicine.* Dorset, England: Grace Publishers; 1995:41–42, 198–199, 215, 270.

Berkow R, ed. *Merck Manual of Diagnosis and Therapy.* 16th ed. Rahway, NJ: The Merck Publishing Group; 1992.

Berkow R, Beers MH, Fletcher AJ, eds. *Merck Manual, Home Edition.* Rahway, NJ: Merck & Co; 1997.

Blumenthal M, ed. *The Complete German Commission E Monographs.* Boston, Mass: Integrative Medicine Communications; 1998:71–72, 135–138, 142–143, 197.

Fauci AS, Braunwald E, Isselbacher KJ et al, eds. *Harrison's Principles of Internal Medicine.* 14th ed. New York, NY: McGraw-Hill; 1998.

Gruenwald J, Brendler T, Jaenicke C et al, eds. *PDR for Herbal Medicines.* Montvale, NJ: Medical Economics Company; 1998:871–873,1219–1222.

Larson DE, ed. *Mayo Clinic Family Health Book.* 2nd ed. New York, NY: William Morrow and Company; 1996.

Miller Alan. Cardiovascular Disease: Toward a unified approach. *Alternative Medicine Review.* September 1996;1:132–147.

Murray MT. *The Healing Power of Herbs: The Enlightened Person's Guide to the Wonders of Medicinal Plants.* Rocklin, Calif: Prima Publishing; 1998:107–113, 118–131.

Murray MT, Pizzorno JE. *Encyclopedia of Natural Medicine.* Rocklin, Calif: Prima Publishing; 1998:156–170.

Raloff J. Why cutting fats may harm the heart. *Science News.* March 20, 1999;155:181.

Ravitsky M. Herbs: Atherosclerosis. *Newlife Magazine.* Jan/Feb 1997:19.

Werbach M. *Nutritional Influences on Illness.* New Canaan, Conn: Keats Publishing; 1988:40–78.

ATTENTION-DEFICIT/HYPERACTIVITY DISORDER

Balch JF, Balch PA. *Prescription for Nutritional Healing.* Garden City Park, NY: Avery Publishing Group; 1997.

Bartram T. *Encyclopedia of Herbal Medicine.* Dorset, England: Grace Publishers; 1995:270, 238.

Blumenthal M, ed. *The Complete German Commission E Monographs.* Boston, Mass: Integrative Medicine Communications; 1998:160, 107.

Gruenwald J, Brendler T et al, eds. *PDR for Herbal Medicines.* Montvale, NJ: Medical Economics Company; 1998:929, 961–963, 967–968, 991–992, 1015–1016.

Morrison R. *Desktop Guide to Keynotes and Confirmatory Symptoms.* Albany, Calif: Hahnemann Clinic Publishing; 1993:33–36, 39–44, 115–117.

Murray MT, Pizzorno JE. *Encyclopedia of Natural Medicine.* Rocklin, Calif: Prima Publishing; 1998:372–377.

Werbach M. *Nutritional Influences on Illness.* New Canaan, Conn: Keats Publishing; 1988:221–226.

BENIGN PROSTATIC HYPERPLASIA

Berkow R, Beers MH et al, eds. *Merck Manual of Medical Information: Home Edition.* Whitehorse Station, NJ: The Merck Publishing Group; 1997.

Blumenthal M, ed. *The Complete German Commission E Monographs.* Boston, Mass: Integrative Medicine Communications; 1998:201.

Morrison R. *Desktop Guide to Keynotes and Confirmatory Symptoms.* Albany, Calif: Hahnemann Clinic Publishing; 1993:119, 141, 286, 341, 388–389.

Murray MT, Pizzorno JE. *Encyclopedia of Natural Medicine.* Rocklin, Calif: Prima Publishing; 1998:480–486.

Prostate Enlargement: Benign Prostatic Hyperplasia. The National Kidney and Urologic Diseases Information Clearinghouse. NIH publication no. 91:3012.

Werbach, M. *Nutritional Influences on Illness.* New Canaan, Conn: Keats Publishing; 1988:82–84.

BRONCHITIS

Allan H, Goroll MD, et al, eds. *Primary Care Medicine.* 3rd ed. Philadelphia, Pa: Lippincott-Raven Publishers; 1995:252–260, 285–294.

Bartram T. *Encyclopedia of Herbal Medicine.* Dorset, England: Grace Publishers; 1995:72–73.

Bone RC, ed. *Pulmonary and Critical Care Medicine.* St. Louis, Mo: Mosby-Year Book, Inc; 1998:G3 1–6.

Cecil RL, Plum F, Bennett JC, eds. *Cecil Textbook of Medicine.* 20th ed. Philadelphia, Pa: WB Saunders Company; 1996:382–389.

Kruzel T. *The Homeopathic Emergency Guide.* Berkeley, Calif: North Atlantic Books; 1992:40–43.

Rakel RE, ed. *Conn's Current Therapy.* 50th ed. Philadelphia, Pa: WB Saunders Company; 1998:211–212.

BURNS

Bartram T. *Encyclopedia of Herbal Medicine.* Dorset, England: Grace Publishers; 1995:77.

Blumenthal M, ed. *The Complete German Commission E Monographs.* Boston, Mass: Integrative Medicine Communications; 1998:423.

Castro M. *The Complete Homeopathy Handbook.* New York, NY: St. Martin's Press; 1991.

Foley D, Nechas E, Perry S, Salmon DK. *The Doctor's Book of Home Remedies for Children.* Emmaus, Pa: Rodale Press; 1994.

Forgey WW, ed. *Wilderness Medical Society Practice Guidelines for Wilderness Emergency Care.* Merrillville, Ind: ICS Books, Inc; 1995.

Kruzel T. *The Homeopathic Emergency Guide.* Berkeley, Calif: North Atlantic Books; 1992:48–50.

Lynn SG, Weintraub P. *Medical Emergency! The St. Luke's-Roosevelt Hospital Center Book of Emergency Medicine.* New York, NY: Hearst Books; 1996.

Noble J, ed. *Textbook Of Primary Care Medicine.* St. Louis, Mo: Mosby-Year Book; 1996.

Tierney Jr LM, McPhee SJ, Papadakis MA, eds. *Current Medical Diagnosis and Treatment.* Norwalk, Conn: Appleton & Lange; 1994.

Tyler VE. *Herbs of Choice: The Therapeutic Use of Phytomedicinals.* New York, NY: Pharmaceutical Products Press; 1994.

BURSITIS

Andreoli TE, Bennett JC, Carpenter CCJ. *Cecil Essentials of Medicine.* 3rd ed. Philadelphia, Pa: W.B. Saunders; 1993.

Barker LR, Burton JR, Zieve PD, eds. *Principles of Ambulatory Medicine.* 4th ed. Baltimore, Md: Williams & Wilkins; 1995:885–894.

Dambro MR, ed. *Griffith's 5 Minute Clinical Consult 1999.* Baltimore, Md: Lippincott Williams & Wilkins; 1999.

Murray MT. *The Healing Power of Herbs: The Enlightened Person's Guide to the Wonders of Medicinal Plants.* Rocklin, Calif: Prima Publishing; 1998.

Stein JH, ed. *Internal Medicine.* 4th ed. St. Louis, Mo: Mosby-Year Book; 1994:2400–2404.

CANDIDIASIS

Bartram T. *Encyclopedia of Herbal Medicine.* Dorset, England: Grace Publishers; 1995:263, 417.

Berkow R, Fletcher AJ, eds. *The Merck Manual of Diagnosis and Therapy.* Rahway, NJ: Merck & Company Inc; 1992.

Blumenthal M, ed. *The Complete German Commission E Monographs.* Boston, Mass: Integrative Medicine Communications; 1998:463.

Coeugniet E, Kühnast R. Recurrent candidiasis: Adjutant immunotherapy with different formulations of Echinacin®. *Therapiewoche.* 1986;36:3352–3358.

Conn RB, Borer WZ, Snyder JW, eds. *Current Diagnosis 9.* Philadelphia, Pa: WB Saunders; 1996.

Gruenwald J, Brendler T, Jaenicke C et al, eds. *PDR for Herbal Medicines.* Montvale, NJ: Medical Economics Company; 1998:728.

Henry JR. *Clinical Diagnosis and Management by Laboratory Methods.* Philadelphia, Pa: WB Saunders Company; 1996.

Morrison R. *Desktop Guide to Keynotes and Confirmatory Symptoms.* Albany, Calif: Hahnemann Clinic Publishing; 1993:68, 115–117, 171–172, 210.

Thierney Jr LM, McPhee SJ, Papadakis MA, eds. *Current Medical Diagnosis and Treatment 1999.* 38th ed. Stamford, Conn: Appleton & Lange; 1999.

CHRONIC FATIGUE SYNDROME

Castro M. *The Complete Homeopathy Handbook.* New York, NY: St. Martin's Press; 1990.

Fukuda K, et al. The chronic fatigue syndrome: a comprehensive approach to its definition and study. *Ann Intern Med.* 1994;121:953–959.

Management of CFS: Pharmacologic therapy and nonpharmacologic therapy. Centers for Disease Control and Prevention. Accessed at www.cdc.gov/ncidod/diseases/cfs/mgmt1.htm on January 4, 1999.

Noble J, ed. *Textbook of Primary Care Medicine.* 2nd ed. St Louis, Mo: Mosby-Year Book, Inc; 1996:918–922.

Scalzo R. *Naturopathic Handbook of Herbal Formulas.* Durango, Colo: 2nd ed. Kivaki Press; 1994:S/A18–S/A19.

Werbach M. *Nutritional Influences on Illness.* New Canaan, Conn: Keats Publishing; 1988:418–421.

CHRONIC OBSTRUCTIVE PULMONARY DISEASE

Blumenthal M, ed. *The Complete German Commission E Monographs.* Boston, Mass: Integrative Medicine Communications; 1998:423, 468.

Bordow RA, Moser KM. *Manual of Clinical Problems in Pulmonary Medicine.* 4th ed. Boston, Mass:Little, Brown; 1996:212–215.

Celli BR. Pulmonary rehabilitation in patients with COPD. *Am J Respir Crit Care Med.* 1995;152:861–864.

Duke JA. *The Green Pharmacy.* Emmaus, Pa: Rodale Press; 1997:93–95, 179–183.

Fauci AS, Braunwald E, Isselbacher KJ et al, eds. *Harrison's Principles of Internal Medicine.* 14th ed. New York, NY: McGraw-Hill; 1998:1451–1457.

Ferguson GT, Cherniack RM. Management of chronic obstructive pulmonary disease. *N Engl J Med.* 1993;328:1017–1022.

Snider GL. *Standards for the Diagnosis and Care of Patients with Chronic Obstructive Pulmonary Disease.* Washington Crossing, Pa: Scientific Frontiers; 1996:1–12.

Woodley M, Whelan A. *Manual of Medical Therapeutics.* 27th ed. Boston, Mass: Little, Brown; 1992:200–202.

CIRRHOSIS OF THE LIVER

Bartram T. *Encyclopedia of Herbal Medicine.* Dorset, England: Grace Publishers; 1995:295.

Bone K. *Clinical Applications of Ayurvedic and Chinese Herbs.* Queensland, Australia: Phytotherapy Press; 1996:69.

Branch WT. *Office Practice of Medicine.* 3rd ed. Philadelphia, Pa: WB Saunders; 1994:326–338.

Fauci AS, Braunwald E, Isselbacher KJ et al, eds. *Harrison's Principles of Internal Medicine.* 14th ed. New York, NY: McGraw-Hill; 1998:1704–1710.

Ferenci P, Dragosics B, Dittrich H, et al. Randomized controlled trial of silymarin treatment in patients with cirrhosis of the liver. *J Hepatol.* 1989;9:105–113.

Gruenwald J, Brendler T et al, eds. *PDR for Herbal Medicines.* Montvale, NJ: Medical Economics Company; 1998:1138–1139.

Marshall AW, Graul RS, Morgan MY, Sherlock S. Treatment of alcohol-related liver disease with thioctic acid: a six month radomized double-blind trial. *Gut.* 1982;23:1088–1093.

Mowrey DB. *The Scientific Validation of Herbal Medicine.* New Canaan, Conn: Keats Publishing; 1986:179.

Murray MT, Pizzorno JE. *Encyclopedia of Natural Medicine.* 2nd ed. Rocklin, Calif: Prima Publishing; 1998:211–220.

Walker LP, Brown EH. *The Alternative Pharmacy.* Paramus, NJ: Prentice Hall; 1998:394.

Wyngaarden JB, Smith Jr LH, Bennett JC, eds. *Cecil Textbook of Medicine.* 19th ed. Philadelphia, Pa: WB Saunders; 1992:786–795.

COMMON COLD

Behrman RE, ed. *Nelson Textbook of Pediatrics.* 15th ed. Philadelphia, Pa: WB Saunders; 1996.

Cummings S, Ullman D. *Homeopathic Medicines.* Los Angeles, Calif: Jeremy P. Tarcher, Inc; 1984.

Dorn M, Knick E, Lewith G. Placebo-controlled, double-blind study of *Echinacea pallidae radix* in upper respiratory tract infections. *Complementary Therapies in Medicine.* 1997;5:40–42.

Eby GA. Zinc ion availability—the determinant of efficacy in zinc lozenge treatment of common colds. *J Antimicrob Chemother.* 1997;40:483–493.

Fauci AS, Braunwald E, Isselbacher KJ et al, eds. *Harrison's Principles of Internal Medicine.* 14th ed. New York, NY: McGraw-Hill; 1998.

Garland ML, Hagmeyer KO. The role of zinc lozenges in treatment of the common cold. *Ann Pharmacother.* 1998;32:63–69.

Gruenwald J, Brendler T, Jaenicke C et al, eds. *PDR for Herbal Medicines.* Montvale, NJ: Medical Economics Company; 1998:817.

Hoheisel O, Sandberg M, Bertram S, Bulitta M, Schäfer M. Echinagard treatment shortens the course of the common cold: a double-blind, placebo-controlled clinical trial. *Eur J Clin Res.* 1997;9:261–269.

Melchart D, Walther E, Linde K, Brandmeier R, Lersch, C. Echinacea root extracts for the prevention of upper respiratory tract infections. *Archives of Family Medicine.* 1998;7:541–545.

Morrison R. *Desktop Guide to Keynotes and Confirmatory Symptoms.* Albany, Calif: Hahnemann Clinic Publishing; 1993:3–6, 13–14, 158, 244–246.

Sazawal S, Black RE, Jalla S, et al. Zinc supplementation reduces the incidence of acute lower respiratory infections in infants and preschool children: a double-blind, controlled trial. *Pediatrics.* 1998;102(part 1):1–5.

Scaglione, et al. Efficacy and safety of the standardized ginseng extract G115 for potentiating vaccination against common cold and/or influenza syndrome. *Drugs Exp Clin Res.* 1996;22:65–72.

Schöneberger D. The influence of immune-stimulating effects of pressed juice from *Echinacea purpurea* on the course and severity of colds. *Forum Immunol.* 1992;8:2–12.

CONGESTIVE HEART FAILURE

Bartram T. *Encyclopedia of Herbal Medicine.* Dorset, England: Grace Publishers; 1995:218–219.

Blumenthal M, ed. *The Complete German Commission E Monographs.* Boston, Mass: Integrative Medicine Communications; 1998:120,142–144,162–163,171–172,197.

Brady JA, Rock CL, Horneffer MR. Thiamin status, diuretic medications, and the management of congestive heart failure. *J Am Diet Assoc.* 1995;95:541–544.

Cecil RL, Plum F, Bennett JC, eds. *Cecil Textbook of Medicine.* 20th ed. Philadelphia, Pa: WB Saunders; 1996.

Gruenwald J, Brendler T, Jaenicke C et al, eds. *PDR for Herbal Medicines.* Montvale, NJ: Medical Economics Company; 1998:779–781,932–923,1101–1103,1175–1176,1185–1187,1219–1221.

Murray MT. *Encyclopedia of Nutritional Supplements.* Rocklin, Calif: Prima Publishing; 1996:378–379.

Schmidt U, Kuhn U, Ploch M, Hubner WD. Efficacy of the hawthorn (Crataegus) preparation LI 132 in 78 patients with chronic congestive heart failure defined as NYHA functional class II. *Phytomedicine.* 1994;1:17-24.

Washington University School of Medicine, Department of Medicine. *Washington Manual*

of Medical Therapeautics. 29th ed. Philadelphia, Pa: Lippincott-Raven Publishers; 1998.

Werbach MR. *Nutritional Influences on Illness.* New Canaan, Conn: Keats Publishing, Inc; 1987:40–78,136–139,227–240.

CONJUNCTIVITIS

Abelson MB, Casey R. How to manage atopic keratoconjunctivitis. *Rev Ophthalmol.* May 1996.

Abelson MB, McGarr, P. How to diagnose and treat inclusion conjunctivitis. *Rev Ophthalmol.* March 1997.

Abelson MB, Richard KP. What we know and don't know about GPC. *Rev Ophthalmol.* August 1994.

Abelson MB, Welch D. How to treat bacterial conjunctivitis. *Rev Ophthalmol.* December 1994.

Acute conjunctivitis. Acupuncture.com. Accessed at www.acupuncture.com/Clinical/Conjunct.htm on January 29, 1999.

Clinical imperatives of ocular infection. *Primary Care Optometry News.* Roundtable. March 1996. Available at www.slackinc.com/eye/pcon/199603/impera.htm.

Friedlaender MH. Update on allergic conjunctivitis. *Rev Ophthalmol.* March 1997.

Homeopathic drops for allergy: ready or not? *Primary Care Optometry News.* May 1996.

Infectious Diseases and Immunization Committee. Canadian Pediatric Society. Recommendations for the prevention of neonatal ophthalmia. *Can Med Assoc J.* 1983; 129:554–555.

Morrison R. *Desktop Guide to Keynotes and Confirmatory Symptoms.* Albany, Calif: Hahnemann Clinic Publishing; 1993:5, 28.

Pascucci S, Shovlin J. How to beat giant papillary conjunctivitis. *Rev Ophthalmol.* June 1994.

Rapoza PA, Francesconi CM. How to diagnose chronic red eye. *Rev Ophthalmol.* October 1997.

CONSTIPATION

Andreoli TE, Bennett JC, Carpenter CCJ. *Cecil Essentials of Medicine.* 3rd ed. Philadelphia, Pa: WB Saunders; 1993.

Ashraf W, Park F, Lof J, Quigley EM. Effects of psyllium therapy on stool characteristics, colon transit and anorectal function in chronic idiopathic constipation. *Aliment Pharmacol Ther.* 1995;9:639–647.

Barker LR, Burton JR, Zieve PD, eds. *Principles of Ambulatory Medicine.* 4th ed. Baltimore, Md: Williams & Wilkins; 1995:476–491.

Dambro MR. *Griffith's 5 Minute Clinical Consult 1999.* Baltimore, Md: Lippincott Williams & Wilkins; 1999.

Hobbs C. *Foundations of Health: The Liver and Digestive Herbal.* Capitola, Calif: Botanica Press; 1992:129–135.

McRorie JW, Daggy BP, Morel JG, Diersing PS, Miner PB, Robinson M. Psyllium is superior to docusate sodium for treatment of chronic constipation. *Aliment Pharmacol Ther.* 1998;12:491–497.

Morrison R. *Desktop Guide to Keynotes and Confirmatory Symptoms.* Albany, Calif: Hahnemann Clinic Publishing; 1993:85, 274, 281, 350.

Stein JH, ed. *Internal Medicine.* 4th ed. St. Louis, Mo: Mosby-Year Book; 1994.

COUGH

American Academy of Family Physicians. Available at: http://www.aafp.org/.

Duke JA. *The Green Pharmacy.* Emmaus, Pa: Rodale Press; 1997.

Fauci AS, Braunwald E, Isselbacher KJ et al, eds. *Harrison's Principles of Internal Medicine.* 14th ed. New York, NY: McGraw-Hill; 1998.

Kruzel T. The Homeopathic Emergency Guide. Berkeley, Calif: North Atlantic Books; 1992.

Newall A, Anderson LA, Phillipson JD. *Herbal Medicines.* London, England: The Pharmaceutical Press; 1996.

Schulz V, Hänsel R, Tyler VE. *Rational Phytotherapy.* 3rd ed. Berlin, Germany: Springer-Verlag, 1998.

Tierney Jr. LM, McPhee SJ, Papadakis MA, eds. *Current Medical Diagnosis & Treatment, 1999.* Stamford, Conn: Appleton & Lange; 1999.

Tyler VE. *Herbs of Choice.* Binghamton, NY: Pharmaceutical Products Press; 1994.

CUTANEOUS DRUG REACTIONS

American Academy of Dermatology. Guidelines of care for cutaneous adverse drug reactions. *J Am Acad Dermatol.* 1996;35:458-461. Available at www.aad.org/guidelinecutaneousdrug.html.

Balch JF, Balch PA. *Prescription for Nutritional Healing.* 2nd ed. Garden City Park, NY: Avery Publishing Group; 1997.

Dambro MR, ed. *Griffith's 5 Minute Clinical Consult.* Baltimore, Md: Lippincott, Williams & Wilkins; 1998.

Fauci AS, Braunwald E, Isselbacher KJ et al, eds. *Harrison's Principles of Internal*

Medicine. 14th ed. New York, NY: McGraw-Hill; 1998.

Morrison R. *Desktop Guide to Keynotes and Confirmatory Symptoms.* Albany, Calif: Hahnemann Clinic Publishing; 1993.

Murray MT, Pizzorno JE. *Encyclopedia of Natural Medicines.* 2nd ed. Rocklin, Calif: Prima Publishing; 1998.

DEMENTIA

American Psychiatric Association. *Diagnostic and Statistical Manual of Mental Disorders.* 4th ed. Washington, DC: American Psychiatric Association; 1994.

Bartram T. *Encyclopedia of Herbal Medicine.* Dorset, England: Grace Publishers; 1995:214, 376.

Blumenthal M, ed. *The Complete German Commission E Monographs.* Boston, Mass: Integrative Medicine Communications; 1998:136, 138, 197.

Gruenwald J, Brendler T, Jaenicke C et al, eds. *PDR for Herbal Medicines.* Montvale, NJ: Medical Economics Company; 1998:967–968, 1101–1102, 1219–1220, 1229–1230.

Hofferberth B. The efficacy of EGb 761 in patients with senile dementia of the Alzheimer type; A double-blind, placebo-controlled study on different levels of investigation. *Hum Psychopharmacol.* 1994;9:215–222.

Kanowski S, Hermann WM, Stephan K, Wierich W, Horr R. Proof of efficacy of the Ginkgo biloba special extract EGb 761 in outpatients suffering from mild to moderate dementia of the Alzheimer's type or multi-infarct dementia. *Pharmacopsychiatry.* 1996;29:47–56.

Le Bars, et al. A placebo-controlled, double-blind, randomized trial of an extract of Gingko biloba for dementia. *JAMA.* 1997;278:1327–1332.

Maurer K. et al. Clinical efficacy of Gingko biloba special extract EGb 761 in dementia of the Alzheimer type. *J Psychiatr Res.* 1997;31:645–655.

Morrison R. *Desktop Guide to Keynotes and Confirmatory Symptoms.* Albany, Calif: Hahnemann Clinic Publishing; 1993:17–17, 32–33, 124–125, 176–177, 248–249.

Morris JC, ed. *Handbook of Dementing Illnesses.* New York, NY: Marcel Dekker Inc; 1994.

National Institutes of Health. Available at http://text.nlm.nih.gov/.

Perry EK, Pickering AT, Wang WW, Houghton P, Perry NS. Medicinal plants and Alzheimer's disease: Integrating ethnobotanical and contemporary scientific evidence. *J Altern Complement Med.* 1998;4:419–428.

Rai GS, Shovlin C, Wesnes KA. A double-blind, placebo controlled study of Ginkgo biloba extract in elderly patients with mild to moderate memory impairment. *Curr Med Res Opin.* 1991;12:350–355.

Rakel RE. *Conn's Current Therapy 1997: Latest Approved Methods of Treatment for the Practicing Physician.* Philadelphia, Pa: WB Saunders; 1997.

Werbach, M. *Nutritional Influences on Illness.* New Canaan, Conn: Keats Publishing; 1988:149–154.

DEPRESSION

Blumenthal M, ed. *The Complete German Commission E Monographs.* Boston, Mass: Integrative Medicine Communications; 1998:422, 425.

Diagnostic and Statistical Manual of Mental Disorders. 4th ed. Washington, DC: American Psychiatric Association; 1994.

Gruenwald J, Brendler T et al, eds. *PDR for Herbal Medicines.* Montvale, NJ: Medical Economics Company; 1998:967–968, 1015.

Hippius H. St John's wort *(Hypericum perforatum)*—a herbal antidepressant. *Curr Med Res Opin.* 1998;14:171–184. In process.

Kaplan HW, ed. *Comprehensive Textbook of Psychiatry.* 6th ed. Baltimore, Md: Williams & Wilkins; 1995.

Linde K, Ramirez G, Mulrow CD, et al. St. John's wort for depression—an overview and meta-analysis of randomized clinical trials. *Br Med J.* 1996;313:253–258.

Rakel RE, ed. *Conn's Current Therapy.* 50th ed. Philadelphia, Pa: WB Saunders Company; 1998.

Reuter HD. St. John's wort as a herbal antidepressant. *Eur J Herbal Med.* Part 1. 1995;1(3):19–24. Part 2. 1995;1(4):15–21.

DERMATITIS

Bartram T. *Encyclopedia of Herbal Medicine.* Dorset, England: Grace Publishers; 1995:144.

Habif TP. *Clinical Dermatology.* 3rd ed. St. Louis, Mo: Mosby-Year Book; 1996.

Middleton E, ed. *Allergy: Principles and Practice.* 5th ed. St. Louis, Mo: Mosby-Year Book; 1998.

Morrison R. *Desktop Guide to Keynotes and Confirmatory Symptoms.* Albany, Calif: Hahnemann Clinic Publishing; 1993:29, 326, 394.

Rakel RE, ed. *Conn's Current Therapy.* 50th ed. Philadelphia, Pa: WB Saunders; 1998.

Scalzo R. *Naturopathic Handbook of Herbal Formulas.* Durango, Colo: 2nd ed. Kivaki Press; 1994:36.

Schulpis KH, Nyalala JO, Papakonstantinou ED, et al. Biotin recycling impairment in phenylketonuric children with seborrheic dermatitis. *Int J Dermatol.* 1998;37:918–921.

Stewart JCM, et al. Treatment of severe and moderately severe atopic dermatitis with evening primrose oil (Epogam): a multi-center study. *J Nut Med.* 1991;2:9–16.

DIABETES MELLITUS

Anderson RA, Cheng N, Bryden NA, et al. Elevated intakes of supplemental chromium improve glucose and insulin variables in individuals with type 2 diabetes. *Diabetes.* 1997;46:1786–1791.

Blumenthal M, ed. *The Complete German Commission E Monographs.* Boston, Mass: Integrative Medicine Communications; 1998:134, 176.

Boden G, Chen X, Igbal N. Acute lowering of plasma fatty acids lowers basal insulin secretion in diabetic and nondiabetic subjects. *Diabetes.* 1998;47:1609–1612.

Cohen N, Halberstam M, Shlimovich P, Chang CJ, Shamoon H, Rossetti L. Oral vanadyl sulfate improves hepatic and peripheral insulin sensitivity in patients with with non-insulin-dependent diabetes mellitus. *J Clin Invest.* 1995;95:2501–2509.

Gruenwald J, Brendler T, Jaenicke C, et al, eds. *PDR for Herbal Medicines.* Montvale, NJ: Medical Economics Company; 1998:1201.

Hirsch IB, Atchley DH, Tsai E, et al. Ascorbic acid clearance in diabetic nephropathy. *J Diabet Complications.* 1998;12:259–263.

Koutsikos D, Agroyannis B, Tzanatos-Exarchou H. Biotin for diabetic peripheral neuropathy. *Biomed Pharmacother.* 1990;44:511–514.

Noble J. *Textbook of Primary Care Medicine.* 2nd ed. St Louis, Mo: Mosby-Year Book; 1996.

Perossini M, et al. Diabetic and hypertensive retinopathy therapy with Vaccinum myrtillus anthocyanosides (Tegens): double blind placebo controlled clinical trial. *Annali di Ottalmaologia e Clinica Ocaulistica.* 1987;CXII.

Poucheret P, Verma S, Grynpas MD, McNeill JH. Vanadium and diabetes. *Mol Cell Biochem.* 1998;188:73–80.

Tandan R, et al. Topical capsaicin in painful diabetic neuropathy. Controlled study with long-term follow-up. *Diabetes Care.* 1992;15:8–14.

Thibodeau GA, Patton KT. *Anatomy and Physiology.* 4th ed. St Louis, Mo: Mosby-Year Book; 1999.

Tierney Jr LM, McPhee SJ, Papadakis MA, eds. *Current Medical Diagnosis and Treatment.* 33rd ed. Norwalk, Conn: Appleton & Lange; 1994.

Ziegler D, Hanefeld M, Ruhnau KJ, et al. Treatment of symptomatic diabetic peripheral neuropathy with the anti-oxidant slpha-lipoc acid. A 3-week randomized controlled trial. *Diabetologia.* 1995;38:1425–1433.

Ziegler D, Schatz H, Conrad F, Gries FA, Ulrich H, Reichel G. Effects of treatment with the antioxidant alpha-lipoic acid on cardiac autonomic neuropathy in NIDDM patients. A 4-month randomized controlled multicenter trial. *Diabetes Care.* 1997;20:369–373.

DIARRHEA

Andreoli TE, Bennett JC, Carpenter CCJ. *Cecil Essentials of Medicine.* 3rd ed. Philadelphia, Pa: WB Saunders; 1993:271–277.

Barker LR, Burton JR, Zieve PD, eds. *Principles of Ambulatory Medicine.* 4th ed. Baltimore, Md: Williams & Wilkins; 1995:481–491.

Bartram T. *Encyclopedia of Herbal Medicine.* Dorset, England: Grace Publishers; 1995:147.

Bensky D, Gamble A. *Chinese Herbal Medicine.* Seattle, Wash: Eastland Press; 1986:47–49.

Blumenthal M, ed. *The Complete German Commission E Monographs.* Boston, Mass: Integrative Medicine Communications; 1998:425, 464.

Berkow R. *The Merck Manual of Medical Information.* Whitehouse Station, NJ: Merck Research Laboratories; 1997:523–525.

Morrison R. *Desktop Guide to Keynotes and Confirmatory Symptoms.* Albany, Calif: Hahnemann Clinic Publishing; 1993:15, 42, 116, 246, 305.

Murray MT. *Encyclopedia of Nutritional Supplements.* Rocklin, Calif: Prima Publishing; 1996:431–439.

Dambro MR. *Griffith's 5-Minute Clinical Consult–1999.* Baltimore, Md: Lippincott Williams & Wilkins; 1999: 316–319.

Gruenwald J, Brendler T, Jaenicke C et al, eds. *PDR for Herbal Medicines.* Montvale, NJ: Medical Economics Company; 1998:617–618, 621–622, 763–766, 1047–1050, 1061–1063, 1078–1079, 1103–1104, 1201–1202, 1226–1227.

Stein JK, ed. *Internal Medicine.* 4th ed. St. Louis, Mo: Mosby-Year Book; 1994:436–440.

Stoller JK, Ahmad M, Longworth DL, eds. *The Cleveland Clinic Intensive Review of Internal Medicine.* Baltimore, Md: Williams & Wilkins; 1998:638–643.

Tyler VE. *Herbs of Choice.* Binghamton, NY: Haworth Press; 1994:51–54.

Walker LP, Brown EH. *The Alternative Pharmacy.* Paramus, NJ: Prentice Hall Press; 1998:147–150.

DYSMENORRHEA

Batchelder HJ, Scalzo R. Allopathic specific condition review: dysmenorrhea. *The Protocol Journal of Botanical Medicine.* 1995;1(1).

Berkow R, ed. *The Merck Manual of Diagnosis and Therapy.* 16th ed. Rahway, NJ: Merck Research Laboratories; 1992.

Branch WT, Jr. *Office Practice of Medicine.* 3rd ed. Philadelphia, Pa: WB Saunders Company; 1994.

Penland JG, Johnson PE. Dietary calcium and manganese effects on menstrual cycle symptoms. *Am J Obstet Gynecol.* 1993;168:1417–1423.

Werbach MR. *Nutritional Influences on Illness.* New Canaan, Conn: Keats Publishing Inc; 1987.

DYSPHAGIA

Andreoli TE, Bennett JC, Carpenter CCJ. *Cecil Essentials of Medicine.* 3rd ed. Philadelphia, Pa: WB Saunders; 1993:284–285.

Barker LR, Burton JR, Zieve PD, eds. *Principles of Ambulatory Medicine.* 4th ed. Baltimore, Md: Williams & Wilkins; 1995:435–447.

Bartram T. *Encyclopedia of Herbal Medicine.* Dorset, England: Grace Publishers; 1995.

Dambro MR, ed. *Griffith's 5-Minute Clinical Consult–1999.* Baltimore, Md: Lippincott Williams & Wilkins; 1999:346–347.

Morrison R. *Desktop Guide to Keynotes and Confirmatory Symptoms.* Albany, Calif: Hahnemann Clinic Publishing; 1993.

Reynolds JEF. *Martindale: the Extra Pharmacopoeia.* 31st ed. London, England: Royal Pharmaceutical Society of Great Britain; 1996:1192.

Snow JA. *Glycyrrhiza glabra L.* (Leguminaceae). *The Protocol Journal of Botanical Medicine.* 1996;1:9.

Stein JK, ed. *Internal Medicine.* 4th ed. St. Louis, Mo: Mosby–Year Book; 1994:361–362.

Stoller JK, Ahmad M, Longworth DL eds. *The Cleveland Clinic Intensive Review of Internal Medicine.* Baltimore, Md: Williams & Wilkins; 1998:592–601.

ECZEMA

The Burton Goldberg Group. *Alternative Medicine: The Definitive Guide.* Tiburon, Calif: Future Medicine Publishing Inc; 1997.

Morse PF, et al. Meta-analysis of placebo-controlled studies of the efficacy of Epogam in the treatment of atopic eczema: Relationship between plasma essential fatty acid changes and clinical response. *Br J Dermatol.* 1989;121:75–90.

Murray MT, Pizzorno JE. *Encyclopedia of Natural Medicine.* Rocklin, Calif: Prima Publishing; 1998:296–300.

Noble J, ed. *Textbook of Primary Care Medicine.* 2nd ed. St Louis, Mo: Mosby-Year Book; 1996:345–365, 368–375, 1064–1084.

Tierney LM Jr, McPhee SJ, Papadakis MA, eds. *Current Medical Diagnosis and Treatment.* Norwalk, Conn: Appleton & Lange; 1994.

Werbach, M. *Nutritional Influences on Illness.* New Canaan, Conn: Keats Publishing; 1988:186–188

EDEMA

Balch JF, Balch PA. *Prescription for Nutritional Healing.* Garden City Park, NY: Avery Publishing Group; 1997.

Bartram T. *Encyclopedia of Herbal Medicine.* Dorset, England: Grace Publishers; 1995:73, 155, 156, 188.

Blumenthal M, ed. *The Complete German Commission E Monographs.* Boston, Mass: Integrative Medicine Communications; 1998:424, 425, 429.

Mayo Foundation for Medical Education and Research. Available at www.healthanswers.com

MDX Health Digest. Available at www.thriveonline.com

Mindell E, Hopkins V. *Prescription Alternatives.* New Canaan, Conn: Keats Publishing Inc; 1998.

Vanderbilt University Medical Center. Available at www.mc.vanderbilt.edu

Weiss RF. *Herbal Medicines.* Beaconsfield, England: Beaconsfield Publishers, Ltd; 1988:188–191, 241.

ENDOCARDITIS

Barker LR, Burton JR, Zieve PD, eds. *Principles of Ambulatory Medicine.* 4th ed. Baltimore, Md: Williams & Wilkins; 1995:379–381.

Bartram T. *Encyclopedia of Herbal Medicine.* Dorset, England: Grace Publishers; 1995:99,167–168,220.

Dambro MR. *Griffith's 5-Minute Clinical Consult–1999.* Baltimore, Md: Lippincott Williams & Wilkins; 1999:358–361.

Endocarditis: a rare but serious disease. *Drug Ther Perspect.* 1998;12(4):6–9.

Gruenwald J, Brendler T, Jaenicke C et al, eds. *PDR for Herbal Medicines.* Montvale, NJ: Medical Economics Company; 1998:772–773, 1130–1131.

Kruzel T. *The Homeopathic Emergency Guide.* Berkeley, Calif: North Atlantic Books; 1992:58–61.

Murray MT. *Encyclopedia of Nutritional Supplements.* Rocklin, Calif: Prima Publishing; 1996:401,404, 463–464.

Snow JM. Hydrastis canadensis L. (Ranunculaceae). *The Protocol Journal of Botanical Medicine.* 1997;2:25–28.

Stein JK, ed. *Internal Medicine.* 4th ed. St. Louis, Mo: Mosby-Year Book; 1994:189–201.

Stoller JK, Ahmad M, Longworth DL, eds. *The Cleveland Clinic Intensive Review of Internal Medicine.* Baltimore, Md: Williams & Wilkins; 1998:137–141,299.

Walker LP, Brown EH. *The Alternative Pharmacy.* Paramus, NJ: Prentice Hall Press; 1998:239–240.

Werbach MR. *Nutritional Influences on Illness.* New Canaan, Conn: Keats Publishing, Inc; 1987:252–262.

ENDOMETRIOSIS

Facts About Endometriosis. U.S. Department of Health and Human Services. National Institutes of Child Health and Human Development. NIH Publication no. 91-2413.

Kruzel T. *The Homeopathic Emergency Guide.* Berkeley, Calif: North Atlantic Books; 1992:112–114.

Medicines from the Earth. Harvard, Mass: Gaia Herbal Research Institute; 1997:182–183.

Protocol Journal of Botanical Medicine. 1996;1:30–46.

Tureck RW. Endometriosis: diagnosis and initial treatment. *Hospital Physician Obstetrics and Gynecology Board Review Manual.* April 1997;3:1–8.

FEVER OF UNKNOWN ORIGIN

Bartram T. *Encyclopedia of Herbal Medicine.* Dorset, England: Grace Publishers; 1995:182.

Berkow R. *Merck Manual, Home Edition.* Rahway, NJ: The Merck Publishing Group; 1997.

Berkow R, Beers MH. *The Merck Manual of Diagnosis and Therapy.* Rahway, NJ: The Merck Publishing Group; 1992.

Blumenthal M, ed. *The Complete German Commission E Monographs.* Boston, Mass: Integrative Medicine Communications; 1998:427.

Duke JA. *The Green Pharmacy.* Emmaus, Pa: Rodale Press, 1997.

Morrison R. *Desktop Guide to Keynotes and Confirmatory Symptoms.* Albany, Calif: Hahnemann Clinic Publishing; 1993:6, 58, 62.

Walker LP, Hodgson Brown E. *The Alternative Pharmacy.* Paramus, NJ: Prentice Hall Press; 1996

FIBROMYALGIA

Abraham GE, Flechas JG. Management of fibromyalgia: rationale for the use of magnesium and malic acid. *J Nutr Med.* 1992;3:49–59.

Caruso I, Sarzi Puttini P, Cazzola M, et al. Double-blind study of 5-hydroxytryptophan versus placebo in the treatment of primary fibromyalgia syndrome. *J Int Med Res.* 1990;18:201–209.

Chaitow L. *Fibromyalgia: the muscle pain epidemic.* Part I. Available at: www.healty.net/library/articles/chaitow/fibromy/fibro1.htm.

Fauci AS, Braunwald E, Isselbacher KJ et al, eds. *Harrison's Principles of Internal Medicine.* 14th ed. New York, NY: McGraw-Hill; 1998:1955–1957.

Holland NW, Gonzalez EB. Soft tissue problems in older adults. *Clin Geriatr Med.* 1998;14:601–603.

Kelley WN, ed. *Textbook of Rheumatology.* 5th ed. Philadelphia, Pa: WB Saunders; 1997:511–518.

Koopman WJ. *Arthritis and Allied Conditions: A Textbook of Rheumatology.* 13th ed. Baltimore, Md: Williams & Wilkins; 1993:1619–1635.

Nicolodi M, Sicuteri F. Fibromyalgia and migraine, two faces of the same mechanism. Serotonin as the common clue for pathogenesis and therapy. *Adv Exp Med Biol.* 1996;398:373–379.

Romano TJ, Stiller JW. Magnesium deficiency in fibromyalgia syndrome. *J Nutri Med.* 1994;4:165–167.

Russell IJ. Fibromyalgia syndrome: formulating a strategy for relief. *J Musculoskel Med.* 1998;November:4–21.

Starlanyl D, Copeland M. *Fibromyalgia and Chronic Myofascial Pain Syndrome: A Survival Manual.* Oakland, Calif: New Harbinger Publications Inc; 1996:215–224, 227–235.

Tyler VE. *Herbs of Choice: The Therapeutic Use of Phytomedicinals.* New York, NY: Haworth Press; 1994.

Wolfe F, Smyth HA, Yunus MB, et al. American College of Rheumatology 1990 Criteria for the Classification of Fibromyalgia: report of the Multicenter Criteria Committee. *Arthritis Rheum.* 1990;33:160–172.

FOOD ALLERGY

American College of Allergy, Asthma and Immunology. Accessed at www.allergy.mcg.edu on January 1, 1999.

Carey CF, Lee HH, Woeltje KF, eds. *The Washington Manual of Medical Therapeutics*. 29th ed. New York, NY: Lippincott-Raven; 1998:216–271, 223–225.

Dambro MD. *Griffith's 5 Minute Clinical Consult*. Philadelphia, Pa: Williams & Wilkins; 1998:400–401.

Fauci AS, Braunwald E, Isselbacher KJ et al, eds. *Harrison's Principles of Internal Medicine*. 14th ed. St. Louis, Mo: McGraw-Hill; 1997.

The Food Allergy Network. Accessed at www.foodallergy.org/ on January 1, 1999.

Klag MJ, ed. *Johns Hopkins Family Health Book*. Harper Resource; 1998.

Murray MT. *Encyclopedia of Nutritional Supplements*. Rocklin, Calif: Prima Health;1996:448–449.

Murray MT, Pizzorno JE. *Encyclopedia of Natural Medicine*. Rocklin, Calif: Prima Publishing; 1998:321.

Murray MT, Pizzorno JE. *Encyclopedia of Natural Medicine*. 2nd ed. Rocklin, Calif: Prima Publishing; 1998:464–475.

National Institute of Allergy and Infectious Diseases. National Institute of Health. Accessed at www.niaid.nih.gov/ on January 1, 1999.

Sampson HA. Food allergy. *JAMA*. 1997; 278:1888–1894.

Werbach M. *Nutritional Influences on Illness*. New Canaan, Conn: Keats Publishing Inc; 1987:23–28.

GALLBLADDER DISEASE

Blumenthal M, ed. *The Complete German Commission E Monographs*. Boston, Mass: Integrative Medicine Communications; 1998:422, 427, 465

Fauci AS, Braunwald E, Isselbacher KJ et al, eds. *Harrison's Principles of Internal Medicine*. 14th ed. New York, NY: McGraw-Hill; 1998.

Morrison R. *Desktop Guide to Keynotes and Confirmatory Symptoms*. Albany, Calif: Hahnemann Clinic Publishing; 1993:118, 139, 230.

Murray MT, Pizzorno JE. *Encyclopedia of Natural Medicine*. 2nd ed. Rocklin, Calif: Prima Publishing, 1998.

Sabiston DC, Lyerly HK. *Textbook of Surgery*. 15th ed. Philadelphia, Pa: WB Saunders, 1998

Weiss RF; Meuss AR, trans. *Herbal Medicine*. Medicina Biologica; 82–89, 94–97.

GASTRITIS

Blumenthal M, ed. *The Complete German Commission E Monographs*. Boston, Mass: Integrative Medicine Communications; 1998:427.

Fauci AS, Braunwald E, Isselbacher KJ et al, eds. *Harrison's Principles of Internal Medicine*. 14th ed. New York, NY: McGraw-Hill; 1998: 941–943,1610–1614.

Murray MT, Pizzorno JE. *Encyclopedia of Natural Medicine*. Rocklin, Calif: Prima Publishing; 1998:522–523.

Sklar M, ed. Gastoenterologic problems. *Clinics in Geriatric Medicine*. 1991;7:235–238.

Sleisenger MH, Fordtran JS, Scharschmidt BF, et al. *Gastrointestinal Disease*. 5th ed. Philadelphia, Pa: WB Saunders; 1993:545–564.

GASTROESOPHAGEAL REFLUX DISEASE

Andreoli TE, Bennett JC, Carpenter CCJ. *Cecil Essentials of Medicine*. 3rd ed. Philadelphia, Pa: WB Saunders; 1993:285–287.

Barker LR, Burton JR, Zieve PD, eds. *Principles of Ambulatory Medicine*. 4th ed. Baltimore, Md: Williams & Wilkins; 1995:443–446.

Bartram T. *Encyclopedia of Herbal Medicine*. Dorset, England: Grace Publishers; 1995:217.

Dambro MR. *Griffith's 5 Minute Clinical Consult–1999*. Baltimore, Md: Lippincott Williams & Wilkins; 1999:422–423.

Kelley WN, ed. *Essentials of Internal Medicine*. Philadelphia, Pa: J.B. Lippincott Company; 1994:104–106.

Morrison R. *Desktop Guide to Keynotes and Confirmatory Symptoms*. Albany, Calif: Hahnemann Clinic Publishing; 1993:39–43, 102–103, 229–231, 272–275.

Stoller JK, Ahmad M, Longworth DL, eds. *The Cleveland Clinic Intensive Review of Internal Medicine*. Baltimore, Md: Williams & Wilkins; 1998:595–599.

Werbach MR. *Nutritional Influences on Illness*. New Canaan, Conn: Keats Publishing Inc; 1987:210.

GOUT

The Burton Goldberg Group, compilers. *Alternative Medicine: The Definitive Guide*. Tiburon, Calif: Future Medicine Publishing; 1997.

Ferri FF. *Ferri's Clinical Advisor: Instant Diagnosis and Treatment*. St Louis, Mo: Mosby-Year Book; 1999.

Larson DE, ed. *Mayo Clinic Family Health Book*. 2nd ed. New York, NY: William Morrow and Company; 1996.

Murray MT, Pizzorno JE. *Encyclopedia of Natural Medicine*. 2nd ed. Rocklin, Calif: Prima Publishing; 1997.

Rose B. *The Family Health Guide To Homeopathy*. Berkeley, Calif: Celestial Arts Publishing; 1992.

Theodosakis J, Adderly B, Fox B. *The Arthritis Cure*. New York, NY: St Martin's Press; 1997.

Tierney LM Jr, McPhee SJ, Papadakis MA, eds. *Current Medical Diagnosis and Treatment 1994*. Norwalk, Conn: Appleton & Lange; 1994.

Werbach MR. *Nutritional Influences on Illness*. New Canaan, Conn: Keats Publishing Inc; 1987.

HEADACHE, MIGRAINE

Berkow R. *The Merck Manual*. 15th ed. Rahway, NJ: Merck Sharp & Dohme Research Laboratories; 1987.

De Weerdt CJ, Bootsma HPR, Hendricks H. Herbal medicines in migraine prevention. Randomized double-blind placebo controlled crossover trial of a feverfew preparation. *Phytomedicine*. 1996;3:225–230.

Gruenwald J, Brendler T, Jaenicke C et al, eds. *PDR for Herbal Medicines*. Montvale, NJ: Medical Economics Company; 1998.

Minirth F. *The Headache Book: Prevention and Treatment for All Types of Headaches*. Nashville, Tenn: Thomas Nelson; 1994.

Morrison R. *Desktop Guide to Keynotes and Confirmatory Symptoms*. Albany, Calif: Hahnemann Clinic Publishing; 1993.

Murphy JJ, Heptinsall S, Mitchell JRA. Randomised double-blind placebo-controlled trial of feverfew in migraine prevention. *Lancet*. 1988;2:189–192.

Murray MT. *Encyclopedia of Nutritional Supplements*. Rocklin, Calif: Prima Publishing; 1996.

Palevitch D, Earon G, Carasso R. Feverfew (Tanacetum parthenium) as a prophylactic treatment for migraine: a double-blind controlled study. *Phytotherapy Res*. 1997;11:508–511.

Pryse-Phillips W. Guideline for the diagnosis and management of migraine in clinical practice. *Can Med Assoc J*. 1997;156:1273–1287.

Walker L, Brown E. *The Alternative Pharmacy: Break The Drug Cycle With Safe Natural Treatment For 200 Everyday Ailments*. Paramus, NJ: Prentice Hall; 1998.

HEADACHE, SINUS

Berkow R. *The Merck Manual*. 15th ed. Rahway, NJ: Merck Sharp & Dohme Research Laboratories; 1987.

Gobel H, Schmidt G, Soyka D. Effect of Peppermint and Eucalyptus oil preparations on neurophysiological and experimental algesimetric headache parameters. *Cephalalgia*. 1994;14:228–234.

National Headache Foundation. Headache Topics: Sinus Headache. Accessed at www.headaches.org/sheets/sinus.html on January 30, 1999.

Pryse-Phillips W. Guideline for the diagnosis and management of migraine in clinical practice. *Canadian Medical Association Journal (CMAJ)*. 1997;156:1273-87.

University of Michigan Health System. Health Topics A to Z: Sinus Headaches. Accessed at www.med.umich.edu/1libr/topics/hdache08.htm on January 30, 1999.

Walker L, Brown E. *The Alternative Pharmacy: Break the Drug Cycle With Safe Natural Treatment for 200 Everyday Ailments*. Paramus, NJ: Prentice Hall; 1998.

HEADACHE, TENSION

Berkow R. *The Merck Manual*. 15th ed. Rahway, NJ: Merck Sharp & Dohme Research Laboratories; 1987.

Scalzo R. *Naturopathic Handbook of Herbal Formulas*. Durango, Colo: 2nd ed. Kivaki Press; 1994.

Walker L, Brown E. *The Alternative Pharmacy: Break the Drug Cycle With Safe Natural Treatment for 200 Everyday Ailments*. Paramus, NJ: Prentice Hall; 1998.

HEMORRHOIDS

Balch JF. *Prescription for Nutritional Healing*. 2nd ed. Garden City Park, NY: Avery Publishing, 1997.

Barker LR, Burton JR, Zieve PD, eds. *Principles of Ambulatory Medicine*. 4th ed. Baltimore, Md: Williams & Wilkins; 1995:1,347–1,361.

Duke JA. *The Green Pharmacy*. Emmaus, Pa: Rodale Press; 1997.

Gruenwald J, Brendler T, Jaenicke C et al, eds. *PDR for Herbal Medicines*. Montvale, NJ: Medical Economics Company; 1998.

Kruzel T. *The Homeopathic Emergency Guide*. Berkeley, Calif: North Atlantic Books; 1992:181–183.

Murray MT, Pizzorno JE. *Encyclopedia of Natural Medicine*. Rocklin, Calif: Prima Publishing; 1998.

Olshevsky M, Noy S, Zwang M. *Manual of Natural Therapy: A Succinct Catalog of Complementary Treatments*. New York, NY: Facts on File; 1989.

Stein JH, ed. *Internal Medicine*. 4th ed. St. Louis, Mo: Mosby-Year Book; 1994:486–492.

United States Pharmacopeial Convention, Inc. *Advice for the Patient*. 15th ed. USPDI; 1995:2.

HEPATITIS, VIRAL

Andreoli TE, Bennett JC, Carpenter CCJ. *Cecil Essentials of Medicine*. 3rd ed. Philadelphia, Pa: WB Saunders; 1993:327–334.

Barker LR, Burton JR, Zieve PD, eds. *Principles of Ambulatory Medicine*. 4th ed. Baltimore: Williams & Wilkins; 1995:507–515.

Batchelder HJ. The Protocol Journal of Botanical Medicine. Ayer, MA: *Herbal Research Publications, Inc.;* 1995: Vol 1, No 2, 133–137.

Batchelder IIJ, Hudson, T." *The Protocol Journal of Botanical Medicine*. 1995;1:138–140.

Dambro MR. *Griffith's 5-Minute Clinical Consult–1999*. Baltimore, Md: Lippincott Williams & Wilkins; 1999:408-409.

Dharmananda S. *The Protocol Journal of Botanical Medicine*. 1995: Vol 1, No 2: 151-158.

Ergil K. *The Protocol Journal of Botanical Medicine*. 1995:Vol 1, No 2:145–150.

Kiesewetter E, et al. Results of two double-blind studies on the effect of silymarin in chronic hepatitis. *Leber Magen Darm*. 1977;7:318–323.

Scalzo R. *Therapeutic Botanical Protocol for Viral Hepatitis*. The Protocol Journal of Botanical Medicine. 1995:Vol 1, No 2, 159-160.

Sodhi V. *The Protocol Journal of Botanical Medicine*. 1995:Vol 1, No 2, 141-144.

Stein JK, ed. *Internal Medicine*. 4th ed. St. Louis: Mosby-Year Book; 1994:586–601.

Stoller JK, Ahmad M, Longworth DL, eds. *The Cleveland Clinic Intensive Review of Internal Medicine*. Baltimore, Md: Williams & Wilkins; 1998:573-756.

Stedman's Medical Dictionary. 26th edition. Baltimore, Md: Williams & Wilkins; 1995:784-786.

Thyagarajan SP. Effect of Phyllanthus amarus on chronic carriers of hepatitis B virus. *Lancet*. October 1, 1988:764–766.

HERPES SIMPLEX VIRUS

Balch JF, Balch PA. *Prescription for Nutritional Healing*. 2nd ed. Garden City Park, NY: Avery Publishing; 1997:317–319.

Bartram T. *Encyclopedia of Herbal Medicine*. Dorset, England: Grace Publishers; 1995:226–227.

Fauci AS, Braunwald E, Isselbacher KJ et al, eds. *Harrison's Principles of Internal Medicine*. 14th ed. New York, NY: McGraw-Hill; 1998:1080–1086.

Holmes KK, Mardh PA, Sparling PF. *Sexually Transmitted Diseases*. 2nd ed. New York, NY: McGraw-Hill; 1995:391–408.

Krugman S, Katz SL, Gershon AA, et al. *Infectious Diseases of Children*. St. Louis, Mo: Mosby-Year Book; 1992:175–188.

Lad VD. *The Complete Book of Ayurvedic Home Remedies*. New York, NY: Harmony Books; 1998:200–201.

Mandell GL, Douglas RG Jr, Bennett JE. *Principles and Practice of Infectious Diseases*. 3rd ed. New York, NY: Churchill Livingstone; 1990:1144–1151.

Milman N, Scheibel J, Jessen O, et al. Lysine prophylaxis in recurrent herpes simplex labialis: a double-bline, controlled crossover study. *Acta Derm Venereol*. 1980;60:85–87.

Morrison R. *Desktop Guide to Keynotes and Confirmatory Symptoms*. Albany, Calif: Hahnemann Clinic Publishing; 1993:29, 171, 172, 289.

Murray MT, Pizzorno JE. *Encyclopedia of Natural Medicine*. 2nd ed. Rocklin, Calif: Prima Publishing; 1998:360, 520–524.

Thein DJ, Hurt WC. Lysine as a prophylactic agent in the treatment of recurrent herpes simplex labialis. *Oral Surg Oral Med Oral Pathol*. 1984;58:659–666.

Tyler VE. *Herbs of Choice: The Therapeutic Use of Phytomedicinals*. New York, NY: Pharmaceutical Products Press; 1994:162–166.

Werbach, M. *Nutritional Influences on Illness*. New Canaan, Conn: Keats Publishing; 1988:213–215.

Wöbling RH, Leonhardt K. Local therapy of herpes simplex with dried extract from *w* 1994;1:25–31.

HERPES ZOSTER (VARICELLA–ZOSTER) VIRUS

Fauci AS, Braunwald E, Isselbacher KJ et al, eds. *Harrison's Principles of Internal Medicine*. 14th ed. New York, NY: McGraw-Hill; 1998:1086–1088.

Krugman S, Katz SL, Gershon AA, et al. *Infectious Diseases of Children*. St. Louis, Mo: Mosby-Year Book; 1992:587–609.

Mandell GL, Douglas RG Jr, Bennett JE. *Principles and Practice of Infectious Diseases*. 3rd ed. New York, NY: Churchill Livingstone; 1995:1153–1158, 2237–2240.

Morrison R. Desktop Guide to *Keynotes and Confirmatory Symptoms*. Albany, Calif: Hahnemann Clinic Publishing; 1993:218, 249, 289.

HIV AND AIDS

Auerbach J, Oleson T, Solomon G. A behavioral medicine intervention as an adjunctive treatment for HIV-related illness. *Psychology and Health*. 1992;6:325–334.

Blumenthal M, ed. *The Complete German Commission E Monographs*. Boston, Mass: Integrative Medicine Communications; 1998:119–120, 134, 169–170.

Dubin J. *HIV Infection and AIDS*. Emergency Medicine Online. 1998. Accessed at www.emedicine.com/emerg/topic253.htm on February 13, 1999.

Dworkin BM. Selenium deficiency in HIV infection and the acquired immunodeficiency syndrome (AIDS). *Chem Biol Interact*. 1994;91:181–186.

Fawzi WW, Mbise RL, Hertzmark E, et al. A randomized trial of vitamin A supplements in relation to mortality among human immunodeficiency virus-infected and uninfected children in Tanzania. *Pediatr Infect Dis J*. 1999;18:127–133.

Gruenwald J, Brendler T, Jaenicke C et al, eds. *PDR for Herbal Medicines*. Montvale, NJ: Medical Economics Company; 1998:626–627, 866–867, 903–904, 1138–1139, 1174–1175.

Guidelines for the use of antiretroviral agents in HIV-infected adults and adolescents. U.S. Department of Health and Human Services. December 1, 1998.

Hamilton Nunnelley EM. *Biochemistry of Nutrition: A Desk Reference*. New York, NY: West Publishing Company; 1987:183–184.

Hanna L. Complementary and alternative medicine: exploring options and making decisions. *Bulletin of Experimental Treatments for AIDS*. January 1998.

Hayashi K, Hayashi T, Kojima I. A natural sulfated polysaccharide, calcium spirulan, isolated from Spirulina platensis: in vitro and ex vivo evaluation of anti-herpes simplex virus and anti-human immunodeficiency virus activities. *AIDS Res Hum Retroviruses*. 1996;12:1463–1471.

Lissoni, P, Vigore L, Rescaldani R, et al. Neuroimmunotherapy with low-dose subcutaneous interleukin-2 plus melatonin in AIDS patients with CD4 cell number below 200/mm3: a biological phase-II study. J Biol Regul Homeost Agents. 1995;9:155–158.

Nerad JL, Gorbach SL, et al. Nutritional aspects of HIV infection. *Infect Dis Clin North Am*. 1994;8:499–515.

Noyer CM, Simon D, Borczuk A, Brandt LJ, Lee MJ, Nehra V. A double-blind placebo-controlled pilot study of glutamine therapy for abnormal intestintal permeability in patients with AIDS. *Am J Gastroenterol*. 1998;93:972–975.

Patarca R, Fletcher MA. Massage therapy is associated with enhancement of the immune system's cytotoxic capacity. *Int J Neurosci*. February 1996;84:205–217.

Remacha AF, Cadafalch J. Cobalamin deficiency in patients infected with the human immunodeficiency virus. *Semin Hematol*. 1999;36:75–87.

HYPERCHOLESTEROLEMIA

Auer W, Eiber A, Hertkorn E, et al. Hypertension and hyperlipidaemia: garlic helps in mild cases. *Br J Clin Pract*. 1990;44:3–9.

Barrie SA, Wright JV, Pizzorno JE. Effects of garlic on platelet aggregation, serum lipids and blood pressure in humans. *J Orthomolec*. 1987;2:15–21.

Bordia A. Effect of garlic on blood lipids in patients with coronary heart disease. *Am J Clin Nutr*. 1981;34:2100–2103.

Bordia A, Bansal HC, Arora SK, et al. Effect of the essential oils of garlic and onion on alimentary hyperlipemia. *Atherosclerosis*. 1975;21:15–19.

Jain AK, Vargas R, et al. Can garlic reduce levels of serum lipids? A controlled clinical study. *Am J Med*. 1993;94:632–635.

Johns Hopkins Health Information. Accessed at http://www.intelihealth.com on January 25, 1999.

Murray MT, Pizzorno JE. *The Encyclopedia of Natural Medicine*. 2nd ed. Rocklin, Calif: Prima Publishing; 1998.

Silagy C, Neil A. Garlic as a lipid lowering agent-a meta-analysis. *JR Coll Physicians Lond*. 1994;28:39–45.

Steiner M, Khan AH, Holbert D, Lin RI. A double-blind crossover study in moderately hypercholesterolemic men that compared the effect of aged garlic extract and placebo administration on blood lipids. *Am J Clin Nutr*. 1996;64:866–870.

Vorberg G, Scheider B. Therapy with garlic: Results of a placebo-controlled, double-blind study. *Br J Clin Pract*. 1990;7–11.

Warshafsky S, Kramer RS, Sivak SL. Effect of garlic on total serum cholesterol: a meta-analysis. *Ann Intern Med*. 1993;119:599–605.

Werbach, M. *Nutritional Influences on Illness*. New Canaan, Conn: Keats Publishing; 1988.

Yamamoto M. Serum HDL-cholesterol increasing and fatty liver improving actions of *Panax ginseng* in high cholesterol diet-fed rats with clinical affect on hyperlipidemia in man. *Am J Chin Med*. 1983;1:96–101.

HYPERKALEMIA

Blumenthal M, ed. *The Complete German Commission E Monographs*. Boston, Mass: Integrative Medicine Communications; 1998:162.

Lee HS, Yu YC, Kim ST, Kim KS. Effects of moxibustion on blood pressure and renal function in spontaneously hypertensive rats. *Am J Chin Med.* 1997;25: 21–26.

Wheeless CR. Management of Hyperkalemia. *Wheeless' Textbook of Orthopaedics.* 1996. Accessed at http://wheeless.belgianorthoweb.be/oo3/24.htm on 2/17/99.

Zwanger M. *Hyperkalemia.* Emergency Medicine Online Text. 1998. Accessed at http://www.emedicine.com/emerg/topic261.htm on 2/13/99.

HYPERTENSION

Barker LR, Burton JR et al, eds. *Principles of Ambulatory Medicine.* 4th ed. Baltimore, Md: Williams & Wilkins; 1995:803–843.

Bartram T. *Encyclopedia of Herbal Medicine.* Dorset, England: Grace Publishers; 1995:240.

Dambro MR. *Griffith's 5 Minute Clinical Consult 1999.* Baltimore, Md: Lippincott Williams & Wilkins; 1999.

Detre Z, Jellinek H, Miskulin R. Studies on vascular permeability in hypertension. *Clin Physiol Bichem.* 1986;4:143–149.

Golik A, Zaidenstein R, Dishi V, et al. Effects of captopril and enalapril on zinc metabolism in hypertensive patients. *J Am Coll Nutri.* 1998;17:75–78.

Kwan CY. Vascular effects of selected antihypertensive drugs derived from traditional medicinal herbs. *Clin Exp Pharmacol Physiol.* 1995;(suppl 1):S297–S299. Review.

Liva R. Naturopathic specific condition review: hypertension. Protocol Journal of Botanical Medicine. 1995;1:222.

Murray MT. *The Healing Power of Herbs.* Rocklin, Calif: Prima Publishing; 1991:90–96, 107–112.

Murray MT, Pizzorno JE. *Encyclopedia of Natural Medicine.* 2nd ed. Rocklin, Calif.:Prima Publishing; 1998.

Stein JH, ed. *Internal Medicine.* 4th ed. St. Louis, Mo: Mosby-Year Book; 1994:302–323.

Werbach M. *Nutritional Influences on Illness.* New Canaan, Conn: Keats Publishing; 1988:227–240.

The fifth report of the joint national committee on detection, evaluation, and treatment of high blood pressure. *Arch Intern Med.* 1993;153:154.

HYPERTHYROIDISM

Bartram T. *Encyclopedia of Herbal Medicine.* Dorset, England: Grace Publishers; 1995:422.

Berkow R. *Merck Manual.* 16th ed. Whitehorse Station, NJ: The Merck Publishing Group; 1992.

Blumenthal M, ed. *The Complete German Commission E Monographs.* Boston, Mass: Integrative Medicine Communications; 1998:432.

Hoffman D. *The New Holistic Herbal.* New York, NY: Barnes & Noble Books; 1995:95.

HYPOGLYCEMIA

Anderson RA, Polansky MM, Bryden NA, Bhathena SJ, Canary JJ. Effects of supplemental chromium on patients with symptoms of reactive hypoglycemia. *Metabolism.* 1987;36:351–355.

Branch WT Jr. *Office Practice of Medicine.* 3rd ed. Philadelphia, Pa: WB Saunders; 1994:574–575.

Fauci AS, Braunwald E, Isselbacher KJ, et al., eds. *Harrison's Principles of Internal Medicine.* 14th ed. New York, NY: McGraw-Hill; 1998:2069–2071.

Mowry DB. *The Scientific Validation of Herbal Medicine.* New Canaan, Conn: Keats Publishing; 1986:25.

Tyler VE. *Herbs of Choice: The Therapeutic Use of Phytomedicinals.* New York, NY: Pharmaceutical Products Press; 1994:141.

Wilson JD, Foster DW. Williams *Textbook of Endocrinology.* 8th ed. Philadelphia, Pa: WB Saunders; 1992:1232–1248.

Wyngaarden JB, Smith LH Jr. *Cecil Textbook of Medicine.* 17th ed. Philadelphia, Pa: WB Saunders; 1985:1342–1348.

HYPOTHYROIDISM

Bartram T. *Encyclopedia of Herbal Medicine.* Dorset, England: Grace Publishers; 1995:304.

Berkow R. *Merck Manual.* 16th ed. Whitehorse Station, NJ: The Merck Publishing Group; 1992.

Murray MT, Pizzorno JE. *Encyclopedia of Natural Medicine.* Rocklin, Calif: Prima Publishing; 1998:386–390.

INFANTILE COLIC

Ayllon T. *Stopping Baby's Colic.* New York, NY: Putnam; 1989.

Boericke W. *Materia Medica.* 9th ed. Santa Rosa, Calif: Boericke and Tafel; 1927:151.

Jones S. *Crying Baby, Sleepless Nights: Why Your Baby Is Crying and What You Can Do About It.* Boston, Mass. The Harvard Common Press; 1992.

Kemper KJ. *The Holistic Pediatrician.* New York, NY: HarperPerennial; 1996.

Kruzel T. *The Homeopathic Emergency Guide.* Berkeley, Calif: North Atlantic Books; 1992:126–128.

Schiff D, Shelov P, eds. *American Academy of Pediatrics: The Official, Complete Home Reference Guide to Your Child's Symptoms, Birth Through Adolescence.* New York, NY: Villard Books; 1997.

Wilen J, Wilen L. *Folk Remedies That Work.* New York, NY. HarperPerennial; 1996.

INFLUENZA

Baron S. *Medical Microbiology.* University of Texas Medical Branch; 1996:58. Available at http://129.109.112.248/microbook/ch058.htm.

Blumenthal M, ed. *The Complete German Commission E Monographs.* Boston, Mass: Integrative Medicine Communications; 1998:446.

Bräunig B, Dorn M, Knick E. *Echinacea purpurea radix* for strengthening the immune response in flu-like infections. *Z Phytotherapie.* 1992;13:7–13.

Dorn M. Mitigation of flu-like effects by means of a plant immunostimulant. *Natur und Ganzheitsmedizin.* 1989; 2:314–319.

Gruenwald J, Brendler T, Jaenicke C et al, eds. *PDR for Herbal Medicines.* Montvale, NJ: Medical Economics Company; 1998:604–605.

Hoffman D. *The New Holistic Herbal.* New York, NY: Barnes & Noble Books; 1995: 191.

Influenza. Centers for Disease Control and Prevention. Accessed at www.cdc.gov/nci-dod/diseases/flu/fluinfo.htm on February 13, 1999.

Kennedy M. Influenza viral infections: presentation, prevention and treatment. *Nurse Pract.* September 1998.

Kruzel T. *The Homeopathic Emergency Guide.* Berkeley, Calif: North Atlantic Books; 1992:190–196.

Murray MT, Pizzorno JE. *Encyclopedia of Natural Medicine.* Rocklin, Calif: Prima Publishing; 1998:66–68.

Ody P. *The Complete Medicinal Herbal.* New York, NY: DK Publishing; 1993.

Roettger B. Homeopathy as an effective treatment for colds and flus. *Nutrition Science News Magazine.* August 1995.

Savtsova ZD, Zalesskii VN, Orlovskii AA. The immunocorrective effect of laser reflexotherapy in experimental influenza infection [in Russian]. *Zh Mikrobiol Epidemiol Immunobiol.* January 1990:75–80.

Scaglione, et al. Efficacy and safety of the standardized ginseng extract G115 for potentiating vaccination against common cold and/or influenza syndrome. *Drugs Exp Clin Res.* 1996;22:65–72.

Tan D. Treatment of fever due to exopathic wind-cold by rapid acupuncture. *J Tradit Chin Med.* 1992;12:267–271.

Wagner H. Herbal immunostimulants for the prophylaxis and therapy of colds and influenza. *Eur J Herbal Med.* 1997;3(1).

INSECT BITES AND STINGS

Habif TP. *Clinical Dermatology.* 3rd ed. St. Louis, Mo: Mosby-Year Book; 1996.

Kruzel T. *The Homeopathic Emergency Guide.* Berkeley, Calif: North Atlantic Books; 1992:198–200.

Middleton E, ed. *Allergy: Principles and Practice.* 5th ed. St. Louis, Mo: Mosby-Year Book; 1998.

Rakel RE, ed. *Conn's Current Therapy.* 50th ed. Philadelphia, Pa: WB Saunders; 1998

INSOMNIA

Blumenthal M, ed. *The Complete German Commission E Monographs.* Boston, Mass: Integrative Medicine Communications; 1998:422, 431.

Bravo SQ, et al. Polysomnographic and subjective findings in insomniacs under treatment with placebo and valerian extract (LI 156). Proceedings of the Second International Congress on Phytomedicine, Munich. *Eur J Clin Pharmacol.* 1996;50:552.

DreBring H. Insomnia: Are valerian/balm combinations of equal value to Benzodiazepine? *Therapiewoche.* 1992;42:726.

Emser W. Phytotherapy of insomnia—a critical overview. *Pharmacopsychiatry.* 1993;26:150.

Fauci AS, Braunwald E, Isselbacher KJ et al, eds. *Harrison's Principles of Internal Medicine.* 14th ed. New York, NY: McGraw-Hill; 1998.

Goroll, Allan H, ed. *Primary Care Medicine.* 3rd ed. Philadelphia, Pa: Lippincott-Raven; 1995.

Rakel RE, ed. *Conn's Current Therapy.* 50th ed. Philadelphia, Pa: WB Saunders; 1998.

INTESTINAL PARASITES

Fauci AS, Braunwald E, Isselbacher KJ et al, eds. *Harrison's Principles of Internal Medicine.* 14th ed. New York, NY: McGraw-Hill; 1998.

Morrison R. *Desktop Guide to Keynotes and Confirmatory Symptoms.* Albany, Calif: Hahnemann Clinic Publishing; 1993:128, 329, 353.

Rakel RE, ed. *Conn's Current Therapy.* 50th ed. Philadelphia, Pa: WB Saunders; 1998.

IRRITABLE BOWEL SYNDROME

Berkow R, ed. *Merck Manual of Diagnosis and Therapy.* 16th ed. Rahway, NJ: The Merck Publishing Group; 1992.

Dambro MR. *Griffith's Five-Minute Clinical Consult.* New York, NY: Lippincott, Williams and Wilkins; 1998.

Koch TR. Peppermint oil and irritable bowel syndrome [In Process Citation]. *Am J Gastroenterol.* 1998;93:2304–2305.

Liu JH, Chen GH, Yeh HZ, Huang CK, Poon SK. Enteric-coated peppermint-oil capsules in the treatment of irritable bowel syndrome: a prospective, randomized trial. *J Gastroenterol.* 1997;32:765–768.

Murray MT, Pizzorno JE. *Encyclopedia of Natural Medicine.* Rocklin, Calif: Prima Publishing; 1998:396–400.

Pittler MH, Ernst E. Peppermint oil for irritable bowel syndrome: a critical review and metaanalysis. *Am J Gastroenterol.* 1998;93:1131–1135.

LARYNGITIS

Berkow R, ed. *Merck Manual of Diagnosis and Therapy.* 16th ed. Rahway, NJ: Merck Research Laboratories; 1992.

Berkow R, Beers MH, Fletcher AJ, eds. *Merck Manual, Home Edition.* Rahway, NJ: Merck & Co; 1997.

Ballenger JJ, Snow JB, eds. *Otorhinolaryngology.* 15th ed. Philadelphia, Pa: Williams and Wilkins; 1996;30:535–555.

Hoffman D. *The New Holistic Herbal.* New York, NY: Barnes & Noble Books; 1995: 47.

Larson DE, ed. *Mayo Clinic Family Health Book.* 2nd ed. New York, NY: William Morrow and Company; 1996.

LOW BACK PAIN

Balch JF, Balch PA. *Prescription for Nutritional Healing.* 2nd ed. Garden City Park, NY: Avery Publishing Group; 1997:149–150.

Bartram T. *Encyclopedia of Herbal Medicine.* Dorset, England: Grace Publishers; 1995:238–239, 277–278.

Blumenthal M, ed. *The Complete German Commission E Monographs.* Boston, Mass: Integrative Medicine Communications; 1998:81–82, 136–137, 183, 197, 222–223, 226–227, 230–231.

Gruenwald J, Brendler T, Jaenicke C et al, eds. *PDR for Herbal Medicines.* Montvale, NJ: Medical Economics Company; 1998:662–663, 786–787, 871–872,

Kitade T, Odahara Y, Shinohara S, et al. Studies on the enhanced effect of acupuncture analgesia and acupuncture anesthesia by D-phenylalanine (2nd report): schedule of administration and clinical effects in low back pain and tooth extraction. *Acupunct Electrother Res.* 1990;15:121–135.

Kruzel T. *The Homeopathic Emergency Guide.* Berkeley, Calif: North Atlantic Books; 1992:30–38.

Morrison R. *Desktop Guide to Keynotes and Confirmatory Symptoms.* Albany, Calif: Hahnemann Clinic Publishing; 1993:36–39, 59–61.

Mowrey D. *The Scientific Validation of Herbal Medicine.* New Canaan, Conn: Keats Publishing; 1986:223–227.

Murray MT, Pizzorno JE. *Encyclopedia of Natural Medicine.* Rocklin, Calif: Prima Publishing; 1998:338.

Snider RK, ed. *Essentials of Musculoskeletal Care.* Rosemont, Ill: American Academy of Orthopaedic Surgeons; 1997.

Werbach M. *Nutritional Influences on Illness.* New Canaan, Conn: Keats Publishing Inc.; 1987:1987: 342-345.

MENOPAUSE

Bartram T. *Encyclopedia of Herbal Medicine.* Dorset, England: Grace Publishers; 1995:291–292.

Blumenthal M, ed. *The Complete German Commission E Monographs.* Boston, Mass: Integrative Medicine Communications; 1998:108, 466.

Devine A, Dick IM, Heal SJ, et al. A 4-year follow-up study of the effects of calcium supplementation on bone density in elderly postmenopausal women. *Osteoporosis Int.* 1997;7:23–28.

Gruenwald J, Brendler T, Jaenicke C et al, eds. *PDR for Herbal Medicines.* Montvale, NJ: Medical Economics Company; 1998:647–648, 871–872.

Kistner RW, ed. *Kistner's Gynecology: Principles and Practice.* 6th ed. St. Louis, Mo: Mosby-Year Book; 1995.

Murray MT. *The Healing Power of Herbs: The Enlightened Person's Guide to the Wonders of Medicinal Plants.* Rocklin, Calif: Prima Publishing; 1995:163–164.

Murray MT, Pizzorno JE. *Encyclopedia of Natural Medicine.* Rocklin, Calif: Prima Publishing; 1998.

Thys-Jacobs S, Starkey P, Bernstein D, Tian J. Calcium carbonate and the premenstrual syndrome: effects on premenstrual and menstrual symptoms. Premenstrual Syndrome Study Group. *Am J Obstet Gynecol.* 1998;179:444–452.

Villa ML, Packer E, Cheema M, et al. Effects of aluminum hydroxide on the parathyroid-vitamin D axis of postmenopausal women. *J Clin Endocrinol Metab.* 1991;73:1256–1261.

Vorberg G. Treatment of menopause symptoms—Successful hormone-free therapy with Remifemin®. *ZFA.* 1984;60:626–629.

Weiss RF. *Herbal Medicines.* Beaconsfield, England: Beaconsfield Publishers; 1998:317–319.

MOTION SICKNESS

Blumenthal M, ed. *The Complete German Commission E Monographs.* Boston, Mass: Integrative Medicine Communications; 1998:429.

Dobie TG, May JG. The effectiveness of a motion sickness counselling programme. *Br J Clin Psychol.* 1995;34 (part 2):301–311.

Gresty MA, Grunwald EA. Medical perspective of motion sickness. Proceedings of the International Workshop on Motion Sickness: Medical and Human Factors; May 1997; Marbella, Spain.

Helling K, Hausmann S, Flottmann T, Scherer H. Individual differences in susceptibility to motion sickness [in German]. *HNO.* 1997;45:210–215.

Hoffman D. *The New Holistic Herbal.* New York, NY: Barnes & Noble Books; 1995:181.

Hu S, Stritzel R, Chandler A, Stern RM. P6 acupressure reduces symptoms of vection-induced motion sickness. *Aviat Space Environ Med.* 1995;66:631–634.

Jozsvai EE, Pigeau RA. The effect of autogenic training and biofeedback on motion sickness tolerance. *Aviat Space Environ Med.* 1996;67:963–968.

Morrison R. *Desktop Guide to Keynotes and Confirmatory Symptoms.* Albany, Calif: Hahnemann Clinic Publishing; 1993:133, 288, 379.

Pray WS. Motion sickness: a sensory conflict. *U.S. Pharmacist.* March 1998.

Ramsey A. Virtual reality induced symptoms and effects: a psychophysiological prespective. Proceedings of the International Workshop on Motion Sickness: Medical and Human Factors. Marbella, Spain, May 1997.

Stern RM, Hu S, Uijtdehaage SH, Muth ER, Xu LH, Koch KL. Asian hypersusceptibility to motion sickness. *Hum Hered.* 1996;46:7–14.

MYOCARDIAL INFARCTION

Iliceto S, Scrutinio D, Bruzzi P, et al. Effects of L-carnitine administration on left ventricular remodeling after acute anterior myocardial infarction: the L-Carnitine Ecocardiografia Digitalizzata Infarto Miocardico (CEDIM) Trial. *J Am Coll Cardiol.* August 1995;26:380.

Kruzel T. *The Homeopathic Emergency Guide.* Berkeley, Calif: North Atlantic Books; 1992:58–60.

Murray MT. *The Healing Power of Herbs: The Enlightened Person's Guide to the Wonders of Medicinal Plants.* Rocklin, Calif: Prima Publishing; 1998:184.

Rakel RE, ed. *Conn's Current Therapy.* 50th ed. Philadelphia, Pa: WB Saunders; 1998.

Singh RB, Niaz MA, Agarwal P, Begom R, Rastogi SS. Effect of antioxidant-rich foods on plasma ascorbic acid, cardiac enzyme, and lipid peroxide levels in patients hospitalized with acute myocardial infarction. *J Am Diet Assoc.* July 1995;95:775–780.

Singh RB, Singh NK, Niaz MA, Sharma JP. Effect of treatment with magnesium and potassium on mortality and reinfarction rate of patients with suspected acute myocardial infarction. *Int J Clin Pharmacol Thera.* 1996;34:219–225.

Washington Manual of Medical Therapeautics. 29th ed. Philadelphia, Pa: Lippincott-Raven Publishers; 1998.

OBESITY

Balch JF, Balch PA. *Prescription for Nutritional Healing.* 2nd ed. Garden City Park, NY: Avery Publishing; 1997:406–412.

Bartram T. *Encyclopedia of Herbal Medicine.* Dorset, England: Grace Publishers; 1995:315.

Blumenthal M, ed. *The Complete German Commission E Monographs.* Boston, Mass: Integrative Medicine Communications; 1998:125–126, 169–170, 179–181.

Branch Jr WT. *Office Practice of Medicine.* 3rd ed. Philadelphia, Pa: WB Saunders; 1994:1053–1065.

Cangiano C, Ceci F, Cascino A, et al. Eating behavior and adherence to dietary prescriptions in obese adult subjects treated with 5-hydroxytryptophan. *J Clin Nutr.* 1992;56:863–867.

Fauci AS, Braunwald E, Isselbacher KJ, et al., eds. *Harrison's Principles of Internal Medicine.* 14th ed. New York, NY: McGraw-Hill; 1998:454–462.

Gruenwald J, Brendler T, Jaenicke C et al, eds. *PDR for Herbal Medicines.* Montvale, NJ: Medical Economics Company; 1998:779–780, 1022–1024, 1138–1139.

Mowrey DB. *The Scientific Validation of Herbal Medicine.* New Canaan, Conn: Keats Publishing; 1986:277–282.

Murray MT, Pizzorno JE. *Encyclopedia of Natural Medicine.* 2nd ed. Rocklin, Calif: Prima Publishing; 1998:437–446, 680–694.

Nestel PJ, et al. Arterial compliance in obese subjects is improved with dietary plant n-3 fatty acid from flaxseed oil despite increased LDL oxidizability. *Arterioscler Thromb Vasc Biol.* 1997;17:1163–1170.

Uusitupa M. New aspects in the management of obesity: operation and the impact of lipase inhibitors. *Curr Opin Lipidol.* 1999;10:3–7.

Wyngaarden JB, Smith LH Jr, Bennett, JC. *Cecil Textbook of Medicine.* 19th ed. Philadelphia, Pa: WB Saunders; 1992:1162–1169.

OSTEOARTHRITIS

Fauci AS, Braunwald E, Isselbacher KJ et al, eds. *Harrison's Principles of Internal Medicine.* 14th ed. New York, NY: McGraw-Hill, 1998:1935–1941.

Kelly WN. *Textbook of Internal Medicine.* 3rd ed. Philadelphia, Pa: Lippincott-Raven; 1997:1121–1124.

Koopman WJ. *Arthritis and Allied Conditions: A Textbook of Rheumatology.* 13th ed. Baltimore, Md:Williams & Wilkins; 1997:1985–2006.

Lockie A, Geddes N. *The Complete Guide to Homeopathy.* New York, NY: DK Publishing, 1995:154–155.

Morrison R. *Desktop Guide to Keynotes and Confirmatory Symptoms.* Albany, Calif: Hahnemann Clinic Publishing; 1993:38,74,314,326.

Murray MT. *Encyclopedia of Nutritional Supplements.* Rocklin, Calif: Prima Publishing; 1996:336–342, 365–373, 475

Murray MT, Pizzorno JE. *Encyclopedia of Natural Medicine.* 2nd ed. Rocklin, Calif: Prima Health; 1998:695–705.

OSTEOMYELITIS

Berkow R, ed. *Merck Manual of Diagnosis and Therapy.* 16th ed. Rahway, NJ: Merck Research Laboratories; 1992.

Dambro MR. *Griffith's Five-Minute Clinical Consult.* New York, NY: Lippincott, Williams and Wilkins; 1998.

Larson DE, ed. *Mayo Clinic Family Health Book.* 2nd ed. New York, NY: William Morrow and Company; 1996.

OSTEOPOROSIS

Chapuy MC, Arlot ME, Duboeuf F, et al. Vitamin D$_3$ and calcium to prevent hip fractures in elderly women. *N Engl J Med.* 1992;327:1637–1642.

Chesney RW. Vitamin D. Can an upper limit be defined? *J Nutr.* 1989;119:1825–1828.

Fauci AS, Braunwald E, Isselbacher KJ et al, eds. *Harrison's Principles of Internal Medicine.* 14th ed. New York, NY: McGraw-Hill; 1998.

Feskanich D, Weber P, Willett WC, Rockett H, Booth SL, Colditz GA. Vitamin K intake and hip fractures in women: a prospective study. *Am J Clin Nutr.* 1999;69:74–79.

Gaby AR. *Preventing and Reversing Osteoporosis: Every Woman's Essential Guide.* Rocklin, Calif: Prima Publishing; 1995.

Goroll AH, ed. *Primary Care Medicine.* 3rd ed. Philadelphia, Pa: Lippincott-Raven; 1995.

Werbach M. *Nutritional Influences on Illness.* New Canaan, Conn: Keats Publishing; 1988:331–340.

OTITIS MEDIA

Bitnun A, Allen UD. Medical therapy of otitis media: use, abuse, efficacy and morbidity. *J Otolaryngol.* 1998;27(suppl 2):26–36.

Bizakis JG, Velegrakis GA, Papadakis CE, Karampekios SK, Helidonis ES. The silent epidural abscess as a complication of acute otitis media in children. *Int J Pediatr Otorhinolaryngol.* 1998;45:163–166.

Cohen R, Levy C, Boucherat M, Langue J, de la Rocque F. A multicenter, randomized, double-blind trial of 5 versus 10 days of antibiotic therapy for acute otitis media in young children. *J Pediatr.* 1998;133:634–639.

Gehanno P, Nguyen L, Barry B, et al. Eradication by ceftriaxone of streptococcus pneumoniae isolates with increased resistance to penicillin in cases of acute otitis media. *Antimicrob Agents Chemother.* 1999;43:16–20.

Kruzel T. *The Homeopathic Emergency Guide.* Berkeley, Calif: North Atlantic Books; 1992:243–245.

Reichenberg-Ullman J, Ullman R. Healing otitis media through homeopathy. 1996. Available at www.healthy.net/library/articles/rbullman/ottis.htm.

Uhari M, Kontiokari T, Koskela M, Niemela M. Xylitol chewing gum in prevention of acute otitis media: double-blind randomised trials. *Br Med J.* 1996;313:1180–1184.

Wright E.D, Pearl AJ, Manoukian JJ. Laterally hypertrophic adenoids as a contributing factor in otitis media. *Int J Pediatr Otorhinolaryngol.* 1998;45:207–214.

PARKINSON'S DISEASE

Bartram T. *Encyclopedia of Herbal Medicine.* Dorset, England: Grace Publishers; 1995:328–329.

Blumenthal M, ed. *The Complete German Commission E Monographs.* Boston, Mass: Integrative Medicine Communications; 1998:138.

Fauci AS, Braunwald E, Isselbacher KJ et al, eds. *Harrison's Principles of Internal*

Medicine. 14th ed. New York, NY: McGraw-Hill; 1998.

Morrison R. *Desktop Guide to Keynotes and Confirmatory Symptoms.* Albany, Calif: Hahnemann Clinic Publishing; 1993:32–33, 111–113, 244–247, 303–304, 401–403.

National Institutes of Health. Accessed at www.ninds.nih.gov/healinfo/disorder/parkinso/pdhtr.htm on January 16, 1999.

Parkinson's Disease Foundation. Accessed at www.pdf.org/ on January 16, 1999.

Perry TL, Godin DV, Dansen S. Parkinson's disease: a disorder due to nigral glutathione deficiency. *Neurosci Lett.* 1982;33:305–310.

Thierney LM Jr, McPhee SJ, Papadakis MA. *Current Medical Diagnosis & Treatment 1999.* 38th ed. Stamford, Conn: Appleton & Lange; 1999.

Werbach M. *Nutritional Influences on Illness.* New Canaan, Conn: Keats Publishing; 1988:346–349.

PEPTIC ULCER

Blumenthal M, ed. *The Complete German Commission E Monographs.* Boston, Mass: Integrative Medicine Communications; 1998:427, 432.

Fauci AS, Braunwald E, Isselbacher KJ et al, eds. *Harrison's Principles of Internal Medicine.* 14th ed. New York, NY: McGraw-Hill; 1998.

Kruzel T. *The Homeopathic Emergency Guide.* Berkeley, Calif: North Atlantic Books; 1992:134–137.

Murray M, Pizzorno JE. *Encyclopedia of Natural Medicine.* 2nd ed. Rocklin, Calif: Prima Publishing; 1998:522–523.

Sabiston DC, ed. *Textbook of Surgery.* 15th ed. Philadelphia, Pa: WB Saunders; 1998.

PERICARDITIS

Andreoli TE, Bennett JC, Carpenter CCJ. *Cecil Essentials of Medicine.* 3rd ed. Philadelphia, Pa: WB Saunders; 1993:110–114.

Dambro MR. *Griffith's 5-Minute Clinical Consult–1999.* Baltimore, Md: Lippincott Williams & Wilkins; 1999:792–793.

Fleming T, Gruenwald J, Brendler T, Jaenicke C, eds. *PDR for Herbal Medicines.* Montvale, NJ: Medical Economics Company; 1998:606–608.

Stein JK, ed. *Internal Medicine.* 4th ed. St. Louis, Mo: Mosby-Year Book; 1994:248–252.

Stoller JK, Ahmad M, Longworth DL, eds. *The Cleveland Clinic Intensive Review of Internal Medicine.* Baltimore, Md: Williams & Wilkins; 1998:759–760.

PERTUSSIS

Bartram T. *Encyclopedia of Herbal Medicine.* Dorset, England: Grace Publishers; 1995:452–453.

Behrman RE, Kliegman R, eds. *Nelson Textbook of Pediatrics.* 15th ed. Philadelphia, Pa: WB Saunders; 1996.

Blumenthal M, ed. *The Complete German Commission E Monographs.* Boston, Mass: Integrative Medicine Communications; 1998:432.

Bove M. *An Encyclopedia of Natural Healing for Children and Infants.* New Canaan, Conn: Keats Publishing; 1996:205–208.

Rakel RE, ed. *Conn's Current Therapy.* 50th ed. Philadelphia, Pa: WB Saunders; 1998.

Rosen P, Barkin R, eds. *Emergency Medicine: Concepts and Clinical Practice.* 4th ed. St. Louis, Mo: Mosby-Year Book; 1996.

Scott J. *Natural Medicine for Children.* London, England: Gaia Books Ltd; 1990:133–134.

PHARYNGITIS

Berkow R, ed. *Merck Manual.* 16th ed. Rahway, NJ: Merck Research Laboratories; 1992.

Larson DE, ed. *Mayo Clinic Family Health Book.* 2nd ed. New York, NY: William Morrow and Company; 1996.

Lewis WH, Elvin-Lewis MPF. *Medical Botany/Plants Affecting Man's Health.* New York, NY: John Wiley & Sons; 1977.

Morrison R. *Desktop Guide to Keynotes and Confirmatory Symptoms.* Albany, Calif: Hahnemann Clinic Publishing; 1993:5, 28.

PREECLAMPSIA

Berkow R, ed. *Merck Manual of Diagnosis and Therapy.* 16th edition. Rahway, NJ: The Merck Publishing Group; 1992.

Berkow R, Beers MH, Fletcher AJ, eds. *Merck Manual, Home Edition.* Rahway, NJ: Merck & Co; 1997.

Klonoff-Cohen HS, Cross JL, Pieper CF. Job stress and preeclampsia. *Epidemiol.* 1996;7:245–249.

Larson DE, ed. *Mayo Clinic Family Health Book.* 2nd ed. New York, NY: William Morrow and Company; 1996.

Murray M. *Encyclopedia of Nutritional Supplements.* Rocklin, Calif: Prima Health; 1996.

Scalzo R. *Naturopathic Handbook of Herbal Formulas.* Durango, Colo: 2nd ed. Kivaki Press; 1994.

PRIMARY PULMONARY HYPERTENSION

Bartram T. *Encyclopedia of Herbal Medicine.* Dorset, England: Grace Publishers; 1995:195, 270, 276, 376.

Bordow RA, Moser KM. *Manual of Clinical Problems in Pulmonary Medicine.* 4th ed. Boston, Mass: Little, Brown; 1996:304–311,353,424, 431–434.

Fauci AS, Braunwald, E, Isselbacher KJ et al, eds. *Harrison's Principles of Internal Medicine.* 14th ed. New York, NY: McGraw-Hill; 1998:1466–1468.

Fishman AP, Elias JA, Fishman JA, et al. *Fishman's Pulmonary Diseases and Disorders.* 3rd ed. New York, NY: McGraw-Hill; l998: 1261–1296.

Hinshaw HC, Murray JF. *Disease of the Chest.* 4th ed. Philadelphia, Pa: WB Saunders; 1980:684–697.

Woodley M, Whelan A. *Washington Manual of Therapeutics.* 27th ed. Boston, Mass: Little, Brown; 1992:211–212.

PROSTATITIS

Bartram T. *Encyclopedia of Herbal Medicine.* Dorset, England: Grace Publishers; 1995:52, 128, 203.

Berkow R, ed. *The Merck Manual of Diagnosis and Therapy.* 16th ed. Rahway, NJ: The Merck Publishing Group; 1992.

Blumenthal M, ed. *The Complete German Commission E Monographs.* Boston, Mass: Integrative Medicine Communications; 1998:75, 201.

Buck AC, Rees RWM, Ebeling L. Treatment of chronic prostatitis and prostadynia with pollen extract. *Br J Urol.* 1989;64:496–499.

Conn RB, Borere WZ, Snyder JW, eds. *Current Diagnosis 9.* Philadelphia, Pa: WB Saunders; 1996.

Driscoll CE, Bope ET, Smith CW JR, Carter BL, eds. *The Family Practice Desk Reference.* 3rd ed. St. Louis, Mo: Mosby-Year Book; 1996.

Gruenwald J, Brendler T et al, eds. *PDR for Herbal Medicines.* Montvale, NJ: Medical Economics Company; 1998:817, 1,229.

Morrison R. *Desktop Guide to Keynotes and Confirmatory Symptoms.* Albany, Calif: Hahnemann Clinic Publishing; 1993:119, 228–231, 341, 388–389.

Murray MT, Pizzorno JE. *Encyclopedia of Natural Medicine.* Rocklin, Calif: Prima Publishing; 1998:480–486.

Thierney Jr LM, McPhee SJ, Papadakis MA, eds. *Current Medical Diagnosis & Treatment 1999.* 38th ed. Stamford, Conn: Appleton & Lange; 1999.

Werbach, M. *Nutritional Influences on Illness.* New Canaan, Conn: Keats Publishing; 1988:82–84.

PSORIASIS

Blumenthal M, ed. *The Complete German Commission E Monographs.* Boston, Mass: Integrative Medicine Communications; 1998:169–170.

The Editors of Time-Life Books. *The Medical Advisor.* Alexandria, Va: Time-Life Books; 1996.

Ergil KV. *Medicines from the Earth: Protocols for Botanical Healing.* Harvard, Mass: Gaia Herbal Research Institute; 1996:207–211.

Gruenwald J, Brendler T et al, eds. *PDR for Herbal Medicines.* Montvale, NJ: Medical Economics Company; 1998:903–904, 114, 1157.

Syed TA, et al. Management of psoriasis with aloe vera extract in a hydrophilic cream: a placebo-controlled, double-blind study. *Trop Med Int Health.* 1996;1:505–509.

Walker JP, Brown EH. *The Alternative Pharmacy.* Paramus, NJ: Prentice Hall Press; 1998.

Werbach MR. *Nutritional Influences on Illness.* New Canaan, Conn: Keats Publishing Inc; 1988:370–373.

PULMONARY EDEMA

Bartram T. *Encyclopedia of Herbal Medicine.* Dorset, England: Grace Publishers; 1995:73, 80, 155, 156.

Blumenthal M, ed. *The Complete German Commission E Monographs.* Boston, Mass: Integrative Medicine Communications; 1998:423, 425.

Dambro MR, ed. *Griffith's 5 Minute Clinical Consult.* Baltimore, Md: Williams & Wilkins; 1998.

Fauci AS, Braunwald E, Isselbacher KJ et al, eds. *Harrison's Principles of Internal Medicine.* 14th ed. New York, NY: McGraw-Hill; 1998.

Thierney LM Jr, McPhee SJ, Papadakis MA, eds. *Current Medical Diagnosis & Treatment 1999.* 38th ed. Stamford, Conn: Appleton & Lange; 1999.

RAYNAUD'S PHENOMENON

Balch JF, Balch PA. *Prescription for Nutritional Healing.* 2nd ed. Garden City Park, NY: Avery Publishing Group; 1997.

Batchelder HJ. Allopathic specific condition review: Raynaud's disease. *The Protocol Journal of Botanical Medicine.* 1996;2:134–137.

Fauci AS, Braunwald E, Isselbacher KJ et al, eds. *Harrison's Principles of Internal Medicine.* 14th ed. New York, NY: McGraw-Hill; 1998.

Mitchell W, Batchelder HJ. Naturopathic specific condition review: Raynaud's disease. *The Protocol Journal of Botanical Medicine.* 1996;2:138–140.

Thierney LM Jr, McPhee SJ, Papadakis MA, eds. *Current Medical Diagnosis & Treatment 1999.* 38th ed. Stamford, Conn: Appleton & Lange; 1999.

REITER'S SYNDROME

Bartram T. *Encyclopedia of Herbal Medicine.* Dorset, England: Grace Publishers; 1995:368–369.

Gruenwald J, Brendler T, Jaenicke C et al, eds. *PDR for Herbal Medicines.* Montvale, NJ: Medical Economics Company; 1998.

Koopman WJ, ed. *Arthritis and Allied Conditions.* 13th ed. Baltimore, Md: Lippincott, Williams & Wilkins; 1996.

Murray MT, Pizzorno JE. *Encyclopedia of Natural Medicine.* 2nd ed. Rocklin, Calif: Prima Publishing; 1998.

Weiss RF. *Herbal Medicines.* Beaconsfield, England: Beaconsfield Publishers; 1998:339.

RHEUMATOID ARTHRITIS

American College of Rheumatology, Clinical Guidelines Committee. Guidelines for rheumatoid arthritis management. *Arthritis Rheum.* 1996;39:713–722.

Blumenthal M, ed. *The Complete German Commission E Monographs.* Boston, Mass: Integrative Medicine Communications; 1998:121, 135, 150–151, 138, 226–227.

Gruenwald J, Brendler T, Jaenicke C et al, eds. *PDR for Herbal Medicines.* Montvale, NJ: Medical Economics Company; 1998:810.

Kelley WN, Harris ED, Sledge CB, eds. *Textbook of Rheumatology.* 5th ed. Philadelphia, Pa: WB Saunders Company; 1997: chap 55.

Mazzetti I, Grigolo B, Borzai RM, Meliconi R, Facchini A. Serum copper/zinc superoxide dismutase levels in patients with rheumatoid arthritis. *J Clin Lab Res.* 1996;26(4):245–249.

Morrison R. *Desktop Guide to Keynotes and Confirmatory Symptoms.* Albany, Calif: Hahnemann Clinic Publishing; 1993:73–75, 85–86, 226, 329–330.

Mulherrin DM, Thurnham DI, Situnayake RD. Glutathione reductase activity, riboflavin status, and disease activity in rheumatoid arthritis. *Ann Rheum Dis.* 1996;55:837–840.

Murray MT, Pizzorno JE. *Encyclopedia of Natural Medicine.* Rocklin, Calif: Prima Publishing; 1998:492–501.

Tierney Jr LM, McPhee SJ, Papadakis MA, eds. *Current Medical Diagnosis & Treatment, 1999.* Stamford, Conn: Appleton & Lange; 1999.

Weisman MH, Weinblatt ME, eds. *Treatment of the Rheumatic Diseases: Companion to the Textbook of Rheumatology.* Philadelphia, Pa: WB Saunders Company; 1995: chap 3.

Wylie G, et al. A comparative study of Tenidap, a cytokine-modulating anti-rheumatic drug, and diclofenac in rheumatoid arthritis: a 24 week analysis of a 1-year clinical trial. *Br J Rheumatol.* 1995;34:554–563.

Zurier RB, Rossetti RG, Jacobson EW, et al. Gamma-linolenic acid treatment of rheumatoid arthritis. A randomized, placebo-controlled trial. *Arthritis Rheum.* 1996;39:1808–1817.

ROSEOLA

Behrman RE, Kliegman RM, Nelson WE, Arvin AM, eds. *Nelson Textbook of Pediatrics.* 15th ed. Philadelphia, Pa: WB Saunders; 1996.

Bove M. *An Encyclopedia of Natural Healing for Children and Infants.* Stamford, Conn: Keats Publishing; 1996:174–176.

Fauci AS, Braunwald E, Isselbacher KJ et al, eds. *Harrison's Principles of Internal Medicine.* 14th ed. New York, NY: McGraw-Hill; 1998.

Morrison R. *Desktop Guide to Keynotes and Confirmatory Symptoms.* Albany, Calif: Hahnemann Clinic Publishing; 1993:3–6, 58–62, 115–117, 310–315.

SEIZURE DISORDERS

Adams RD, Victor M, Ropper AH. *Principles of Neurology.* 6th ed. New York, NY: McGraw-Hill; 1997:313–341.

Bartram T. *Encyclopedia of Herbal Medicine.* Dorset, England: Grace Publishers; 1995:170–171.

Fauci AS, Braunwald E, Isselbacher KJ et al, eds. *Harrison's Principles of Internal Medicine.* 14th ed. New York, NY: McGraw-Hill Book Company; 1998:2311–2325.

Gruenwald J, Brendler T, Jaenicke C et al, eds. *PDR for Herbal Medicines.* Montvale, NJ: Medical Economics Company; 1998:1128, 1135, 1204, 1219.

Morrison R. *Desktop Guide to Keynotes and Confirmatory Symptoms.* Albany, Calif: Hahnemann Clinic Publishing; 1993:46,76,111–114,124,146–147,276.

Murray MT. *Encyclopedia of Nutritional Supplements.* Rocklin, Calif: Prima Publishing; 1996:84.

Murray MT. *The Healing Power of Herbs.* 2nd ed. Rocklin, Calif: Prima Publishing; 1995:40,91.

Rowland LP. *Merritt's Textbook of Neurology.* 9th ed. Media, Pa: Williams & Wilkins; 1995:845–868.

Werback MR. *Nutritional Influences on Illness.* New Canaan, Conn: Keats Publishing, Inc; 1987:189–193.

SEXUAL DYSFUNCTION

American Psychiatric Association. *Diagnostic and Statistical Manual of Mental Disorders.* 4th ed. Washington, DC: American Psychiatric Association; 1994.

Blumenthal M, ed. *The Complete German Commission E Monographs.* Boston, Mass: Integrative Medicine Communications; 1998:383.

Conn RB, Borer WZ, Snyder JW. *Current Diagnosis* (No. 9). Philadelphia, Pa: WB Saunders; 1996:9.

Hoffman D. *The New Holistic Herbal.* New York, NY: Barnes & Noble Books; 1995:195.

Murray MT. *The Healing Power of Herbs: The Enlightened Person's Guide to the Wonders of Medicinal Plants.* Rocklin, Calif: Prima Publishing; 1995:127, 149–150.

Scalzo R. *Naturopathic Handbook of Herbal Formulas.* Durango, Colo: 2nd ed. Kivaki Press; 1994:66.

Tierney LM, McPhee SJ, Papadakis, MA, eds. *Current Medical Diagnosis & Treatment 1999.* Stamford, Conn: Appleton & Lange; 1999.

SINUSITIS

Barkin R, Rosen P, eds. *Emergency Medicine: Concepts and Clinical Practice.* 4th ed. St. Louis, Mo: Mosby-Year Book; 1996.

Blumenthal M, ed. *The Complete German Commission E Monographs.* Boston, Mass: Integrative Medicine Communications; 1998:122–123.

Gruenwald J, Brendler T, et. al, eds. *PDR for Herbal Medicines.* Montvale, NJ: Medical Economics Company; 1998:684–685.

Kruzel T. *The Homeopathic Emergency Guide.* Berkeley, Calif: North Atlantic Books; 1992:286–290.

Middleton E, ed. *Allergy: Principles and Practice.* 5th ed. St. Louis, Mo: Mosby-Year Book; 1998.

Rakel RE. *Conn's Current Therapy.* 50th ed. Philadelphia, Pa: WB Saunders; 1998.

SLEEP APNEA

Caldwell JP. *Sleep: Everything You Need to Know.* Buffalo, NY: Firefly Books; 1997.

Dunkell S. *Goodbye Insomnia, Hello Sleep.* New York, NY: Carol Publishing Group; 1994

Lipman DS. *Snoring From A to ZZZZ: Proven Cures for the Night's Worst Nuisance.* Portland, Ore: Spencer Press; 1996.

Morrison R. *Desktop Guide to Keynotes and Confirmatory Symptoms.* Albany, Calif: Hahnemann Clinic Publishing; 1993.

Pascualy RA, Soest SW. *Snoring and Sleep Apnea: Personal and Family Guide to Diagnosis and Treatment.* 2nd ed. New York, NY: Demos Vermande; 1996.

Smolley LA, Bruce DF. *Breathe Right Now: A Comprehensive Guide to Understanding and Treating the Most Common Breathing Disorders.* New York, NY: WW Norton & Co; 1998.

SPRAINS AND STRAINS

Balch JF, Balch PA. *Prescription for Nutritional Healing.* Garden City Park, NY: Avery Publishing Group; 1997.

Birrer RB, ed. *Sports Medicine for the Primary Care Physician.* Boca Raton, Fla: CRC Press; 1994.

Blumenthal M, ed. *The Complete German Commission E Monographs.* Boston, Mass: Integrative Medicine Communications; 1998:429.

Brown DJ. *Herbal Prescriptions for Better Health.* Rocklin, Calif: Prima Health; 1996.

Kibler WB, Herring S, Press J, Lee P. *Functional Rehabilitation of Sports and Musculoskeletal Injuries.* Gaithersburg, Md: Aspen Publishers; 1998.

Morrison R. *Desktop Guide to Keynotes and Confirmatory Symptoms.* Albany, Calif: Hahnemann Clinic Publishing; 1993:38, 326, 330.

Null G. *The Clinician's Handbook of Natural Healing.* New York, NY: Kensington Publishing Corp; 1997.

Olshevsky M, Noy S, Zwang M, Burger R. *Manual of Natural Therapy.* New York, NY: Facts on File; 1989.

Strauss RH, ed. *Sports Medicine.* Philadelphia, Pa: WB Saunders Company; 1991.

Ullmann D. *The Consumer's Guide to Homeopathy.* New York, NY: G. P. Putnam's Sons; 1995.

Zachazewski JE, Magee DJ, Quillen WS. *Athletic Injuries and Rehabilitation.* Philadelphia, Pa: WB Saunders Company; 1996.

TENDINITIS

Balch JF, Balch PA. *Prescription for Nutritional Healing.* 2nd ed. Garden City Park, NY: Avery Publishing; 1997:174–175.

Duke JA. *The Green Pharmacy.* Emmaus, Pa: Rodale Press; 1997:106–109.

Kelly WN, Harris Jr ED, Ruddy S, Sledge CB. *Textbook of Rheumatology.* 5th ed. Philadelphia, Pa:WB Saunders Company; 1997:372–373, 386, 422–429, 462–463, 486, 558–559, 598–599, 603–606, 642.

Koopman WJ. *Arthritis and Allied Conditions: A Textbook of Rheumatology.* 13th ed. Baltimore, Md:Williams & Wilkins; 1997:44,1769–1771, 1795, 1894–1896.

Millar AP. *Sports Injuries and Their Management.* Sydney, Australia: Maclennan & Petty; 1994:10–14, 84–85, 101–103, 111–112,118–119, 8830–8831.

Morrison R. *Desktop Guide to Keynotes and Confirmatory Symptoms.* Albany, Calif: Hahnemann Clinic Publishing; 1993:72–74, 298.

Murray MT, Pizzorno JE. *Encyclopedia of Natural Medicine.* 2nd ed. Rocklin, Calif: Prima Publishing; 1998:805–809.

Noble J. *Textbook of General Medicine and Primary Care.* Boston, Mass: Little, Brown; 1987:228–229, 288–290, 293–296.

Vinger PF, Hoener EF, eds. *Sports Injuries: The Unthwarted Epidemic.* Boston, Mass: John Wright; 1982:227, 255.

THYROIDITIS

Blumenthal M, ed. *The Complete German Commission E Monographs.* Boston, Mass: Integrative Medicine Communications; 1998:432.

The Burton Goldberg Group, compilers. *Alternative Medicine: The Definitive Guide.* Tiburon, Calif: Future Medicine Publishing Inc; 1997.

Ferri FF. *Ferri's Clinical Advisor: Instant Diagnosis and Treatment.* St Louis, Mo: Mosby-Year Book;1999.

Hoffman D. *The New Holistic Herbal.* New York, NY: Barnes & Noble Books; 1995:95.

Murray MT, Pizzorno JE. *Encyclopedia of Natural Medicine.* Rocklin, Calif: Prima Publishing; 1998:386–390.

Noble J, ed. *Textbook of Primary Care Medicine.* 2nd ed. St Louis, Mo: Mosby-Year Book; 1996.

Tierney Jr LM, McPhee SJ, Papadakis MA, eds. *Current Medical Diagnosis and Treatment.* Norwalk, Conn: Appleton & Lange; 1994.

ULCERATIVE COLITIS

Berkow R, ed. *The Merck Manual of Diagnosis and Therapy.* 16th ed. Rahway, NJ: Merck Research Laboratories; 1992.

Blumenthal M, ed. *The Complete German Commission E Monographs.* Boston, Mass: Integrative Medicine Communications; 1998:427–428, 432.

Greenfield, S.M. et al. A randomized controlled study of evening primrose oil and fish oil in ulcerative colitis. *Aliment Pharmacol Ther.* 1993;7:159–166.

Roediger WE, Moore J, Babidge W. Colonic sulfide in pathogenesis and treatment of ulcerative colitis. *Dig Dis Sci.* 1997;42:1571–1579.

Weatherall DJ, Ledingham JGG, Warrell DA, eds. *Oxford Textbook of Medicine.* 3rd ed. New York, NY: Oxford University Press; 1996.

Werbach, M. *Nutritional Influences on Illness.* New Canaan, Conn: Keats Publishing; 1988:424–427.

Wyngaarden JB, Smith LH, Bennett JC, eds. *Cecil Textbook of Medicine.* Philadelphia, Pa: WB Saunders; 1992.

URETHRITIS

Bartram T. *Encyclopedia of Herbal Medicine.* Dorset, England: Grace Publishers; 1995:436–437.

Berkow R, Beers MH. *The Merck Manual of Diagnosis and Therapy.* Rahway, NJ: Merck and Company; 1992.

Blumenthal M, ed. *The Complete German Commission E Monographs.* Boston, Mass: Integrative Medicine Communications; 1998:432.

Bowie WR. Approach to men with urethritis and urologic complications of sexually trans- mitted diseases. *Med Clin North Am.* 1990;74:1543–1557. Accessed at www.thriveonline.com.

Hoffman D. *The New Holistic Herbal.* New York, NY: Barnes & Noble Books; 1995:109–110.

Kruzel T. *The Homeopathic Emergency Guide.* Berkeley, Calif: North Atlantic Books; 1992:98–102.

Shealy CN. *The Illustrated Encyclopedia of Healing Remedies.* Boston, Mass: Element Books Limited; 1998.

Tierney LM, et al, eds. *Current Medical Diagnosis & Treatment 1999.* 38th ed. Stamford, Conn: Appleton & Lange; 1999.

Virtual Hospital: University of Iowa Family Practice Handbook. 3rd ed. Available at www.vh.org.

URINARY INCONTINENCE

Bartram T. *Encyclopedia of Herbal Medicine.* Dorset, England: Grace Publishers; 1995:247.

Blumenthal M, ed. *The Complete German Commission E Monographs.* Boston, Mass: Integrative Medicine Communications; 1998:432.

Dambro MR. *Griffith's 5 Minute Clinical Consult:* Baltimore, Md: Williams & Wilkins; 1998.

Fauci AS, Braunwald, E, Isselbacher KJ et al, eds. *Harrison's Principles of Internal Medicine.* 14th ed. New York, NY: McGraw-Hill; 1998:1466–1468.

Morrison R. *Desktop Guide to Keynotes and Confirmatory Symptoms.* Albany, Calif: Hahnemann Clinic Publishing; 1993:111–113, 258–261, 286, 402.

Olshevsky M, Noy S, Zwang M, et al. *Manual of Natural Therapy.* New York, NY: Facts on File Inc; 1989.

Thom DH, Van den Eedcn SK, Brown JS. Evaluation of parturition and other reproductive variable as risk factors for urinary incontinence. *Obstet Gynecol.* 1997;90:983–989.

Ullman D. *The Consumer's Guide to Homeopathy.* New York, NY: The Putnam Publishing Group; 1995.

URINARY TRACT INFECTION IN WOMEN

Avorn J, Monane M, Gurwitz JH, Glynn RJ, Choodnovskiy I, Lipsitz LA. Reduction of bacteriuria and pyuria after ingestion of cranberry juice. *JAMA.* 1994; 271:751–754.

Berkow R, ed. *The Merck Manual.* 16th ed. Rahway, NJ: Merck and Company Inc; 1992.

Blumenthal M, ed. *The Complete Commission E Monographs, American Botanical Council.* Boston, Mass: Integrative Medicine Communications; 1998:432.

Engel JD, Schaeffer AJ. Evaluation of and antimicrobial therapy for recurrent urinary tract infections in women. *Urol Clin N Am.* 1998;25: 685–701.

Goodman-Gilman A, Rall T, Nies A, Palmer T. *The Pharmacological Basis of Therapeutics.* 8th ed. New York, NY: Pergamon Press; 1990.

Howell A, Vorsa N, Der Marderosian A, Foo Lai Yeap. Inhibition of the adherence of P-fimbriated Escherichia cola to uroepithelia-cell surfaces by proanthocyanidin extracts in cranberries. *N Engl J Med.* 1998;339:1085–1086. Letter.

Kruzel T. *The Homeopathic Emergency Guide.* Berkeley, Calif: North Atlantic Books; 1992:98–102.

Murray M, Pizzorno J. *Encyclopedia of Natural Medicine.* Rocklin, Calif: Prima Publishing; 1990.

Ofek I, Goldhar J, Zafriri D, Lis H, Adar R, Sharon N. Anti-Escherichia coli adhesion activity of cranberry and blueberry juices. *N Engl J Med.* 1991;324:1599. Letter.

Schmidt DR, Sobota AE. An examination of the anti-adherence activity of cranberry juice on urinary and nonurinary bacterial isolates. *Microbios.* 1988;55:173–181.

Schultz V, Hansel R, Tyler VE. *Rational Phytotherapy: A Physician's Guide to Herbal Medicine.* New York, NY: Springer; 1997.

Sobel JD. Pathogenesis of urinary tract infection: role of host defenses. *Infect Dis Clin of North Am.* 1997;11:531–549.

Sobota AE. Inhibition of bacterial adherence by cranberry juice: potential use for the treatment of urinary tract infections. *J Urol.* 1984;131:1013–1016.

Ullman D. The Consumer's Guide to Homeopathy. Tarcher/Putnam; 1996.

Werbach M, Murray M. *Botanical Influences on Illness: A Sourcebook of Clinical Research.* Tarzania, Calif: Third Line Press; 1994.

Zafriri D, Ofek I, Adar R, Pocino M, Sharon N. Inhibitory activity of cranberry juice on adherence of type 1 and type P fimbriated Escherichia coli to eucaryotic cells. *Antimicrob Agents Chemother.* 1989;33:92–98.

UROLITHIASIS

Ferri FF. *Ferri's Clinical Advisor: Instant Diagnosis and Treatment.* St Louis, Mo: Mosby-Year Book; 1999.

Tierney LM Jr, McPhee SJ, Papadakis MA, eds. *Current Medical Diagnosis and Treatment 1994.* Norwalk, Conn: Appleton & Lange; 1994.

Grases F, et al. Urolithiasis and phytotherapy. *Int Urol Nephrol.* 1994;26:507–511.

Larson DE, ed. *Mayo Clinic Family Health Book.* 2nd ed. New York, NY: William Morrow and Company; 1996.

Scalzo R. *Naturopathic Handbook of Herbal Formulas.* Durango, Colo: 2nd ed. Kivaki Press; 1994.

The Burton Goldberg Group, compilers. *Alternative medicine: The Definitive Guide.* Tiburon, Calif: Future Medicine Publishing; 1997.

VAGINITIS

Dambro MR. *Griffith's 5-Minute Clinical Consult–1999.* Baltimore, Md: Lippincott Williams & Wilkins; 1999:358–361.

Fauci AS, Braunwald E, Isselbacher KJ et al, eds. *Harrison's Principles of Internal Medicine.* 14th ed. New York, NY: McGraw-Hill; 1998.

Habif TP. *Clinical Dermatology.* 3rd ed. St. Louis, Mo: Mosby-Year Book; 1996.

Morrison R. *Desktop Guide to Keynotes and Confirmatory Symptoms.* Albany, Calif:

Hahnemann Clinic Publishing; 1993:43, 69, 85, 171, 346.

Murray MT, Pizzorno JE. *Encyclopedia of Natural Medicine.* 2nd ed. Rocklin, Calif: Prima Publishing; 1998:530–535

WARTS

Barker LR, et al, eds. *Principles of Ambulatory Medicine.* 4th ed. Baltimore, Md: Williams and Wilkins; 1995:1467–1469.

Berkow R, Beers MH. *The Merck Manual of Medical Information.* Whitehouse Station, NJ: Merck Research Laboratories; 1997:984–985.

Brodell RT. *Infect Med.* SCP Communications, Inc.; 1996:13:56–60, 66.

Dambro MR. *Griffith's 5-Minute Clinical Consult–1999.* Baltimore, Md: Lippincott Williams and Wilkins; 1999:1166–1169.

Duke JA. *The Green Pharmacy.* Emmaus, Pa: Rodale Press; 1997: 452–455.

Ewald GA, McKenzie CR, eds. *Manual of Medical Therapeutics.* 28th ed. Boston, Mass: Little, Brown and Company; 1995:20–21.

Lockie A, Deddes N. *The Complete Guide to Homeopathy.* New York, NY: DK Publishing Inc; 1995:187, 189, 227.

Ody P. *The Complete Medicinal Herbal.* New York, NY: DK Publishing Inc; 1993:160–161.

Pray WS. *Nonprescription Product Therapeutics.* Baltimore, Md: Lippincott Willliams & Wilkins, in press.

Scalzo R. *Naturopathic Handbook of Herbal Formulas.* 2nd ed. Durango, Colo: Kivaki Press; 1994:73.

Walker LP, Brown EH. *The Alternative Pharmacy.* Paramus, NJ: Prentice Hall Press; 1998:353–354.

■ RESOURCES - HERBS

ALOE

Blitz JJ, et al. Aloe vera gel in peptic ulcer therapy: preliminary report. *J Am Osteopath Assoc.* 1963;62:731–735.

Blumenthal M, ed. *The Complete German Commission E Monographs.* Boston, Mass: Integrative Medicine Communications. 1998.

Castleman M. *The Healing Herbs.* New York, NY: Bantam Books. 1991.

Danhof I. Potential benefits from orally-injested internal aloe vera gel. International Aloe Science Council Tenth Annual Aloe Scientific Seminar; 1991; Irving, Texas.

Duke J. *The Green Pharmacy.* Emmaus, Penn: Rodale Press. 1997.

Fahim MS, Wang M. Zinc acetate and lyophilized *Aloe barbadensis* as vaginal contraceptive. *Contraception.* 1996;53:231–236.

Fulton JE Jr. The stimulation of postdermabrasion wound healing with stabilized aloe vera gel-polyethylene oxide dressing. *J Dermatol Surg Onco.* 1990;16:460.

Grindlay D, Reynolds T. The aloe vera phenomenon: a review of the properties and modern uses of the leaf parenchyma gel. *J Ethnopharmacol.* 1986;16:117–151.

Gruenwald J, Brendler T, Jaenicke C et al, eds. *PDR for Herbal Medicines.* Montvale, NJ: Medical Economics Company. 1998.

Heggers J, et al. Beneficial effects of aloe in wound healing. *Phytother Res.* 1993;7:S48–S52.

Murray M, Pizzorno J. *Encyclopedia of Natural Medicine.* Rocklin, Calif: Prima Publishing. 1991.

Murray M. *Healing Power of Herbs.* Rocklin, Calif: Prima Publishing. 1995.

Newall C, et al. *Herbal Medicines.* London, England: Pharmaceutical Press. 1996.

Plemmons JM, et al. Evaluation of acemannan in the treatment of aphthous stomatitis. *Wounds.*1994;6.

Saoo K, et al. Antiviral activity of aloe extracts against cytomegalovirus. *Phytother Res.* 1996;10:348–350.

Schmidt JM, Greenspoon JS. Aloe vera dermal wound gel is associated with a delay in wound healing. *Ostet Gynecol.* 1991;78(1).

Shida, T. et al. 1985. Effect of aloe extract on peripheral phagocytosis in adult bronchial asthma. Planta Med 51.

Syed TA, et al. Management of psoriasis with aloe vera extract in a hydrophilic cream: a placebo-controlled, double-blind study. *Trop Med Int Health.* 1996;1:505–509.

Tyler VE. *The Honest Herbal.* New York, NY: Pharmaceutical Products Press. 1993.

Vazquez B, et al. Anti-inflammatory activity of extracts from aloe vera gel. *J Ethnopharmacol.* 1996;55:69–75.

BARBERRY

Amin AH, Subbaiah, TV, Abbasi KM. Berberine sulfate: antimicrobial activity, bioassay, and mode of action. *Can J Microbiol.* 1969;15:1067–1076.

Bergner P. Goldenseal and the common cold; goldenseal substitutes. *Medical Herbalism: A Journal for the Clinical Practitioner.* Winter 1996–1997;8:1.

Blumenthal M, ed. *The Complete German Commission E Monographs.* Boston, Mass: Integrative Medicine Communications; 1998.

Foster S, Duke JA. *A Field Guide to Medicinal Plants: Eastern and Central North America.* Boston, Mass: Houghton Mifflin; 1990.

Harborn, J, Baxter H. *Phytochemical Dictionary: A Handbook of Bioactive Compounds from Plants.* Washington DC: Taylor & Francis; 1993.

Ivanovska N, Philipov S. Study on the antiinflammatory action of *Berberis vulgaris* root extract, alkaloid fractions, and pure alkaloids. *Int J Immunopharmacol.* 1996;18:552–561.

Kowalchik C,Hylton W, eds. *Rodale's Illustrated Encyclopedia of Herbs.* Emmaus Pa: Rodale Press; 1998.

Leung A, Foster S. *Encyclopedia of Common Natural Ingredients Used in Food, Drugs, and Cosmetics.* 2nd ed. New York, NY: John Wiley & Sons; 1996.

McGuffin M, Hobbs C, Upton R, Goldberg A. *American Herbal Products Associations's Botanical Safety Handbook.* Boca Raton, Fla: CRC Press; 1996.

Muller K, et al. The antipsoriatic Mahonia aquifolium and its active constituents; I. Pro- and antioxidant properties and inhibition of 5-lipoxygenase. *Planta Med.* 1994;60:421–424.

Murray M. *The Healing Power of Herbs: the Enlightened Person's Guide to the Wonders of Medicinal Plants.* Rocklin, Calif: Prima Publishing; 1995.

Murray MT, Pizzorno JE. *Encyclopedia of Natural Medicine.* 2nd ed. Rocklin, Calif: Prima Publishing; 1998:310.

Shamsa F, et al. Antihistaminic and anticholinergic activity of barberry fruit *(Berberis vulgaris)* in the guinea-pig ileum. *J Ethnopharmacol.* 1999;64:161–166.

Sotnikova R, et al. Relaxant properties of some aporphine alkaloids from Mahonia aquifolium. *Methods Find Exp Clin Pharmacol.* 1997;19:589–597.

Sun D, Courtney HS, Beachey EH. Berberine sulfate blocks adherence of Streptococcus pyogenes to epithelial cells, fibronectin, and hexadecane. *Antimicrob Agents Chemother.* 1988;32:1370–1374.

BILBERRY

Blumenthal M, ed. *The Complete German Commission E Monographs.* Boston, Mass: Integrative Medicine Communications; 1998.

Bomser J, et al. In vitro anti-cancer activity of fruit extracts from *Vaccinium* species. *Planta Med.* 1996;62:212–216.

Brown D. *Herbal Prescriptions for Better Health.* Rocklin, Calif: Prima Publishing; 1996.

Detre Z, Jellinek H, Miskulin R. Studies on vascular permeability in hypertension. *Clin Physiol Bichem.* 1986;4:143–149.

Duke J. *The Green Pharmacy.* Emmaus, Pa: Rodale Press; 1997.

Gruenwald J, Brendler T, Jaenicke C et al, eds. *PDR for Herbal Medicines.* Montvale, NJ: Medical Economics Company Inc; 1998.

Havsteen B. Flavonoids, a class of natural products of high pharmacological potency. *Biochem Pharmacol.* 1983;32:1141–1148.

Morazzoni P, Bombardelli E. *Vaccinium myrtillus L. Fitoterapia.* 1996;LXVII:3–29.

Murray M. *The Healing Power of Herbs.* Rocklin, Calif: Prima Publishing; 1995.

Orsucci PL, et al. Treatment of diabetic retinopthy with anthocyanosides: a preliminary report. *Clin Oc.* 1983;5:377.

Perossini M, et al. Diabetic and Hypertensive retinopathy therapy with Vaccinium myrtillus anthocyanosides (Tegens): Double blind placebo controlled clinical trial. *Annali di Ottalmaologia e Clinica Ocaulistica.* 1987;CXII.

Schulz V et al. *Rational Phytotherapy.* Berlin, Germany: Springer-Verlag; 1998.

Tyler V. *Herbs of Choice.* New York, NY: Haworth Press Inc; 1994.

BLACK COHOSH

Beuscher N. *Cimicifuga racemosa L.*—Black Cohosh. *Z Phytotherapie.* 1995;16:301–310.

Blumenthal M, ed. *The Complete German Commission E Monographs.* Boston, Mass: Integrative Medicine Communications; 1998.

Daiber W. Climacteric Complaints: success without using hormones. *Ärztliche Praxis.* 1983;35:1946–1947.

Lieberman S. A review of the effectiveness of *Cimicifuga racemosa* (black cohosh) for the symptoms of monopause. *J Womens Health.* 1998;5:525–529.

Murray MT, Pizzorno JE. *Encyclopedia of Natural Medicine.* 2nd ed. Rocklin, Calif: Prima Publishing; 1998.

Newall CA, Anderson LA, Phillipson DJ. *Herbal Medicines: A Guide for Health-Care Professionals.* London, England: The Pharmaceutical Press; 1996.

Ringer DL, ed. *Physicians' Guide to Nutriceuticals.* Omaha, Neb: Nutritional Data Resources LP; 1998.

Schulz V, Hänsel R, Tyler VE. *Rational Phytotherapy.* Berlin, Germany: Springer-Verlag; 1998.

Stoll W. Phytopharmacon influences atrophic vaginal epithelium: Double blind-study—cimicifuga vs. estrogenic substances. *Therapeuticum.* 1987;1:23–31.

Taylor M. Alternatives to Hormone Replacement Therapy. *Comprehensive Therapy.* 1997;23:514–532.

Tyler VE. *Herbs of Choice: The Therapeutic Use of Phytomedicinals.* New York, NY: Pharmaceutical Products Press; 1994.

Warnecke G. Influencing menopausal symptoms with a phytotherapeutic agent: successful therapy with *Cimicifuga* mono-extract. *Med Welt.* 1985;36:871–874.

BURDOCK

Blumenthal M, ed. *The Complete German Commission E Monographs.* Boston, Mass: Integrative Medicine Communications; 1998:318.

Bradley P, ed. *British Herbal Compendium.* Dorset, England: British Herbal Medicine Association; 1992:1:46–49.

British Herbal Pharmacopoeia. 4th ed. Dorset, England: British Herbal Medicine Association; 1996:47–49.

De Smet PAGM, Keller K, Hänsel R, Chandler RF, eds. *Adverse Effects of Herbal Drugs.* Berlin, Germany: Springer-Verlag; 1997:231–237.

Dombradi CA, et al. Screening report on the antitumor activity of purified *Arctium Lappa* extracts. *Tumori.*1966;52:173–175.

Grases F, et al. Urolithiasis and phytotherapy. *Int Urol Nephrol.* 1994;26:507–511.

Grieve M. *A Modern Herbal.* New York, NY: Dover; 1971:1:143–145.

Gruenwald J, Brendler T, Jaenicke C. *PDR for Herbal Medicines.* Montvale, NJ: Medical Economics Company; 1998:656–657

Hutchens A. *Indian Herbalogy of North America.* Boston, Mass: Shambhala Publications; 1991:62–65.

Ito Y, et al. Suppression of 7,12-dimethylbenz(a)anthracene-induced chromosome aberrations in rat bone marrow cells by vegetable juices. *Mutat Res.* 1986;172:55–60.

Lapinina L, Sisoeva T. Investigation of some plants to determine their sugar lowering action. *Farmatevt Zh.* 1964;19:52–58.

Lin CC, et al. Anti-inflammatory and radical scavenge effects of *Arctium lappa.* *Am J Chin Med.* 1996;24:127–137.

Millspaugh C. *American Medicinal Plants*. New York, NY: Dover Publications; 1974:360–362.

Mowry D. *The Scientific Validation of Herbal Medicine*. New Canaan, Conn: Keats Publishing; 1986:3–6, 57–63.

Newall C, Anderson L, Phillipson J. *Herbal Medicines: A Guide for Health-care Professionals*. London, England: Pharmaceutical Press; 1996:52–53.

Swanston-Flatt SK, Day C, Flatt PR, Gould BJ, Bailey CJ. Glycaemic effects of traditional European plant treatments for diabetes. Studies in normal and streptozotocin diabetic mice. *Diabetes Res*. 1989;413:69–73.

Tyler V. *The Honest Herbal: A Sensible Guide to the Use of Herbs and Related Remedies*. 3rd ed. Binghamton, NY: Pharmaceutical Products Press; 1993:63–64.

CAT'S CLAW

Aquino R, De Simone F, Pizza C, Conti C, Stein ML. Plant metabolites. Structure and in vitro activity of quinovic acid glycosides from *Uncaria tomentosa* and Guettarda platypoda. *J Nat Prod*. 1989;52:679–685.

Aquino R, De Simone F, Vincieri FF, Pizza C, Gacs-Baitz C. New polyhydroxylated triterpenes from *Uncaria tomentosa. J Nat Prod*. 1990;53: 559–564.

Blumenthal M, ed. *The Complete German Commission E Monographs*. Boston, Mass: Integrative Medicine Communications; 1998.

Blumenthal M. Herbal update: Una de gato (cat's claw): Rainforest herb gets scientific and industry attention. *Whole Foods Magazine*. 1995: 62–68, 78.

Blumenthal M, Riggins C. *Popular Herbs in the U.S. Market: Therapeutic Monographs*. Austin, Tex: The American Botanical Council; 1997.

Davis BW. A "new" world class herb for applied kinesiology practice: *Uncaria tomentosa*—a.k.a. Una de Gato (UDG). Collected Papers of the International College of Applied Kinesiology. 1992.

de Matta SM, Monache FD, Ferrari F, Marini-Bettolo GB. Alkaloids and procyanidine of an Uncaria sp. from Peru. *Farmaco* [Sci]. 1976;31:527–535.

Keplinger K, et al. *Uncaria tomentosa* (Willd.) DC.—ethnomedicinal use and new pharmacological, toxicological and botanical results. *J Ethnopharmacol*. 1999;64:23–34.

Lemaire I, et al. Stimulation of interleukin-1 and -6 production in alveolar macrophages by the neotropical liana, *Uncaria tomentosa. J Ethnopharmacol*. 1999;64:109–115.

Lininger S, Wright J, Austin S, Brown D, Gaby A. *The Natural Pharmacy*. Rocklin, Calif: Prima Health; 1998:246.

McGuffin M, Hobbs C, Upton R, Goldberg A. *American Herbal Products Association's Botanical Safety Handbook*. Boca Raton, Fla: CRC Press; 1997.

Ozaki Y. Pharmacological studies of indole alkaloids obtained from domestic plants, Uncaria rhynchophylla Miq. And Amsonia elliptica Roem. et Schult. *Nippon Yakurigaku Zasshi*. 1989;94:17–26.

Sandoval-Chacon M, et al. Anti-inflammatory actions of cat's claw: the role of NF-kappaB. *Aliment Pharmacol Ther*. 1998;12:1,279–1,289.

Senatore A, Cataldo A, Iaccarino FP, Elberti MG. Phytochemical and biological study of *Uncaria tomentosa. Boll Soc Ital Biol Sper*. 1989;65:517–520.

Sheng Y, et al. Induction of apoptosis and inhibition of proliferation in human tumor cells treated with extracts of *Uncaria tomentosa. Anticancer Res*. 1998;18:3,363–3,368.

Steinberg PN. Cat's claw: medicinal properties of this Amazon vine. *Nutrition Science News*. 1995.

Wurm M, et al. Pentacyclic oxindole alkaloids from *Uncaria tomentosa* induce human endothelial cells to release a lymphocyte-proliferation-regulating factor. *Planta Med*. 1998;64:701–704.

Yepez AM, de Ugaz OL, Alvarez CM, De Feo V, Aquino R, De Simone F, Pizza C. Quinovic acid glycosides from *Uncaria guianensis. Phytochemistry*. 1991;30:1,635–1,637.

CAYENNE

Boone CW, Kelloff GJ, Malone WE. Identification of candidate cancer chemopreventive agents and their evaluation in animal models and human clinical trials: a review. *Cancer Res*. 1990;50:2–9.

Chevallier A. *The Encyclopedia of Medicinal Plants*. London, England: DK Publishing Inc; 1996.

Duke J. *The Green Pharmacy*. Emmaus, Pa: Rodale Press; 1997.

Hot peppers and substance P. *Lancet*. 1983;I:1198. Editorial.

Gruenwald J, Brendler T, Jaenicke C et al, eds. *PDR for Herbal Medicines*. Montvale, NJ: Medical Economics Company; 1998.

Heinerman J. *Heinerman's Encyclopedia of Fruits, Vegetables and Herbs*. Englewood Cliffs, NJ: Prentice Hall; 1988.

Kowalchik C, Hylton W, eds. *Rodale's Illustrated Encyclopedia of Herbs*. Emmaus, Pa: Rodale Press; 1998.

Locock RA. Capsicum. *Can Pharm J*. 1985;517–519.

Munn SE, et al. The effect of topical capsaicin on substance P immunoreactivity: A clinical trial and immuno-hisochemical analysis [letter]. *Acta Derm Venereol (Stockb)*. 1997;77:158–159.

Murray M. *The Healing Power of Herbs*. Rocklin, Calif: Prima Publishing; 1995.

Newall C, et al. *Herbal Medicines*. London, England: Pharmaceutical Press; 1996.

Tandan R, et al. Topical capsaicin in painful diabetic neuropathy. Controlled study with long-term follow-up. *Diabetes Care*. 1992;15:8–14.

Tyler V. *The Honest Herbal*. New York, NY: Pharmaceutical Products Press; 1993.

Visudhiphan S, et al. The relationship between high fibrinolytic activity and daily capsicum ingestion in Thais. *Am J Clin Nutr*. 1982;35:1452–1458.

Vogl T. Treatment of hunan hand. *N Engl J Med*. 1982;306:178.

Yeoh KG, et al. Chili protects against aspirin-induced gastroduodenal mucosal injury in humans. *Dig Dis Sci*. 1995;40:580–583.

CELERY SEED

Appel LJ, Moore TJ et al. A clinical trial of the effects of dietary patterns on blood pressure. *N Engl J Med*. 1997;336:1117–1124. Abstract.

Atta AH, et al. Anti-nociceptive and anti-inflammatory effects of some Jordanian medicinal plant extracts. *J Ethnopharmacol*. 1998;60:117–124.

Balch J, Balch P. *Prescription for Nutritional Healing: A-to-Z Guide to Drug-Free Remedies Using Vitamins, Minerals, Herbs, & Food Supplements*. New York, NY: Avery Publishing Group; 1990.

Banerjee S, Sharma R, Kale RK, Rao AR. Influence of certain essential oils on carcinogen-metabolizing enzymes and acid-soluble sulfhydryls in mouse liver. *Nutr Cancer*. 1994;21:263–269. Abstract.

Duke JA. *Handbook of Phytochemical Constituents of GRAS Herbs and Other Economic Plants*. Boca Raton, Fla: CRC Press; 1992.

Ko FN, et al. Vasodilatory action mechanisms of apigenin isolated from *Apium graveolens* in rat thoracic aorta. Biochim Biophys Acta. November 14; 1991;1115:69–74.

Lewis, DA, et al. The anti-inflammatory activity of celery *Apium graveolens* L. *Int J Crude Drug Res*. 1985;23.

Mills SY. *Dictionary of Modern Herbalism: A Comprehensive Guide to Practical Herbal Therapy*. Rochester, Vt: Healing Arts Press; 1988.

Singh A, Handa SS. Hepatoprotective activity of Apium graveolens and Hygrophila auriculata against paracetamol and thioacetamide intoxication in rats. *J Ethnopharmacol*. 1995;49:119–126.

Steinmetz KA, Potter JD. Vegetables, fruit, and cancer. II. Mechanisms. *Cancer Causes Control*. 1991;2:427–442. Abstract.

Tsi D, et al. Effects of aqueous celery (*Apium graveolens*) extract on lipid parameters of rats fed a high fat diet. *Planta Med*. 1995;61:18–21.

Zheng GQ, et al. Chemoprevention of benzo[a]pyrene-induced forestomach cancer in mice by natural phthalides from celery seed oil. *Nutr Cancer*. 1993;19:77–86.

Zheng GQ, Kenney PM, Zhang J, Lam LK. Chemoprevention of benzo[a]pyrene-induced forestomach cancer in mice by natural phthalides from celery seed oil. *Nutr Cancer*. 1993;19:77–86.

CHAMOMILE, GERMAN

Achterrath-Tuckermann U, et al. Pharmacological investigations with compounds of chamomile. V. Investigations on the spasmolytic effect of compounds of chamomile and Kamillosan on the isolated guinea pig ileum. *Planta Med*. 1980;39:38–50.

Blumenthal M, ed. *The Complete German Commission E Monographs*. Boston, Mass: Integrative Medicine Communications; 1998.

de la Motte S, Bose-O'Reilly S, Heinisch M, Harrison F. Doppelblind-vergleich zwischen einem apfelpektin/kamillenextrakt-präparat und plazebo bei kindern mit diarrhoe. *Arzneimittelforschung*. 1997;47:1247–1249.

Duke JA. *The Green Pharmacy*. Emmaus, Pa: Rodale Press; 1997.

Foster S. *Herbal Renaissance: Growing, Using and Understanding Herbs in the Modern World*. Salt Lake City, Utah: Gibbs-Smith; 1993.

Glowania HJ, Raulin C, Swoboda M. Effect of chamomile on wound healing - a clinical double-blind study. *Z Hautkr*. 1987; 62:1262, 1267–1271.

Kowalchik C, Hylton W, eds. *Rodale's Illustrated Encyclopedia of Herbs*. Emmaus, Pa: Rodale Press; 1998.

McGuffin M, Hobbs C, Upton R, Goldberg A. *American Herbal Products Associations's Botanical Safety Handbook*. Boca Raton, Fla: CRC Press; 1996.

Newall CA, Anderson LA, Phillipson JD. *Herbal Medicines: A Guide for Health Care Professionals*. London, England: The Pharmaceutical Press; 1996.

Salamon I. Chamomile: A medicinal plant. *Herb, Spice, and Medicinal Plant Digest*. 1992;10:1–4.

Schultz V, Hansel R, Tyler V. *Rational Phytotherapy: A Physician's Guide to Herbal Medicine*. Heidelberg: Springer; 1998.

Viola H, et al. Apigenin, a component of *Matricaria recutita* flowers, is a central benzo-diazepine receptors-ligand with anxiolytic effects. *Planta Med*. 1995;61:213–216.

CHAMOMILE, ROMAN

Achterrath-Tuckermann U, et al. Pharmacologisch untersuchungen von kamillen-inhal-testoffen. *Planta Med.* 1980;39:38-50.

Berry M. The chamomiles. *Pharm J.* 1995;254:191–193.

Blumenthal M, ed. *The Complete German Commission E Monographs.* Boston, Mass: Integrative Medicine Communications; 1998.

Bradley PR. *British Herbal Compendium.* Dorset, England: British Herbal Medicine Association; 1992:1.

DeSmet PAGM, Keller K, Hansel R, Chandler RF. *Adverse Effects of Herbal Drugs.* New York, NY: Springer-Verlag; 1992:2.

Evans WC. *Trease and Evans' Pharmacognosy.* 13th ed. London, England: Bailliere Tindall; 1989.

Foster S. *Herbal Renaissance: Growing, Using and Understanding Herbs in the Modern World.* Salt Lake City, Utah: Gibbs-Smith; 1993.

Harborne J, Baxter H. *Phytochemical Dictionary: A Handbook of Bioactive Compounds from Plants.* Washington, DC: Taylor and Francis; 1993.

Harris B, Lewis R. Chamomile part 1. *Int J Alt Comp Med.* September 1994;12.

Hausen BM, et al. The sensitizing capacity of Compositae plants. *Planta Med.* 1984;50.

Leung A, Foster S. *Encyclopedia of Common Natural Ingredients Used in Food, Drugs, and Cosmetics.* 2nd ed. New York, NY: Wiley & Sons; 1996.

McGuffin M, Hobbs C, Upton R, Goldberg A. *American Herbal Products Associations's Botanical Safety Handbook.* Boca Raton, Fla: CRC Press; 1996.

Newall CA, Anderson LA, Phillipson JD. *Herbal Medicines: A Guide for Health Care Professionals.* London, England: The Pharmaceutical Press; 1996:72–73.

Opdyke DLJ. Chamomile oil roman. *Food Cosmet Toxicol.* 1974;12:853.

Weiss RF. *Herbal Medicines.* Beaconsfield, England: Beaconsfield Publishers, Ltd; 1988.

COMFREY

Behninger C, et al. Studies on the effect of an alkaloid extract of *Symphytum officinale* on human lymphocyte cultures. *Planta Med.* 1989;55:518–522.

Blumenthal M, ed. *The Complete German Commission E Monographs.* Boston. Mass: Integrative Medicine Communications; 1998:115–116.

Bradley P. ed. *British Herbal Compendium. Vol. I.* Dorset, England: British Herbal Medicine Association; 1992:66–68.

Dorland's Illustrated Medical Dictionary. 25th ed. Philadelphia, Pa: WB Saunders; 1974.

Furmanowa M, et al. Mutagenic effects of aqueous extracts of *Symphytum officinale* L. and of its alkaloidal fractions. *J Appl Toxico.* 1983;Jun;3(3):127-30.

Goldman RS, et al. Wound healing and analgesic effect of crude extracts of *Symphytum officinale. Fitoterapi.* 1985;(6):323–329.

Gruenwald J, Brendler T, Jaenicke C, eds. *PDR for Herbal Medicines.* Montvale, NJ: Medical Economics Co.; 1998:1163–1166.

Heinerman J. *Heinerman's Encyclopedia of Fruits, Vegetables and Herbs.* Englewood Cliffs, NJ: Prentice Hall; 1988:112–113.

Newall CA, Anderson LA, Phillipson JD. eds. *Herbal Medicines: A Guide for Health-care Professionals.* London: Pharmaceutical Press; 1996:87–89.

Olinescu A, et al. Action of some proteic and carbohydrate components of *Symphytum officinale* upon normal and neoplastic cells. *Roum Arch Microbiol Immunol.* 1993;52:73–80.

Ridker PM, et al. Hepatic venocclusive disease associated with the consumption of pyrrolizidine-containing dietary supplements. *Gastroenterology.* 1985;(88):1050–1054.

Schulz V, Hänsel R, Tyler VE. *Rational Phytotherapy: A Physician's Guide to Herbal Medicine.* 3rd ed. Berlin: Springer; 1998:262.

Shealy C. *The Illustrated Encyclopedia of Healing Remedies.* Dorset, UK: Element Books; 1998:132.

Tyler VE. *Herbs of Choice: The Therapeutic Use of Phytomedicinals.* Binghamton, NY: Pharmaceutical Products Press; 1994:158–169.

Tyler VE. *The Honest Herbal: A Sensible Guide to the Use of Herbs and Related Remedies.* 3rd Ed. Binghamton, NY: Pharmaceutical Products Press; 1993:97–100.

DEVIL'S CLAW

Baghdikian B, Lanhers M, Fleurentin J, et al. An analytical study, anti-inflammatory and analgesic effects of *Harpagophytum procumbens* and *Harpagophytum zeyheri. Planta Med.* 1997;63:171–176.

Blumenthal M, ed. *The Complete German Commission E Monographs.* Boston, Mass: Integrative Medicine Communications; 1998.

Bradley P, ed. *British Herbal Compendium.* Dorset, England: British Herbal Medicine Association; 1992:1:96–98.

British Herbal Pharmacopoeia 1996. 4th ed. Dorset, England: British Herbal Medicine Association; 1996.

Costa de Pasquale R, Busa G, Circosta C, et al. A drug used in traditional medicine: *Harpagophytum procumbens DC.* III. Effects on hyperkinetic ventricular arrhythmias by reperfusion. *J Ethnopharmacology.* 1985;(13):193-9.

Grahame R, Robinson B. Devil's claw (*Harpagophytum procumbens*): pharmacological and clinical studies. *Ann Rheum Dis.* 1981;40:632.

Guyader M. 1984. Les plantes antirhumatismales. Etude historique et pharmacologique, et etude clinique du nebulisat *d'Harpagophytum procumbens* DC chez 50 patients arthrosiques sivis en service hospitalier. Paris: Universite Pierre et Marie Curie.

Lanhers MC, Fleurentin J, Mortier F, Vinche A, Younos C. Anti-inflammatory and analgesic effects of an aqueous extract of *Harpagophytum procumbens. Planta Med.* 1992;58:117–123.

Mabberley DJ. *The Plant-Book: A Portable Dictionary of the Higher Plants.* Cambridge, England: Cambridge University Press; 1987.

McLeod D, et al. Investigations of *Harpagophytum procumbens* (Devil's Claw) in the treatment of experimental inflammation and arthritis in the rat. *Br J Pharmacol.* 1979;66:140P

Moussard C, Alber D, Toubin M, Thevenon N, Henry JC. A drug used in traditional medicine, *Harpagophytum procumbens:* no evidence for NSAID-like effect on whole blood eicosanoid production in human. *Prostaglandins Leukot Essent Fatty Acids.* 1992;46:283–286.

Newall C, Anderson L, Phillipson J. *Herbal Medicines: A Guide for Health-care Professionals.* London, England: Pharmaceutical Press; 1996.

Occhiuto F, Circosta C, Ragusa S, Ficarra P, Costa De Pasquale R. A drug used in traditional medicine: *Harpagophytum procumbens* DC. IV. Effects on some isolated muscle preparations. *J Ethnopharmacol.* 1985;13:201–208.

Schulz V, Hänsel R, Tyler VE. *Rational Phytotherapy: A Physician's Guide to Herbal Medicine.* 3rd ed. Berlin, Germany: Springer-Verlag; 1998.

Tyler VE. *The Honest Herbal: A Sensible Guide to the Use of Herbs and Related Remedies.* 3rd ed. Binghampton, NY: Pharmaceutical Products Press; 1993.

Whitehouse L, et al. Devil's Claw *(Harpagophytum procumbens):* no evidence for anti-inflammatory activity in the treatment of arthritic disease. *Can Med Assoc J.* 1983;129:249–251.

ECHINACEA

Berman S. Dramatic increase in immune-mediated HIV killing activity induced by *Echinacea angustifolia. Int Conf AIDS* 12 (582). Abstract 32309.

Blumenthal M, ed. *The Complete German Commission E Monographs.* Boston, Mass: Integrative Medicine Communications; 1998.

Bräunig B, Dorn M, Knick E. *Echinacea purpurea radix* for strengthening the immune response in flu-like infections. *Z Phytotherapie.* 1992;13:7–13.

Dorn M, Knick E, Lewith G. Placebo-controlled, double-blind study of *Echinacea pallidae radix* in upper respiratory tract infections. *Complementary Therapies in Medicine.* 1997;5:40–42.

Hobbs C. Echinacea: a literature review. *Herbalgram* 1994;30:33–47.

Hoheisel O, Sandberg M, Bertram S, Bulitta M, Schäfer M. Echinagard treatment shortens the course of the common cold: a double-blind, placebo-controlled clinical trial. *European Journal of Clinical Research.* 1997;9:261–269.

Hyman R, Pankhurst R. *Plants and Their Names: A Concise Dictionary.* New York, NY: Oxford University Press; 1995.

McGuffin M, Hobbs C, Upton R, Goldberg A, eds. *American Herbal Products Association's Botanical Safety Handbook.* Boca Raton, Fla: CRC Press; 1996.

Melchart D, Walther E, Linde K, Brandmaier R, Lersch C. Echinacea root extracts for the prevention of upper respiratory tract infections: a double-blind, placebo-controlled randomized trial. *Arch Fam Med.* 1998;7:541–545.

Melchart D, Linde IK, Worku F, Sarkady L, Holzmann M, Jurcic K, et al. Results of Five Randomized Studies on the Immunomodulatory Activity of Preparations of Echinacea. *J Alt Comp Med.* 1995;1(2):145–160.

Murray MT. *The Healing Power of Herbs: The Enlightened Person's Guide to the Wonders of Medicinal Plants.* Rocklin, Calif: Prima Publishing; 1995.

Newall CA, Anderson LA, Phillipson JD. *Herbal Medicines: A Guide for Health-Care Professionals.* London: The Pharmaceutical Press; 1996.

Schulz V, Hänsel R, Tyler VE. *Rational Phytotherapy: A Physicians' Guide to Herbal Medicine.* 3rd ed. Berlin: Springer; 1998.

Snow JM. *Echinacea. Protocol J Botanical Medicine.* 1997;2:18–24.

Thompson KD. Antiviral activity of Viracea against acyclovir susceptible and acyclovir resistant strains of herpes simplex virus. *Antiviral Res.* 1998;39:55–61.

Tyler VE. *Herbs of Choice: The Therapeutic Use of Phytomedicinals.* Binghamton, NY: Pharmaceutical Products Press; 1994.

Verhoef MJ, Hagen N, Pelletier G, Forsyth P. Alternative therapy use in neurologic disease: use in brain tumor patients. *Neurology* 1999;52:617–622.

EUCALYPTUS

Belzner S. [Eucalyptus oil dressings in urinary retention] Eukalyptusol-kompresse bei harnverhalten. *Pflege Aktuell.* 1997;51:386–387.

Benouda A, Hassar M, Menjilali B. In vitro antibacterial properties of essential oils, tested against hospital pathogenic bacteria. *Fitoterapia.* 1988;59:115119.

Blumenthal M, ed. *The Complete German Commission E Monographs.* Boston, Mass: Integrative Medicine Communications; 1998.

Bremness L. *Herbs.* New York, NY: DK Publishing; 1994.

Burrow A, Eccles R, Jones AS. The effects of camphor, eucalyptus and menthol vapour on nasal resistance to airflow and nasal sensation. *Acta Otolaryngol (Stockh).* 1983;96(1-2):157–161.

Castleman M. *The Healing Herbs.* Emmaus, Pa: Rodale Press; 1991.

El-keltawi NEM, Megalla SE, Ross SA. Antimicrobial activity of some Egyptian aromatic plants. *Herba Pol.* 1980;26:245250.

Evans WC. *Trease and Evans' Pharmacognosy.* 13th ed. London, England: Bailliere Tindall; 1989.

Gruenwald J, Brendler T et al, eds. *PDR for Herbal Medicines.* Montvale, NJ: Medical Economics Company Inc; 1998.

Kumar A, et al. Antibacterial properties of some *Eucalyptus* oils. *Fitoterapia.* 1988;59:141-144.

Leung A, Foster S. *Encyclopedia of Common Natural Ingredients Used in Food, Drugs, and Cosmetics.* 2nd ed. New York, NY: Wiley & Sons; 1996.

McGuffin M, Hobbs C, Upton R, Goldberg A. *American Herbal Products Associations's Botanical Safety Handbook.* Boca Raton, Fla: CRC Press; 1996.

Newall CA, Anderson LA, Phillipson JD. *Herbal Medicines: A Guide for Health Care Professionals.* London, England: The Pharmaceutical Press; 1996:72–73.

Nichimura H, Calvin M. Essential oil of Eucalyptus globulus in California. *J Agr Food Chem.* 1979;27:432–435.

Osawa K, et al. Macrocarpals H, I, and J from the Leaves of *Eucalyptus globulus. J Nat Prod.* 1996;59:823–827.

Tovey ER, McDonald LG. Clinical aspects of allergic disease: A simple washing procedure with eucalyptus oil for controlling house dust mites and their allergens in clothing and bedding. *J Allergy Clin Immunol.* 1997;100:464–467.

Whitman BW, Ghazizadeh H. Eucalyptus oil: therapeutic and toxic aspects of pharmacology in humans and animals [letter; comment]. *J Paediatr Child Health.* 1994;30(2):190–191.

EVENING PRIMROSE

Belch JJR, Ansell D, Madhok R, O'Dowd A, Sturrock RD. Effects of altering dietary essential fatty acids on requirements for NSAIDs in patients with rheumatoid arthritis. *Ann Rheum Dis.* 1988;47:96–104.

Blumenthal M, Riggins C. *Popular Herbs in the U.S. Market: Therapeutic Monographs.* Austin, Tex: The American Botanical Council; 1997.

Brehler R, Hildebrand A, Luger TA. Clinical reviews: recent developments in the treatment of atopic eczema. *J Am Acad Dermatol.* 1997; 36: 989–990.

Foster S. *Herbal Renaissance: Growing, Using and Understanding Herbs in the Modern World.* Salt Lake City, Utah: Gibbs-Smith; 1993.

Fugh-Berman A. Complementary and Alternative Therapies in Primary Care: Clinical trials of herbs. *Primary Care: Clinics in Office Practice.* 1997; 24: 889–903.

Graham-Brown R. Psychodermatology: Managing adults with atopic dermatitis. *Dermatologic Clinics.* 1996;14: 536.

Greenfield S.M, et al. A randomized controlled study of evening primrose oil and fish oil in ulcerative colitis. *Aliment Pharmacol Ther.* 1993;7:159–166.

Horrobin DF. Interactions between n-3 and n-6 essential fatty acids (EFAs) in the regulation of cardiovascular disorders and inflammation. *Prostaglandins Leukot Essent Fatty Acids.* 1991;44:127–131.

Horrobin DF. The relationship between schizophrenia and essential fatty acid and eicosanoid metabolism. *Prostaglandins Leukot Essent Fatty Acids.* 1992;46:71–77.

Jamal GA, Carmichael H. The effect of y-linolenic acid on human diabetic peripheral neuropathy: A double-blind placebo-controlled trial. *Diabetic Med.* 7:319-323.

Khoo SK, Munro C, Battistutta, D. 1990. Evening primrose oil and treatment of premenstrual syndrome. *Med J Aust.* 153.

Leung A, Foster S. *Encyclopedia of Common Natural Ingredients Used in Food, Drugs, and Cosmetics.* 2nd ed. New York, NY: Wiley & Sons; 1996.

McGuffin M, Hobbs C, Upton R, Goldberg A. *American Herbal Products Associations' Botanical Safety Handbook.* Boca Raton, Fla: CRC Press; 1996.

Murray M. *The Encyclopedia of Nutritional Supplements.* Rocklin, Calif: Prima Publishing; 1996.

Newall CA, Anderson LA, Phillipson JD. *Herbal Medicines: A Guide for Health Care Professionals.* London, England: The Pharmaceutical Press; 1996.

Scarff DH, Lloyd DH. Double-blind, placebo-controlled crossover study of evening primrose oil in the treatment of canine atopy. *Veterinary.* 1992.

Schultz V, Hansel R, Tyler V. Rational Phytotherapy: *A Physician's Guide to Herbal Medicine.* Heidelberg: Springer-Verlag; 1998.

Stewart JCM, et al. Treatment of severe and moderately severe atopic dermatitis with evening primrose oil (Epogam): a multi-center study. *J Nut Med.* 1991;2:9–16.

FEVERFEW

Blumenthal M, ed. *The Complete German Commission E Monographs. Therapeutic Guide to Herbal Medicines.* Boston, Mass: Integrative Medicine Communications; 1998:12.

Bradley P, ed. *British Herbal Compendium.* Dorset, England: British Herbal Medicine Association; 1992:1:96–98

Brown D. *Herbal Prescriptions for Better Health.* Rocklin, Calif: Prima Publishing; 1996:91–95

De Weerdt CJ, Bootsma HPR, Hendriks H. Herbal Medicines in migraine prevention. Randomized double-blind placebo controlled crossover trial of a feverfew preparation. *Phytomedicine.* 1996;3:225–230.

Grieve M. *A Modern Herbal.* New York, NY: Dover; 1971:1:309–310.

Gruenwald J, Brendler T, Jaenicke C et al, eds. *PDR for Herbal Medicines.* Montvale, NJ: Medical Economics Company; 1998:1171–1173.

Heptinstall S, Groenewegen W, Spangenberg P, Lösche W. Inhibition of platelet behavior by feverfew: a mechanism of action involving sulfhydryl groups. *Folia Haematol Int Mag Klin Morphol Blutforsch.* 1988;43:447–449.

Johnson ES, Kadam NP, Hylands DM, Hylands PJ. Efficacy of feverfew as prophylactic treatment of migraine. *Br Med J.* 1985;291:569–573.

Johnson ES. Patients who chew chrysanthemum leaves. *MIMS Magazine* May 15, 1983:32–35.

Murphy JJ, Heptinstall S, Mitchell JR. Randomised double-blind placebo-controlled trial of feverfew in migraine prevention. *Lancet.* 1988;2:189–192.

Murray MT. *The Healing Power of Herbs: The Enlightened Person's Guide to the Wonders of Medicinal Plants.* 2nd ed. Rocklin, Calif: Prima Publishing; 1995.

Newall CA, Anderson LA, Phillipson JD. *Herbal Medicines: A Guide for Health-care Professionals.* London, England: Pharmaceutical Press; 1996:119–120.

Palevitch D, Earon G, Carasso R. Feverfew *(Tanacetum parthenium)* as a prophylactic treatment for migraine: a double-blind controlled study. *Phytotherapy Res.* 1997;11:508–511.

Pattrick M, Heptinstall S, Doherty M. Feverfew in rheumatoid arthritis: a double-blind, placebo controlled study. *Ann Rheum Dis.* 1989;48:547–549.

Tyler VE. *Herbs of Choice: The Therapeutic Use of Phytomedicinals.* Binghamton, NY: Pharmaceutical Products Press; 1994:126–134.

Tyler VE. *The Honest Herbal: A Sensible Guide to the Use of Herbs and Related Remedies.* 3rd ed. Binghamton, NY: Pharmaceutical Products Press; 1993.

FLAXSEED

Allman MA, Pena MM, Pang D. Supplementation with flaxseed oil versus sunflowerseed oil in healthy young men consuming a low fat diet: effects on platelet composition and function. *Eur J Clin Nutr.* 1995;49:169–178.

Bierenbuam ML, Reichstein R, Watkins TR. Reducing atherogenic risk in hyperlipemic humans with flax seed supplementation: a preliminary report. *J Am Coll Nutr.* 1993;12:501–504.

Blumenthal M, ed. *The Complete German Commission E Monographs. Therapeutic Guide to Herbal Medicines.* Boston, Mass: Integrative Medicine Communications; 1998:47,132.

British Herbal Pharmacopoeia. 4th ed. Dorset, England: British Herbal Medicine Association; 1996.

Clark WF, et al. Flaxseed: a potential treatment of lupus nephritis. *Kidney International.* 1995;48:475–480.

Cunnane SC, et al. High alpha-linolenic acid flaxseed *(Linum usitatissimum):* some nutritional properties in humans. *Br J Nutr.* 1993;69:443–453.

Cunnane SC. Nutritional attributes of traditional flaxseed in healthy-young adults. *Am J Clin Nutr.* 1995;61:62–68.

De Smet P. *Adverse Effects of Herbal Drugs.* New York, NY: Springer-Verlag; 1997.

Grieve M. *A Modern Herbal.* New York, NY: Dover; 1971:1:309–310.

Gruenwald J, Brendler T, Christof J. *PDR for Herbal Medicines.* Montvale, NJ: Medical Economics Company; 1998:940–941.

Prasad K, Mantha S, Muir A, Westcott N. Reduction of hypercholesterolemic arteriosclerosis by CDC-flaxseed with very low alpha-linolenic acid. *Arteriosclerosis.* 1998;434:367–375.

Serraino M, Thompson L. The effect of flaxseed supplementation on the initiation and promotional stages of mammary tumorigenesis. *Nutr Cancer.* 1992;25:153–159.

Sung M, Lautens M, Thompson L. Mammalian lignans inhibit the growth of estrogen-independent human colon tumor cells. *Anticancer Research.* 1998;1346:1405–1408.

Thompson L, Richard S, Orcheson L, Seidl M. Flaxseed and its lignan and oil components reduce mammary tumor growth at a late stage of carcinogenesis. *Carcinogenesis.* 1996;434:1373–1376.

Yan L, Yee J, Li D, McGuire M, Thompson L. Dietary flaxseed supplementation and experimental metastasis of melanoma cells in mice. *Cancer Lett.* 1998;61:181–186.

GARLIC

Berthold HK, et al. Effect of a garlic oil preparation on serum lipoproteins and cholesterol metabolism. *JAMA.* 1998;279.

Bradley PR, ed. *British Herbal Compendium.* Dorset, England: British Herbal Medicine Association; 1992:1:105–108.

DeSmet PAGM, Keller K, Hänsel R, Chandler RF, eds. *Adverse Effects of Herbal Drugs.* Berlin, Germany: Springer-Verlag; 1997:235–236.

Gruenwald J, Brendler T, Jaenicke C et al, eds. *PDR for Herbal Medicines.* Montvale, NJ: Medical Economics Company 1998:940–941.

Kiesewetter, H; Jung F, Mrowietz C, et al. Effects of garlic on blood fluidity and fibrinolytic activity: a randomised, placebo-controlled, double-blind study. *Br J Clin Pract.* 1990;44:24–29.

Mader FH. Treatment of hyperlipidaemia with garlic-powder tablets. Evidence from the German Association of General Practitioners' multicentric placebo-controlled double-blind study. *Arzneimittelforschung.* October 1990;40:1111–1116.

Murray MT. *The Healing Power of Herbs: The Enlightened Person's Guide to the Wonders of Medicinal Plants.* Second Ed. Rocklin, Calif: Prima Publishing; 1995:121–131.

Newall C, Anderson L, Phillipson J. *Herbal Medicines: A Guide for Health-care Professionals.* London, England: Pharmaceutical Press; 1996:129–133.

Orekhov A, Tertov V, Sobenin I, Pivovorava E. Direct antiatherosclerosis-related effects of garlic. *Ann Med.* 1995;37:63–65.

Schulz V, Hansel R, Tyler V. *Rational Phytotherapy: A Physician's Guide to Herbal Medicine.* 3rd ed. Berlin, Germany: Springer-Verlag; 1998:107–123.

Silagy C, Neil A. Garlic as a lipid lowering agent-a meta-analysis. *JR Coll Physicians Lond.* 1994;28:39–45.

Steiner M, Khan AH, Holbert D, Lin RI. A double-blind crossover study in moderately hypercholesterolemic men that compared the effect of aged garlic extract and placebo administration on blood lipids. *Am J Clin Nutr.* 1996;64:866–870.

Tyler V. *Herbs of Choice: The Therapeutic Use of Phytomedicinals.* Binghamton, NY: Pharmaceutical Products Press; 1994:104–115.

Tyler V. *The Honest Herbal: A Sensible Guide to the Use of Herbs and Related Remedies.* 3rd ed. Binghamton, NY: Pharmaceutical Products Press; 1993:139–143.

Warshafsky S, Kramer RS, Sivak SL. Effect of garlic on total serum cholesterol. *Ann Intern Med.* 1993;119:599–605.

GINGER ROOT

Awang DVC. Ginger. *Can Pharma J.* 1992:309–311.

Blumenthal M, ed. *The Complete German Commission E Monographs: Therapeutic Guide to Herbal Medicine.* Boston, Mass: Integrative Medicine Communications; 1998.

Blumenthal M, Riggins CW. *American Botanical Council's Popular Herbs in the U.S. Market: Therapeutic Monographs.* Austin, Texas: ABC; 1997:33–240.

Bremness L. *Herbs: The Visual Guide to More than 700 Herb Species from around the World.* London: Dorling Kindersley Limited; 1994.

Duke JA. *The Green Pharmacy.* Emmaus, Pa: Rodale Press; 1997.

USP publishes information monographs on ginger and valerian. *HerbalGram.* 1998;43:30, 57, 71.

Grontved A, et al. Ginger root against seasickness: a controlled trial on the open sea. *Acta Otolaryngol.* 1988;105:45-49.

Kowalchik C, Hylton W, ed. *Rodale's Illustrated Encyclopedia of Herbs.* Emmaus, Pa: Rodale Press; 1998.

McGuffin M, Hobbs C, Upton R, Goldberg A, eds. *American Herbal Products Association's Botanical Safety Handbook.* Boca Raton, Fla: CRC Press; 1997.

Nagabhushan M, Amonkar AJ, Bhide SV. Mutagenicity of gingerol and shogoal and antimutagenicity of zingerone in salmonella/microsome assay. *Cancer Lett.* 1987;36:221-233.

Nakamura H, Yamamoto T. Mutagen and anti-mutagen in ginger, *Zingiber officinale.* *Mutat Res.* 1982;103:119-126.

Newall CA, Anderson LA, Phillipson JD. *Herbal Medicines: A Guide for Health-care Professionals.* London: The Pharmaceutical Press; 1996:157–159.

Schulick P. The many roles of ginger. *Natural Foods Merchandiser's Nutrition Science News.* 1995:6–7.

Schulz V, Hänsel R, Tyler VE. *Rational Phytotherapy: A Physicians' Guide to Herbal Medicine.* 3rd ed. Berlin, Germany: Springer; 1998.

Yeung H. *Handbook of Chinese Herbs and Formulas.* Los Angeles, Calif: Los Angeles Institute of Chinese Medicine; 1985:1.

GINKGO BILOBA

Bauer U. Six-month double-blind randomized clinical trial of *Ginkgo biloba* extract versus placebo in two parallel groups of patients suffering from peripheral arterial insufficiency. *Arzneimittelforschung.* 1984;34:716–720.

Blumenthal M, ed. *The Complete German Commission E Monographs: Therapeutic Guide to Herbal Medicines.* Boston, Mass: Integrative Medicine Communications; 1998.

Brown D. *Herbal Prescriptions for Better Health.* Rocklin, Calif: Prima Publishing; 1996.

Carper J. *Miracle Cures.* New York, NY: HarperCollins, 1997.

DeSmet PAGM, Keller K, Hänsel R, Chandler RF, eds. *Adverse Effects of Herbal Drugs.* Berlin, Germany: Springer-Verlag; 1997.

Kinghorn A, Ed. *Human Medicinal Agents from Plants.* Washington, DC: American Chemical Society, 1993.

Le Bars PL, Katz MM, Berman N, Itil TM, Freedman AM, Schatzberg AF. A placebo-controlled, double-blind, randomized trial of an extract of *Ginkgo biloba* for dementia. *JAMA.* 1997;278:1327–1332.

Murray M. *The Healing Power of Herbs: The Enlightened Person's Guide to the Wonders of Medicinal Plants.* 2nd ed. Rocklin, Calif: Prima Publishing; 1995.

Newall C, et al. *Herbal Medicines: A Guide for Health-care Professionals.* London, England: Pharmaceutical Press; 1996.

Peters H, Kieser M, Holscher U. Demonstration of the efficacy of *Ginkgo biloba* special extract Egb 761 on intermittent claudication a placebo-controlled, double-blind trial. *Vasa.* 1998;27:105–110.

Schulz V, Hänsel R, Tyler VE. *Rational Phytotherapy: A Physicians' Guide to Herbal Medicine.* Berlin, Germany: Springer-Verlag; 1998.

GINSENG, AMERICAN

Bahrke M, Morgan P. Evaluation of the ergogenic properties of ginseng. *Sports Medicine.* 1994;18:229–248.

Blumenthal M, ed. *The Complete German Commission E Monographs.* Boston, Mass: Integrative Medicine Communications; 1998.

Blumenthal M, Riggins C. *Popular Herbs in the U.S. Market: Therapeutic Monographs.* Austin, Tex: The American Botanical Council; 1997.

Chen X, et al. The effects of Panax quinquefolium saponin (PQS) and its monomer ginsenoside on heart. *Chung Kuo Chung Yao Tsa Chih.* 1994;19:617–20, 640.

Foster S. *Herbal Renaissance: Growing, Using and Understanding Herbs in the Modern World.* Salt Lake City, Utah: Gibbs-Smith; 1993.

Huang KC. *The Pharmacology of Chinese Herbs.* Boca Raton, Fla: CRC Press; 1993.

Kowalchik C, Hylton W, eds. *Rodale's Illustrated Encyclopedia of Herbs.* Emmaus, Pa: Rodale Press; 1998.

Kwan CY. Vascular effects of selected antihypertensive drugs derived from traditional medicinal herbs. *Clin Exp Pharmacol Physiol.* 1995;(suppl 1):S297–S299. Review.

Li J, et al. Panax quinquefolium saponins protects low density lipoproteins from oxidation. *Life Sci.* 1999;64:53–62.

McGuffin M, Hobbs C, Upton R, Goldberg A. *American Herbal Products Association's Botanical Safety Handbook.* Boca Raton, Fla: CRC Press; 1996.

Murphy LL, et al. Effect of American ginseng (Panax quinquefolium) on male copulatory behavior in the rat. *Physiol Behav.* 1998;64:445–450.

Murray M. *The Healing Power of Herbs: the Enlightened Person's Guide to the Wonders of Medicinal Plants.* Rocklin, Calif: Prima Publishing; 1995.

Newall CA, Anderson LA, Phillipson JD. *Herbal Medicines: A Guide for Health Care Professionals.* London, England: The Pharmaceutical Press; 1996.

Oshima Y. Isolation and hypoglycemic activity of quinquefolans A, B, and C, glycans of *Panax quinquefolium* roots. J Nat Prod. 1987;50:188–190.

Schultz V, Hansel R, Tyler V. *Rational Phytotherapy: A Physicians' Guide to Herbal Medicine.* New York, NY: Springer; 1998.

Thornton L. The ethics of wildcrafting. *The Herb Quarterly.* 1998:41–46.

Waki I. Effects of a hypoglycemic component of Ginseng radix on insulin biosynthesis in normal and diabetic animals. *J Pharmacobiodyn.* 1982;5:547–554.

Yuan CS, et al. Modulation of American ginseng on brainstem GABAergic effects in rats. *J Ethnopharmacol.* 1998;62:215–222.

GINSENG, ASIAN

Bahrke M, Morgan P. Evaluation of the ergogenic properties of ginseng. *Sports Medicine.* 1994;18:229–248.

Blumenthal M, ed. *The Complete German Commission E Monographs.* Boston, Mass: Integrative Medicine Communications; 1998.

Blumenthal M, Riggins C. *Popular Herbs in the U.S. Market: Therapeutic Monographs.* Austin, Tex: The American Botanical Council; 1997.

Choi HK, Seong DH, Rha KH. Clinical Efficacy of Korean red ginseng for erectile dysfunction. *Int J Impotence Res.* 1995;7:181–186.

D'Angelo L, et al. A double-blind, placebo-controlled clinical study on the effect of a standardized ginseng extract on psychomotor performance in healthy volunteer. *J Ethnopharmacol.* 1986;16:15–22.

Dega H, Laporte JL, Frances C, Herson S, Chosidow O. Ginseng as a cause for Stevens-Johnson Syndrome? *Lancet.* 1996;347:1344.

De Smet PAGM, Keller K, Hansel R, Chandler RF, eds. *Adverse Effects of Herbal Drugs.* New York, NY: Springer-Verlag; 1992:1.

Dorling E. Do ginsenosides influence the performance? Results of a double-blind study. *Notabene medici.* 1980;10:241–246.

Foster S. *Asian Ginseng.* Austin, Tex: The American Botanical Council; 1996.

Gross D, Krieger D, Efrat R, Dayan M. Ginseng extract G115 for the treatment of chronic respiratory diseases. *Schweizerische Zeitschrift fur Ganzheits Medizin.* 1995;1(95):29–33.

Huang KC. *The Pharmacology of Chinese Herbs.* Boca Raton, Fla: CRC Press; 1993.

Kowalchïk C, Hylton W, eds. *Rodale's Illustrated Encyclopedia of Herbs.* Emmaus, Pa: Rodale Press; 1998.

McGuffin M, Hobbs C, Upton R, Goldberg A. *American Herbal Products Association's Botanical Safety Handbook.* Boca Raton, Fla: CRC Press; 1996.

Murray M. *The Healing Power of Herbs: the Enlightened Person's Guide to the Wonders of Medicinal Plants.* Rocklin, Calif: Prima Publishing; 1995.

Newall CA, Anderson LA, Phillipson JD. *Herbal Medicines: A Guide for Health-Care Professionals.* London, England: The Pharmaceutical Press; 1996.

Quiroga HA, Imbriano AE. The effect of *Panax ginseng* extract on cerebrovascular deficits. *Orientacion Medica.* 1979;1208:86–87.

Quiroga HA. Comparative double-blind study of the effect of Ginsana Gii5 and Hydergin on cerebrovascular deficits. *Orientacion Medica.* 1982;1281:201–202.

Schulz V, Hansel R, Tyler V. *Rational Phytotherapy: A Physicians' Guide to Herbal Medicine.* New York, NY: Springer; 1998.

Sun XB, Matsumoto T, Yamada H. Purification of immune complexes clearance enhancing polysaccharide from the leaves of *Panax ginseng*, and its biological activities. *Phytomedicine.* 1994;1:225–231.

Tang W, Eisenbrand G. *Chinese Drugs of Plant Origin: Chemistry, Pharmacology, and Use in Traditional and Modern Medicine.* New York, NY: Springer; 1992.

You JS, Hau DM, Chen KT, Huang HF. Combined effects of ginseng and radiotherapy on experimental liver cancer. *Phytotherapy Research.* 1995;9:331–335.

GINSENG, SIBERIAN

Asano K, et al. Effect of *Eleutherococcus senticosus* extract on human physical working capacity. *Planta Medica.* 1986;3:175–177.

Awang D. Siberian ginseng toxicity may be case of mistaken identity. *Can Med Assoc J.* 1996;155:1237.

Blumenthal M, Riggins C. *Popular Herbs in the U.S. Market: Therapeutic Monographs.* Austin, Tex: The American Botanical Council; 1997.

Blumenthal M, ed. *The Complete German Commission E Monographs.* Boston, Mass: Integrative Medicine Communications; 1998.

Farnsworth N, Wagner H, Kikino H. *Economic and Medicinal Plant Research.* London, England: Academic Press Inc; 1985:1.

Foster S. *Siberian Ginseng (Eleutherococcus senticosus).* Austin, Tex: American Botanical Council; 1990.

Hacker B, Medon P. Cytotoxic effects of *E. sentococcus aqueous* extract against L1210 leukemia cells. *J Pharm Sci.* 1984;73:270–272.

Hebel S, ed. Eleutherococcus. *The Lawrence Review of Natural Products.* Facts and Comparisons; 1996:1–3.

Kaloeva ZD. Effect of glycosides from *Eleutherococcus senticosus* on the parameters of hemodynamics in patients with hypotension. *Farmakol Toksikol.* 1986;49:73.

Leung A, Foster S. *Encyclopedia of Common Natural Ingredients Used in Food, Drugs, and Cosmetics.* 2nd ed. New York, NY: John Wiley & Sons, Inc; 1996.

McGuffin M, Hobbs C, Upton R, Goldberg A. *American Herbal Products Association's Botanical Safety Handbook.* Boca Raton, Fla: CRC Press; 1996.

Murray M. *The Healing Power of Herbs: the Enlightened Person's Guide to the Wonders of Medicinal Plants.* Rocklin, Calif: Prima Publishing; 1995.

Newall CA, Anderson LA, Phillipson JD. *Herbal Medicines: A Guide for Health-Care Professionals.* London, England: The Pharmaceutical Press; 1996.

Novozhilov GN, Sil'chenko KI. The mechanism of adaptogenic action of *Eleutherococcus senticosus* extract on the human body under thermal stress. *Fiziol Cheloveka.* 1985;11:303–306.

Schulz V, Hansel R, Tyler V. *Rational Phytotherapy: A Physicians' Guide to Herbal Medicine.* New York, NY: Springer; 1998.

Wu Jia Seng: Acanthopanax senticosus [in Chinese]. Heilungkiang Institute of Traditional Chinese Medicine. [No date].

Xiao P-G, et al. Immunological aspects of Chinese medicinal plants as antiaging drugs. *J Ethnopharmacol.* 1993;38:167–175.

GOLDENSEAL

Balch J, Balch P. *Prescription for Nutritional Healing: A-to-Z Guide to Drug-Free Remedies Using Vitamins, Minerals, Herbs, & Food Supplements.* New York, NY: Avery Publishing Group; 1990.

Duke JA. *Handbook of Phytochemical Constituents of GRAS Herbs and Other Economic Plants.* Boca Raton, Fla: CRC Press; 1992.

Foster S. Goldenseal. *American Botanical Council: Botanical Series No. 309.*

Genest K, Hughes DW. Natural products in Canadian pharmaceuticals, *Hydrastis canadensis. Can J Pharm Sci.* 1969;4.

Kaneda Y, Tanaka T, Saw T. Effects of berberine, a plant alkaloid, on the growth of anaerobic protozoa in axenic culture. *Tokai J Exp Clin Med.* 1990;15:417–423.

Mills SY. *Dictionary of Modern Herbalism: A Comprehensive Guide to Practical Herbal Therapy.* Rochester, Vt: Healing Arts Press; 1988.

Nishino H, et al. Berberine sulfate inhibits tumor-promoting activity of teleocidin in two-stage carcinogenesis on mouse skin. *Oncology.* 1986;43:131–134.

Shideman FE. A review of the pharmacology and therapeutics of Hydrastis and its alkaloids, hydrastine, berberine and canadine. *Comm on Nat Formulary Bull.* 1950;18:3–19.

Sun D, Courtney HS, Beachey EH. Berberine sulfate blocks adherence of Streptococcus pyogenes to epithelial cells, fibronectin, and hexadecane. *Antimicrob Agents Chemother.* 1988;32:1370–1374.

Swanston-Flatt SK, et al. Evaluation of traditional plant treatments for diabetes: studies in streptozotocin diabetic mice. *Acta Diabetol Lat.* 1989;26:51–55.

Zhu B, Ahrens FA. Effect of berberine on intestinal secretion mediated by Escherichia coli heat-stable enterotoxin in jejunum of pigs. *Am J Vet Res.* 1982; 43:1594–1598.

GRAPE SEED EXTRACT

Amsellem M, et al. Endotelon in the treatment of venolymphatic problems in premenstrual syndrome: multi-center study on 165 patients. *Tempo Medical.* 1987;282.

Ariga TK, Hamano M. Radical scavenging action and its mode in procyanidins B-1 and B-3 from azuki beans to peroxyl radicals. *Agricultural Biological Chemistry.* 1990;54:2499–2504.

Baruch J. Effect of grape seed extract in postoperative edema [in French]. *Ann Chir Plast Esthet.* 1984;4.

Blumenthal M, Riggins C. *Popular Herbs in the U.S. Market: Therapeutic Monographs.* Austin, Tex: American Botanical Council; 1997.

Bombardelli E, Morazzoni P. *Vitis vinifera L. Fitoterapia.* 1995; 66:291–317.

Chang WC, Hsu FL. Inhibition of platelet aggregation and arachidonate metabolism in platelets by procyanidins. *Prostagland Leukotri Essential Fatty Acids.* 1989;38:181–188.

Corbe C, Boissin JP, Siou A. Light vision and chorioretinal circulation: study of the effect of procyanidolic oligomers (Endotelon) [in French]. *J Fr Ophthalmol.* 1988;11:453–460.

Delacrois P. Double-blind study of grape seed extract in chronic venous insufficiency. *La Revue De Med.* 1981;28–31.

Fromantin M. Les oligomeres procyanidoliques dans le traitement de la fragilite capillaire et de la retinopathie chez les diabetiques: a propos de 26 cas. *Med Int.* 1982;16.

Kashiwada Y, et al. Antitumor agents, 129: tannins and related compounds as selective cytotoxic agents. *J Nat Prod.* 1992;55:1033–1043.

Lagrua G, et al. A study of the effects of procyanidol oligomers on capillary resistance in hypertension and in certain nephropathis. *Sem Hop.* 1981;57:1399–1401.

Maffei FR, Carini M, Aldini G, Bombardelli E, Morazzoni P, Morelli R. Free radical scavenging action and anti-enzyme activities of procyanidins from *Vitis vinifera*: a mechanism for their capillary protective action. *Arzneimittelfarichung.* May 1994; 44:592–601.

Maffei FR, Carini M, Aldini G, Bombardelli E, Morazzoni P. Sparing effect of procyanidins from *Vitis vinifera* on vitamin E: in vitro studies. *Planta Med.* 1998;64:343–347.

Masquelier J. Comparative action of various vitamin P related factors on the oxidation of ascorbic acid by cupric ions. *Bulletin de la Societe de Chimie Biologique.* 1951;33:304–305.

Masquelier J. Natural products as medicinal agents. *Planta Med.* 1980;242S–256S.

Meunier, M.T., et al. Inhibition of angiotensin I converting enzyme by flavonolic compounds: in vitro and in vivo studies. *Planta Med.* 1987;53: 12–15.

Murray M. *The Healing Power of Herbs: the Enlightened Person's Guide to the Wonders of Medicinal Plants.* Rocklin, Calif: Prima Publishing; 1995.

Schulz V, Hänsel R, Tyler V. *Rational Phytotherapy: A Physician's Guide to Herbal Medicine.* New York, NY: Springer-Verlag; 1998.

Schwitters B, Masquelier J. *OPC in Practice: The Hidden Story of Proanthocyanidins, Nature's Most Powerful and Patented Antioxidant.* Rome, Italy: Alfa Omega Publishers; 1995.

Tebib, K, et al. Dietary grape seed tannins affect lipoproteins, lipoprotein lipases, and tissue lipids in rats fed hypercholesterolemic diets. *J Nutr.* 1994; 124: 2451–2457.

Tebib K, et al. Polymeric grape seed tannins prevent plasma cholesterol changes in high-cholesterol-fed rats. *Food Chem.* 1994;49:403–406.

Walker, Morton. The nutritional therapeutics of Masquelier's oligomeric proanthocyanidins (OPCs). *Townsend Letter for Doctors and Patients.* 1996;175/76: 84–92.

Zafirov D, Bredy-Dobreva G, Litchev V, Papasova M. Antiexudative and capillaritonic effects of procyanidines isolated from grape seeds *(V. vinifera)*. *Acta Physiol Pharmacol Bulg.* 1990;16:50–54.

GREEN TEA

Ali M, et al. A potent thromboxane inhibitor in green tea. *Prostaglandins Leukot Essent Fatty Acids.* 1990;40:281–283.

Blumenthal M, ed. *The Complete German Commission E Monographs.* Therapeutic Guide to Herbal Medicines. Boston, Mass: Integrative Medicine Communications; 1998:47, 132.

Bradley P, ed. *British Herbal Compendium.* Dorset, England: British Herbal Medicine Association; 1992:1:96–98.

Heinerman J. *Heinerman's Encyclopedia of Fruits, Vegetables and Herbs.* Englewood Cliffs, NJ: Prentice Hall; 1988:112–113.

Imai K, Nakachi K. Cross sectional study of effects of drinking green tea on cardiovascular and liver diseases. *BMJ.* 1995;310:693–696.

Murray M. *The Healing Power of Herbs: The Enlightened Person's Guide to the Wonders of Medicinal Plants.* Second Ed. Rocklin, Calif: Prima Publishing; 1995.

Poppel Piet A, van den Brandt. Consumption of black tea and cancer risk: a prospective cohort study. *J Natl Cancer Inst.* 1996;88:93–100.

Shim JH, Kang MG, Kim YH, Roberts J, Lee IP. Chemopreventive effect of green tea (Camellia sinensis) among cigarette smoke. *Cancer-Epidemio-Biomarkers-Prev.* 1995;Jun; 4(4): 387-91.

Sirving K. Drinking black tea may cut risk of stroke. *AMA Arch Intern Med.* March 25, 1998.

Snow J. Camellia sinensis (L.) Kuntze (Theaceae). *The Protocol Journal of Botanical Medicine.* 1995;1:47–51.

Tamozawa H, et al. Natural antioxidants I. Antioxidant components of tea leaf (Thea sinensis L.). *Chem Pharm Bull.* 1984;32:2011–2014.

Tyler V. *Herbs of Choice: The Therapeutic Use of Phytomedicinals.* Binghamton, NY: Haworth; 1994.

Wang Z, et al. Antimutagenic activity of green tea polyphenols. *Mutation Research.* 1989;223:273–285.

Windridge C. *The Fountain of Health. An A-Z of Traditional Chinese Medicine.* London, England: Mainstream Publishing; 1994:259.

HAWTHORN

Bahorun T, Gressier B, Trotin F, et al. Oxygen species scavenging activity of phenolic extracts from hawthorn fresh plant organs and pharmaceutical preparations. *Arzneimittelforschung.* 1996;46:1086–1089.

Blumenthal M, ed. *The Complete German Commission E Monographs: Therapeutic Guide to Herbal Medicines.* Boston, Mass: Integrative Medicine Communications; 1998.

Blumenthal M, Riggins C. *American Botanical Council's Popular Herbs in the U.S. Market. Therapeutic Monographs.* Austin Tex: ABC; 1997.

Chaterjee SS. In vitro and in vivo studies on the cardioprotective action of oligomeric procyanidins in a crataegus extract of leaves and blooms. *Arzneimittelforschung.* 1997;47:821–825.

The Criteria Committee of the New York Heart Association I. *Diseases of the Heart and Blood Vessels: Nomenclature and Criteria for Diagnosis.* 6th ed. Boston, Mass: Little, Brown; 1964.

Hoffmann D. Hawthorn: The Heart Helper. *Alternative & Complementary Therapies.* 1995;4:191–192.

Kowalchik C, Hylton W, eds. *Rodale's Illustrated Encyclopedia of Herbs.* Emmaus, Pa: Rodale Press; 1998.

Leuchtgens H. Crataegus special extract WS 1442 in NYHA II heart failure. A placebo controlled randomized double-blind study [in German]. *Fortschr Med.* 1993;111:352–354.

Loew D, Albrecht M, Podzuweit H. Efficacy and tolerability of a Hawthorn preparation in patients with heart failure stage I and II according to NYHA—a surveillance study. Presented at the Second International Congress on Phytomedicine; 1996; Munich, Germany.

McGuffin M, Hobbs C, Upton R, Goldberg A. *American Herbal Products Association's Botanical Safety Handbook.* Boca Raton, Fla: CRC Press; 1997.

Nasa Y, Hashizume AN, Hoque E, Abiko Y. Protective effect of crataegus extract on the cardiac mechanical dysfunction in isolated perfused working rat heart. *Arzneimittelforschung.* 1993;42II(9):945–949.

Newall CA, Anderson LA, Phillipson JD. *Herbal Medicines: A Guide for Health-Care*

Professionals. London, England: The Pharmaceutical Press; 1996.

Nikolov N, Wagner H, Chopin J, Della Monica G, Chari VM, Seligmann O. Recent investigations of crataegus flavonoids. Proceedings of the International Bioflavonoid Symposium; 1981; Munich, Germany.

Popping S, Rose H, Ionescu I, Fischer Y, Kammermeier H. Effect of a hawthorn extract on contraction and energy turnover of isolated rat cardiomyocytes. *Arzneimittelforschung.* 1995;45:1157–1161.

Schmidt U, Kuhn U, Ploch M, Hubner WD. Efficacy of the hawthorn (crataegus) preparation LI 132 in 78 patients with chronic congestive heart failure defined as NYHA functional class II. *Phytomedicine.* 1994;1:17–34.

Schultz V, Hansel R, Tyler V. *Rational Phytotherapy: A Physician's Guide to Herbal Medicine.* Heidelberg: Springer; 1998.

Schussler M, Holzl J, Fricke U. Myocardial effects of flavonoids from crataegus species. *Arzneimittelforschung.* 1995;45:842–845.

Tauchert M, Ploch M, Hubner WD. Effectiveness of hawthorn extract LI 132 compared with the ACE inhibitor Captopril: Multicenter double-blind study with 132 NYHA stage II. *Muench Med Wochenschr.* 1994;136 (suppl):S27–S33.

Vibes J, Lasserre B, and Gleye J. Effects of a methanolic extract from *Crataegus oxycantha* blossoms on TXA2 and PGI2 synthesizing activities of cardiac tissue. *Med Sci Res.* 1993;21:534–436.

Vibes J, Lasserre B, Gleye J, Declume C. Inhibition of thromboxane A2 biosynthesis I vitro by the main components of *Crataegus oxyacantha* (hawthorn) flower heads. *Prostaglandins, Leukotrienes and Essential Fatty Acids.* 1994;50:174–175.

Weikl A, Assmus KD, Neukum-Schmidt A, et al. Crataegus special extract WS 1442. Assessment of objective effectiveness in patients with heart failure. *Fortschr Med.* 1996;114:291–296.

Weiss R F. *Herbal Medicine.* Beaconsfield, England: Beaconsfield Publishers, Ltd; 1988:162–169.

Werbach M. *Botanical Influences on Illness.* Tarzana, Calif: Third Line Press; 1994.

Zapfe G, Assmus KD, Noh HS. Placebo-controlled multicenter study with Crataegus special extract WS 1442: clinical results in the treatment of NYHA II cardiac insufficiency. Presented at the Fifth Congress on Phytotherapy; June 11, 1993; Bonn, Germany.

KAVA KAVA

Blumenthal M, ed. *The Complete German Commission E Monographs: Therapeutic Guide to Herbal Medicines.* Boston, Mass: Integrative Medicine Communications; 1998.

Foster S. *101 Medicinal Herbs.* Loveland, Colo: Interweave Press; 1998.

Kinzler E, Kromer J, Lehmann E. Effect of a special kava extract in patients with anxiety-, tension, and excitation states of non-psychotic genesis. Double blind study with placebos over four weeks [in German]. *Arzneimforsch.* 1991;41:584–588.

Lehmann E, et al. Efficacy of special kava extract *(Piper methysticum)* in patients with states of anxiety, tension and excitedness of non-mental origin—A double blind placebo controlled study of four weeks treatment. *Phytomedicine.* 1996;3:113–119.

Lindenberg Von D, Pitule-Schodel H. D, I-Kavain in comparison with oxazepam in anxiety states. Double-blind clinical trial. *Forscbr Med.* 1990;108:50–54.

McGuffin M, Hobbs C, Upton R, Goldberg A. *American Herbal Products Associations's Botanical Safety Handbook.* Boca Raton, Fla: CRC Press; 1996.

Munte TE, Heinze HJ, Matzke M, et al. Effects of oxazepam and an extract of kava roots *(Piper methysticum)* on event-related potentials in a word recognition task. *Neuropsychobiology.* 1993;27:46–53.

Schulz V, Hänsel R, Tyler V. *Rational Phytotherapy: A Physicians' Guide to Herbal Medicine.* New York, NY: Springer-Verlag; 1998.

Singh YD, Blumenthal M. Kava: An overview. *HerbalGram.* 39:34–55.

Volz HP, Kieser M. Kava-kava extract WS 1490 versus placebo in anxiety disorders—a randomized placebo-controlled 25-week outpatient trial. *Pharmacopsychiatry.* 1997;30:1–5.

Warnecke G. Psychosomatic dysfunction in the female climacteric. Clinical effectiveness and tolerance of kava extract WS 1490 [in German]. *Fortschr Med.* 1991;109:119–122.

LEMON BALM

Auf'mkolk M, Ingbar JC, Kubota K, et al. Extracts and auto-oxidized constituents of certain plants inhibit the receptor-binding and the biological activity of Graves' immunoglobulins. *Endocrinology.* 1985;116:1687–1693.

Auf'mkolk M, Hesch H, Ingbar RD, Ingbar SH, Amir JC, Winterhoff SM, Sourgens H. Inhibition by certain plant extracts of the binding and adenylate cyclase stimulatory effect of bovine thyrotropin in human thyroid membranes. *Endocrinology.* 1984;115:527–534.

Blumenthal M, ed. *The Complete German Commission E Monographs.* Boston, Mass: Integrative Medicine Communications; 1998.

Bremness L. *Herbs.* New York, NY: DK Publishing, 1994.

Castleman M. *The Healing Herbs*. Emmaus, Pa: Rodale Press; 1991.

Duke JA. *The Green Pharmacy*. Emmaus, Pa: Rodale Press; 1997.

Foster S. *Herbal Renaissance: Growing, Using and Understanding Herbs in the Modern World*. Salt Lake City, Utah: Gibbs-Smith; 1993.

Kowalchik C and Hylton W, eds. *Rodale's Illustrated Encyclopedia of Herbs*. Emmaus, Pa: Rodale Press; 1998.

Leung A, Foster S. *Encyclopedia of Common Natural Ingredients Used in Food, Drugs, and Cosmetics*. 2nd ed. New York, NY: Wiley & Sons; 1996.

May G, Willuhn G. Antiviral effect of aqueous plant extracts in tissue culture [In German]. *Arzneimittelforschung*. 1978;28:1–7.

McCaleb R. Melissa relief for herpes sufferers. *HerbalGram*. 1995;34.

McGuffin M, Hobbs C, Upton R, Goldberg A. *American Herbal Products Associations's Botanical Safety Handbook*. Boca Raton, Fla: CRC Press; 1996.

Perry EK, et al. Medicinal plants and Alzheimer's disease: Integrating ethnobotanical and contemporary scientific evidence. *J Altern Complement Med*. 1998;4:419–428.

Schulz V, Hansel R, Tyler V. *Rational Phytotherapy: A Physician's Guide to Herbal Medicine*. New York, NY: Springer-Verlag; 1998.

Soulimani R, et al. Neurotropic action of the hydroalcoholic extract of *Melissa officinalis* in the mouse. *Planta Med*. 1991;57:105–109.

Tagashira M, Ohtake Y. New Antioxidative 1,3-Benzodioxole from *Melissa officinalis*. *Planta Med*. 1988;64:555–558.

Taylor L. *Herbal Secrets of the Rainforest*. Rocklin, Calif: Prima Publishing; 1998.

Tyler VE. Phytomedicines in Western Europe: their potential impact on herbal medicine in the United States. Presented at: Human Medicinal Agents from Plants, The American Chemical Society, 1992. *HerbalGram* 30, 67.

Vogt HJ, Tausch I, Wöbling RH, Kaiser PM. Melissenextrakt bei Herpes simplex. *Der Allgemeinarzt*. 1991;13:832–841.

Wöbling RH, Leonhardt K. Local therapy of herpes simplex with dried extract from *Melissa officinalis*. *Phytomedicine*. 1994;1:25–31.

LICORICE

Acharya SK, Dasarathy S, Tandon A, Joshi YK, Tandon BN. A preliminary open trial on interferon stimulator (SNMC) derived from *Glycyrrhiza glabra* in the treatment of subacute hepatic failure. Indian *J Med Res*. 1993;98:69–74.

Arase Y, et al. The long term efficacy of glycyrrhizin in chronic hepatitis C. *Cancer*. 1997;79:1494–1500.

Blumenthal M, ed. *The Complete German Commission E Monographs: Therapeutic Guide to Herbal Medicines*. Boston, Mass: Integrative Medicine Communications; 1998:161–162.

Bradley P, ed. *British Herbal Compendium*. Dorset, England: British Herbal Medicine Association; 1992:1:145–148.

Chen M, et al. Effect of glycyrrhizin on the pharmokinetics of prednisolone following low dosage of prednisolone hemisuccinate. *J Clin Endocrinol Metab*. 1990;70:1637–1643.

De Smet PAGM, Keller K, Hänsel R, Chandler RF, eds. *Adverse Effects of Herbal Drugs*. Berlin, Germany: Springer-Verlag; 1997:67–87.

Gruenwald J, Brendler T, Christof J, Jaenicke C, eds. *PDR for Herbal Medicines*. Montvale, NJ: Medical Economics Co.; 1998:875–879.

Hattori T, et al. Preliminary evidence for inhibitory effect of glycyrrhizin on HIV replication in patients with aids. *Antiviral Research*. 1989;II:255–262.

Heinerman J. *Heinerman's Encyclopedia of Fruits, Vegetables and Herbs*. Englewood Cliffs, NJ: Prentice Hall; 1988.

Kinghorn A, Balandrin M, eds. *Human Medicinal Agents from Plants*. Washington DC: American Chemical Society; 1993: chap 3.

Mori, K. et al. Effects of glycyrrhizin (SNMC: stronger neo-minophagen C) in hemophilia patients with HIV-I infection. Tohoku *J. Exp. Med*. 1990;162:183–193.

Murray MT. *The Healing Power of Herbs: The Enlightened Person's Guide to the Wonders of Medicinal Plants*. 2nd ed. Rocklin, Calif: Prima Publishing; 1995:228–239.

Newall CA, Anderson LA, Phillipson JD, eds. *Herbal Medicines: A Guide for Health-care Professionals*. London: Pharmaceutical Press; 1996:183–186.

Ohuchi K, et al. Glycyrrhizin inhibits prostaglandin E2 formation by activated peritoneal macrophages from rats. *Prostagland Med*. 1981; 7:457–463.

Snow JM. Glycyrrhiza glabra L. (Leguminacaee). *Protocol J Botan Med*. 1996;1:9–14.

Turpie A, Runcie J, Thomson T. Clinical trial of deglycyrrhizinate liquorice in gastric ulcer. *Gut*. 1969;10:299–303.

Tyler VE. *Herbs of Choice: The Therapeutic Use of Phytomedicinals*. Binghamton, NY: Pharmaceutical Products Press; 1994:197–199.

MILK THISTLE

Alarcón de la Lastra A, Martín M, Motilva V, et al. Gastroprotection induced by silymarin, the hepatoprotective principle of Silybum marianum in ischemia-reperfusion mucosal

injury: role of neutrophils. *Planta Med*. 1995;61:116–119.

Dorland Newman WA, ed. Dorland's Illustrated Medical Dictionary. 25th ed. Philadelphia, Pa: WB Saunders. 1974.

Feher J, Deak G, Muzes G, Lang I, Neiderland V, Nekan K, et al. Hepatoprotective activity of silymarin therapy in patients with chronic alcoholic liver disease. *Orv Hetil*. 1990;130:51.

Ferenci P, Dragosics B, Dittrich H, Frank H., Benda L, Lochs H, et al. Randomized controlled trial of silymarin treatment in patients with cirrhosis of the liver. *J Hepatol*. 1989;9:105-13.

Flora K, Hahn M, Rosen H, Benner K. Milk thistle (Silybum marianum) for the therapy of liver disease. *Am J Gastroenterol*. 1998;93:139–43.

Hobbs C. *Milk Thistle: The Liver Herb*. 2nd ed. Capitola, Calif: Botanica Press; 1992.

Hocking G. A Dictionary of Natural Products. Medford, NJ: Plexus; 1997.

Kinghorn A, Balandrin M, eds. *Human Medicinal Agents from Plants*. Washington, DC: American Chemical Society; 1993.

Magliulo E, Gagliardi B, Fiori GP. Results of a double blind study on the effect of silymarin in the treatment of acute viral hepatitis, carried out at two medical centres. *Med Klinik*. 1978;73:1060–1065.

Morazzoni P, Bombardelli E. *Silybum marianum (Carduus marianus)*. Fitoterapia. 1995;LXVI.

Murray MT. *The Healing Power of Herbs: The Enlightened Person's Guide to the Wonders of Medicinal Plants*. 2nd ed. Rocklin, Calif: Prima Publishing; 1995.

Murray MT, Pizzorno JE. *Encyclopedia of Natural Medicine*. 2nd ed. Rocklin, Calif: Prima Publishing; 1998.

Palasciano G, Portincasa P, Palmieri V, Ciani D, Vendemiale G, Altomare E. The effect of silymarin on plasma levels of malon-dialdehyde in patients receiving long-term treatment with psychotropic drugs. *Curr Therapeut Res*. 1994;55(5):537-545.

Schulz V, Hansel R, Tyler V. *Rational Phytotherapy: A Physicians's Guide to Herbal Medicine*. 3rd ed. Berlin, Germany: Springer-Verlag; 1998.

Tyler V. *The Honest Herbal: A Sensible Guide to the Use of Herbs and Related Remedies*. 3rd ed. New York, NY: Pharmaceutical Products Press; 1993:chap 3.

PAU D'ARCO

Anesini C, et al. Screening of plants used in Argentine folk medicine for antimicrobial activity. *J Ethnopharmacol*. 1993;39:119–128.

Block J, Sterpick A, Miller W; Wiernik P. Early clinical studies with lapachol (NSC-11905). *Cancer Chemother Rep*. 1974;4(part 2):27–28.

Gershon H, Shanks L. Fungitoxicity of 1,4-naphthoquinones to *Candida albicans* and *Trichophyton mentagrophytes*. *Can J of Microbio*. 1975;21:1317–1321.

Duke J, Vasquez R. *Amazonian Ethnobotanical Dictionary*. Boca Raton, Fla: CRC Press; 1994:164.

Kinghorn AD, Balandrin MA, eds. *Human Medicinal Agents from Plants*. Washington, DC: American Chemical Society; 1993:16–17.

Murray MT. *The Healing Power of Herbs: The Enlightened Person's Guide to the Wonders of Medicinal Plants*. 2nd ed. Rocklin, Calif: Prima Publishing; 1995:220–227.

Nakona K, et al. Iridoids From *Tabebuia Avellanedae*. Phytochemisty. 1993;32:371–373.

Perez H, et al. Chemical Investigations and in Vitro Antimalarial Activity of *Tabebuia ochracea* ssp. Neochrysanta. *International Journal of Pharmacognosy*. 1997;35:227–231.

Schultes RE, Raffauf RF. *The Healing Forest: Medicinal and Toxic Plants of the Northwest Amazonia*. Portland, Ore: Dioscorides Press; 1990:107–109.

Shealy CN. *The Illustrated Encyclopedia of Healing Remedies*. Dorset UK: Element Books; 1998:132.

Tyler VE. *Herbs of Choice: The Therapeutic Use of Phytomedicinals*. Binghamton, NY: Pharmaceutical Products Press; 199:180.

Tyler VE. *The Honest Herbal: A Sensible Guide to the Use of Herbs and Related Remedies*. 3rd ed. Binghamton, NY: Pharmaceutical Products Press; 1993:239–240.

Ueda S, et al. Production of anti-tumour-promoting furanonaphthoquinones in *Tabebuia avellanedae* cell cultures. *Phytochemistry*. 1994;36:323–325.

PEPPERMINT

Blumenthal M, ed. *The Complete German Commission E Monographs*. Boston, Mass: Integrative Medicine Communications; 1998.

Castleman M. *The Healing Herbs*. New York, NY: Bantam Books; 1991.

Dew MJ, Evans BK, Rhodes J. Peppermint oil for the irritable bowel syndrome: a multi-centre trial. *Br J Clin Pract*. 1984;(11–12):394, 398.

Duke J. *The Green Pharmacy*. Emmaus, Pa: Rodale Press; 1997.

Feng XZ. Effect of Peppermint oil hot compresses in preventing abdominal distension in postoperative gynecological patients [In Chinese]. *Chung Hua Hu Li Tsa Chih.* 1997; 32:577–578.

Hills J. The mechanism of action of peppermint oil on gastrointestinal smooth muscle. *Gastroenterology.* 1991;101:55–65.

Koch TR. Peppermint oil and irritable bowel syndrome [In Process Citation]. *Am J Gastroenterol.* 1998;93:2304–2305.

Kowalchik C, Hylton W, eds. *Rodale's Illustrated Encyclopedia of Herbs.* Emmaus, Pa: Rodale Press; 1987.

Lawson MJ, Knight, RE, Tran K, Walker G, Robers-Thompson, IC. Failure of enteric-coated peppermint oil in the irritable bowel syndrome: a randomized double-blind crossover study. *J Gastroent Hepatol.* 1988;3:235-238.

Mowrey D. *The Scientific Validation of Herbal Medicine.* New Canaan, Conn: Keats Publishing, Inc; 1986.

Murray MT. *The Healing Power of Herbs.* Rocklin, Calif: Prima Publishing; 1995.

Pittler MH, Ernst E. Peppermint oil for irritable bowel syndrome: a critical review and metaanalysis. *Am J Gastroenterol.* 1998;93:1131–1135.

Rees W. Treating irritable bowel syndrome with peppermint oil. *Br Med J.* 1979;II:835–836.

Schulz V, Hänsel R, Tyler V. *Rational Phytotherapy.* Berlin, Germany: Springer; 1998.

Tyler V. *Herbs of Choice: The Therapeutic Use of Phytomedicinals.* New York, NY: Pharmaceutical Products Press; 1994.

SAW PALMETTO

Blumenthal M, ed. *The Complete German Commission E Monographs:Therapeutic Guide to Herbal Medicine.* Boston, Mass: Integrative Medicine Communications; 1998.

Braeckman J. The extract of *Serenoa repens* in the treatment of benign prostatic hyperplasia: A multicenter open study. *Curr Therapeut Res* 1994;55:776–785.

Carilla E, Briley M, Fauran F, et al. Binding of Permixon, a new treatment for prostatic benign hyperplasia, to the cytosolic androgen receptor in the rat prostate. *J Steroid Biochem* 1984;20:521-523.

Carraro JC, et al. Comparison of phytotherapy (Permixon) with finasteride in the treatment of benign prostate hyperplasia: a randomized international study of 1,098 patients. *The Prostate.* 1996;29(4):231-240.

Champault G, Patel JC, Bonnard AM. A double-blind trial of an extract of the plant *Serenoa repens* in benign prostatic hyperplasia. *Br J Clin Pharmacol.* 1984;18:461-462.

Di Silverio F, D'Eramo G, Lubrano C, et al. Evidence that *Serenoa repens* extract displays an antiestrogenic activity in prostatic tissue of benign prostatic hypertrophy patients. *Eur Uro.*1992;21:309-314.

el-Sheikh M, Dakkak MR, Saddique A. The effect of permixon on androgen receptors. *Acta Obstet Gynecol Scand.* 1988;67:397–399.

Hutchens AR. *Indian Herbalogy of North America.* Boston, Mass: Shambhala Publications; 1973:243–244.

Leung A, Foster S. *Encyclopedia of Common Natural Ingredients Used in Food, Drugs, and Cosmetics.* 2nd ed. New York, NY: John Wiley & Sons; 1996:467–468.

McGuffin M, Hobbs C, Upton R, Goldberg A. *American Herbal Products Association's Botanical Safety Handbook.* Boca Raton, Fla: CRC Press; 1996.

Murray MT. *The Healing Power of Herbs: The Enlightened Person's Guide to the Wonders of Medicinal Plants.* Rocklin, Calif: Prima Publishing; 1995.

Newall CA, Anderson LA, Phillipson JD. *Herbal Medicines: A Guide for Health-Care Professionals.* London, England: The Pharmaceutical Press; 1996.

Schulz V, Hänsel R, Tyler VE. *Rational Phytotherapy: A Physicians' Guide to Herbal Medicine.* Berlin, Germany: Springer-Verlag; 1998.

Sökeland J, Albrecht J. A combination of *Sabal* and *Urtica* extracts vs. finasteride in BHP (stage I to II acc. to Alken): A comparison of therapeutic efficacy in a one-year double-blind study. *Urologe A.* 1997;36:327–333.

Mandressi A, et al. Treatment of uncomplicated benign prostatic hypertrophy BPH by an extract of *Serenoa Repens* clinical results. *J Endocrinol Invest.* 1987;10(suppl 2):49.

Wilt TJ, Ishani A, Stark G, et al. Saw palmetto extracts for treatment of benign prostatic hyperplasia: a systematic review. *JAMA.* 1998;280:1604–1609.

Wood HC, Osol A. *United States Dispensatory.* 23rd ed. Philadelphia, Pa: J.B. Lippincott; 1943;971–972.

ST. JOHN'S WORT

Bombardelli E, Morazzoni P. *Hypericum perforatum. Fitoterapia.* 1995;LXVI:43–68.

Cott JM. In vitro receptor binding and enzyme inhibition by *Hypericum perforatum* extract. *Pharmacopsychiatry.* 1997;30(suppl 2):108–112.

Degar S, et al. Inactivation of the human immunodeficiency virus by hypericin: Evidence for phytochemical alterations of p24 and a block in uncoating. *AIDS Res Hum Retroviruses.* 1992;8:1929–1936.

De Smet P, Peter AGM, Nolen WA. St. John's wort as an antidepressant. *Br Med J.* 1996;313:241–247.

Furner V, Bek M, Gold JA. A phase I/II unblinded dose ranging study of hypericin in HIV-positive subjects. *Int Conf AIDS.* 1991;7:199.

Gulick R, et al. Human hypericism: A photosensitivity reaction to hypericin (St. John's wort). *Int Conf AIDS.* 1992; 8:B90.

Lavie G, et al. Studies of the human mechanism of action of the antiviral agents hypericin and pseudohypericin. *Proc Natl Acad Sci USA.* 1989;86:5963–5967.

Linde K, Ramirez G, Mulrow CD, et al. St. John's wort for depression: an overview and meta-analysis of randomised clinical trials. *BMJ.* 1996;313:253–257.

Martinez B, Kasper S, Ruhrmann S, Moller HJ. Hypericum in the treatment of seasonal affective disorders. *J Geriatr Psychiatry Neurol.* 1994;7(Suppl 1):S29–33.

Meruelo D, Lavie G, Lavie D. Therapeutic agents with dramatic antiretroviral activity and little toxicity at effective doses: Aromatic polycyclic diones hypericin and pseudohypericin. *Proc Natl Acad Sci USA.* 1988;85:5230–5234.

Muller WE, Rolli M, Schafer C, Hafner, U. Effects of *hypericum* extract (LI 160) in biochemical models of antidepressant activity. *Pharmacopsychiatry.* 1997;30(suppl):102–107.

Murray MT. *The Healing Power of Herbs: The Enlightened Person's Guide to the Wonders of Medicinal Plants.* Rocklin, Calif: Prima Publishing; 1995.

Rasmussen P. St. John's wort: a review of its use in depression. *Australian Journal of Medical Herbalism.* 1998;10:8–13.

Tyler VE. *The Honest Herbal: A Sensible Guide to the Use of Herbs and Related Remedies.* Binghamton, NY: Pharmaceutical Products Press; 1993.

STINGING NETTLE

Balzarini J, Neyts J, Schols D, Hosoya M, Van Damme E, Peumans W, De Clercq E. The mannose-specific plant lectins from Cymbidium hybrid and Epipactis helleborine and the (N-acetylglucosamine) n-specific plant lectin from *Urtica dioica* are potent and selective inhibitors of human immunodeficiency virus and cytomegalovirus replication in vitro. *Antiviral Research.* 1992;18:191–207.

Belaiche P, Lievoux O. Clinical Studies on the Palliative Treatment of Prostatic Adenoma with Extract of Urtica Root. *Phytotherapy Research.* 1991;5:267-269.

Blumenthal M, ed. *The Complete German Commission E Monographs. Therapeutic Guide to Herbal Medicines.* Boston, Mass: Integrative Medicine Communications; 1998:47, 132.

Bradley P, ed. *British Herbal Compendium.* Dorset, England: British Herbal Medicine Association; 1992;1:166–167.

Chrubasik S, Enderlein W, Bauer R, Grabner W. Evidence for antirheumatic effectiveness of Herba *Urticae dioica* in acute arthritis: A pilot study. *Phytomedicine.* 1997;4:105–108.

Grieve M. A Modern Herbal. New York, NY: Dover; 1971;2:574-579

Gruenwald J, Brendler T, Christof J. *PDR for Herbal Medicines.* Montvale, NJ: Medical Economics Company; 1998:1197–1199.

Hutchens A. *Indian Herbalogy of North America.* Boston, Mass: Shambhala; 1991:204–206.

Krzeski T, Kazon M, Borkowski A, Witeska A, Kuczera J. Combined extracts of *Urtica dioica* and *Pygeum africanum* in the treatment of benign prostatic hyperplasia: double-blind comparison of two doses. *Clin Ther.* 1993;15:1011–1020.

Millspaugh C. *American Medicinal Plants.* New York, NY: Dover; 1974:611–614.

Newall C, Anderson L, Phillipson J. *Herbal Medicines: A Guide for Health-Care Professionals.* London, England: Pharmaceutical Press; 1996:201–202.

Oliver F, Amon E, Breathnach A, Francis D, Sarathchandra P, Black A, Greaves M. Contact urticaria due to the common stinging nettle (*Urtica dioica*—histological, ultrastructural and pharmacological studies. *Clin Exp Dermatology.* 1991;267:1–7.

Schneider H, Honold E, Masuhr T. Treatment of benign prostatic hyperplasia. Results of a treatment study with the phytogenic combination of Sabal extract WS 1473 and Urtica extract WS 1031 in urologic specialty practices. *Fortschr Med.* 1995;267:37–40.

Schulz V, Hänsel R, Tyler VE. *Rational Phytotherapy: A Physician's Guide to Herbal Medicine.* Third ed. Berlin, Germany: Springer-Verlag; 1998:228–238.

Sökeland J, Albrecht J. Lignans from the roots of *Urtica dioica* and their metabolites bind to human sex hormone binding globulin (SHBG). *Planta Med.* 1997;36:529–532.

Tyler VE. *Herbs of Choice: The Therapeutic Use of Phytomedicinals.* Binghamton, NY: Haworth; 1994:84–85.

Wylie G, et al. A comparative study of Tenidap, a cytokine-modulating anti-rheumatic drug, and diclofenac in rheumatoid arthritis: a 24 week analysis of a 1-year clinical trial. *Br J Rheumatol.* 1995;34:554–563.

VALERIAN ROOT

Balderer G, Borbely AA. Effect of valerian on human sleep. *Psychopharmacol.* 1985;87:406–409.

Blumenthal M, ed. *The Complete German Commission E Monographs.* Boston, Mass: Integrative Medicine Communications; 1998.

Blumenthal M, Riggins C. *Popular Herbs in the U.S. Market: Therapeutic Monographs.* Austin, Tex: The American Botanical Council; 1997.

Brown D. *Herbal Prescriptions for Better Health.* Rocklin, Calif: Prima Publishing; 1996.

DeSmet PAGM, ed. *Adverse Effects of Herbal Drugs.* New York, NY: Springer-Verlag; 1997:3.

Diefenbach K, et al. Valerian effects on microstructure of sleep in insomniacs. (2nd Congress of the European Assoc. for Clinical Pharmacology and Therapeutics, Berlin, Germany, Sept. 17-20.) *Eur J Clin Pharmacol.* 1997;52 (suppl):A169.

Hobbs C. *The Herbal Prescriber.* Santa Cruz, Calif. Botanica Press; 1995.

Kowalchik C, Hylton W, eds. *Rodale's Illustrated Encyclopedia of Herbs.* Emmaus, Pa: Rodale Press; 1998:495–496.

Leathwood PD. Aqueous extract of valerian root (*Valeriana officinalis* L.) improves sleep quality in man. *Pharmacol Biochem Behav.* 1982;17:65–71.

Leung A, Foster S. *Encyclopedia of Common Natural Ingredients Used in Food, Drugs, and Cosmetics.* 2nd ed. New York, NY: John Wiley and Sons; 1996.

Lindahl O, Lindwall L. Double-blind study of a valerian preparation. *Pharmacol Biochem Behav.* 1989;32:1065–1066.

Lindahl O, Lindwall L. Double–blind study of valopotriates by hairy root cultures of *Valeriana officinalis* var. sambucifolia. *Planta Med.* 1992;58:A614.

McGuffin M, Hobbs C, Upton R, Goldberg A. *American Herbal Products Association's Botanical Safety Handbook.* Boca Raton, Fla: CRC Press; 1997:120.

Murray, MT. *The Healing Power of Herbs: The Enlightened Person's Guide to the Wonders of Medicinal Plants.* Rocklin, Calif: Prima Publishing; 1995.

Newall CA, Phillipson JD. Interactions of Herbs with Other Medicines. Kings Centre for Pharmacognosy, the School of Pharmacy, University of London. *The European Phytojournal.* 1998; 1. Available at: www.ex.ac.uk/phytonet/phytojournal.

Petkov V. Plants with hypotensive, antiatheromatous and coronarodilating actions. *Am J Chin Med.* 1979;7:197–236.

Samuelsson G. *Drugs of Natural Origin: A Textbook of Pharmacognosy.* Stockholm, Sweden: The Swedish Pharmaceutical Press; 1992.

Santos MS. Synaptosomal GABA release as influenced by valerian root extract—involvement of the GABA carrier. *Arch Int Pharmacodyn Ther.* 1994; 327:220–231.

Schultz V, Hansel R, Tyler V. *Rational Phytotherapy: A Physician's Guide to Herbal Medicine.* New York, NY: Springer-Verlag; 1998.

Seifert T. Therapeutic effects of valerian in nervous disorders: a field study. *Therapeutikon.* 1988;2(94).

Schultz H, Stolz C, Muller J. The effect of valerian extract on sleep polygraph in poor sleepers: a pilot study. *Pharmacopsychiatry.* 1994;27:147–151.

Wagner et al. Comparative studies on the sedative action of valeriana extracts, valepotriates, and their degradation products. *Planta Med.* 1980;39:358–365.

RESOURCES - SUPPLEMENTS
5-HYDROXYTRYPTOPHAN (5-HTP)

Angst J, et al. The treatment of depression with L-5-hydroxytryptophan versus imipramine. Results of two open and one double-blind study. *Arch Psychiatr Nervenkr.* 1977;224:175–186.

Birdsall TC. 5-Hydroxytryptophan: a clinically-effective serotonin precursor. *Altern Med Rev.* 1998;3:271–280.

Byerley WF, et al. 5-Hydroxytryptophan: a review of its antidepressant efficacy and adverse effects. *J Clin Psychopharmacol.* 1987;7:127–137.

Cangiano C, et al. Effects of oral 5-hydroxy-tryptophan on energy intake and macronutrient selection in non-insulin dependent diabetic patients. *Int J Obes Relat Metab Disord.* 1998; 22:648–654.

Cangiano C, Ceci F, Cascino A, et al. Eating behavior and adherence to dietary prescriptions in obese adult subjects treated with 5-hydroxytryptophan. *J Clin Nutr.* 1992;56:863–867.

Caruso I, Sarzi Puttini P, Cazzola M, et al. Double-blind study of 5-hydroxytryptophan versus placebo in the treatment of primary fibromyalgia syndrome. *J Int Med Res.* 1990;18:201–209.

Ceci F, Cangiano C, Cairella M, Cascino A, et al. The effects of oral 5-hydroxytryptophan administration on feeding behavior in obese adult female subjects. *J Neural Transm.* 1989;76:109–117.

DeBenedittis G, Massei R. Serotonin precursors in chronic primary headache. A double-blind cross-over study with L-5-hydroxytryptophan vs. placebo. *J Neurosurg Sci.* 1985; 29:239–248.

DeGiorgis, G, et al. Headache in association with sleep disorders in children: a psychodiagnostic evaluation and controlled clinical study—L-5-HTP versus placebo. *Drugs Exp Clin Res.* 1987;13:425–433.

Ganong WF. *Review of Medical Physiology.* 13th ed. San Mateo, Calif: Appleton & Lange; 1987.

Juhl JH. Primary fibromyalgia syndrome and 5-hydroxy-L-tryptophan: a 90-day open study. *Altern Med Rev.* 1998;3:367–375.

Magnussen I, Nielson-Kudsk F. Bioavailability and related pharmacokinetics in man of orally administered L-5-Hydroxytryptophan in steady state. *Acta Pharmacol et Toxicol.* 1980;46:257–262.

Martin TG. Serotonin syndrome. *Ann Emerg Med.* 1996;28:520–526.

Murray MT, Pizzorno JE. *Encyclopedia of Natural Medicine.* 2nd ed. Rocklin, Calif: Prima Publishing; 1998.

Nicolodi M, Sicuteri F. Fibromyalgia and migraine, two faces of the same mechanism. Serotonin as the common clue for pathogenesis and thearpy. *Adv Exp Med Biol.* 1996;398:373–379.

Puttini PS, Caruso I. Primary fibromyalgia and 5-hydroxy-L-tryptophan: a 90-day open study. *J Int Med Res.* 1992;20:182–189.

Reibring L, Agren H, Hartvig P, et al. Uptake and utilization of [beta-11c] 5-hydroxytryptophan (5-HTP) in human brain studied by positron emission tomography. *Pyschiatry Research.* 1992;45:215–225.

Shils ME, Olson JA, Shike M, eds. *Modern Nutrition in Health and Disease.* 8th ed. Media, Pa: Williams & Wilkins; 1994:1.

Takahashi S, et al. Measurement of 5-hydroxindole compounds during L-5-HTP treatment in depressed patients. *Folia Psychiatr Neurol Jpn.* 1976;30:461–473.

Van Hiele IJ. L-5-hydroxytryptophan in depression: the first substitution therapy in psychiatry? *Neuropsychobiology.* 1980; 6:230–240.

Van Praag HM. Management of depression with serotonin precursors. *Biol Psychiatry.* 1981;16:291–310.

Zmilacher K, et al. L-5-hydroxytryptophan alone and in combination with a peripheral decarboxylase inhibitor in the treatment of depression. *Neuropsychobiology.* 1988;20:28–33.

ALPHA-LINOLENIC ACID (ALA)

Ando H, Ryu A, Hashimot A, Oka M, Ichihashi M. Linoleic acid and alpha-linolenic acid lightens ultraviolet-induced hyperpigmentation of the skin. *Arch Dermatol Res.* 1998;290:375–381.

Billeaud C, Bougle D, Sarda P, et al.. Effects of preterm infant formula supplementation with alpha-linolenic acid with a linoleate/alpha-linoleate ration of 6. *Eur J Clin Nutr.* August 1997;51:520–527.

DeDeckere EA, Korver O, Verschuren PM, Katan MB. Health aspects of fish and n-3 polyunsaturated fatty acids from plant and marine origin. *Eur J Clin Nutr.* 1998;52:749–753.

Edwards R, Peet M, Shay J, Horrobin D. Omega-3 polyunsaturated fatty acid levels in the diet and in red blood cell membranes of depressed patients. *J Affect Disord.* 1998;48:149–155.

Ensminger AH, Ensminger ME, Konlande JE, Robson JRK. *Foods & Nutrition Encyclopedia.* 2nd ed. Baton Rouge, Fla: CRC Press, Inc; 1994:1:684–708.

Ferretti A, Flanagan VP. Antithromboxane activity of dietary alpha-linolenic acid. *Prostaglandins Leukot Essent Fatty Acids.* 1996;54:451–455.

Freese R, Mutanen M. Alpha-linolenic acid and marine long-chain n-3 fatty acids differ only slightly in their effects on hemostatic factors in healthy subjects. *Am J Clin Nutr.* 1997;66:591–598.

Garrison Jr RH, Somer E. *The Nutrition Desk Reference.* 3rd ed. New Canaan, Conn: Keats Publishing, Inc; 1995:23–64.

Haas EM. *Staying Healthy with Nutrition.* Berkley, Calif: Celestial Arts Publishing; 1992:65–79.

Harris WS. N-3 fatty acids and serum lipoproteins: human studies. *Am J Clin Nutr.* 1997;65:1645S (10).

de Lorgeril M, Renaud S, Mamelle N, et al. Mediterranean alpha-linolenic acid-rich diet in secondary prevention of coronary heart disease. *Lancet.* 1994;343:1454–1459.

Mantzioris E., James MJ, Gibson RA, Cleland LG. Dietary subsitutions with an alpha-linolenic acid-rich vegetable oil increases eicosapentaenoic acid concentrations in tissues. *Am J Clin Nutr.* 1994;59:1304–1309.

Murray MT. *Encyclopedia of Nutritional Supplements.* Rocklin, Calif: Prima Publishing; 1996:239–278.

Nestel PJ, Pomeroy SE, Sasahara T, et al. Arterial compliance in obese subjects is improved with dietary plant n-3 fatty acid from flaxseed oil despite increased LDL oxidizability. *Arterioscler Thromb Vasc Biol.* 1997;17:1163–1170.

Newstrom H. *Nutrients Catalog.* Jefferson, NC: McFarland & Co, Inc; 1993:103–105.

Simon JA, Fong J, Bernert JT Jr, Browner WS. Serum fatty acids and the risk of stroke. *Stroke.* 1995;26:778–782.

Shils ME, Olson JA, Shike M, Ross AC. *Modern Nutrition in Health and Disease.* 9th ed. Baltimore, Md: Williams & Wilkins; 1999:90–92, 1377–1378.

Voskuil DW, Feskens EJM, Katan MB, Kromhout D. Intake and sources of alpha-linolenic acid in Dutch elderly men. *Eur J Clin Nutr.* 1996;50:784–787.

Wapnir RA. Copper absorption and bioavailability. *Am J Clin Nutr.* 1998;67:1054s.

Wagner W, Nootbaar-Wagner U. Prophylactic treatment of migraine with gamma-linolenic and alpha-linolenic acids. *Cephalalgia.* April 1997;17:127–130.

Werbach MR. *Nutritional Influences on Illness.* 2nd ed. Tarzana, Calif: Third Line Press; 1993:13–22; 655–671.

Yehuda S, Rabinovitz S, Carasso RL, Mostofsky DI. Fatty acids and brain peptides. *Peptides.* 1998;19:407–419.

ALPHA-LIPOIC ACID

Hocking GM. *A Dictionary of Natural Products.* Medford, NJ: Plexus Publishing; 1997:39;449,797.

Mindell E, Hopkins V. *Prescription Alternatives.* New Canaan, Conn: Keats Publishing; 1998:55–56.

Packer J, Tritschler HJ, Wessel K. Neuroprotection by the metabolic antioxidant alpha-linoic acis. *Free Radic Biol Med.* 1997;22:359–378.

Walker LP, Brown E. *The Alternative Pharmacy.* Paramus, NJ: Prentice Hall; 1998:36, 78, 216, 326, 362, 375.

Ziegler D, Gries FA. Alpha-lipoic acid in the treatment of diabetic peripheral and cardiac autonomic neuropathy. *Diabetes.* 1997;46 (suppl 2):S62–66.

BREWER'S YEAST

Balch J, Balch P. *Prescription for Nutritional Healing.* Garden Park City, NY: Avery Publishing Group; 1997.

Bentley JP, Hunt TK, Weiss JB, et al. Peptides from live yeast cell derivative stimulate wound healing. *Arch Surg.* 1990;125:641–646.

Chromium necessary to regulate blood sugar. *Conscious Choice: The Journal of Ecology and Natural Living.* June 1998;11:33.

Hegoczki J, Suhajda A, Janzso B, Vereczkey G. Preparation of chromium enriched yeasts. *Acta Alimentaria.* 1997;26:345–358.

Li Y-C. Effects of brewer's yeast on glucose tolerance and serum lipids in Chinese adults. *Biol Trace Elem Res.* 1994;41:341–347.

McCarty MF. Insulin resistance in Mexican Americans: a precursor to obestity and diabetes? *Med Hypotheses.* 1993;41:308–315.

Murray M. Biotin: An overlooked essential B vitamin. *The America Journal of Natural Medicine.* May 1996;3:5–6.

Murray M. The chromium connection. *Health Counselor.* March 1997;9:48–59.

Rabinowitz MB, Gonick HC, Levin SR, Davidson MB. Effects of chromium and yeast supplements on carbohydrate and lipid metabolism in diabetic men. *Diabetes Care.* 1983;6:319–327.

BROMELAIN

Bromelain. *Alternative Medicine Review.* August 1998;3:302–305.

Desser L, Rehberger A, Kokron E, Paukovits W. Cytokine synthesis in human peripheral blood mononuclear cells after oral administration of polyenzyme preparations. *Oncology.* 1993;50:403–407.

Haas EM. *Staying Healthy with Nutrition: The Complete Guide to Diet and Nutritional Medicine.* Berkeley, Calif: Celestial Arts; 1992:257–258.

Harborne J, Baxter H, eds. *Phytochemical Dictionary: A Handbook of Bioactive Compounds from Plants.* London, England: Taylor & Francis; 1993:376.

Masson M. Bromelain in blunt injuries of the locomotor system. A study of observed applications in general practice. *Fortschr Med.* 1995;113:303–306.

Murray MT. *Encyclopedia of Nutritional Supplements: The Essential Guide for Improving Your Health Naturally.* Rocklin, Calif: Prima Publishing; 1996:429.

Murray MT, Pizzorno JE. *Encyclopedia of Natural Medicine.* 2nd ed. Rocklin, Calif: Prima Publishing; 1998:208,297–298,568,807,829–830.

Reynolds JEF, ed. *Martindale: The Extra Pharmacopoeia.* 31st ed. London, England: Royal Pharmaceutical Society; 1996:1681.

Taussig SJ, Batkin S. Bromelain, the enzyme complex of pineapple (Ananas comosus) and its clinical application. An update. *J Ethnopharmacol.* 1998;22:191–203.

Uhlig G, Seifert J. The effect of proteolytic enzymes (traumanase) on posttraumatic edema. *Fortschr Med.* 1981;99:554–556.

Walker JA, Cerny FJ, Cotter JR, Burton HW. Attenuation of contraction-induced skeletal muscle injury by bromelain. *Med Sci Sports Exerc.* 1992;24:20–25.

Werbach MR. *Nutritional Influences on Illness: A Sourcebook of Clinical Research.* New Canaan, Conn: Keats Publishing; 1987:64–65,268–269,386.

CALCIUM

Cappuccio FP, Elliott P, Allender PS, et al. Epidemiologic association between dietary calcium intake and blood pressure: a meta-analysis of published data. *Am J Epidemiol.* 1995;142:935–945.

Devine A, Dick IM, Heal SJ, et al. A 4-year follow-up study of the effects of calcium supplementation on bone density in elderly postmenopausal women. *Osteoporosis Int.* 1997;7:23–28.

Ensminger AH, Ensminger ME, Konlande JE, Robson JRK. *Foods and Nutrition Encyclopedia.* 2nd ed. Baton Rouge, Fla: CRC Press Inc; 1994;2:1338–1341.

Garrison Jr RH, Somer E. *The Nutrition Desk Reference.* 3rd ed. New Canaan, Conn: Keats Publishing Inc; 1995:158–165.

Hardman JG, Gilman AG, Limbird LE, eds. *Goodman and Gilman's Pharmacological Basis of Therapeutics.* 9th ed. New York, NY: McGraw-Hill; 1996:839–874.

Heinerman J. *Heinerman's Encyclopedia of Nature's Vitamins and Minerals.* Paramus, NJ: Prentice Hall Inc; 1998:296–302.

Murray MT. *Encyclopedia of Nutritional Supplements.* Rocklin, Calif: Prima Publishing; 1996:159–175.

Nicar MJ, Pak CY. Calcium bioavailability from calcium carbonate and calcium citrate. *J Clin Endocrinol Metab.* 1985;61(2):391–393.

Rodrâiguez JA, Novik V. Calcium intake and bone density in menopause. Data of a sample of Chilean women followed-up for 5 years with calcium supplementation. *Rev Med Chil.* 1998;126:145–150.

Shils ME, Olson JA, Shike M, Ross AC. *Modern Nutrition in Health and Disease.* 9th ed. Baltimore, Md: Williams & Wilkins; 1999:169–192, A127–A128.

Thys-Jacobs S, Starkey P, Bernstein D, Tian J. Calcium carbonate and the premenstrual syndrome: effects on premenstrual and menstrual symptoms. Premenstrual Syndrome Study Group. *Am J Obstet Gynecol.* 1998;179:444–452.

Werbach MR. *Nutritional Influences on Illness.* 2nd ed. Tarzana, Calif: Third Line Press; 1993:655–680.

CARTILAGE

Balch J, Balch P. *Prescription for Nutritional Healing.* 2nd ed. Garden City Park, NY: Avery Publishing Group; 1997.

Burton Goldberg Group. *Alternative Medicine: The Definitive Guide.* Puyallup, Wash: Future Medicine Publishing, Inc; 1994.

Cassileth BR. *The Alternative Medicine Handbook.* New York, NY: W. W. Norton & Company; 1998.

Dupont E, Savard PE, Jourdain C, et al. Antiangiogenic properties of a novel shark cartilage extract: potential role in the treatment of psoriasis. *J Cutan Med Surg.* 1998;2:146–152.

Horsman MR, Alsner J, Overgaard J. The effect of shark cartilage extracts on the growth and metastatic spread of the SCCVII carcinoma. *Acta Oncol.* 1998;37:441–445.

Kriegal H, John Prudden and Bovine Tracheal Cartilage Research. *Alternative & Complementary Therapies.* April/May 1995.

Miller DR, Anderson GT, Stark JJ, Granick JL, Richardson D. Phase I/II trial of the safety and efficacy of shark cartilage in the treatment of advanced cancer. *J Clin Oncol.* 1998;16:3649–3655.

Moss R. *Cancer Therapy.* Brooklyn, NY: Equinox Press Inc; 1992.

Murray M. *Encyclopedia of Nutritional Supplements.* Rocklin, Calif: Prima Publishing; 1996.

Prudden JF. The treatment of human cancer with agents prepared from bovine cartilage. *Biol Response Mod.* 1985;4:551–584.

Romano CF, Lipton A, Harvey HA, Simmonds MA, Romano PJ, Imboden SL. A phase II study of Catrix-S in solid tumors. *J Biol Response Mod.* 1985;4:585–589.

Sheu JR, Fu CC, Tsai Ml, Chung WJ. Effect of U-995, a potent shark cartilage-derived angiogenesis inhibitor, on anti-angiogenesis and anti-tumor activities. *Anticancer Res.* 1998;18:4435–4441.

CHROMIUM

Anderson RA, Cheng N, Bryden NA, et al. Elevated intakes of supplemental chromium improve glucose and insulin variables in individuals with type 2 diabetes. *Diabetes.* 1997;46:1,786–1,791.

Anderson RA, Polansky MM, Bryden NA, Bhathena SJ, Canary JJ. Effects of supplemental chromium on patients with symptoms of reactive hypoglycemia. *Metabolism.* 1987;36:351–355.

Bahadori B, Wallner S, Schneider H, Wascher TC, Toplak H. Effect of chromium yeast and chromium picolinate on body composition of obese, non-diabetic patients during and after a formula diet. *Acta Med Austriaca.* 1997;24:185–187.

Friedman E, ed. *Biochemistry of the Essential Ultratrace Elements.* New York, NY: Plenum Press; 1984.

Fujimoto S. Studies on the relationships between blood trace metal concentrations and the clinical status of patients with cerebrovascular disease, gastric cancer, and diabetes mellitus. *Hokkaido Igaku Zasshi.* 1987;62:913–932.

Krause MV, Mahan LK. *Food, Nutrition, and Diet Therapy.* 7th ed. Philadelphia, Pa: WB Saunders Co; 1984.

McCarty MF. Anabolic effects of insulin on bone suggests a role for chromium picolinate in preservation of bone density. *Med Hypotheses.* 1995;45:241–246.

Murray MT, Pizzorno JE. *Encyclopedia of Natural Medicine.* 2nd ed. Rocklin, Calif: Prima Publishing; 1998.

Shils ME, Olsen JA, Shike M, eds. *Modern Nutrition in Health and Disease.* 8th ed. Media, Pa: Williams and Wilkins Co; 1994:1.

Somer E. *The Essential Guide to Vitamins & Minerals.* New York, NY: HarperCollins Publishers; 1992

Urberg M, Zemel MB. Evidence for synergism between chromium and nicotinic acid in the control of glucose tolerance in elderly humans. *Metabolism.* 1987;36:896–899.

Wilson BE, Gondy A. Effects of chromium supplementation on fasting insulin levels and lipid parameters in healthy, non-obese young subjects. *Diabetes Res Clin Pract.* 1995;28:179–184.

COPPER

Asseth J, Haugen M, et al. Rheumatoid arthritis and metal compounds—perspectives on the role of oxygen radical detoxification. *Analyst.* 1998;123:3–6.

Ensminger AH, Ensminger ME, Konlande JE, Robson JRK. *Foods and Nutrition Encyclopedia.* 2nd ed. Baton Rouge, Fla: CRC Press Inc; 1994;1:476–479.

Garrison Jr RH, Somer E. *The Nutrition Desk Reference.* 3rd ed. New Canaan, Conn: Keats Publishing Inc; 1995:188–192.

Haas EM. *Staying Healthy With Nutrition.* Berkley, Calif: Celestial Arts Publishing; 1992:190–194.

Hardman JG, Gilman AG, Limbird LE, eds. *Goodman and Gilman's Pharmacological Basis of Therapeutics.* 9th ed. New York, NY: McGraw-Hill; 1996:1325–1326.

Heinerman J. *Heinerman's Encyclopedia of Nature's Vitamins and Minerals.* Paramus, NJ: Prentice Hall Inc; 1998:250–255.

Mazzetti I, Grigolo B, Borzai RM, Meliconi R, Facchini A. Serum copper/zinc superoxide dismutase levels in patients with rheumatoid arthritis. *J Clin Lab Res.* 1996;26(4):245–249.

Murray MT. *Encyclopedia of Nutritional Supplements.* Rocklin, Calif: Prima Publishing, 1996:199–203.

Newstrom H. *Nutrients Catalog.* Jefferson, NC: McFarland & Co. Inc; 1993:141–151.

Olivares M, Uauy R. Copper as an essential nutrient. *Am J Clin Nutr.* 1996;63:791S–796S.

Pennington JA, Schoen SA. Total diet study: estimated dietary intakes of nutritional elements. *Int J Vitam Nutr Res.* 1996;66:350–362.

Shils ME, Olson JA, Shike M, Ross AC. *Modern Nutrition in Health and Disease.* 9th ed. Baltimore, Md: Williams & Wilkins; 1999:241–252.

Uauy R, Olivares M, Gonzalez M. Essentiality of copper in humans. *Am J Clin Nutr.* 1998;67(5 suppl):952S–959S.

Wapnir RA. Copper absorption and bioavailability. *Am J Clin Nutri.* May 1998;67;5:1054s.

Werbach MR. *Nutritional Influences on Illness.* 2nd ed. Tarzana, Calif: Third Line Press; 1993:655–680.

CREATINE

Bosco C, et al. Effect of oral creatine supplementation on jumping and running performance. *Int J Sports Med.* 1997;18:369–372.

Earnets, CP, Almada AL, Mitchell TL. High-performance capillary electrophoresis: pure creatine monohydrate reduces blood lipids in men and women. *Clin Sci.* 1996;91:113–118.

Grindstaff PD, et al. Effects of creatine supplementation on repetitive sprint performance and body composition in competitive swimmers. *Int J Sport Nutr.* 1997;7:330–346.

Juhn MS, Tarnopolsky M. 1998. Potential side effects of oral creatine supplementation: a critical review. *Clin J Sport Med.* 1998;8:298–304.

Juhn MS, Tarnopolsky M. Oral creatine supplementation and athletic performance: a critical review. *Clin J Sport Med.* 1994;8:286–297.

Kreider RB, Ferreira M, et al. Effects of creatine supplementation on body composition, strength and sprint performance. *Med Sci Sports Exerc.* 1998;30(1):73–82.

Kreider RB, Rasmussen C, Ransom J, Almada AL. Effects of creatine supplementation during training on the incidence of muscle cramping, injuries and GI distress. Presented at the National Strength and Conditioning Association Convention; June 24–28, 1998; Nashville, Tenn. Accessed at www.eas.com/research/creatine/0698.html on February 21, 1999.

Kreider RB, Ferreira M, Wilson M, et al. Effects of creatine supplementation on body composition, strength, and sprint performance. *Med Sci Sports Exerc.* 1998;30:73–82

Lawrence SR, et al. The effect of oral creatine supplementation on maximal exercise performance in competitive rowers. *Sports Medicine, Training and Rehabilitation.* 1997;7:243–253.

McNaughton LR, Dalton B, Tarr J. The effects of creatine supplementation on high–intensity exercise performance in elite performers. *Eur J Appl Physiol.* 1998;78:236–240.

Odland LM, et al. Effect of oral creatine supplementation on muscle [PCr] and short-term maximum power output. *Med Sci Sports Exerc.* 1997;29:216–219.

Poortmans JR, et al. Effect of short-term creatine supplementation on renal responses in men. *Eur J Appl Physiol.* 1997;76:566–567.

Prevost MC, Nelson AG, Morris GS. Creatine supplementation enhances intermittent work performance. *Res Q Exerc Sport.* 1997;68:233–240.

Schneider DA, et al. Creatine supplementation and the total work performed during 15-s and 1-min bouts of maximal cycling. *Aust J Sci Med Sport.* 1997;29:65–68.

Smith JC, et al. Effect of oral creatine ingestion on paarameters of the work rate-time relationship and time to exhaustion in high-intensity cycling. *Eur J Appl Physiol.* 1998;77:360–365.

Thompson CH, et al. Effect of creatine on aerobic and anaerobic metabolism in skeletal muscles in swimmers. *Br J Sports Med.* 1996;30:222–225.

Vandenberghe K, et al. Caffeine counteracts the ergogenic action of muscle creatine loading. *J Appl Physiol.* 1996;80:452–457.

Vandebuerie F, Vanden Eynde B, Vandenberghe K, Hespel P, et al. Effects of creatine loading on endurance capacity and sprint power in cyclists. *Int J Sports Med.* 1998;19:490–495.

Vandenberghe K, et al. Long-term creatine intake is beneficial to muscle performance during resistance training. *J Appl Physiol.* 1997;83:2055–2063.

Volek JS, et al. Creatine supplementation enhances muscular performance during high-intensity resistance exercise. *J Am Diet Assoc.* 1997;97:765–770.

Werbach MR. *Nutritional Influences on Illness: A Sourcebook of Clinical Research.* New Canaan, Conn: Keats Publishing, Inc; 1988.

DEHYDROEPIANDROSTERONE (DHEA)

Balch JF, Balch PA. *Prescription for Nutritional Healing.* 2nd ed. Garden City Park, NY: Avery Publishing; 1997:544–555.

Mindell E, Hopkins V. *Prescriptions Alternatives.* New Canaan, Conn: Keats Publishing; 1998:473–476.

Reynolds JE. *Martindale: The Extra Pharmacopoeia.* 31st ed. London, England: Royal Pharmaceutical Society; 1996:1504.

Shealy CN. *The Illustrated Encyclopedia of Healing Remedies.* Shaftesbury, England: Element Books; 1998:273.

Thompson G. Doctors warn of dangers of muscle-building drugs. *The New York Times.* March 2, 1999.

ETHYLENEDIAMINETETRAACETIC ACID (EDTA)

Burns CB, Currie B. The efficacy of chelation therapy and factors influencing mortality in lead intoxicated petrol sniffers. *Aust N Z J Med.* 1995;25:197–203.

Chappell LT, Stahl JP. The correlation between EDTA chelation therapy and improvement in cardiovascular function: a meta-analysis. *J Adv Med.* 1993;6:139–160.

Carey C, Lee H, and Woeltje K, eds. *Washington Manual of Medical Therapeutics.* 29th ed. Philadelphia, Penn: Lippincott-Raven; 1998.

Cranton E, Brecher A. *Bypassing Bypass.* Norfolk, Va: Donning Co; 1989.

Cranton E. *A Textbook on EDTA Chelation.* New York, NY: Humay Sciences Press; 1989.

Guldager B, Brixen KT, Jorgensen SJ, Nielsen HK, Mosekilde L, Jelnes R. Effects of intra-venous EDTA treatment on serum parathyroid hormone (1-84) and biochemical markers of bone turnover. *Dan Med Bull.* 1993;40:627–630.

Hancke C, Flytlie K. Benefits of EDTA chelation therapy on arteriosclerosis. *J Adv Med.* 1993;6:161–172.

Lin JL, Ho HH, Yu CC. Chelation therapy for patients with elevated body lead burden and progressive renal insufficiency. A randomized, controlled trial. *Ann Intern Med.* 1999;130:7–13.

Murray M. *Encyclopedia of Nutritional Supplements: The Essential Guide for Improving Your Health Naturally.* Rocklin, CA: Prima Publishing; 1996:435–436.

Olszewer E, Sabag FC, Carter JP. A pilot double-blind study of sodium-magnesium EDTA in peripheral vascular disease. *J Natl Med Assoc.* 1990;82:173–177.

Olszewer E, Carter JP. EDTA chelation therapy in chronic degenerative disease. *Med Hypotheses.* 1988;27:41–49.

Reynolds JEF, ed. *Martindale: The Extra Pharmacopoeia.* 31st ed. London, England: Royal Pharmaceutical Society; 1996.

Sloth-Nielson J, Guldager B, Mouritzen C, et al. Arteriographic findings in EDTA chelation therapy on peripheral arteriosclerosis. *Am J Surg.* 1991;162:122–125.

FLAXSEED OIL

Allman-Farinelli MA, Hall D, Kingham K, Pang D, Petocz P, Favaloro EJ. Comparison of the effects of two low fat diets with different alpha-linolenic acid ratios on coagulation and fibrinolysis. *Atherosclerosis.* 1999;142:159–168.

Bierenbuam ML, Reichstein R, Watkins TR. Reducing atherogenic risk in hyperlipemic humans with flaxseed supplementation: a preliminary report. *J Am Coll Nutr.* 1993;12:501–504.

Clark WF, Parbtani A, Hugg MW, et al. Flaxseed: a potential treatment of lupus nephritis. *Kidney Int.* 1995;48:475–480.

Cunnane SC, Ganguli S, Menard C, et al. High alpha-linolenic acid flaxseed (Linum usitatissimum): some nutritional properties in humans. *Br J Nutr.* 1993;69:443–453.

Cunnane SC, Hamadeh MJ, Liede AC, Thompson LU, Wolever TM, Jenkins DJ. Nutritional attributes of traditional flaxseed in healthy-young adults. *Am J Clin Nutr.* 1995;61:62–68.

Das UN, Madhavi N, Sravan KG, Padma M, Sangeetha P. Can tumor cell drug resistance be reversed by essential fatty acids and their metabolites? *Prostaglandins Leukot Essent Fatty Acids.* 1998;58:39–54.

Dox IG, Melloni BJ, Eisner GM. *The HarperCollins Illustrated Medical Dictionary.* New York, NY: HarperCollins Publishers; 1993.

Gerster H. Can adults adequately convert alpha-linolenic acid (18:3n-3) to eicosapentaenoic acid (20:5n-3) and docosahexaenoic acid (22:6n-3)? *Int J Vitam Nutr Res.* 1998;68:159–173.

Harris WS. N-3 fatty acids and serum lipoproteins: human studies. *Am J Clin Nutr.* May 1997;65(5 suppl):1645S–1654S.

Heller A, Koch T, Schmeck J, Van Ackern K. Lipid mediators in inflammatory disorders. *Drugs.* 1998;55:487–496.

Ingram AJ, Parbtani A, Clark WF, Spanner E, Huff MW, Philbrick DJ, Holub BJ. Effects of flax oil diets in a rat-5/6 renal ablation model. *Am J Kidney Dis.* 1995;25:320–329.

Kaminskas A, Levaciov, Lupinovic V, Kuchinskene Z. The effect of linseed oil on the fatty acid composition of blood plasma low- and very low-density lipoproteins and cholesterol in diabetics [in Russian]. *Vopr Pitan.* 1992;5–6:13–14.

Leece EA, Allman MA. The relationships between dietary alpha-linolenic: linoleic acid and rat platelet eicosapentaenoic and arachidonic acids. *Br J Nutr.* 1996;76:447–452.

Mantzioris E, James MJ, Gibson RA, Cleland LG. Differences exist in the relationships between dietary linoleic and alph-linolenic acids and their respective long-chain metabolites. *Am J Clin Nutr.* 1995;61:320–324.

Mayser P, Mrowietz U, Arenberger P, et al. Omega-3 fatty acid-based lipid infusion in patients with chronic plaque psoriasis: results of a double-blind, randomized, placebo-controlled, multicenter trial. *J Am Acad Dermatol.* 1998;38:539–547

Murray MT, Pizzorno JE. *Encyclopedia of Natural Medicine.* 2nd ed. Rocklin, Calif: Prima Publishing; 1998.

Nestel PJ, et al. Arterial compliance in obese subjects is improved with dietary plant n-3 fatty acid from flaxseed oil despite increased LDL oxidizabilty. *Arterioscler Thromb Vasc Biol.* 1997;17:1163–1170.

Norman AW, Litwack G. *Hormones.* Orlando, Fla: Academic Press, Inc; 1987.

Orten JM, Neuhaus OW, eds. *Human Biochemistry.* 10th ed. St. Louis, Mo: The C.V. Mosby Company; 1982.

Prasad K. Dietary flaxseed in prevention of hypercholesterolemic atherosclerosis. *Atherosclerosis.* 1997;132:69–76.

Shils ME, Olson JA, Shike M, eds. *Modern Nutrition in Health and Disease.* 8th ed. Media, Pa: Williams and Wilkins Co; 1994:1.

Schmidt MA. *Smart Fats: How Dietary Fats and Oils Affect Mental, Physical and Emotional Intelligence.* Berkeley, Calif: Frog, Ltd; 1997.

Valsta LM, Salminen I, Aro A, Mutanen M. Alpha-linolenic acid in rapeseed oil partly compensates for the effect of fish restriction on plasma long chain n-3 fatty acids. *Eur J Clin Nutr.* 1996;50:229–235.

GAMMA-LINOLENIC ACID (GLA)

Bolton-Smith C, Woodward M, Tavendale R. Evidence for age-related differences in the fatty acid composition of human adipose tissue, independent of diet. *Eur J Clin Nutr.* 1997;51:619–624.

Brzeski M, Madhok R, Capell HA. Evening primrose oil in patients with rheumatoid arthritis and side-effects of non-steroidal anti-inflammatory drugs. *Br J Rheumatol.* 1991;30:370–372.

Brown NA, Bron AJ, Harding JJ, Dewar HM. Nutrition supplements and the eye. *Eye.* 1998;12(pt 1):127–133.

Ensminger AH, Ensminger ME, Konlande JE, Robson JRK. *Foods & Nutrition Encyclopedia.* 2nd ed. Baton Rouge, Fla: CRC Press, Inc; 1994:1:684–708.

Fan YY, Chapkin RS. Importance of dietary gamma-linolenic acid in human health and nutrition. *J Nutr.* 1998;128:1411–1414.

Garrison RH Jr, Somer E. *The Nutrition Desk Reference.* 3rd ed. New Canaan, Conn: Keats Publishing, Inc; 1995:23–64.

Haas EM. *Staying Healthy with Nutrition.* Berkley, Calif: Celestial Arts Publishing; 1992:65–79.

Jamal GA, Carmichael H. The effects of gamma-linolenic acid on human diabetic peripheral neuropathy: a double-blind placebo-controlled trial. *Diabet Med.* 1990;7:319–323.

Jiang WG, Hiscox S, Bryce RP, Horrobin DF, Mansel RE. The effects of n-6 polyunsaturated fatty acids on the expression of nm-23 in human cancer cells. *Br J Cancer.* 1998;77:731–738.

Jiang WG, Hiscox S, Bryce RP, Horrobin DF, Mansel RE. Gamma linolenic acid regulates expression of maspin and the motility of cancer cells. *Biochem Biophys Res Commun.* 1997;237:639–644.

Kruger MC, Coetzer H, deWinter R, Gericke G, Papendorp DH. Calcium, gamma-linolenic acid and eicosapentaenoic acid supplementation in senile osteoporosis. *Aging (Milano).* 1998;10:385–394.

Leventhal LJ, Boyce EG, Zurier Rb. Treatment of rheumatoid arthritis with blackcurrant seed oil. *Br J Rheumatol.* 1994;33:847–852.

Murray MT. *Encyclopedia of Nutritional Supplements.* Rocklin, Calif: Prima Publishing; 1996:239-278.

Newstrom H. Nutrients Catalog. Jefferson, NC: McFarland & Co., Inc; 1993:103–105.

Puolakka J, Makarainen L, Viinikka L, Ylikorkala O. Biochemical and clinical effects of treating the premenstrual syndrome with prostaglandin synthesis precursors. *J Reprod Med.* 1985;30:149–153.

Shils ME, Olson JA, Shike M, Ross AC. *Modern Nutrition in Health and Disease.* 9th ed. Baltimore, Md: Williams & Wilkins; 1999:90–92; 1377–1378.

Wagner W, Nootbaar-Wagner U. Prophylactic treatment of migraine with gamma-linolenic and alpha-linolenic acids. *Cephalalgia.* 1997;17:127–130.

Werbach MR. *Nutritional Influences on Illness.* 2nd ed. Tarzana, Calif: Third Line Press; 1993:13–22; 655–671.

Zurier RB, Rossetti RG, Jacobson EW, et al. Gamma-Linolenic acid treatment of rheumatoid arthritis. A randomized, placebo-controlled trial. *Arthritis Rheum.* 1996;39:1808–1817.

GLUTAMINE

Balch J, Balch P. *Prescription for Nutritional Healing.* 2nd ed. Garden City Park, NY: Avery Publishing Group; 1997.

Castell LM, Newsholme EA. The effects of oral glutamine supplementation on athletes after prolonged, exhaustive exercise. *Nutrition.* 1997;13:738–742.

Den Hond E. Hiele M, Peeters M, Ghoos Y, Rutgeerts P. Effect of long-term oral glutamine supplements on small intestinal permeability in patients with Crohn's disease. *J Parenter Enteral Nutr.* 1999;23:7–11.

Giller R, Matthews K. *Natural Prescriptions.* New York, NY: Carol Southern Books/Crown Publishers; 1994.

Gottlieb B. *New Choices in Natural Healing.* Emmaus, Pa.: Rodale Press, Inc.; 1995.

Haas R. *Eat Smart, Think Smart.* New York, NY: HarperCollins; 1994.

Kirschmann G, Kirschmann J. *Nutrition Almanac.* 4th ed. New York, NY: McGraw Hill; 1996.

LaValle J. Natural agents for a healthy GI tract. *Drug Store News.* January 12, 1998;20.

Li J, Langkamp-Henken B, Suzuki K, Stahlgren LH. Glutamine prevents paranteral nutrition-induced increases intestinal permeability. *J Parenter Enteral Nutr.* 1994;18:303–307.

Napoli M. Chemo effect alleviated. *Health Facts.* October 1998;23:6.

Noyer CM, Simon D, Borczuk A, Brandt LJ, Lee MJ, Nehra V. A double-blind placebo-controlled pilot study of glutamine therapy for abnormal intestintal permeability in patients with AIDS. *Am J Gastroenterol.* 1998;93:972–975.

Shabert JK, Wilmore DW. Glutamine deficiency as a cause of human immunodeficiency virus wasting. *Med Hypotheses.* March 1996; 46:252–256.

Yoshida S, Matsui M, Shirouzu Y, Fujita H, Yamana H, Shirouzu K. Effects of glutamine supplements and radiochemotherapy on systemic immune and gut barrier function in patients with advanced esophageal cancer. *Ann Surg.* 1998;227:485–491.

IRON

Belton N. Iron deficiency in infants and young children. *Professional Care of Mother and Child.* 1995;5:69–71.

Cook JD, Skikne BS. Intestinal regulation of body iron. *Blood Rev.* 1987;1:267–272.

Ekhard ZE, Filer LJ, eds. *Present Knowledge in Nutrition.* 7th ed. Washington, DC: ILSI Press; 1996:191–201.

Fleming DJ, Jacques PF, Dallal GE, et al. Dietary determinants of iron stores in a free-living elderly population: the Framingham Heart Study. *Am J Clin Nutr.* 1998;67:722–733.

Hardman JG, Limbird LE, eds. *Goodman and Gillman's The Pharmacological Basis of Therapeutics.* 9th ed. New York: McGraw-Hill; 1996:1326–1333.

Mahan LK, Arlin MT, eds. *Krause's Food, Nutrition, and Diet Therapy.* 8th ed. Philadelphia, Pa: WB Saunders Co.; 1992:96–97.

National Research Council. *Recommended Dietary Allowances.* 10th ed. Washington, DC: National Academy Press; 1989:158–165.

Mason P. *Nutrition and Dietary Advice in the Pharmacy.* Oxford, UK: Blackwell Scientific; 1994:234–235.

Recommendations to Prevent and Control Iron Deficiency in the United States. Atlanta, Ga: Centers for Disease Control and Prevention. Morbidity and Mortality Weekly Report; April 3, 1998;47(RR-3):1–29.

The Food and Nutrition Information Center. National Agricultural Library (NAL), United States Department of Agriculture's (USDA) Agricultural Research Service (ARS). Accessed at *www.nal.usda.gov/fnic/Dietary/rda.html* on January 8, 1999.

Tzonou A, Lagiou P, Trichopoulou A, et al. Dietary iron and coronary heart disease: a study from Greece. *Am J Epidemiol.* 1998;147:161–166.

LIPASE

Berkow R, ed. *The Merck Manual of Medical Information.* Home Ed. Whitehouse Station, NJ: Merck Research Laboratories; 1997.

Mahan KL, Marian A. *Krause's Food Nutrition and Diet Therapy.* 8th ed. Philadelphia, Pa: WB Saunders Co; 1993.

Murray MT. *Encyclopedia of Nutritional Supplements.* Rocklin, Calif: Prima Publishing; 1986.

Shils ME, Olson JA, Shike M, eds. *Modern Nutrition in Health and Disease.* 8th ed. Philadelphia, Pa.: Lea and Febiger; 1994

LYSINE

Bruzzese N, Sica G, Iacopino F, et al. Growth inhibition of fibroblasts from nasal polyps and normal skin by lysine acetylsalicylate. *Allergy.* 1998;53:431–434.

De los Santos AR, Marti MI, Espinosa D, Di Girolamo G, Vinacur JC, Casadei A. Lysine clonixinate vs. paracetamol/codeine in postepisiotomy pain. *Acta Physiol Pharmacol. Ther Latinoam.* 1998;48:52–58.

Ensminger AH, Ensminger ME, Konlande JE, Robson JRK. *Foods & Nutrition Encyclopedia.* 2nd ed. Baton Rouge, Fla: CRC Press, Inc; 1994:1,2:60–64, 1,748.

Flodin NW. The metabolic roles, pharmacology, and toxicology of lysine. *J Am Coll Nutr.* 1997;16:7–21.

Garrison Jr RH, Somer E. *The Nutrition Desk Reference.* 3rd ed. New Canaan, Conn: Keats Publishing, Inc; 1995:39–52.

Haas EM. *Staying Healthy With Nutrition.* Berkeley, Calif: Celestial Arts Publishing; 1992.

Hugues FC, Lacoste JP, Danchot J, Joire JE. Repeated doses of combined oral lysine acetyl-salicylate and metoclopramide in the acute treatment of migraine. *Headache.* 1997;37:452–454.

Newstrom H. *Nutrients Catalog.* Jefferson, NC: McFarland & Co; 1993:303–312.

Shils ME, Olson JA, Shike M, Ross AC. *Modern Nutrition in Health and Disease.* 9th ed. Baltimore, Md: Williams & Wilkins; 1999:41, 1,010.

Werbach MR. *Nutritional Influences on Illness.* 2nd ed. Tarzana, Calif: Third Line Press; 1993:159–160, 384, 434, 494–495, 506, 580, 613–614, 636.

MAGNESIUM

Britton J, Pavord I, Richards K, Wisniewski A, Knox A, Lewis S. Dietary magnesium, lung function, wheezing, and airway hyperactivity in a random adult population sample. *Lancet.* 1994; 344:357–362.

Ensminger AH, Ensminger ME, Konlande JE, Robson JRK. *Foods and Nutrition Encyclopedia.* 2nd ed. Baton Rouge, Fla: CRC Press Inc; 1994;2:1338–1341.

Garrison Jr RH, Somer E. *The Nutrition Desk Reference.* 3rd ed. New Canaan, Conn: Keats Publishing Inc; 1995:158–165.

Hardman JG, Gilman AG, Limbird LE, eds. *Goodman and Gilman's Pharmacological Basis of Therapeutics.* 9th ed. New York, NY: McGraw-Hill; 1996:839–874.

Heinerman J. *Heinerman's Encyclopedia of Nature's Vitamins and Minerals.* Paramus, NJ: Prentice Hall Inc; 1998:296–302.

Murray MT. *Encyclopedia of Nutritional Supplements.* Rocklin, Calif: Prima Publishing; 1996:159–175.

Posaci C, Erten O, Uren A, Acar B. Plasma copper, zinc and magnesium levels in patients with premenstrual tensions syndrome. *Obstetricia et Gynecologica Scandinavica.* 1994; 73:452–455.

Romano TJ. Magnesium deficiency in systemic lupus erythematosus. *J Nutr Environ Med.* 1997;7:107–111.

Romano TJ, Stiller JW. Magnesium deficiency in fibromyalgia syndrome. *J Nutr Med.* 1994;4:165–167.

Sacks FM, Willett WC, Smith A, Brown LB, Rosner B, Moore TJ. Effect on blood pressure of potassium, calcium, and magnesium in women with low habitual intake. *Hypertension.* 1998;31:131–138.

Shils ME, Olson JA, Shike M, Ross AC. *Modern Nutrition in Health and Disease.* 9th ed. Baltimore, Md: Williams & Wilkins; 1999:169–192, A127–A128.

Werbach MR. *Nutritional Influences on Illness.* 2nd ed. Tarzana, Calif: Third Line Press; 1993:655–680.

MANGANESE

Davis CD, Greger JL. Longitudinal changes of manganese-dependent superoxide dismu-tase and other indexes of manganese and iron status in women. *Am J Clin Nutr.* 1992;55:747–752.

el-Yazigi A, Hannan N, Raines DA. Urinary excretion of chromium, copper, and man-ganese in diabetes mellitus and associated disorders. *Diabetes Res.* 1991;18:129–134.

Fell JM, Reynolds AP, Meadows N, et al. Manganese toxicity in children receiving long-term parenteral nutrition. *Lancet.* 1996;347:1218–1221.

Friedman E, ed. *Biochemistry of the Essential Ultratrace Elements.* New York, NY: Plenum Press; 1984.

Goering PL, Haassen CD. Mechanism of manganese-induced tolerance to cadmium lethal-ity and hepatotoxicity. *Biochem. Pharmacol.* 1985;34:1371-1379.

Itokawa Y. Trace elements in long-term total parenteral nutrition [in Japanese]. *Nippon Rinsho.* 1996;54:172–178.

Johnson MA, Smith MM, Edmonds JT. Copper, iron, zinc, and manganese in dietary sup-plements, infant formulas, and ready-to-eat breakfast cereals. *Am J Clin Nutr.* 1998;67(suppl):1035S–1040S.

Krause, MV., & Mahan, L.K. *Food, Nutrition, and Diet Therapy.* 7th ed. Philadelphia, Pa: WB Saunders Co., 1984.

Orten JM., Neuhaus OW, eds. *Human Biochemistry.* 10th ed. St. Louis, MO: The C.V. Mosby Co; 1982.

Pasquier C, Mach PS, Raichvarg D, Sarfati G, Amor B, Delbarre F. Manganese-containing superoxide-dismutase deficiency in polymorphonuclear leukocytes of adults with rheumatoid arthritis. *Inflammation.* 1984;8:27–32.

Saltman PD, Strause LG. The role of trace minerals in osteoporosis. *J Am Coll Nutr.* 1993;12:384–389.

Shils ME, Olson JA, Shike M, eds. *Modern Nutrition in Health and Disease.* 8th ed. Media, Pa: Williams and Wilkins Co; 1994:1.

Shvets NV, Kramarenko LD, Vydyborets SV, Gaidukova SN. Disordered trace element con-tent of the erythrocytes in diabetes mellitus [in Russian]. *Lik Sprava.* 1994;1:52–55.

Somer E. *The Essential Guide to Vitamins & Minerals.* New York, NY: HarperCollins Publishers; 1992.

Whitney EN, Hamilton EN. *Understanding Nutrition.* 3rd ed. St. Paul, Minn: West Publishing Co; 1984.

MELATONIN

Atkins R. *Dr. Atkin's Vita-Nutrient Solution.* New York, NY: Simon and Schuster. 1998.

Balch J, Balch P. *Prescription for Nutritional Healing.* Garden City Park, NY: Avery Publishing Group; 1997.

Lissoni P, Vigore L, Rescaldani R, et al. Neuroimmunotherapy with low-dose subcutaneous interleukin-2 plus melatonin in AIDS patients with CD4 cell number below 200/mm3: a biological phase-II study. *J Biol Regul Homeost Agents.* 1995;9:155–158.

MacIntosh A. Melatonin: clinical monograph. *Q Rev Nat Med.* 1996; 47–60.

Mindell E, Hopkins V. *Prescription Alternatives.* New Canaan, Conn: Keats Publishing, Inc.; 1998.

Murphy P, Myers B, Badia P. NSAIDs suppress human melatonin levels. *Am J Nat Med.* 1997; iv: 25.

Murray MT. *Encyclopedia of Nutritional Supplements.* Rocklin, Calif: Prima Publishing; 1996.

Petrie K, Conaglen JV, Thompson L, Chamberlain K. Effect of melatonin on jet lag after long haul flights. *BMJ.* 1989;298:705–707.

Rosenfeld I. *Dr. Rosenfeld's Guide to Alternative Medicine.* New York, NY: Random House; 1996.

Tzischinsky O, Lavie P. Melatonin possesses time-dependent hypnotic effects. *Sleep.* 1994;17:638–645.

Zhdanova IV, Wurtman RJ, Morabito C, Piotrovska VR, Lynch HJ. Effects of low oral doses of melatonin, given 2-4 hours before habitual bedtime, on sleep in normal young humans. *Sleep.* 1996;19:423–431.

Zhdanova IV, Wurtman RJ, Lynch HJ, et al. Sleep-inducing effects of low doses of melatonin ingested in the evening. *Clin Pharmacol Ther.* 1995; 57:552–558.

PHENYLALANINE

Bugard P, Bremer HJ, Buhrdel P, et al. Rationale for the German recommendations for phenylalanine level control in phenylketonuria 1997. *Eur J Pediatr.* 1999;158:46–54.

Ensminger AH, Ensminger ME, Konlande JE, Robson JRK. *Foods & Nutrition Encyclopedia.* 2nd ed. Baton Rouge, Fla: CRC Press, Inc; 1994:1,2:60–64, 1,748.

Garrison Jr RH, Somer E. *The Nutrition Desk Reference.* 3rd ed. New Canaan, Conn: Keats Publishing, Inc; 1995:39–52.

Haas EM. Staying Healthy With Nutrition. Berkeley, Calif: Celestial Arts Publishing; 1992.

Herbert V, Subak-Sharpe GJ, eds. *Total Nutrition (Mount Sinai School of Medicine).* New York, NY: St. Martin's Press; 1995:318–320.

Newstrom H. *Nutrients Catalog.* Jefferson, NC: McFarland & Co; 1993:303–312.

Pietz J. Neurological aspects of adult phenylketonuria. *Curr Opin Neurol.* 1998;11:679–688.

Pietz J, Dunckelmann R, Rupp A, et al. Neurological outcome in adult patients with early-treated phenylketonuria. *Eur J Pediatr.* 1998;157:824–830.

Shils ME, Olson JA, Shike M, Ross AC. *Modern Nutrition in Health and Disease.* 9th ed. Baltimore, Md: Williams & Wilkins; 1999:41, 1,010.

Start K. Treating phenylketonuria by a phenylalanine-free diet. *Prof Care Mother Child.* 1998;8:109–110.

Werbach MR. *Nutritional Influences on Illness.* 2nd ed. Tarzana, Calif: Third Line Press; 1993:159–160, 384, 434, 494–495, 506, 580, 613–614, 636.

PHOSPHORUS

Anderson JJB. Calcium, phosphorus, and human bone development. *J Nutr.* 1996;126:1153S–1158S.

Berner YN, Shike M. Consequences of phosphate imbalance. *Annu Rev Nutr.* 1988;8:121–148.

Carey CF, Lee HH, Woeltje KF, eds. *The Washington Manual of Medical Therapeutics.* 29th ed. New York, NY: Lippincott-Raven; 1998:230–237,444–448.

da Cunha DF, dos Santos VM, Monterio JP, de Carvalho da Cunha SF. Miner *Electrolyte Metab.* 1998;24:337–340.

Kuntziger H, Altman JJ. Hyperphosphoremia and hypophosphoremia [in French]. *Rev Prat.* 1989;39:949–953.

Metz JA, Anderson JJB, Gallagher Jr PN. Intakes of calcium, phosphorus, and protein, and physical activity level are related to radial bone mass in young adult women. *Am J Clin Nutr.* 1993;58: 537–542.

Mindell E, Hopkins V. *Prescription Alternatives.* Canaan, Conn: Keats Publishing Inc; 1998:495–496.

Reynolds JEF, ed. *Martindale: The Extra Pharmacopoeia.* 31st ed. London, Great Britain: Royal Pharmaceutical Society; 1996:1181–1182, 1741.

Shires R, Kessler GM. The absorption of tricalcium phosphate and its acute metabolic effects. *Calcif Tissue Int.* 1990;47:142–144.

Villa ML, Packer E, Cheema M, et al. Effects of aluminum hydroxide on the parathyroid-vitamin D axis of postmenopausal women. *J Clin Endocrinol Metab.* 1991;73:1256–1261.

Walker LP, Brown EH. *The Alternative Pharmacy.* NJ: Prentice-Hall; 1998:97.

Werbach MR. *Nutritional Influences on Illness: A Sourcebook of Clinical Research.* Canaan, Conn: Keats Publishing Inc; 1987.

POTASSIUM

Apstein C. Glucose-Insulin-Potassium for accute mycocardial infraction: remarkable results from a new prospective, randomized trial. *Circulation.* 1998;98:2223–2226.

Ascherio A, Rimm EB, Hernan MA, et al. Intake of potassium, magnesium, calcium, and fiber and risk of stroke among U.S. men. *Circulation.* 1998;98:1198–1204.

Brancati FL, Appel LJ, Seidler AJ, Whelton PK. Effect of potassium supplementation on blood pressure in African Americans on a low-potassium diet. *Arch Intern Med.* 1996;156:61–72.

Luft F, Ekhard ZE, Filer LJ, eds. *Present Knowledge in Nutrition.* 7th ed. Washington, DC: ILSI Press; 1996:272–276.

Mahan LK, Arlin MT, eds. *Krause's Food, Nutrition, and Diet Therapy.* 8th ed. Philadelphia, Pa: WB Saunders Co.; 1992:147, 390.

National Research Council: Recommended Dietary Allowances. 10th ed. Washington, DC: National Academy Press; 1989:255–257.

Ganong WF. *Review of Medical Physiology.* 18th ed. Stamford, Conn: Appleton & Lange; 1997: 677.

Perazella M, Mahnensmith R. Hyperkalemia in the elderly. *J Gen Intern Med.* 1997;12:646–656.

Sacks FM, Willett WC, Smith A, et al. Effect on blood pressure of potassium, calcium, and magnesium in women with low habitual intake. *Hypertension.* 1998;31(1):131–138

Singh RB, Singh NK, Niaz MA, Sharma JP. Effect of treatment with magnesium and potassium on mortality and reinfarction rate of patients with suspected acute myocardial infarction. *Int J Clin Pharmacol Thera.* 1996;34:219–225.

Suter PM. Potassium and Hypertension. *Nutrition Reviews.* 1998;56:151–133.

Young DB, Lin H, McCabe RD. Potassium's cardiovascular protective mechanisms. *Am J Physiology.* 1995;268(part 2):R825–R837.

PSYLLIUM

Alabaster O, Tang ZC, Frost A, Sivapurkar N. Potential synergism between wheat brain and psyllium: enhanced inhibition of colon cancer. *Cancer Lett.* 1993;75:53–58.

Ashraf W, Park F, Lof J, Quigley EM. Effects of psyllium therapy on stool characteristics, colon transit and anorectal function in chronic idiopathic constipation. *Aliment Pharmacol Ther.* 1995;9:639–647.

Balch J, Balch P. *Prescription for Nutritional Healing.* 2nd ed. Garden City Park, NY: Avery Publishing Group; 1997.

Fernandez-Banares F, Hinojosa J, Sanchez-Lombrana JL, et al. Randomized clinical trials of Platago ovata seeds (dietary fiber) as compared with mesalaminein maintaining remission in ulcerative colitis. *Am J Gastroenterol.* 1999;94:427–433.

Giller R, Matthews K. *Natural Prescriptions.* New York, NY: Carol Southern Books; 1994.

Kirschmann G, Kirschman J. *Nutrition Almanac.* 4th ed. New York, NY: McGraw-Hill; 1996.

McRorie JW, Daggy BP, Morel JG, Diersing PS, Miner PB, Robinson M. Psyllium is superior to docusate sodium for treatment of chronic constipation. *Aliment Pharmacol Ther.* 1998;12:491–497.

Moss R. *Cancer Therapy.* Brooklyn, NY: Equinox Press, Inc.; 1992.

Murray MT. *Encyclopedia of Nutritional Supplements.* Rocklin, Calif: Prima Publishing; 1996.

The Review of Natural Products. St. Louis, Mo: Facts and Comparisons; 1998.

Rodrigues-Moran M, Guerrero-Romero F, Lazcano-Burciaga G. Lipid- and glucose-lowering efficacy of Plantago Psyllium in type II diabetes. *J Diabetes Complications.* 1998;12:273–278.

SELENIUM

Balch JF, Balch PA. *Prescription for Nutritional Healing.* 2nd ed. Garden City Park, NY: Avery Publishing Group; 1997:28.

Clark LC, Combs GF Jr, Turnbull BW, et al. Effects of selenium supplementation for cancer prevention in patients with carcinoma of the skin. *JAMA.* 1996;276:1957–1963.

Combs GF, Clark LC. Can dietary selenium modify cancer risk? *Nutr Rev.* 1985;43:325–331.

Dworkin BM. Selenium deficiency in HIV infection and the acquired immunodeficiency syndrome (AIDS). *Chem Biol Interact.* 1994;91:181–186.

Garland M, Morris JS, Stampfer MJ, et al. Prospective study of toenail selenium levels and cancer among women. *J Natl Cancer Inst.* 1995;8:497–505.

Haas EM. *Staying Healthy with Nutrition: The Complete Guide to Diet and Nutritional Medicine.* Berkeley, Calif: Celestial Arts; 1992:211–216.

Murray MT. *Encyclopedia of Nutritional Supplements: The Essential Guide for Improving Your Health Naturally.* Rocklin, Calif: Prima Publishing; 1996:10–13, 222–228.

National Research Council, Diet and Health. *Implications for Reducing Chronic Disease Risk.* Washington, DC: National Academy Press; 1989:376–379.

Prasad K, ed. *Vitamins, Nutrition and Cancer.* New York, NY: Karger; 1984.

Walker LP, Hodgson Brown E. *The Alternative Pharmacy.* Paramus, NJ: Prentice Hall Press; 1998:313.

Wasowicz W. Selenium concentration and glutathione peroxidase activity in blood of children with cancer. *J Trace Elem Electrolytes Health Dis.* 1994;8:53–57.

Werbach MR. *Nutritional Influences on Illness: A Sourcebook of Clinical Research.* New Canaan, Conn: Keats Publishing; 1988.

Yang GQ, Xia YM. Studies on human dietary requirements and safe range of dietary intakes of selenium in China and their application in the prevention of related endemic diseases. *Biomed Environ Sci.* 1995;8:187–201.

Yoshizawa K, Willett WC, Morris SJ, et al. Studies of prediagnostic selenium level in toenails and the risk of advanced prostrate cancer. *J Natl Cancer Inst.* 1998;90:1219–1224.

SPIRULINA

Annapurna VV, Deosthale YG, Bamji MS. Spirulina as a source of vitamin A. *Plant Foods Hum Nutr.* 1991;41:125–134.

Chamorro G, Salazar M, Favila L, Bourges H. Pharmacology and toxicology of Spirulina alga. *Rev Invest Clin.* 1996;48:389–399. *Abstract.*

Chamorro G, Salazar M. Teratogenic study of spirulina in mice. *Arch Latinoam Nutr.* 1990;40:86–94.

Spirulina: good source of beta-carotene, but no miracle food. *Environ Nutr.* 1995;18:7.

Gonzalez R, Rodriguez S, Romay C, et al. Anti-inflammatory activity of phycocyanin extract in acetic acid-induced colitis in rats. *Pharmacol Res.* 1999;39:1055–1059.

Hayashi K, Hayashi T, Kojima I. A natural sulfated polysaccharide, calcium spirulan, isolated from *Spirulina platensis*: in vitro and ex vivo evaluation of anti-herpes simplex virus and anti-human immunodeficiency virus activities. *AIDS Res Hum Retroviruses.* 1996;12:1463–1471.

Mathew B, Sankaranarayanan R, Nair PP, et al. Evaluation of chemoprevention of oral cancer with *Spirulina fusiformis. Nutr Cancer.* 1995;24:197–202.

Qureshi MA, Garlich JD, Kidd MT. Dietary *Spirulina platensis* enhances humoral and cell-mediated immune functions in chickens. *Immunopharmacol Immunotoxicol.* 1996;18:465–476.

Romay C, Armesto J, Remirez D, Gonzalez R, Ledon N, Garcia I. Antioxidant and anti-inflammatory properties of C-phycocyanin from blue-green algae. *Inflamm Res.* 1998;47:36–41.

Salazar M, Martinez E, Madrigal E, Ruiz LE, Chamorro GA. Subchronic toxicity study in mice fed *Spirulina maxima. J Ethnopharmacol.* 1998;62:235–241.

Shealy NC. *The Illustrated Encyclopedia of Healing Remedies.* Boston, Mass: Element Books; 1998:277.

Walker LP, Brown EH. *The Alternative Pharmacy.* Paramus, NJ: Prentice Hall Press; 1998:51–53.

SULFUR

Balch J, Balch P. *Prescription for Nutritional Healing.* 2nd ed. Garden City, NY: Avery Publishing Group; 1997.

Eades MD. *The Doctor's Complete Guide to Vitamins and Minerals.* New York, NY: Dell Publishing; 1994.

Haas EM. *Staying Healthy with Nutrition.* Berkeley, Calif: Celestial Arts; 1992.

Lockie A, Geddes N. *The Complete Guide to Homeopathy.* New York, NY: DK Publishing; 1995.

Lester MR. Sulfite sensitivity: significance in human health. *J Am Coll Nutr.* 1995;14(3):229-32.

Mahan LK, Arlin MT. *Krause's Food, Nutrition and Diet Therapy.* 8th ed. Philadelphia, Pa: WB Saunders Company (Harcourt, Brace, Jovanovich, Inc.); 1992.

Martensson J. The effect of fasting on leucocyte and plasma glutathione and sulfur amino acid concentrations. *Metabolism.* 1986;35:118–121.

Midell E, Hopkins V. *Prescription Alternatives.* New Canaan, Conn: Keats Publishing; 1998.The Mineral Connection website. MSM, Biologicial Sulfur supplements. Accessed at *www.mineralconnection.com/msm.htm* on March 5, 1999.

Murray MT, Pizzorno JE. *Encyclopedia of Natural Medicine.* Rev. 2nd edition. Rocklin, Calif: Prima Publishing; 1998.

Nutrition Search, Inc.. *Nutrition Almanac.* Rev. ed. New York, NY: McGraw-Hill; 1979.

Pratsel HG, Eigner UM, Weinert D, Limbach B. The analgesic efficacy of sulfur mud baths in treating rheumatic diseases of the soft tissues [In Russian]. *Vopr Kurortol Fizioter Lech Fiz Kult.* 1992;1992:37–41.

Roediger WE, Moore J, Babidge W. Colonic sulfide in pathogenesis and treatment of ulcerative colitis. *Dig Dis Sci.* 1997;42:1571–1579.

Rossi A, Kaitila I, Wilcox WR, et al. Proteoglycan sulfation in cartilage and cell cultures from patients with sulfate transporter chondrodysplasias: relationship to clinical severity and indications on the role of intracellular sulfate production. *Matrix Biol.* 1998;17:361–369.

Shealy CN. *The Illustrated Encyclopedia of Healing Remedies.* Boston, Mass: Element Books, Inc; 1998.

Smith SM, McDonald A, Webb D. *Complete Book of Vitamins and Minerals.* Lincolnwood, Ill: Publications International, Ltd; 1998.

Smirnova OV, Saliev VP, Klemparskaia NN, Dobronravova NN. Purified sulfur as an agent to relieve the side effects in the radiation therapy of cervical cancer [In Russian]. *Med Radiol Mosk.* 1991;36:16–19.

Somer E. *The Essential Guide to Vitamins and Minerals.* New York, NY: Harper Collins Publishers Inc; 1995.

Sukenik S, Giryes H, Halevy, et al. Treatment of psoriatic arthritis at the Dead Sea. *J Rheumatol.* 1994;21:1305–1309.

Weiner M. *The Complete Book of Homeopathy.* New York, NY: MJF Books; 1989.

Werbach MR. *Nutritional Influences on Illness: A Sourcebook of Clinical Research.* New Canaan, Conn: Keats Publishing, Inc; 1988.

TYROSINE

Balch JF, Balch PA. *Prescriptions for Nutritional Healing.* 2nd ed. Garden City Park, NY: Avery Publishing; 1997:42.

Haas EM. *Staying Healthy with Nutrition.* Berkeley, Calif: Celestial Arts; 1992:51.

Mindell E, Hopkins V. Prescription Alternatives. New Canaan, Conn: Keats Publishing; 1998:398.

Shealy CN. *The Illustrated Encyclopedia of Healing Remedies.* Shaftesbury, England: Element; 1998:269

Werbach MR. *Nutritional Influences on Illness.* New Canaan, Conn: Keats Publishing, 1987:162.

VANADIUM

Balch JF, Balch PA. *Prescription for Nutritional Healing.* Garden City Park, NY: Avery Publishing; 1997:29.

Bender DA, Bender AE. *Nutrition: A Reference Handbook.* New York, NY: Oxford University Press; 1997:424.

Murray MT. *Encyclopedia of Nutritional Supplements.* Rocklin, Calif: Prima Publishing, 1996:232–234.

Murray MT, Pizzorno JE. *Enclyclopedia of Natural Medicine.* 2nd ed. Rocklin, Calif: Prima Publishing; 1998:283–284.

Shealy CN. *The Illustrated Encyclopedia of Healing Remedies.* Boston, Mass: Element Books; 1998:268.

Role of vanadium as a mimic of insulin. *Nutri Res Newslett.* 1998;17:11.

Werbach MR. *Nutritional Influences on Illness.* New Canaan, Conn: Keats Publishing; 1987:87–88, 159.

Yale J-F, Lachance D, Bevan AP. Hypoglycemic effects of peroxovanadium compounds in Sprague-Dawley and diabetic BB rats. *Diabetes.* 1995;44:1274–1276.

VITAMIN A (RETINOL)

Eades MD. *The Doctor's Complete Guide to Vitamins and Minerals.* New York, NY: Dell Publishing; 1994:48.

Fawzi WW. Vitamin A supplementation and child mortality. *JAMA.* 1993;269:898–903.

Fawzi WW, Mbise RL, Hertzmark E, et al. A randomized trial of vitamin A supplements in relation to mortality among human immunodeficiency virus-infected and uninfected children in Tanzania. *Pediatr Infect Dis J.* 1999;18:127–133.

Fortes C, Forastiere F, Agabiti N, et al. The effect of zinc and vitamin A supplementation on immune response in an older population. *J Am Geriatr Soc.* 1998;46:19–26.

Futoryan T, Gilchrest BA. Retinoids and the skin. *Nutr Rev.* 1994;52:299–310.

Kindmark A, Rollman O, Mallmin H, et al. Oral isotretinoin therapy in severe acne induces transient suppression of biochemical markers of bone turnover and calcium homeostasis. *Acta Derma Venereol.* 1998;78:266–269.

Melhus H, Michaelsson K, Kindmark A, et al. Excessive dietary intake of vitamin A is associated with reduced bone mineral density and increased risk for hip fracture. *Ann Intern Med.* 1998;129:770–778.

Murray MT. *Encyclopedia of Nutritional Supplements.* Rocklin, Calif: Prima Publishing; 1996.

Nursing '93 Drug Handbook. Springhouse, Pa: Springhouse Corporation; 1993.

Semba RD. Vitamin A, immunity and infection. *Clin Infect Dis.* 1994;19:489–499.

Whitney E, Cataldo C, Rolfes S. *Understanding Normal and Clinical Nutrition.* St. Paul, Minn: West Publishing Company; 1987.

VITAMIN B₁ (THIAMINE)

Boros LG, Brandes JL, Lee W-N P, et al. Thiamine supplementation to cancer patients: a double-edged sword. *Anticancer Res.* 1998;18:595–602.

Ekhard ZE, Filer LJ, eds. *Present Knowledge in Nutrition.* 7th ed. Washington, DC: ILIS Press; 1996:160–166.

Hardman JG, Limbird LE, eds. *Goodman and Gilman's The Pharmacological Basis of Therapeutics.* 9th ed. New York, NY: McGraw-Hill; 1996:1555–1558.

Leslie D, Gheorghiade M. Is there a role for thiamine supplementation in the management of heart failure? *Am Heart J.* 1996;131:1248–1250.

Lindberg MC, Oyler RA. Wernick's encephalopathy. *Am Fam Physician.* 1990;41:1205–1209.

Mahan LK, Arlin MT, eds. *Krause's Food, Nutrition and Diet Therapy.* 8th ed. Philadelphia, Pa: WB Saunders;1992:85–87.

Mason P. *Nutrition and Dietary Advice in the Pharmacy.* Oxford, UK: Blackwell Scientific; 1994:269–271.

National Academy of Science. Recommended Daily Allowances. Accessed at www.nal.usda.gov/fnic/dietary/rda.html on January 4, 1999.

VITAMIN B₂ (RIBOFLAVIN)

1999 Drug Facts and Comparisons. New York, NY: J.B. Lippincott Company; 1998.

Christenson, H. Riboflavin can protect tissues from oxidative injury. *Nutr Rev.* May 1993;51:149–150.

Duyff R. *The American Dietary Association Complete Food and Nutrition Guide.* Minneapolis, Minn: Cronimed Publishing; 1996.

Food and Nutrition Board, Institute of Medicine. Dietary Reference Intakes for Thiamin, Riboflavin, Niacin, Vitamin B6, Folate, Vitamin B12, Pantothenic Acid, Biotin, and Choline. Washington, DC: National Academy Press; 1998.

Matarese L, Gottschlich M. *Contemporary Nutrition Support Practice. A Clinical Guide.* Philadelphia, Pa: WB Saunders Company; 1998.

Murray MT. *Encyclopedia of Nutritional Supplements.* Rocklin, Calif: Prima Health; 1996.

Realey N. *Vitmains Etc.* Melbourne, Australia: Bookman Press; 1998.

Schoenen J, Jacquy J, Lenaerts M. Effectiveness of high-dose riboflavin in migraneprophi-laxis. A randomized controlled trial. *Neurology.* February 1998;50:466–470.

VITAMIN B₃ (NIACIN)

Aronov DM, Keenan JM, Akhmedzhanov NM, Perova NV, Oganove RY, Kiseteva NY. Clinical trial of wax-matrix sustained-release niacin in a Russian population with hypercholes-terolemia. *Arch Fam Med.* 1996;5:567–575.

Berge KG, Canner PL. Coronary drug project: experience with niacin. Coronary Drug Project Research Group. *Eur J Clin Pharmacol.* 1991;40(suppl 1):S49–S51.

Boden G, Chen X, Igbal N. Acute lowering of plasma fatty acids lowers basal insulin secretion in diabetic and nondiabetic subjects. *Diabetes.* 1998;47:1609–1612.

Capuzzi DM, Guyton JR, Morgan JM, et al. Efficacy and safety of an extended-release niacin (Niaspan): a long-term study. *Am J Cardiol.* Dec 17, 1998;82:74U–81U.

Chojnowska-Jezierska J, Adamska-Dyniewska H. Prolonged treatment with slow-release nicotinic acid in patients with type II hyperlipidemia. *Pol Arch Med Wewn.* 1997;98:391–399.

Eades MD. *The Doctor's Complete Guide to Vitamins and Minerals.* New York, NY: Dell Publishing; 1994.

Gardner SF, Schneider EF, Granberry MC, Carter IR. Combination therapy with low-dose lovastatin and niacin is as effective as higher-dose lovastatin. *Pharmacotherapy.* 1996;16:419–423.

Guyton JR. Effect of niacin on atherosclerotic cardiovascular disease. *Am J Cardiol.* Dec 17, 1998;82:18U–23U.

Guyton JR, Capuzzi DM. Treatment of hyperlipidemia with combined niacin-statin regimens. *Am J Cardiol.* Dec 17, 1998;82:82U–84U.

Hendler SS. *The Doctor's Vitamin and Mineral Encyclopedia.* New York, NY: Simon and Schuster; 1990.

Hocking GM. *A Dictionary of Natural Products.* Medford, NJ: Plexus Publishing, Inc; 1997.

Harborne JB, Baxter H, eds. *Phytochemical Dictionary: A Handbook of Bioactive Compounds from Plants.* Rev. ed. London, England: Taylor & Francis; 1995.

Lieberman S, Bruning N. *The Real Vitamin and Mineral Book.* Garden City Park, NY: Avery Publishing Group, Inc; 1990.

Lomnicky Y, Friedman M, Luria MH, Raz I, Hoffman A. The effect of the mode of adminis-tration on the hypolipidaemic activity of niacin: continuous gastrointestinal administra-tion of low-dose niacin improves lipid-lowering efficacy in experimentally-induced hyperlipidaemic rats. *J Pharm Pharmacol.* 1998;50:1233–1239.

Mostaza JM, Schulz I, Vega GL, Grundy SM. Comparison of pravastatin with crystalline nicotinic acid monotherapy in treatment of combined hyperlipidemia. *Am J Cardiol.* 1997;79:1298–1301.

Murray MT. *Encyclopedia of Nutritional Supplements.* Rocklin, Calif: Prima Publishing; 1996.

Nursing 93 Drug Handbook. Springhouse, Pa: Springhouse Corporation; 1993.

Nutrition Search, Inc. *Nutrition Almanac.* Rev. ed. New York, NY: McGraw-Hill, 1979.

O'Keefe Jr JH, Harris WS, Nelson J, Windsor SL. Effects of pravastatin with niacin or mag-nesium on lipid levels and postprandial lipemia. *Am J Cardiol.* 1995;76:480–484.

Smith SM, McDonald A, Webb D. *Complete Book of Vitamins and Minerals.* Lincolnwood, Ill: Publications International, Ltd; 1998.

Somer E. *The Essential Guide to Vitamins and Minerals.* New York, NY: Harper Collins Publishers Inc; 1995.

Vacek J, Dittmeier G, Chiarelli T, White J, Bell HH. Comparison of lovastatin (20 mg) and nicotinic acid (1.2 mg) with either drug alone for type II hyperlipoproteinemia. *Am J Cardiol.* 1995;76:182–184.

Werbach MR. *Nutritional Influences on Illness: A Sourcebook of Clinical Research.* New Canaan, Conn: Keats Publishing, Inc; 1988.

Whitney E, Cataldo C, Rolfes S. *Understanding Normal and Clinical Nutrition.* 2nd ed. St. Paul, Minn: West Publishing Co; 1987.

Zeman F. *Clinical Nutrition and Dietetics.* 2nd ed. New York, NY: Macmillan Publishing Company; 1991.

VITAMIN B₅ (PANTOTHENIC ACID)

Arsenio L, et al. Effectiveness of long-term treatment with pantethine in patients with dyslipidemia. *Clin Ther.* 1986;8:537–545.

Bertolini S, Donati C, Elicio N, et al. Lipoprotein changes induced by pantethine in hyper-lipoproteinemic patients: adults and children. *Int J Clin Pharmacol Ther Toxicol.* 1986;24:630–637.

Binaghi P, Cellina G, Lo Cicero G, et al. Evaluation of the cholesterol-lowering effective-ness of pantethine in women in perimenopausal age [in Italian]. *Minerva Med.* 1990;81:475–479.

Coronel F, Tornero F, Torrente J, et al. Treatment of hyperlipemia in diabetic patients on dialysis with a physiological substance. *Am J Nephrol.* 1991;11:32–36.

Gaddi A, et al. Controlled evaluation of pantethine, a natural hypolipidemic compound in patients with different forms of hyperlipoproteinemia. *Atherosclerosis.* 1984;50:73–83.

Gensini GF, et al. Changes in fatty acid composition of the single platelet phospholipids induced by pantethine treatment. *Int J Clin Pharmacol Res.* 1985;5:309–318.

Haas E. *Staying Healthy with Nutrition: The Complete Guide to Diet and Nutritional Medicine.* Berkeley, Calif: Celestial Arts Publishing; 1992.

Hendler SS. *The Doctors' Vitamin and Mineral Encyclopedia.* New York, NY: Fireside Press; 1991.

Lieberman S, Bruning N. *The Real Vitamin and Mineral Book.* 2nd ed. New York, NY: Avery Publishing Group; 1997.

Murray M. *Encyclopedia of Nutritional Supplements.* Rocklin, Calif: Prima Publishing; 1996.

Prisco D, Rogasi PG, Matucci M, et al. Effect of oral treatment with pantethine on platelet and plasma phospholipids in IIa hyperlipoproteinemia. *Angiology.* 1987;38:241–247.

Somer E. *The Essential Guide to Vitamins and Minerals.* New York, NY: HarperCollins Publishers, Inc; 1995.

Vaxman F, Olender S, Lambert A, et al. Effect of pantothenic acid and ascorbic acid sup-plementation on human skin wound healing process. A double-blind, prospective and randomized trial. *Eur Surg Res.* 1995;27:158–166.

VITAMIN B₆ (PYRIDOXINE)

Ballal RS, Jacobsen DW, Robinson K. Homocysteine: update on a new risk factor. *Cleve Clin J Med.* 1997;64:543–549.

Berger AR, Schaumburg HH, Schroeder C, Apfel S, Reynolds R. Dose response, coasting and differential fiber vulnerability in human toxic neuropathy: a prospective study of pyridoxine neurotoxicity. *Neurology.* 1992;42:1367–1370.

Brush MG, Bennett T, Hansen K. Pyridoxine in the treatment of premenstrual syndrome: a retrospective survey in 630 patients. *Br J Clin Pract.* 1998;42:448–452.

Diegoli MS, da Fonseca AM, Diegoli CA, Pinoltti JA. A double-blind trial of four medica-tions to treat severe premenstrual syndrome. *Int J Gynaecol Obstet.* 1998;62:63–67.

Ekhard ZE, Filer LJ, eds. *Present Knowledge in Nutrition.* 7th ed. Washington, DC: ILSI Press; 1996:191–201.

Folsom AR, Nieto FJ, McGovern PG, et al. Prospective study of coronary heart disease incidence in relation to fasting total homocysteine, related genetic polymorphisms, and B vitamins: the atherosclerosis risk in communities. *Circulation.* 1998;98:204–210.

Gospe SM. Current perspectives on pyridoxine-dependent siezures. *J Pediatr.* 1998;132:919–923.

Hardman JG, Limbird LE, eds. *Goodman and Gillman's Pharmacological Basis of Therapeutics.* 9th ed. New York: McGraw-Hill; 1996:1326–1333.

Keniston RC, Nathan PA, Leklem JE, Lockwood RS. Vitamin B6, vitamin C, and carpal tunnel syndrome. A cross-sectional study of 441 adults. *J Occup Environ Med.* 1997;39:949–959.

Mahan LK, Arlin MT, eds. *Krause's Food, Nutrition, and Diet Therapy.* 8th ed. Philadelphia, Pa: WB Saunders Co; 1992:96–97.

Murphy PA. Alternative therapies for nausea and vomiting of pregnancy. *Obstet Gynecol.* 1998; 91:149-155.

National Research Council: Recommended Dietary Allowances. 10th ed. Washington, DC: National Academy Press; 1989: 158–165.

O'Connell BJ. The pediatrician and the sexually active adolescent: treatment of common menstrual disorders. *Pediatr Clin North Am.* 1997;44:1391–1404.

Recommended Dietary Allowance. American Academy of Sciences. Accessed at www.nal.usda.gov/fnic/Dietary/rda.html on January 8, 1999.

VITAMIN B₉ (FOLIC ACID)

Bendich A, Deckelbaum R, eds. *Prevention Nutrition: The Comprehensive Guide for Health Professionals.* Totowa, NJ: Humana Press; 1997.

Bronstrup A, Hages M, Prniz-Langenohl R, Pietrzik K. Effects of folic acid and combina-tions of folic acid and vitamin B12 on plasma homocysteine concentrations in healthy, young women. *Am J Clin Nutr.* 1998;68:1104–1110.

Cancers, Nutrition and Food. Washington, DC: World Cancer Research Fund/American Institute for Cancer Research; 1997.

Ebly EM, Schaefer JP, Campbell NR, Hogan DB. Folate status, vascular disease and cognition in elderly Canadians. *Age Ageing.* 1998;27:485–491.

1999 Drug Facts and Comparisons. Facts and Comparisons; 1998.

Giles WH, Kittner SJ, Croft JB, Anda RF, Casper ML, Ford ES. Serum folate and risk for coronary heart disease: Results from a cohort of US adults. *Ann Epidemiol.* 1998;8:490–496.

Lewis DP, Van Dyke DC, Stumbo PJ, Berg MJ. Drug and environmental factors associated with adverse pregnancy outcomes. Part II: Improvement with folic acid. *Ann Pharmacother.* 1998;32:947–961.

Malinow MR, Duell PB, Hess DL, et al. Reduction of plasma homocyst(e)ine levels by breakfast cereal fortified with folic acid in patients with coronary heart disease. *N Engl J Med.* 1998;338:1009–1015.

Morgan SL, Baggott JE, Lee JY, Alarcon GS. Folic acid supplementation prevents deficient blood folate levels and hyperhomocysteinemia during long-term, low-dose methotrexate therapy for rheumatoid arthritis: implications for cardiovascular disease prevention. *J Rheumatol.* 1998;25:441–446.

Murray MT. *Encyclopedia of Nutritional Supplements.* Rocklin, Calif: Prima Health; 1996.

Ortiz Z, Shea B, Suarez-Almazor ME, et al. The efficacy of folic acid and folinic acid in reducing methotrexate gastrointestinal toxicity in rheumatoid arthritis. A metaanalysis of randomized controlled trials. *J Rheumatol.* 1998;25:36–43.

Reavley N. *Vitamins, etc.* Melbourne, Australia: Bookman Press; 1998.

Rimm EB, Willett WC, Hu FB, et al. Folate and vitamin B6 from diet and supplements in relation to risk of coronary heart disease among women. *JAMA.* 1998;279:359–364.

Ringer D, ed. *Physician's Guide to Nutriceuticals.* St. Joseph, Mich: Nutritional Data Resources; 1998.

Watkins ML. Efficacy of folic acid prophylaxis for the prevention of neural tube defects. *Ment Retard Dev Disab Res Rev.* 1998;4:282–290.

Wolf PA. Prevention of stroke. *Lancet.* 1998;352 (suppl III):15–18.

VITAMIN B$_{12}$ (COBALAMIN)

Ballal RS, Jacobsen DW, Robinson K. Homocysteine: update on a new risk factor. *Cleve Clin J Med.* 1997;64:543–549.

Committee on Dietary Allowances. *Recommended Dietary Allowances.* National Academy of Sciences. Accessed at *www.nal.usda.gov/fnic/Dietary/rda.html* on January 8, 1999.

Ekhard ZE, Filer LJ, eds. *Present Knowledge in Nutrition.* 7th ed. Washington, DC: ILSI Press; 1996:191–201.

Hardman JG, Limbird LE, eds. *Goodman and Gillman's The Pharmacological Basis of Therapeutics.* 9th ed. New York, NY: McGraw-Hill; 1996:1326–1333.

Mahan LK, Arlin MT, eds. *Krause's Food, Nutrition, and Diet Therapy.* 8th ed. Philadelphia, Pa: WB Saunders Co; 1992:96–97.

Dorland Newman WA, ed. *Dorland's Illustrated Medical Dictionary.* 28th ed. Philadelphia, Pa: WB Saunders Co; 1994:73.

Ingram CF, Fleming AF, Patel M, Galpin JS. The value of intrinsic factor antibody test in diagnosing pernicious anaemia. *Cent Afr J Med.* 1998;44:178–181.

Lobo A, Naso A, Arheart K, et al. Reduction of homocysteine levels in coronary artery disease by low-dose folic acid combined with levels of vitamins B$_6$ and B$_{12}$. *Am J Cardiol.* 1999;83:821–825.

Lee AJ. Metformin in noninsulin-dependent diabetes mellitus. *Pharmacotherapy.* 1996;16:327–351.

National Research Council. *Recommended Dietary Allowances.* 10th ed. Washington, DC: National Academy Press; 1989:158–165.

Nilsson-Ehle H. Age-related changes in cobalamin (vitamin B$_{12}$) handling. Implications for therapy. *Drugs Aging.* 1998;12:277–292.

Remacha AF, Cadafalch J. Cobalamin deficiency in patients infected with the human immunodeficiency virus. *Semin Hematol.* 1999;36:75–87.

van Asselt DZ, van den Broek WJ, Lamers CB, et al. Free and protein-bound cobalamin absorption in healthy middle-aged and older subjects. *J Am Geriatr Soc.* 1996;44:949–953.

VITAMIN C (ASCORBIC ACID)

Cohen H, Neuman I, Nahum H. Blocking effect of Vitamin C in exercise-induced asthma. *Arch Pediatr Adolesc Med.* 1997;151:367–370.

Eades MD. *The Doctor's Complete Guide to Vitamins and Minerals.* New York, NY: Dell Publishing; 1994.

Eberlein-Konig B, Placzek M, Przybilla B. Protective effect against sunburn of combined systemic ascorbic acid (vit.C) and D-alpha-tocopherol (vit.E). *J Am Acad Dermatol.* 1998;38:45–48.

Galley HF, Thornton J, et al. Combination oral antioxidant supplementation reduces blood pressure. *Clin Sci.* 1997;92:361–365.

Hendler SS. *The Doctors' Vitamin and Mineral Encyclopedia.* New York, NY: Fireside Press, 1991.

Lieberman S, Bruning N. *The Real Vitamin & Mineral Book.* 2nd ed. New York, NY: Avery Publishing Group; 1997.

Mahan K, Arlin M, eds. *Krause's Food, Nutrition and Diet Therapy.* 8th ed. Philadelphia, Pa: WB Saunders Company; 1992.

Mosca L, et al. Antioxidant nutrient supplementation reduces the susceptibility of low density lipoprotein to oxidation in patients with coronary artery disease. *J Am Coll Cardiol.* 1997;30:392–399.

Murray MT. *Encyclopedia of Nutritional Supplements.* Rocklin, Calif: Prima Publishing; 1996.

Watanabe H, Kakihana M, Ohtsuka S, Sugishita Y. Randomized, double blind, placebo-controlled study of ascorbate on the preventive effect of nitrate tolerance in patients with congestive heart failure. *Circulation.* 1998;97:886–891.

Whitney E,Cataldo C, Rolfes S. *Understanding Normal and Clinical Nutrition.* St. Paul, Minn: West Publishing Company; 1987

VITAMIN D

American Academy of Sciences. *Dietary Reference Intakes: Calcium Phosphorus, Magnesium, Vitamin D, and Fluoride.* National Academy Press; 1997.

Bendich A, Deckelbaum R, eds. *Preventive Nutrition: The Comprehensive Guide for Health Professionals.* Totowa, NJ: Humana Press; 1997.

Brenner RV, Shabahang M, Schumaker LM, et al. The antiproliferation effect of vitamin D analogs on MCF-7 human breast cancer cells. *Cancer Lett.* 1995;92:77–82.

Dawson-Hughes B, Harris SS, Dallal GE. Plasma calcidiol, season, and serum parathyroid hormone concentrations in healthy elderly men and women. *Am J Clin Nutr.* 1997;65:67–71.

Dawson-Hughes B, Harris SS, Krall EA, etal. Effect of calcium and vitamin D supplementation on bone density in men and women 65 years of age and older. *N Engl J Med.* 1997;337:670–676.

Deroisy R, Collette J, Chevallier T, et al. 1998. Effects of two 1-year calcium and vitamin D$_3$ treatments on bone remodeling markers and femoral bone density in elderly women. *Curr Thera Res.* 59(12):850–862.

Drug Facts and Comparisons 1999. St. Louis, Mo: A. Wolters Kluwer Company; 1998.

Heikkinen AM, Tuppurainen MT, Niskanen L, et al. Long-term vitamin D$_3$ supplementation may have adverse effects on serum lipids during menopause hormone replacement therapy. *J Endocrinology.* 1997;137:495–502.

Kizaki M, Ikeda Y, Simon KJ, et al. Effect of 1,25-dihydroxyvitamin D$_3$ and its analogs on human immunodeficiency virus infection in monocytes-macrophages. *Leukemia.* 1993;7:1525–153.

Kitch BT, Vamvakas EC, Dick IM, et al. Hypovitaminosis D in medical implants. *N Engl J Med.* 1998;338:777–783.

Langman M, Boyle P, et al. Chemoprevention of colorectal cancer. *Gut.* 1998;43:578–585.

Mahan K, Arlin M. *Krause's Food, Nutrition and Diet Therapy.* 8th ed. Philadelphia, Pa: WB Saunders Company; 1992.

Martinez ME, Giovannucci EL Colditz GA, et al. Calcium, vitamin D, and the occurrence of colorectal cancer among women. *JNCI.* 1996;88:1375–1382.

Reavley N. *Vitamins, Etc.* Melbourne, Australia: Bookman Press; 1998.

Thomas MK, Lloyd-Jones DM, Thadhani RI, et al. Hypovitaminosis D in medical inpatients. *N Engl J Med.* 1998;338:777–783.

VITAMIN E

Balch J, Balch, P. *Prescription for Nutritional Healing: A-to-Z Guide to Supplements.* New York, NY: Avery Publishing Group; 1998.

Chan AC. Vitamin E and atherosclerosis. *J Nutr.* 1998;128:(10):1593–1596.

Feltman J. *Prevention's Food & Nutrition.* Emmaus, Pa: Rodale Press; 1993.

Klatz R. Vitamin E. *Total Health.* Sept/Oct 97: 28.

Leske MC, Chylack Jr LT, He Q, et al. Antioxidant vitamins and nuclear opacities: the longitudinal study of cataract. *Ophthalmology.* 1998;105:831–836.

Lieberman S, Bruning N. *The Real Vitamin & Mineral Book.* 2nd ed. New York, NY: Avery Publishing Group; 1997.

Liebman B. Vitamin E and Fat. *Nutrition Action Healthletter.* Jul/Aug 96:10

Mahan K, Arlin M, eds. *Krause's Food, Nutrition and Diet Therapy.* 8th ed. Philadelphia, Pa: WB Saunders Company; 1992.

Meydani SN, Meydani M, Blumberg JB, et al. Assessment of the safety of supplementation with different amounts of vitamin E in healthy older adults. *Am J Clin Nutr.* 1998;68:311–318.

Meydani SN, Meydani M, Blumberg JB, et al. Vitamin E supplementation and in vivo immune response in healthy elderly subjects. A randomized controlled trial. *JAMA.* 1997;277:1380–1386.

Nursing 93 Drug Handbook. Springhouse, Pa: Springhouse Corporation; 1993.

Pronsky Z. *Food-Medication Interactions.* 9th ed. Pottstown, Pa: 1995.

Whitney E, Cataldo C, Rolfes S. *Understanding Normal and Clinical Nutrition.* St. Paul, Minn: West Publishing Co; 1987.

VITAMIN H (BIOTIN)

Bendich A, Deckelbaum R. *Preventive Nutrition: The Comprehensive Guide for Health Professionals.* Totowa, NJ: Humana Press; 1997.

Houchman LG, et al. Brittle nails: response to biotin supplementation. *Cutis.* 1993;51:303–307.

Jung U, Helbich-Endermann M, Bitsch R, et al. Are patients with chronic renal failure (CRF) deficient in biotin and is regular biotin supplementation required? *Z Ernahrungswiss.* 1998;37:363–367.

Koutsikos D, Agroyannis B, Tzanatos-Exarchou H. Biotin for diabetic peripheral neuropathy. *Biomed Pharmacother.* 1990;44:511–514.

Koutsikos D, Fourtounas C, Kapetanaki A, et al. Oral glucose tolerance test after high-dose i.v. biotin administration in normoglucemic hemodialysis patients. *Ren Fail.* 1996;18:131–137.

Messina M. *The Dietitian's Guide to Vegetarian Diets: Issues and Applications.* Gaithersburg, Md: Aspen Publishers, Inc; 1996.

Murray MT. *Encyclopedia of Nutritional Supplements.* Rocklin, Calif: Prima Publishing; 1997.

Reavley N. *Vitamins etc.* Melbourne, Australia: Bookman Press; 1998.

Ringer DL. *Physicians Guide to Nutraceuticals.* Omaha, Neb: Nutritional Data Resources; 1998.

Schulpis KH, Nyalala JO, Papakonstantinou ED, et al. Biotin recycling impairment in phenylketonuric children with seborrheic dermatitis. *Int J Dermatol.* 1998;37:918–921.

Zempleni J, Mock DM. Advanced analysis of biotin metabolites in body fluids allows a more accurate measurement of biotin bioavailability and metabolism in humans. *J Nutr.* 1999;129:494–497.

VITAMIN K

Bendich A, Decklebaum R. *Preventive Nutrition: The Comprehensive Guide for Health Professionals.* Totowa, NJ: Humana Press; 1997.

Drug Facts and Comparisons 1999. St. Louis, Mo: Facts and Comparisons; 1998:270–272.

Craciun AM, Wolf J, Knapen MH, Brouns F, Vermeer C. Improved bone metabolism in female elite athletes after vitamin K supplementation. *Int J Sports Med.* 1998;19:479–484.

Feskanich D, Weber P, Willett WC, Rockett H, Booth SL, Colditz GA. Vitamin K intake and hip fractures in women: a prospective study. *Am J Clin Nutr.* 1999;69:74–79.

Jatoi A, Lennon C, O'Brien M, Booth SL, Sadowski J, Mason JB. Protein-calorie malnutrition does not predict subtle vitamin K depletion in hospitalized patients. *Euro J Clin Nutri.* 1998; 52:934–937.

Jie KG, Bots ML, Vermeer C, Witteman JC, Grobbee DE. Vitamin K status and bone mass in women with and without aortic atherosclerosis: a population-based study. *Calcif Tissue Int.* 1996;59:352–356.

Kohlmeier M, Saupe J, Shearer MJ, Schaefer K, Asmus G. Bone health of adult hemodialysis patients is related to vitamin K status. *Kidney Int.* 1997;51:1218–1221.

Krummel D, Kris-Etherton P. *Nutrition in Women's Health.* Gaithersburg, Md: Aspen Publishers; 1996:434–435.

Lubetsky A, Dekel-Stern E, Chetrit A, Lubin F, Halkin H. Vitamin K intake and sensitivity to warfarin in patients consuming regular diets. *Thromb Haemost.* 1999;8:396–399.

Murray MT. *Encyclopedia of Nutritional Supplements.* Rocklin, Calif: Prima Publishing; 1996:54–58.

Novel form of vitamin K may stop liver cancer cell growth. *Oncology.* 1998;12:1541.

Reavley N. *Vitamins, Etc.* Melbourne, Australia: Bookman Press; 1998

Shils ME, Olson JA, Shike M, Ross CA, eds. *Modern Nutrition in Health and Disease.* 9th ed. New York, NY: Lippincott, Williams & Wilkins; 1998.

Tamatani M, Morimoto S, Nakajima M, et al. Decreased circulating levels of vitamin K and 25-hydroxyvitamin D in osteopenic elderly men. *Metabolism.* 1998;47:195–199.

Which vitamin K preparation for the newborn? *Drug Ther Bull.* March 1998;36:17–19.

ZINC

Eby GA. Zinc ion availability—the determinant of efficacy in zinc lozenge treatment of common colds. *J Antimicrob Chemother.* 1997;40:483–493.

Feltman J. *Prevention's Food & Nutrition.* Emmaus, Pa: Rodale Press; 1993.

Fortes C, Forastiere F, Agabiti N, et al. The effect of zinc and vitamin A supplementation on immune response in an older population. *J Am Geriatr Soc.* 1998;46:19–26.

Garland ML, Hagmeyer KO. The role of zinc lozenges in treatment of the common cold. *Ann Pharmacother.* 1998;32:63–69.

Golik A, Zaidenstein R, Dishi V, et al. Effects of captopril and enalapril on zinc metabolism in hypertensive patients. *J Am Coll Nutr.* 1998;17:75–78.

Haas E. *Staying Healthy with Nutrition, The Complete Guide to Diet and Nutritional Medicine.* Berkeley, Calif: Celestial Arts Publishing; 1992.

Hendler SS. *The Doctors' Vitamin and Mineral Encyclopedia.* New York, NY: Fireside Press; 1991.

Lieberman S, Bruning N. *The Real Vitamin & Mineral Book.* 2nd ed. New York, NY: Avery Publishing Group; 1997.

Murray MT. *Encyclopedia of Nutritional Supplements.* Rocklin, Calif: Prima Publishing; 1996.

Pronsky Z. *Food-Medication Interactions.* 9th ed. Pottstown, Pa: Food-Medicine Interactions; 1995.

Sazawal S, Black RE, Jalla S, et al. Zinc supplementation reduces the incidence of acute lower respiratory infections in infants and preschool children: a double-blind, controlled trial. *Pediatrics.* 1998;102(part 1):1–5.

Shealy CN. *The Illustrated Encyclopedia of Healing Remedies.* Boston, Mass: Element Books Inc.; 1998.

Somer E. *The Essential Guide to Vitamins and Minerals.* New York, NY: HarperCollins Publishers, Inc.; 1995.

Whitney E, Cataldo C, Rolfes S. *Understanding Normal and Clinical Nutrition.* St. Paul, Minn: West Publishing Co.; 1987.

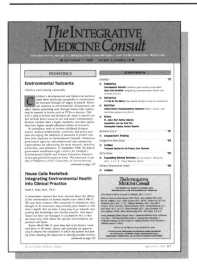
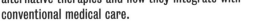
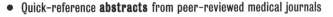
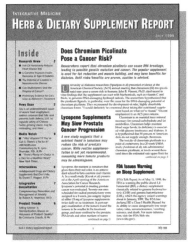